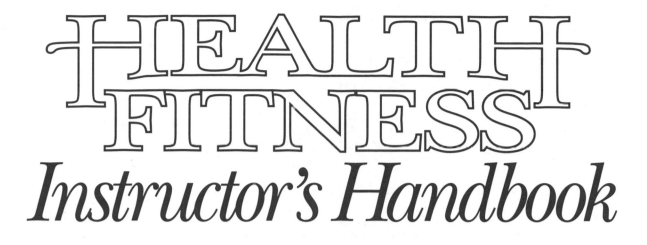

HEALTH FITNESS
Instructor's Handbook

Second Edition

Edward T. Howley
University of Tennessee at Knoxville

B. Don Franks
Louisiana State University at Baton Rouge

Human Kinetics Books
Champaign, Illinois

Library of Congress Cataloging-in-Publication Data

Howley, Edward T., 1943-
    Health fitness instructor's handbook / Edward T. Howley, B. Don
Franks.--2nd ed.
        p.   cm.
    Includes bibliographical references (p.) and index.
    ISBN 0-87322-335-7
    1. Physical fitness.   2. Physical fitness--Testing.   3. Exercise-
-Physiological aspects.   4. Health.   I.   Franks, B. Don.   II.   Title.
    GV481.H734   1992
    613.7'1--dc20   91-686
                                                            CIP

ISBN: 0-87322-335-7

Acquisitions Editor: Rick Frey, PhD
Developmental Editors: Marie Roy and Larret Galasyn-Wright
Assistant Editors: Dawn Levy, Julia Anderson, and Kari Nelson
Copyeditor: Wendy Nelson
Proofreaders: Stephani Day and Terry Olive
Production Director: Ernie Noa
Typesetter: Yvonne Winsor, Sandra Meier, and Kathy Boudreau-Fuoss
Text Design: Keith Blomberg
Text Layout: Denise Lowry, Denise Peters, and Tara Welsch
Cover Design: Jack Davis
Cover Photo: Will Zehr
Interior Art: Keith Blomberg and Gretchen Walters
Printer: Braun-Brumfield

Note. Objectives at the beginning of each chapter were adapted from *Guidelines for Exercise Testing and Prescription* (4th ed.) by American College of Sports Medicine, 1991, Philadelphia: Lea & Febiger. Copyright 1991 by Lea & Febiger. Adapted by permission.

ECG tracings on pp. 282-285 provided by Marquette Electronics, Inc., Milwaukee, WI.

Human Kinetics books are available at special discounts for bulk purchase for sales promotions, premiums, fund-raising, or educational use. Special editions or book excerpts can also be created to specification. For details, contact the Special Sales Manager at Human Kinetics.

Printed in the United States of America

10 9 8 7 6 5 4 3 2 1

Human Kinetics Books
A Division of Human Kinetics Publishers, Inc.
Box 5076, Champaign, IL 61825-5076
1-800-747-4457

Canada Office:
Human Kinetics Publishers, Inc.
P.O. Box 2503, Windsor, ON N8Y 4S2
1-800-465-7301 (in Canada only)

UK Office:
Human Kinetics Publishers (UK) Ltd.
P.O. Box 18
Rawdon, Leeds LS19 6TG
England
(0532) 504211

Dedicated
to
Ann and Liz

└The tw

Contents

Coordinated Texts for Health Fitness Instructors, Leaders, and Participants

Written by fitness experts Don Franks and Edward Howley, the three handbooks in this set provide health/fitness program administrators with a coordinated set of resources to enhance fitness instruction.

- *Health Fitness Instructor's Handbook* (2nd edition) is for advanced fitness instructors and supervisors.
- *Fitness Leader's Handbook* is for the exercise leader with little previous formal training who is responsible for leading safe and effective fitness classes.
- *Fitness Facts: The Healthy Living Handbook* is for the participants in these fitness classes.

These coordinated resources are especially helpful in providing consistently high quality instruction and information in programs where many fitness leaders are coordinated by a fitness supervisor. This series of handbooks complements the American College of Sports Medicine fitness certification program. *Health Fitness Instructor's Handbook* includes all the compe-

tencies for the ACSM Health Fitness Instructor certification, and has been widely used to prepare for this examination.

Fitness Leader's Handbook emphasizes more of the "how to" and less of the "why" to provide leaders with the practical competencies needed for effective instruction. This book contains the *practical* competencies for the ACSM exercise leader certification.

Fitness Facts is an especially useful handbook for students because it concisely and accurately expresses the information in the instructor and leader texts. Each handbook can certainly be used alone for its specific purpose, but supervisors of fitness programs in commercial fitness centers, the workplace, YMCAs, and universities will find the greatest value in using these books as a coordinated set. Instructors preparing for any fitness instructor certification will discover these handbooks to be indispensable as will instructors or leaders looking for review materials.

Preface

Over the past 10 years we have come to distinguish *performance-based fitness*, which is needed for success at specific sports, from *health-related fitness* that is needed by everyone to have a low risk of preventable diseases. As in the first edition, this second edition of the *Health Fitness Instructor's Handbook* deals with health-related fitness. It is now recognized, on the basis of good scientific research, that regular participation in physical activity and the achievement of higher levels of cardiovascular function are associated with lower risks of disease and lower death rates. Simply put, exercise is good for us!

Although this is not too surprising for those who are involved in the delivery of health and fitness programs, such evidence has resulted in major policy statements from health organizations and the federal government on the importance of physical activity in the achievement of dynamic health and in the *prevention* of a variety of diseases or conditions such as high blood pressure, adult-onset diabetes, obesity, coronary heart disease, low-back pain, and osteoporosis (thinning of bones). Health-related fitness goals of achieving appropriate levels of cardiorespiratory function, body fat, muscular strength and endurance, and low-back flexibility are consistent with these policy statements.

As in the first edition, we address these fitness goals. But, this new edition has been completely revised to include

- new chapters on measurement and evaluation, nutrition, and computer software;
- expanded coverage of exercise leadership, stress reduction, and cardiac medications;
- 1991 ACSM objectives for both Health Fitness Instructor and Exercise Leader certifications;
- key points in each chapter;
- more case studies and illustrations; and
- updated and expanded references and readings.

The fitness professional must be able to deliver fitness testing and programming to individuals of different ages who vary in fitness and health status. The fitness instructor must be prepared to select appropriate tests for school-age children as well as those with age-related orthopedic limitations, and be aware of the special concerns when working with the diabetic and the asthmatic. To do this, one must have an appropriate educational and experiential background.

The recent growth of college and university programs designed to prepare students for careers in health and fitness will facilitate the implementation of health-related fitness programs. To undertake the responsibilities associated with these programs, the interested student must possess knowledges and skills found in a wide variety of courses: anatomy, biomechanics, physiology, psychology, exercise physiology, nutrition, athletic training, exercise testing, exercise prescription, and exercise leadership.

This book is written to facilitate the education of potential fitness professionals and to encourage them to seek formal certification, such as the Health Fitness Instructor (HFI) certification by the American College of Sports Medicine (ACSM). The ACSM has provided a leadership role in certifying individuals involved in exercise testing, prescription, and administration of preventive and clinical exercise programs. The certifications from ACSM are recognized as the ''gold standards'' to achieve, and confirm that the individual possesses the necessary knowledges, skills, and abilities to take on appropriate responsibilities.

The second edition of the *Health Fitness Instructor's Handbook* has been organized around the 1991 behavioral objectives developed by the American College of Sports Medicine for those wishing to be certified as Health Fitness Instructors. The *Health Fitness Instructor's Handbook* is meant to go beyond the college classroom and be an appropriate source for those taking workshops or simply using it as a personal reference. The book is divided into five parts. Part I (Fitness and Health) describes the areas of knowledge and competence needed by the HFI, the relationship of physical activity to optimal health, and how to evaluate health status. Part II (Scientific Foundations) reviews the basics of exercise physiology, anatomy and biomechanics, and measurement and evaluation. Part III (Physical Fitness) focuses on nutrition and health, achieving optimal levels of body fatness, cardiorespiratory fitness, muscular strength, endurance and flexibility for a healthy low back, and the interaction of personality, stress, and fitness. Part IV (Activity Recommendations) delineates the principles of behavior modification, how to develop and implement exercise prescriptions for achieving cardiovascular fitness in diverse populations, and the application of techniques of exercise leadership. It also provides a summary of electrocardiographic changes and medications associated with exercise. Part V (Safe and Effective Programs) describes how to prevent and treat injuries associated with exercise, how to deal with daily and long-term concerns associated with running a fitness program, and finally, where to find appropriate computer software to help provide better services to the fitness participant. The second edition of the *Health Fitness Instructor's Handbook*, then, represents a major revision. It uses the new ACSM behavioral objectives and includes more case studies and illustrations and updated and expanded references, and it is coordinated with the *Fitness Leader's Handbook* and *Fitness Facts*.

A formal college education and certification as a Health Fitness Instructor are the first steps in the process of becoming a fitness professional. The fitness professional must be committed to the process of continuing education to stay abreast of the art and science of exercise testing and programming. We encourage you to join appropriate professional organizations, attend meetings, and read the professional literature. Our involvement in such organizations facilitated both the development and the revision of this book.

Introduction

The Health Fitness Instructor

OBJECTIVE

The reader will be able to:

- List the general competencies needed by Health Fitness Instructors

Health Fitness Instructors (HFIs) play a very important role, because many individuals need help in exercising safely and in achieving higher levels of fitness. The HFI should be aware of the year-2000 health objectives for the nation (2), including specific goals for improved health status, reduced risk factors, increased public awareness, improved services and protection, and improved surveillance and evaluation services. Specifically, these goals for the year 2000 include increases in

- the percentage of people involved in both low- and moderate-intensity exercise,
- muscular strength/endurance and flexibility activities,
- knowledge about the role of exercise in health and fitness,
- knowledge about types of exercise for cardiorespiratory fitness,
- physical education in the schools and fitness programs at work, and
- exercise facilities and programs.

The HFI educates fitness participants about health, fitness, and performance, and helps in the establishment of healthy lifestyles. The HFI needs to be aware of the broad range of factors included in total fitness (see chapter 1). However, the focus of this book and of most of the HFI's activity is on physical fitness.

To accomplish these responsibilities, the HFI needs to possess certain competencies and provide a good role model. This book is meant to provide, in a single source, descriptions of all the competencies needed by the health/fitness professional.

COMPETENCIES FOR HEALTH/ FITNESS PROFESSIONALS

The health/fitness professional must understand a wide variety of fields related to fitness. One of the first of several certification programs for fitness professionals was developed by the American College of Sports Medicine (ACSM). Following are the general ACSM objectives for health/fitness professionals (specifically, for the **Exercise Leader** and the **Health Fitness Instructor**). The chapters dealing with each objective are indicated in parentheses.

ACSM PREVENTIVE TRACT: GENERAL BEHAVIORAL OBJECTIVES FOR EXERCISE LEADER AND HEALTH FITNESS INSTRUCTOR*

Functional Anatomy and Biomechanics
(Chapters 4, 16)

The candidate will demonstrate an understanding of human functional anatomy and biomechanics.

---

*Note. This information appears on pages 230-239, 242-246, and 248 of *Guidelines for Exercise Testing and Prescription* (4th ed.) by American College of Sports Medicine, 1991, Philadelphia: Lea and Febiger. Copyright 1991 by Lea and Febiger. Reprinted by permission.

The candidate will demonstrate a knowledge of the role of biomechanical factors in the development of injuries.

The candidate will describe common exercise movements and identify the major muscle groups involved in each.

Exercise Physiology

(Chapters 3, 10)

The candidate will demonstrate a knowledge of basic exercise physiology.

The candidate will demonstrate an understanding of the basic principles involved in muscular strength, endurance, and flexibility training.

Human Development/Aging

(Chapters 1, 3, 4, 13)

The candidate will demonstrate an understanding of the special problems of human development and aging . . . and (HFI) of the effect of the aging process on the structure and function of the human organism at rest, during exercise, and during recovery.

Human Behavior/Psychology

(Chapters 11, 12)

The candidate will be able to list several motivational techniques used to promote behavior change in the initiation, adherence or return to exercise and other healthy lifestyle behaviors . . . and (HFI) an understanding of basic behavioral psychology, group dynamics, and learning techniques.

Pathophysiology/Risk Factors

(Chapters 1, 2)

The candidate will identify risk factors which may require consultation with medical or allied health professionals prior to participation in physical activity . . . and (HFI) an understanding of the pathophysiology of the major chronic diseases and how these processes are influenced by physical activity.

Health Appraisal and Fitness Testing

(Chapters 2, 5)

The candidate will demonstrate and identify appropriate techniques for health appraisal and use of fitness evaluations.

Emergency Procedures/Safety

(Chapters 1, 13, 16, 17)

The candidate will demonstrate competence in basic life support and implementation of first aid procedures which may be necessary during or after exercise.

The candidate will demonstrate an understanding of the risks associated with exercise participation . . . and (HFI) knowledge of emergency procedures, first aid, and evacuation plans.

Exercise Programming

(Chapters 1, 10, 13, 14)

The candidate will demonstrate an understanding of the concepts of exercise.

The candidate will demonstrate an understanding of exercise for improving flexibility, muscular strength, and muscular endurance.

The candidate will demonstrate a knowledge of class organization and exercise leadership . . . and (HFI) design and implement individualized and group exercise programs.

Nutrition and Weight Management

(Chapters 6, 7)

The candidate will demonstrate an understanding of the principles of weight management and nutrition.

Program Administration

(Chapter 17)

The Health Fitness Instructor will understand his/her supportive role in administration and program management.

KEY POINT.   The role of the Health Fitness Instructor is to help individuals achieve the highest possible fitness levels through a healthy lifestyle. Competencies needed for this role include an understanding of exercise from many perspectives and the ability to implement this knowledge in practical situations.

SUMMARY

The general competencies for fitness professionals, and the role of the HFI in promoting those aspects of physical fitness that can be improved through appropriate physical activity, are listed in the Introduction. This book is aimed at helping you understand and achieve these competencies.

REFERENCES

1. American College of Sports Medicine (1991)
2. U.S. Public Health Service (1990)

See the Bibliography at the end of the book for a complete source listing.

Part I

Fitness and Health

Chapter 1

Goals of Fitness and Health

OBJECTIVES

The reader will be able to:
- Define and differentiate among terms related to health, fitness, performance, and physical activity
- Describe the goals and characteristics of health, fitness, and performance
- Describe healthy behaviors related to fitness
- Describe the atherosclerotic process
- List the risk factors associated with heart disease
- Describe the role of exercise and fitness in the prevention of major health problems
- Describe the components of physical fitness and of performance
- Identify the advantages and disadvantages of exercise

TERMS

The reader will be able to define or describe:

Arteriosclerosis	Low-back problems
Atherosclerosis	Low-intensity exercise
Conditioning	Moderate-intensity exercise
Coronary artery thrombosis	Myocardial infarction
Coronary heart disease (CHD)	Performance
Embolism	Physical activity
Exercise	Physical fitness
Health	Risk factors
Healthy behavior	Stroke
Heart attack	Thrombosis
High-intensity exercise	Total fitness
Hypertension	

Many fitness books begin by describing heart disease as the major cause of death and proceed to define the role of exercise in prevention and rehabilitation programs. The relationship of exercise and fitness to heart disease is not unimportant, but the prevention of heart disease and other major health problems is only one of the goals of regular exercise and only part of achieving a high fitness status. Obtaining the optimal quality of life involves much more than preventing health problems! It also involves having healthy behaviors and high levels of fitness as normal, lifelong goals. This chapter begins by defining terms needed to discuss these concepts. The definitions are followed by a description of the goals, characteristics, and behaviors essential for health, fitness, and performance.

KEY POINT. Exercise and fitness are important for prevention of heart disease as well as for many other aspects of life that allow individuals to achieve the highest quality of life.

There has been increasing differentiation among related areas of physical activity, fitness testing, and health concepts during the past decade. Although many slightly different terms and definitions are used, there appears to be

3

agreement (1, 2, 6, 8, 16) that the following need to be defined and distinguished:

Healthy behavior—Activities and habits that are related to total fitness and low risk of developing major health problems. These behaviors include exercising regularly, maintaining a healthy diet, getting adequate sleep, relaxing and coping with stressors, practicing safety habits, and abstaining from tobacco, alcohol, and nonessential drugs.

Physical activity—Any movement of the body (or substantial parts of the body) produced by skeletal muscles and resulting in energy expenditure.

Exercise—Physical activity whose purpose is to improve some component(s) of physical fitness.

Low-intensity—Exercise at less than 50% of functional capacity, with little increase in respiration and no discomfort. This exercise can be universally recommended, except for individuals with extreme disease or physical impairment, to expend calories and lower risk of health problems. Also called moderate exercise by ACSM (2).

Moderate-intensity—Exercise, at 60% to 85% of functional capacity, that causes mild breathlessness and some perspiration. Individuals who are unaccustomed to it may experience some discomfort and later soreness. After health status evaluation this activity may be recommended for optimal cardiorespiratory benefits. Also called vigorous exercise by ACSM (2).

High-intensity—Activity at 80% to 120% of functional capacity, recommended only for those interested in high-level performance after medical screening. Also called vigorous exercise (2).

Conditioning—Exercise conducted on a regular basis over a period of time. Also called training.

Health—Being alive with no major health problem. Also called apparently healthy.

Total fitness—Striving for optimal quality of life including social, mental, spiritual, and physical components. Also called wellness, or positive health.

Physical fitness—Striving for optimal physical quality of life, including obtaining criterion levels of physical fitness test scores, and low risk of developing health problems. Also called health-related physical fitness, or physiological fitness.

Performance—Ability to perform a task or sport at a desired level. Also called motor fitness, or physical fitness.

Although these concepts are distinct, they are also interrelated. As Paffenbarger, Hyde, and Wing (14) point out, persons who exercise and exhibit other healthy behaviors are more likely to be fit. Achieving fitness standards leads to a healthy, longer life. On the other hand, sedentary existence is related to low levels of fitness and major health problems that shorten life.

KEY POINT. One should exercise at low intensity for health, at moderate intensity for physical fitness, and at high intensity for performance. The status of the individual may include being alive without disease (health), striving for optimal quality of life (fitness), and possessing the ability to compete in a sport at a desired level (performance).

TOTAL FITNESS

Total fitness is the optimal quality of life. This dynamic, multidimensional state has a positive health base and includes individual performance goals. The highest quality of life includes intellectual, social, spiritual, and physical components. Mental alertness and curiosity, emotional feelings, meaningful relations with other humans, awareness and involvement in societal strivings and problems, and the physical capacity to accomplish personal goals with vigor appear to be essential elements of a healthy life. These aspects of total fitness are interrelated; a high level in one of the areas enhances the other areas, and conversely, a low level in any area restricts the accomplishments possible in other areas.

Inherited Limits

Individuals can achieve fitness goals up to their genetic potential, but it is not possible to establish the relative portion of a person's health or performance that is determined by heredity and development. Even though heredity influences physical activity, fitness status, and health (7), most people can lead healthy or unhealthy lives regardless of their inheritances. Thus, genetic background neither dooms a person to poor health nor guarantees a high fitness level.

Environmental Factors

We are born not only with fixed genetic potentials, but into environments that affect our development in many ways. An environment includes physical factors (e.g., climate, altitude, pollution) and social factors (e.g., networks of friends, characteristics of workplace) that affect activity, fitness, and health (8). Some elements, such as nutrition, the air we breathe and water we drink, affect us directly. Other elements, such as the values and behaviors of persons we admire, influence our life-styles indirectly.

Certain aspects of our environments can be controlled—many of the mental and physical activities we do are a matter of choice. However, we are all limited in various ways by our past and current environments. For example, some children have inadequate food as a part of their environments and obviously cannot think about other aspects of fitness until that basic need is fulfilled.

Dynamic Development

An optimal quality of life requires a person to strive, grow, and develop, but the highest level of fitness may never be achieved. The totally fit person continually approaches the highest quality of life possible.

KEY POINT. Total fitness is striving for the highest level of existence, including mental, social, spiritual,

and physical components. It is dynamic, multidimensional, and related to heredity, environment, and individual interests.

PHYSICAL FITNESS, HEALTH, AND PERFORMANCE

Having defined fitness and related terms, we now present the goals and characteristics of health, performance, and physical fitness.

Health Goals

The two primary health goals are to delay death and to avoid disease. It should be noted that these goals provide for a minimum basis for lack of disease, not the optimal goals for positive health. These goals are desirable first steps but fall far short of the optimal level of fitness. Each goal has several components.

Health, Physical Fitness, and Performance Goals

Area	Goal
Health	To delay death To avoid disease
Physical fitness	To lower risks of developing health problems To maintain a positive physical health base
Performance	To complete daily tasks efficiently To achieve desired levels in selected sports

Health Goals

Goal	Components
To delay death	Good inherited characteristics Healthy habits Safe habits Healthy environment
To avoid disease	Good inherited characteristics Preventive actions Aware of signs and symptoms Healthy fitness status Healthy diet

To Delay Death

The death rate for humans is 100%! Death cannot be avoided, but beyond one's inherited characteristics, there are some things that one can do to help postpone it for a period of time. Most generally, one can practice a healthy and safe lifestyle in a healthy environment. The behaviors to be adopted are discussed in the later section of this chapter dealing with the role of the Health Fitness Instructor.

To Avoid Disease

Along with delaying death, the other minimum goal for all of us is to obtain a medical diagnosis that we are free from disease (that we are "apparently healthy"). We try to prevent sickness, illness, and known diseases through awareness, health checks, and healthy habits. You have probably assisted at or attended health fairs that help people identify signs, symptoms, and test scores that might be indicative of possible medical problems.

KEY POINT.   The health goals are to avoid premature death and to avoid preventable disease. Components related to these goals include heredity, environment, habits, and health status.

Physical Fitness Goals

The physical fitness goals are to lower risks of developing health problems and to maintain a positive physical health base. You are undoubtedly familiar with the components of these goals.

To Lower Risks of Health Problems

Many of the health problems responsible for premature deaths can be prevented with careful screening and preventive action (e.g., immunization). There are still many people in the world who need this basic health care, and medical science can provide this service. The solution to this aspect of health care is finding the resources and political will to make it available to everyone.

In more affluent sectors of societies, where preventive health care is routine, another set of health problems has emerged, causing premature death or disability. These health problems are related to characteristics that can be modified with one's lifestyle; they include angina (17), atherosclerosis (22), back pain (13), cancer (10), diabetes (21), hypertension (11), poor mental health (19), obesity (9), osteoporosis (18), and stroke (22).

Cardiovascular Problems.   Cardiovascular problems cause the majority of premature deaths in our society

Physical Fitness Goals

Goal	Components

To lower risks of health problems	Good inherited characteristics
	Healthy levels of
	  Cholesterol
	  Blood pressure
	  Body fat
	  Glucose tolerance
	  Functional capacity
	  Substance use
	  Stress

To maintain a positive physical health base	Healthy levels of
	  Body fat
	  Functional capacity
	  Substance use
	  Stress
	  Midtrunk flexibility
	  Abdominal endurance
	  Flexibility
	  Muscular strength and endurance

(3). In addition, many who survive with these problems have severe limitations in their lives. There are many different forms of these health problems—we will deal only with the most common [see (15) for a comprehensive description of the various cardiovascular diseases].

Arteriosclerosis—An arterial disease characterized by the hardening and thickening of vessel walls

Atherosclerosis—A form of arteriosclerosis in which fatty substances deposit in the inner walls of the arteries

Embolism—Sudden obstruction of a blood vessel by a solid body such as a clot carried in the bloodstream

Thrombosis—A blood clot in a blood vessel

Coronary artery thrombosis—Occlusion of a coronary artery by a blood clot

Coronary heart disease (CHD)—Atherosclerosis of the coronary arteries, also called coronary artery disease (CAD)

Myocardial infarction (MI)—Death to a section of heart tissue where the blood supply has been cut off

Heart attack—Common name for myocardial infarction

Hypertension—Abnormally high blood pressure (BP)

Stroke—A vascular accident (embolism, hemorrhage, or thrombosis) in the brain, often resulting in sudden loss of body function

Coronary heart disease (CHD) is the single leading cause of premature death in the United States (3). Cholesterol is predominant in the plaques that clog up the arteries. As the coronary arteries become narrowed and hardened, the arteries may not be able to supply the oxygen needed by the heart muscle (myocardium). This inability to supply myocardial oxygen is likely to occur when more oxygen is needed (e.g., during stress or strenuous activity). This imbalance between need and supply of oxygen may lead to pain in the chest (angina), neck, jaw, or left shoulder and arm. The narrowed section of the artery may close or become totally occluded, which will lead to a myocardial infarction.

High blood pressure (hypertension) is the most common cardiovascular disease (3). See chapter 2 for standards that define abnormal levels of blood pressure. Hypertension is related to CHD and stroke. Stroke is the result of obstructions in or hemorrhages of blood vessels in the brain. It usually results in an abrupt disruption of bodily function and loss of consciousness, and may cause partial paralysis.

Large-population epidemiological studies of cardiovascular problems have found that several characteristics are highly related to the premature development of cardiovascular disease. [See the comprehensive reviews of epidemiological studies and risk factors in (6, 8, 15).] In the past, the health risks have been divided into primary and secondary **risk factors**. *Primary* risk factors are those characteristics that are highly associated with a particular health problem (e.g., heart disease), independent of all other variables. For example, smoking (a primary risk factor) puts an individual at high risk for heart disease even if no other risk factors are present (e.g., the individual is female, young, white, active, and lean, has no family history of heart disease, copes well with stress, and has normal levels of blood pressure and cholesterol). *Secondary* risk factors, on the other hand, have a high relationship with the health problem only when other risk factors are present. For example, being under stress (a secondary risk factor), an individual would not be at high risk if no other risk factors were present. However, inability to cope with stress does increase the risk of heart disease when other risk factors are present. Although this distinction has been helpful in the past, the differentiation between primary and secondary is increasingly difficult to maintain. For example, earlier reviews concluded that physical inactivity was a secondary risk factor, and cardiorespiratory fitness was not even listed as a risk factor. Recent studies (5, 14) have found strong evidence that both physical inactivity and low levels of cardiorespiratory fitness are primary risk factors. For our purposes, the HFI should know all the risk factors, and more importantly, what individuals need to know to lower their risks of health problems.

Another way to classify risk factors is to distinguish inherited risk factors that cannot be altered from lifestyle behaviors that can be modified. The risk factors that cannot be altered include family history of premature cardiovascular disease, gender (males having higher risk), race (African-Americans having higher risk), and age (the risk increases for all of us as we grow older). Part of the risk associated with family history and age cannot be changed. However, part of the family history risks include unhealthy diet, smoking, and stress behaviors that tend to be transmitted from parents to children. These are the types of behaviors that can be corrected with proper attention throughout life, especially in early childhood. In terms of aging, many fitness characteristics (e.g., maximum cardiovascular function and amount of fat) get worse with age; that is, if people from 20 to 80 years of age were tested, and the results were plotted, a steady deterioration (i.e., decreased cardiovascular function, increased fat) would occur with each decade. This decline, starting in the middle 20s, has been called the aging curve. However, a portion of the deterioration seen in aging curves is caused by less activity in older individuals—not by aging itself. People who maintain active lifestyles slow down the fitness decline seen in typical aging curves.

Other characteristics that increase risk include smoking, high levels of serum cholesterol, high blood pressure, glucose intolerance, fat, inability to cope with stressors, and low levels of physical activity and cardiorespiratory fitness. The good news is that many of these characteristics can be favorably altered with healthy habits.

Numerous studies have shown that more active persons have a lower risk of heart disease than sedentary individuals; however, physical inactivity has been viewed as less important than control of serum cholesterol, blood pressure, and smoking. Recent studies (5, 14) indicate that both physical activity (such as expending 2,000 kcal per week in exercise) and cardiorespiratory fitness levels (such as being able to go longer on a treadmill test) are major factors related to the prevention of heart disease. Physical inactivity and low levels of fitness deserve to be included with the same emphasis as the traditional primary risk factors. Regular exercise also affects many of the CHD risk factors, resulting in an improvement in serum cholesterol levels, blood pressure, glucose tolerance, fatness, and ability to cope with stressors (8).

Although these risk factors normally have been linked with some form of cardiovascular disease, many of them are also related to pulmonary (e.g., chronic obstructive pulmonary disease) and metabolic (e.g., diabetes, see chapter 13) health problems.

Low-Back Problems.   Clinical evidence indicates that several risk factors are associated with **low-back problems** (see chapter 10):

- Lack of abdominal muscle endurance
- Lack of flexibility in the midtrunk and hamstrings
- Poor posture—lying, sitting, standing, and moving
- Poor lifting habits
- Inability to cope with stressors

To Maintain a Positive Physical Health Base

Many of the same characteristics that lower our risk for developing serious health problems also provide a higher quality of life. In other words, having high levels of functional capacity and optimal levels of body fat and stress help us feel good and have the energy to do things that enrich our lives. In addition, having good muscular endurance and flexibility in the midtrunk area is related to a healthy low back. The quality of life continuum illustrates this point (see Figure 1.1).

KEY POINT.   The goals of physical fitness are to have a positive physical health base with a low risk of health problems, characterized by favorable inherited characteristics and healthy levels of serum cholesterol, blood pressure, body fat, cardiorespiratory fitness, flexibility, strength and endurance, and ability to cope with stress.

Performance

The primary performance goals are to complete daily tasks efficiently and to achieve desired levels in selected sports. These goals also involve a number of components.

Daily Tasks

To get through the day efficiently, we must have fundamental motor skills to be able to accomplish various tasks. We must be able to move the body from place to place and push, pull, pick up, carry, and do a number of other tasks requiring use of the hands. Minimum levels of muscular strength and endurance, flexibility, and cardiorespiratory fitness are essential. In addition, we need special abilities to perform the unique activities related to work or home.

Sports

Many individuals also engage in particular games and sports. These activities require specific kinds and levels of motor abilities (such as agility, balance, coordination,

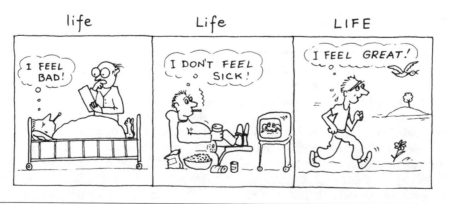

Figure 1.1   Quality of life continuum.

Performance Goals

Goal	Components
To complete daily tasks efficiently	Adequate levels of 　Strength and endurance 　Flexibility 　Aerobic power 　Locomotor skills
To achieve desired levels in selected sports	Specific levels of 　Agility 　Coordination 　Speed 　Strength, endurance, and power 　Dynamic balance 　Aerobic and anaerobic power Specific skills of sport Mental readiness

---

endurance, power, and speed related to the sport), as well as the particular skills of the sport.

Risks of Exercise

Exercise and fitness tests involve risk of injury, cardiovascular problems, or death. High-intensity exercise and competition in many sports place extreme demands on the cardiovascular system and include increased risk of injury. In addition, some fitness participants become obsessed with exercise and overtrain, ending up with decreased fitness and frequent injuries.

Low-intensity exercise is a very low-risk activity. For exercise testing (including postcardiac patients) there are about 5 incidents resulting in hospital treatment and 1 death per 10,000 tests, and there is about 1 exercise-related death per year for every 15,000 to 20,000 active persons. Because of the decreased risk of heart disease in active or fit persons, the overall risk of a cardiovascular problem is greater for those who maintain sedentary habits (12, 20).

The tendency is to deal with this question of risk by identifying various classes of individuals for whom a certain type of medical examination or test is recommended before initiating an exercise program (see chapter 2). Per Olaf Åstrand, a well-known Swedish physiologist, has offered another view. He states that consulting a physician is advisable if there are any doubts about health, but that "there is less risk in activity than in continuous inactivity." He continues, "It is more advisable to pass a careful medical examination if

one intends to be sedentary in order to establish whether one's state of health is good enough to stand the inactivity!" (4). This view is consistent with recent evidence that physical activity and a high level of cardiorespiratory fitness are directly related to a lower risk of heart disease and death (5, 14).

KEY POINT. There is some risk of injury, cardiovascular problems, and death with exercise. However, the health risk of an inactive lifestyle is higher than the risk associated with the kind of fitness activities and tests recommended in this book.

GOAL-RELATED BEHAVIORS

The first two sections of this chapter have discussed definitions, goals, and characteristics related to health, physical fitness, and performance. This section will discuss the behaviors needed to achieve these goals.

Health

The Goal-Related Behaviors list indicates what one must do to acquire the components of the primary health goals. Chapter 18 evaluates computer software that can help participants identify healthy and unhealthy behaviors.

Health Components and Goal-Related Behaviors

Component	Behaviors
Good heredity	Wise selection of parents(!)
Healthy habits	Regular physical activity
	Healthy diet
	No smoking or drugs
	Limited alcohol use
	Relaxation
	Sleep
	Coping with stressors
Safe habits	Use of seat belts
	Avoidance of high-risk activities
Healthy environment	Living where there is clean air and water
Preventive actions	Regular medical and dental exams
	Immunization
	Awareness of signs and symptoms, such as pain and tension
Healthy fitness status	Regular moderate activity
Healthy diet	Choice of proper proportions of different foods
	Choice of low levels of fat, cholesterol, and salt
	Balance of caloric intake and expenditure
	Choice of high % of complex carbohydrates

Fitness

The Physical Fitness Goal-Related Behaviors list indicates what one must do to achieve the components of physical fitness.

Performance

The Performance Goal-Related Behaviors list indicates how one can achieve components of the primary performance goals.

Health and Fitness Behaviors Recommended for All

You have probably noticed that there is some repetition in the behaviors recommended for delaying death, avoiding disease, providing low risk of major health problems, and the development of high levels of positive health. Although individuals need to be educated about signs, symptoms, risk factors, and so on, the ma-

jor emphasis of a fitness program should be on the behaviors on the Health and Fitness Behaviors list.

KEY POINT. Although there are some differences between health and fitness goals, there are many common behaviors to be recommended, including regular exercise and sleep, nutritious diet, no smoking or drugs, limited alcohol, ability to cope with stressors, ability to relax, preventive checkups, and safe habits.

SETTING FITNESS GOALS

Persons entering your fitness class have taken an important first step toward improving their fitness levels. It is your responsibility to help them

- **understand the components of fitness,**
- **analyze current fitness status,**
- **begin or continue appropriate exercise habits,**

Physical Fitness Components and Goal-Related Behaviors

Component	Behaviors
Good heredity	Wise selection of parents
Healthy levels of cholesterol, blood pressure, body fat	Healthy diet, low fat and salt; balanced caloric intake and expenditure
Cardiorespiratory fitness	Regular moderate exercise
Stress	Coping with stressors
	Getting adequate sleep and learning to relax
Substance use	No smoking or drugs
	Limited use of alcohol
Midtrunk flexibility	Static stretching, low back and legs
Abdominal endurance	Abdominal curl-ups
Flexibility	Static stretching
Muscular strength and endurance	Resistance exercises

Performance Components and Goal-Related Behaviors

Component	Behaviors
Adequate levels of	
Strength and endurance	Resistance exercises
Flexibility	Static stretching
Aerobic power	Regular vigorous exercise
Locomotor skills	Walking
Specific levels of	Practicing particular movements related to sport
Agility	
Coordination	
Speed	
Strength, endurance, and power	
Dynamic balance	
Aerobic and anaerobic power	Appropriate interval training
Specific skills of sport	Practice skills in gamelike conditions
Mental readiness	

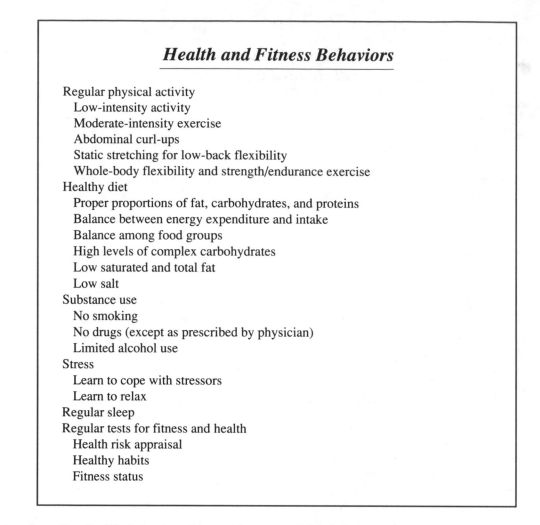

Health and Fitness Behaviors

Regular physical activity
   Low-intensity activity
   Moderate-intensity exercise
   Abdominal curl-ups
   Static stretching for low-back flexibility
   Whole-body flexibility and strength/endurance exercise
Healthy diet
   Proper proportions of fat, carbohydrates, and proteins
   Balance between energy expenditure and intake
   Balance among food groups
   High levels of complex carbohydrates
   Low saturated and total fat
   Low salt
Substance use
   No smoking
   No drugs (except as prescribed by physician)
   Limited alcohol use
Stress
   Learn to cope with stressors
   Learn to relax
Regular sleep
Regular tests for fitness and health
   Health risk appraisal
   Healthy habits
   Fitness status

- **determine other health behaviors that need to be changed, and**
- **take appropriate steps to change behavior.**

Chapter 12 suggests ways to help participants start changing unhealthy behaviors.

PERSONAL CONTROL OF HEALTH STATUS

One of the most frustrating and exciting aspects of dealing with current health problems is that individuals can modify their health status and control major health risks. The frustrating aspect is that many people find it difficult to change unhealthy lifestyles. The exciting element is that they can gain control of their health. The HFI is at the cutting edge of health, in much the same way in which the scientist discovering vaccines for major health problems was at the turn of the 20th century.

This opportunity to provide assistance to people who wish to alter their unhealthy lifestyles carries the responsibility to make recommendations based on the best evidence available. The HFI can help people gain control of their lives through an evaluation of their risk factors and behaviors related to health. Chapter 2 deals with this type of health appraisal.

SUMMARY

Physical fitness consists of aspects of an optimal quality of life that are related to positive physical health. Physical fitness is a necessary ingredient of fitness, but fitness includes much more than the physical aspects. A person cannot achieve total fitness without a good physical base, but a person with a high level of physical fitness without the other aspects of fitness would live a sterile existence. Risk factors associated with heart disease and low-back problems are identified. Recognizing the characteristics and behaviors associated with health problems is a first step in gaining personal control over the factors contributing to health.

REFERENCES

1. American Alliance for Health, Physical Education, Recreation and Dance (1988)
2. American College of Sports Medicine (1991)
3. American Heart Association (1989)
4. Åstrand and Rodahl (1970)
5. Blair et al. (1989)
6. Blair, Painter, Pate, Smith, and Taylor (1988)
7. Bouchard (1990)
8. Bouchard, Shephard, Stephens, Sutton, and McPherson (1990b)
9. Bray (1990)
10. Calabrese (1990)
11. Hagberg (1990)
12. Hanson (1988)
13. Nachemson (1990)
14. Paffenbarger, Hyde, and Wing (1990)
15. Pollock and Wilmore (1990)
16. *Public Health Reports* (1985)
17. Rechnitzer (1990)
18. Smith, Smith, and Gilligan (1990)
19. Stephens (1990)
20. Thompson, P.D. (1988)
21. Vranic and Wasserman (1990)
22. Wood and Stefanick (1990)

See the Bibliography at the end of the book for a complete source listing.

Chapter 2

Evaluation of Health Status

OBJECTIVES

The reader will be able to:
- Evaluate the health status of potential fitness participants
- Make recommendations for the type of fitness program based on health status
- List the conditions and test scores for medical referral
- List the conditions and test scores for supervised programs
- List the conditions that may need special attention during exercise
- Identify individuals who need educational material
- Identify conditions that would cause a shift in exercise recommendations

TERMS

The reader will be able to define or describe:

Emergency information
Forced expiratory volume
High-density lipoprotein cholesterol (HDL-C)
Low-density lipoprotein cholesterol (LDL-C)
Medical history
Medical referral

Supervised programs
Total cholesterol
Total cholesterol/HDL-C ratio
Unsupervised program
Very low-density lipoproteins (VLDL)
Vital capacity (VC)

An important responsibility of the HFI is to help potential fitness participants determine their current health status. If the person has a major health problem that has been diagnosed and is being treated, then you must rely on guidance from the fitness program director and medical professionals for appropriate fitness programs. If health status has been carefully analyzed by physicians and health professionals and there are no health problems or unhealthy behaviors, then the individual can continue a fitness program, making modifications based on interest. However, most people are in between those two extremes. They do not have a known major health problem, but they have not thoroughly checked their health status.

SCREENING FOR LOW-INTENSITY EXERCISE

The Physical Activity Readiness Questionnaire (PAR-Q) (7) can be used as a simple screening for persons beginning low-intensity exercise. It has been shown to be useful in referring those who need additional medical screening while *not* excluding the majority of people who will benefit from participation in regular low-intensity exercise.

SCREENING FOR MODERATE-INTENSITY EXERCISE

The rest of this chapter deals primarily with the screening procedures to be used for persons interested in moderate-intensity exercise. The HFI can assist individuals in evaluating their health status. (See chapter 18 for an evaluation of computer software that can be used for health-risk appraisal.) Health status includes five major categories:

1. Diagnosed medical problems
2. Characteristics that increase the risk of health problems

Physical Activity Readiness
Questionnaire (PAR-Q)*

NAME OF PARTICIPANT _____

DATE _____

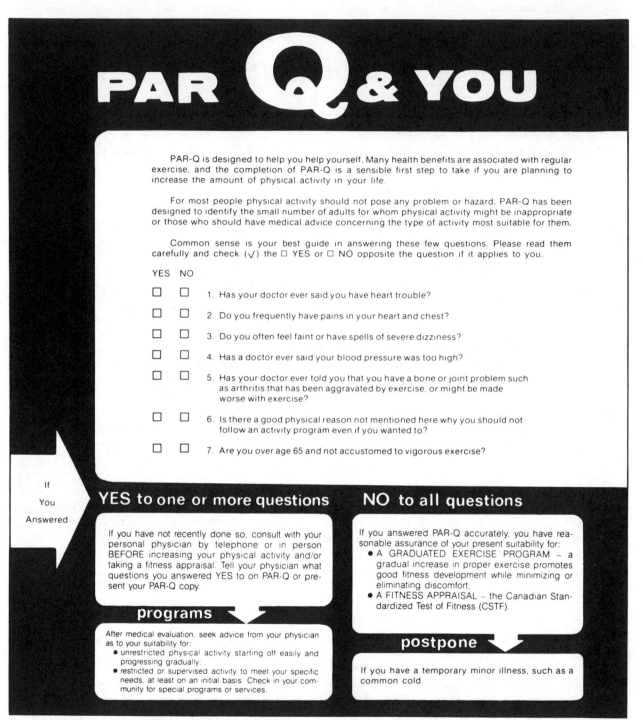

PAR Q & YOU

PAR-Q is designed to help you help yourself. Many health benefits are associated with regular exercise, and the completion of PAR-Q is a sensible first step to take if you are planning to increase the amount of physical activity in your life.

For most people physical activity should not pose any problem or hazard. PAR-Q has been designed to identify the small number of adults for whom physical activity might be inappropriate or those who should have medical advice concerning the type of activity most suitable for them.

Common sense is your best guide in answering these few questions. Please read them carefully and check (√) the ☐ YES or ☐ NO opposite the question if it applies to you.

YES   NO

☐   ☐   1. Has your doctor ever said you have heart trouble?

☐   ☐   2. Do you frequently have pains in your heart and chest?

☐   ☐   3. Do you often feel faint or have spells of severe dizziness?

☐   ☐   4. Has a doctor ever said your blood pressure was too high?

☐   ☐   5. Has your doctor ever told you that you have a bone or joint problem such as arthritis that has been aggravated by exercise, or might be made worse with exercise?

☐   ☐   6. Is there a good physical reason not mentioned here why you should not follow an activity program even if you wanted to?

☐   ☐   7. Are you over age 65 and not accustomed to vigorous exercise?

If You Answered

YES to one or more questions

If you have not recently done so, consult with your personal physician by telephone or in person BEFORE increasing your physical activity and/or taking a fitness appraisal. Tell your physician what questions you answered YES to on PAR-Q or present your PAR-Q copy.

programs

After medical evaluation, seek advice from your physician as to your suitability for:
• unrestricted physical activity starting off easily and progressing gradually;
• restricted or supervised activity to meet your specific needs, at least on an initial basis. Check in your community for special programs or services.

NO to all questions

If you answered PAR-Q accurately, you have reasonable assurance of your present suitability for:
• A GRADUATED EXERCISE PROGRAM – a gradual increase in proper exercise promotes good fitness development while minimizing or eliminating discomfort;
• A FITNESS APPRAISAL – the Canadian Standardized Test of Fitness (CSTF).

postpone

If you have a temporary minor illness, such as a common cold.

Developed by the British Columbia Ministry of Health. Conceptualized and critiqued by the Multidisciplinary Advisory Board on Exercise (MABE). Translation, reproduction and use in its entirety is encouraged. Modifications by written permission only. Not to be used for commercial advertising in order to solicit business from the public.
Reference PAR-Q Validation Report British Columbia Ministry of Health 1978.
Produced by the British Columbia Ministry of Health and the Department of National Health & Welfare.

3. Signs or symptoms indicative of health problems
4. Lifestyle behaviors related to positive or negative health
5. Fitness test results

The Health Status Questionnaire (HSQ) provides information concerning the first four categories. Part 1 of the HSQ provides personal and **emergency information** about the individual. You should keep the emergency information readily available in case you need to call the participant's physician or family. Part 2 of the HSQ includes a **medical history** of the participant and her or his family. This information will aid the director of the fitness program in deciding the appropriate exercise and educational programs. Part 3 deals with *behaviors* known to be related to safety and health. You might be able to help the participant modify these behaviors for a healthier lifestyle. Part 4 includes one of the *psychological aspects* of fitness that is associated with the healthy life. Individual questions and parts of questions are coded to help the HFI utilize the information.

Forms and charts are included in the Fitness Participant Handbook (*Fitness Facts*). Encourage the fitness participants to complete these forms and submit them to you so you can assist them in their programs. These tables and figures are included in this book for your information. You have permission to copy and use the forms in this book for educational purposes.

KEY POINT.   Low-intensity exercise can be recommended for anyone who has self-screened with the PAR-Q. All aspects of health status—medical problems, health-related characteristics, signs, symptoms, behaviors, and fitness tests—should be evaluated prior to moderate-intensity exercise.

MEDICAL EXAMINATIONS

Regular medical examinations are encouraged for everyone. Obviously, seeing a physician is appropriate whenever there are special medical problems. The following guidelines for the frequency of medical examinations are recommended by the National Conference on Preventive Medicine [see (6, p. 166)]:

Age	Frequency of medical examination
0 to 1	At least 4 times
2, 5, 8, 15, 18, 25	At each age listed
35 to 65	Every 5 years
Over 65	Every 2 years

TESTING

Testing is the other source of information concerning an individual's health status. Items included in fitness testing are listed in the Physical Fitness Test Items table. Chapters 7, 9, and 10 in Part III of this book include detailed recommendations for fitness testing.

Table 2.1   Physical Fitness Test Items

Minimum battery	Additional variables
REST	
Heart rate (beats · min^{-1})	12-lead ECG[a]
Blood pressure (mmHg)	Blood profile[b]
% fat	Flexibility for specific joints
Waist-to-hip ratio	Pulmonary function
Sit-and-reach (cm)	
SUBMAXIMAL	
HR	ECG
BP	Blood profile
Rating of perceived exertion (RPE)	
MAXIMAL	
BP	$\dot{V}O_2$
RPE	Blood profile
Time to max (min)	ECG
Functional capacity (METs)	Modified pull-ups (no. up to 25)
Curl-ups (no. up to 35)	

[a]ECG abnormalities are medically evaluated to determine appropriate referral or placement.

[b]Includes total cholesterol, HDL cholesterol, triglycerides, and glucose.

The American College of Sports Medicine (1) recommends that all men over 40 years of age and women over 50 years of age have a maximal graded exercise test (GXT), with a physician present, before beginning moderate-intensity exercise. The maximal GXT, with physician present, is also recommended for those who have a high risk of heart disease. Submaximal tests, without a physician, can be administered by qualified testers to individuals without disease or symptoms.

These guidelines are reasonable for persons who are planning to begin an exercise program with moderate to strenuous intensity, such as jogging, aerobic dance, racquetball, or tennis. However, there is increasing evidence that regular light-intensity activity, such as walking done without any discomfort, can have some health benefits with extremely low risk. Persons of any age with varying levels of fitness can be encouraged to engage in these low-intensity activities (self-screened with PAR-Q) without having to have either medical clearance or fitness testing. The walking program found in chapter 14 is a good example of the type of exercise that can be almost universally recommended.

KEY POINT.   Graded exercise tests are recommended prior to beginning moderate- or high-intensity exercise. The ACSM has guidelines, according to age

Health Status Questionnaire

Instructions

Complete each question accurately. All information provided is confidential if you choose to submit this form to your fitness instructor.

Part 1. Information about the individual

1. _____   _____
   Social sec. no.   Date

2. _____   _____
   Legal name   Nickname

3. _____   _____
   Mailing address   Home phone

   _____   _____
                                                             Business phone

4. *EI* _____   _____
   Personal physician   Phone

   _____   _____
   Address

5. *EI* _____   _____
   Person to contact in emergency   Phone

6. Gender (circle one):   Female   Male (*RF*)

7. *RF* Date of birth: _____
                       Month   Day   Year

8. Number of hours worked per week: Less than 20   20-40   41-60   Over 60

9. *SLA* More than 25% of time spent on job (circle all that apply)

   Sitting at desk   Lifting or carrying loads   Standing   Walking   Driving

Part 2.   Medical history

10. *RF* Circle any who died of heart attack before age 50:

    Father   Mother   Brother   Sister   Grandparent

11. Date of

    Last medical physical exam: _____
                                Year
    Last physical fitness test: _____
                                Year

12. Circle operations you have had:

    Back *SLA*   Heart *MC*   Kidney *SLA*   Eyes *SLA*   Joint *SLA*   Neck *SLA*

    Ears *SLA*   Hernia *SLA*   Lung *SLA*   Other _____

13. Please circle any of the following for which you have been diagnosed or treated by a physician or health professional:

Alcoholism *SEP*	Diabetes *SEP*	Kidney problem *MC*
Anemia, sickle cell *SEP*	Emphysema *SEP*	Mental illness *SEP*
Anemia, other *SEP*	Epilepsy *SEP*	Neck strain *SLA*
Asthma *SEP*	Eye problems *SLA*	Obesity *RF*
Back strain *SLA*	Gout *SLA*	Phlebitis *MC*
Bleeding trait *SEP*	Hearing loss *SLA*	Rheumatoid arthritis *SLA*
Bronchitis, chronic *SEP*	Heart problem *MC*	Stroke *MC*
Cancer *SEP*	High blood pressure *RF*	Thyroid problem *SEP*
Cirrhosis, liver *MC*	Hypoglycemia *SEP*	Ulcer *SEP*
Concussion *MC*	Hyperlipidemia *RF*	Other _____
Congenital defect *SEP*	Infectious mononucleosis *MC*	

Cont.

14. Circle all medicine taken in last 6 months:

Blood thinner *MC*	Epilepsy medication *SEP*	Nitroglycerin *MC*
Diabetic pill *SEP*	Heart-rhythm medication *MC*	Other _____
Digitalis *MC*	High-blood-pressure medication *MC*	
Diuretic *MC*	Insulin *MC*	

15. Any of these health symptoms that occurs frequently is the basis for medical attention. Circle the number indicating how often you have each of the following:

   5 = Very often
   4 = Fairly often
   3 = Sometimes
   2 = Infrequently
   1 = Practically never

   a. Cough up blood *MC*
   1 2 3 4 5
   b. Abdominal pain *MC*
   1 2 3 4 5
   c. Low back pain *SLA*
   1 2 3 4 5
   d. Leg pain *MC*
   1 2 3 4 5
   e. Arm or shoulder pain *MC*
   1 2 3 4 5

   f. Chest pain *RF MC*
   1 2 3 4 5
   g. Swollen joints *MC*
   1 2 3 4 5
   h. Feel faint *MC*
   1 2 3 4 5
   i. Dizziness *MC*
   1 2 3 4 5
   j. Breathless with slight exertion *MC*
   1 2 3 4 5

Part 3. Health-related behavior

16. *RF* Do you now smoke?   Yes   No

17. If you are a smoker, indicate number smoked per day:

   Cigarettes: 40 or more   20-39   10-19   1-9
   Cigars or pipes only: 5 or more or any inhaled   Less than 5, none inhaled

18. *RF* Do you exercise regularly?   Yes   No

19. How many days per week do you normally spend at least 20 minutes in moderate to strenuous exercise?

   0 1 2 3 4 5 6 7   days per week

20. Can you walk 4 miles briskly without fatigue?   Yes   No

21. Can you jog 3 miles continuously at a moderate pace without discomfort?   Yes   No

22. Weight now: _____ lb.   One year ago: _____ lb.   Age 21: _____ lb.

Part 4. Health-related attitudes

23. *RF* These are traits that have been associated with coronary-prone behavior. Circle the number that corresponds to how you feel:

   6 = Strongly agree
   5 = Moderately agree
   4 = Slightly agree
   3 = Slightly disagree
   2 = Moderately disagree
   1 = Strongly disagree

   I am an impatient, time-conscious, hard-driving individual.
   1 2 3 4 5 6

24. List everything not already included on this questionnaire that might cause you problems in a fitness test or fitness program:

```
┌─────────────────────────────────────────────────────────────────────────┐
│                   Code for Health Status Questionnaire                    │
│                                                                           │
│  The following code will help you evaluate the information in the Health Status Questionnaire. │
│                                                                           │
│  EI = Emergency Information—must be readily available.                    │
│  MC = Medical Clearance needed—do not allow exercise without physician's permission. │
│  SEP = Special Emergency Procedures needed—do not let participant exercise alone; make sure the person's │
│     exercise partner knows what to do in case of an emergency.            │
│  RF = Risk Factor for CHD (educational materials and workshops needed).   │
│  SLA = Special or Limited Activities may be needed—you may need to include or exclude specific exercises. │
│                                                                           │
│  OTHER (not marked) = Personal information that may be helpful for files or research. │
└─────────────────────────────────────────────────────────────────────────┘
```

and health status, for when a physician's supervision of the test is required.

FITNESS PROGRAM DECISIONS

A fitness program might not use all of the items on the HSQ—the program director should decide what items are relevant for a specific fitness program. The health status form and fitness testing allow the fitness program director to recommend one of the following actions concerning the person's request to enter a fitness program:

- Denial of request for entry to fitness program, and/or immediate referral for medical attention
- Admission to one of the following fitness programs:

  Low-intensity exercise
  Medically supervised exercise
  Exercise carefully prescribed and supervised by exercise leader
  Any fitness activity offered by fitness center

- Recommend educational information, workshops, or professional help

This chapter outlines procedures for appropriately placing individuals based on their health status.

Medical Referral

The fitness director needs to decide whether a potential fitness participant should get medical clearance before beginning a fitness program. The standards in this area are changing. Several years ago, it was recommended that everyone get a complete medical examination prior to beginning a fitness program. However, three factors have caused that standard to change. In the first place,

it is increasingly recognized that being active is healthier than being inactive (some have suggested it is the folks who plan to remain inactive that need a complete physical examination). Secondly, there is increasing evidence that beginning a good fitness program involves a very low risk of health problems for the vast majority of people. And thirdly, the expense of time and money cannot be justified for healthy individuals and physicians that are needed for persons with known or suspected health problems.

Each fitness program should determine its policy with regard to medical clearance and testing before beginning an exercise program. We suggest the following guidelines:

- **Recommend regular medical checkups and health screening as part of public health policy.**
- **Recommend low-intensity exercise [called moderate exercise by ACSM (1)] for everyone who can do it without symptoms or discomfort.**
- **Require medical clearance before moderate- or high-intensity exercise for those with**
  - **known health problems or signs or symptoms indicative of potential health problems, or**
  - **intentions of engaging in very strenuous activities (in athletic performance where the intensity is much higher than that needed for fitness gains).**
- **Require health status screening and fitness testing prior to moderate-intensity exercise [called vigorous exercise by ACSM (1)].**
- **Recommend maximal GXT, with physician interpretation of ECG, for**
  - **those with known cardiovascular disease,**
  - **those with symptoms related to cardiovascular disease,**
  - **those with high risk of cardiovascular disease, or**
  - **men over 40 years of age and women over 50 years of age.**

KEY POINT.   Regular medical examinations and low-intensity exercise are recommended for everyone. Based on evaluation of their health status, persons are advised to seek medical attention, begin low-intensity exercise, or participate in moderate-intensity exercise with or without supervision. Graded exercise tests are recommended as the first part of a fitness program. Older individuals, or those with symptoms of or at high risk for CHD, should have GXT with physician-interpreted exercise ECG.

All persons indicating illness, characteristics, or symptoms coded MC (medical clearance) in the HSQ are referred to appropriate medical personnel. With permission of the appropriate physician, the individual can be placed in a medically supervised, or HFI-supervised, fitness program. The items that fall into those categories, as well as the test scores from the fitness tests that would be the basis for **medical referral**, are shown in the Basis for Medical Referral table.

Table 2.2   Basis for Medical Referral

CONDITIONS

Heart operation, disease, or problem
Cirrhosis
Concussion
Phlebitis
Stroke
Current medication for heart, blood pressure, or diabetes
Cough up blood
Pain in the abdomen, leg, arm, shoulder, or chest
Swollen joints
Faintness or dizziness
Breathlessness with slight exertion

TEST SCORES[a]

Rest HR > 100
Rest SBP > 160
Rest DBP > 100
% Fat > 40 female; > 30 men
Cholesterol > 260
Cholesterol /HDL > 5
Triglycerides > 200
Glucose > 120
Vital cap < 75 % predicted
FEV_1 < 75%

Note. Any condition or test value that causes the person or the HFI to be concerned for the person's health or safety is the basis for medical referral.

[a]Any of these individual scores would be the basis for referral. A person might also be referred if more than one test score approached these values.

General Measurements

The values selected for medical referral or supervised programs are somewhat arbitrary, but they are based on the recommendations of experts in these areas. All of the variables [with the exception of high heart rate (HR)] have been listed as risk factors for CHD at these levels. The values for medical referral are considered very high (with substantial risk of CHD). The "minimal" level indicating problems in these areas (with greater risk of CHD than normal values) are reflected in our values for supervised programs.

A high resting heart rate indicates severe stress, which may have physical or emotional bases. Extreme amounts of fat put the individual at high risk for a variety of health problems (see chapter 7). A high level of serum glucose is related to diabetes. High blood pressure has been the subject of numerous reports and conferences. For example, a 1987 report (2) selected a diastolic blood pressure (DBP) of 90 mmHg as mild, 105 mmHg as moderate, and 115 mmHg as severely hypertensive. If DBP is below 90 mmHg then systolic blood pressure was considered borderline if 140 mmHg and hypertensive if 160 mmHg or greater. These values represent repeat measurements.

The role of serum lipids in the atherosclerotic process has been extensively investigated. Cholesterol and triglycerides are carried in the blood stream in lipoproteins, with the following subdivisions.

Very low-density lipoproteins (VLDL)—Mainly triglycerides, a secondary risk factor for CHD. *High* levels are a high risk of CHD.

Low-density lipoprotein cholesterol (LDL-C)—This is the form of cholesterol that is responsible for the buildup of plaque in the inner walls of the arteries (atherosclerosis). Thus, *high* levels of LDL-C are related to a high risk of CHD.

High-density lipoprotein cholesterol (HDL-C)—This form of cholesterol is protective in the development of CHD, in that it helps transport cholesterol to the liver, where it is eliminated. Thus, *low* levels of HDL-C are related to a high risk of CHD.

Total cholesterol—This is the sum of all forms of cholesterol. Because LDL-C is usually the primary factor in the total amount, a *high* level of total cholesterol is also a risk factor for CHD.

Ratio of total cholesterol/HDL-C—This is one of the best determinants of CHD risk in terms of cholesterol. *High* ratios of total cholesterol to HDL-C are indicative of a high risk of CHD.

The National Cholesterol Education Program (3) selected 200 mg/dl and below as desirable total cholesterol, with 240 mg/dl and higher as high risk. LDL-C levels 160 mg/dl and over are high risk, with 130 mg/dl and below being low risk. HDL-C values 35 mg/dl and below are considered a high risk for CHD. Values of 5 or over for the total cholesterol/HDL-C ratio are high risk, where values less than 3.5 are low risk (5).

Pulmonary Measurements

Pulmonary function is frequently evaluated as a part of the screening aspect of a fitness program. Although many of these variables change little during a typical fitness program, the HFI can provide a service to participants by suggesting that people with low values participate in additional testing.

Vital capacity (VC) is the maximal volume of air expelled after a maximal inspiration. A person whose VC is less than 75% of the value predicted for her or his age, gender, and height should be referred to a physician for further testing. **Forced expiratory volume in 1 s (FEV$_1$)** is the ratio of the volume of air expelled in 1 s compared to the total VC. A person who can expel less than 75% of his or her VC in 1 s should be referred to a physician.

Supervised Program

The conditions and test scores listed in the Basis for a Supervised Program table may be the basis for medical referral if they are severe; however, individuals with mild or moderate levels can participate in low-intensity exercise or in carefully **supervised** fitness **programs**. A person indicating items on the HSQ coded SEP (special emergency procedure) or with risk factors for CHD (coded RF) can be placed in a carefully supervised fitness program, with the necessary emergency procedures, or participate in low-intensity exercise with education about what to do in case of emergency. It is important that the program director determine whether any of the participants have these or other conditions that might affect their ability to exercise.

On the Basis for Special Attention table, there are numerous problems and fitness-test scores listed that would call for special or limited activities. Your recommended adaptation of activities will be based on common sense regarding the condition, talking with the participant about how to deal with the situation, and consulting with the fitness director or physician about appropriate limitations. You should encourage these individuals to include special activities aimed at improving the fitness component(s) for which they obtained the low score(s).

Although we recommend that all fitness participants be screened prior to participation in a moderate-intensity exercise program, we know that exercise leaders are often in a position to lead moderate-intensity exer-

Table 2.3   Basis for a Supervised Program

MEDICAL CONDITIONS
(Currently under control)[a]

Alcoholism	Diabetes
Allergy	Emphysema
Anemia	Epilepsy
Asthma	Hypoglycemia
Bleeding trait	Mental illness
Bronchitis	Peptic ulcer
Cancer	Pregnancy
Colitis	Thyroid problem

TEST SCORES

Condition	Level
Hypertension	140-155/90-95 mmHg[b]
Hyperlipidemia (cholesterol)	240-255 mg/dl[b]
Cholesterol/HDL	4.5-4.8[b]
Obesity	32%-38% for women[b]
	25%-28% for men[b]
Waist-to-hip ratio	> 0.8 for women
	> 0.9 for men
Smoking	> 20 cigarettes/day
Exercise	< 1-1/2 hours/week at or above moderate intensity

[a]Severe or uncontrolled levels should be referred for medical attention.

[b]Persons with higher scores should be referred for medical attention.

cise (such as an aerobic dance class) for persons who have not been screened. A simple checklist (Checklist for Walk-In, Moderate-Intensity Exercisers) can be done either by each individual prior to exercise (in writing or orally), or by the exercise leader asking for answers from the group as the first part of the exercise session. We suggest that you refer all those who answer *yes* to any of these questions to the director of the fitness program prior to exercise. The director should decide whether to make a medical referral, recommend low-intensity exercise, or allow participation in the moderate-intensity supervised program. For example, individuals who have been active in the past without problems may be allowed in the exercise program even if they have high cholesterol or smoke, whereas previously sedentary individuals with the same risk factors might be directed to a walking and stretching program.

Unsupervised Program

Persons without any of the above problems coded under MC, SEP, or RF in the HSQ can have an **unsupervised program** and be admitted to any of the fitness activities.

Table 2.4 Basis for Special Attention

Lengthy time spent	Operations	Other problems
Driving	Back	Arthritis
Lifting	Eyes	Eye problems
Sitting	Joint(s)	Gout
Standing	Lungs	Hearing loss
	Neck	Hernia
		Low-back pain

Test results

Values of risk factors approaching those in supervised
  programs
Any of the reasons for stopping a maximal test that occur at
  light to moderate work[a]
Max RPE < 5 (15 on 6-20 scale)[a]
Max METs < 8 for males, 6 for females[a]
Max $\dot{V}O_2$ < 30 for males, 20 for females[a]
Percent fat < 15% or > 30% for females[b]
Percent fat < 6% or > 25% for males[b]
Curl-ups < 10[c]
Sit-and-reach < 15 cm[c]
Modified pull-ups < 5[c]

[a]See chapter 9.

[b]Participants who have either too little fat (less than 15% for
females and less than 6% for males), as well as those who
have too much fat (greater than 30% for females and greater
than 25% for males) may have health problems that need
special attention. If there is any question, refer them to the
program director.

[c]See chapter 10.

If they have not been active in the past few months,
it is recommended that they begin with low-intensity
activities, but they will be able to progress quickly to
other activities of interest.

Guidelines

Selecting specific test scores as an indication of high,
moderate, or low risk is somewhat arbitrary. In most
cases, it would be more accurate to view the variable
as going from low to high risk. For example, it is better
to have lower total cholesterol. Although 240 mg/dl has
been set as a high-risk level, a person with 239 mg/dl
is not really different from someone with 242 mg/dl.
Nor is a person with 202 mg/dl really different from
someone with 198 mg/dl, even though 200 mg/dl is
set as a target goal. We should encourage everyone to
decrease their total cholesterol; as it decreases, they
will have lower risk. There is nothing magical about

getting below 240 mg/dl or 200 mg/dl—these are only
goals that have been set along the continuum of high to
low risk.

Note that the values listed for medical referral and
for supervised programs are guidelines to be used along
with other information by the individual and fitness program director. Consider the cholesterol example, for
instance. The risk of the same total cholesterol would
be viewed differently for persons with different levels
of HDL. Some of the variables may be influenced by
pretest activities and reaction to the testing situation
itself (especially in persons not accustomed to being
tested). Borderline scores, especially at rest and during
light work, should be replicated before medical referral. For example, if a high resting heart rate or blood
pressure is measured, it may have been due to the participant's having eaten, smoked, or participated in physical exercise just before the test. Was the person anxious
about taking the test itself? Were there unusual conditions during the test (lots of people, noise, etc.)? The
individual should relax for a few minutes, be reassured
about the purpose and safety of the test, and then be
measured again. On the other hand, a test session might
be scheduled for another day. If the questionable test
result is repeated, the program director may refer that
individual to a physician.

There may be other factors that would cause a person
with the characteristics we have listed under "supervised" programs to be medically referred (e.g., multiple risk factors close to the referral value). Or the
medical consultant may recommend that someone in
our "refer" category be in the supervised program,
based on a recent medical examination or conversation
with the personal physician. Programs with excellent
and accessible medical and emergency personnel may
want to use higher values for referral than the program
that is isolated from medical and emergency facilities.
It is recommended that each program, in consultation
with its medical advisors, establish its own standards.

Education

The HSQ and fitness-test results also provide the fitness
leader with information about needed education and
workshops. All persons with risk factors (RF) for CHD
should have information about their increased risk.
Chapter 18 includes some computer programs that can
be used to describe the individual's health-risk profile.
Sufficient evidence allows you to indicate areas of potential health problems, assisting individuals in becoming aware of the risk characteristics that cannot be
changed, and helping persons with those health-related
behaviors that can be modified. Chapter 12 will assist
the fitness leader in using behavior modification for

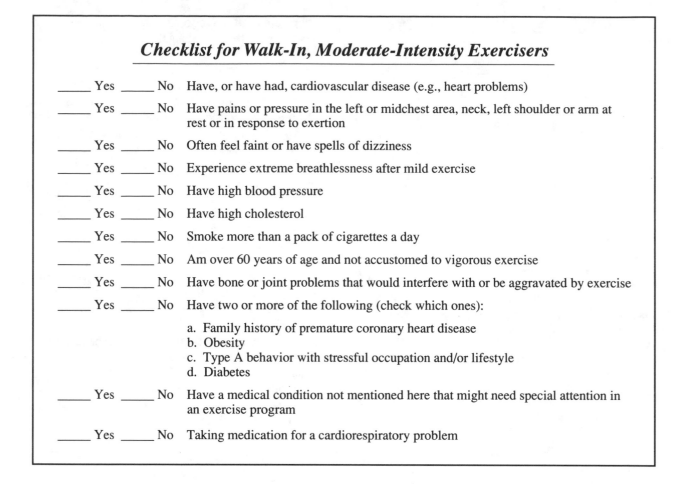

Checklist for Walk-In, Moderate-Intensity Exercisers

_____ Yes _____ No   Have, or have had, cardiovascular disease (e.g., heart problems)

_____ Yes _____ No   Have pains or pressure in the left or midchest area, neck, left shoulder or arm at rest or in response to exertion

_____ Yes _____ No   Often feel faint or have spells of dizziness

_____ Yes _____ No   Experience extreme breathlessness after mild exercise

_____ Yes _____ No   Have high blood pressure

_____ Yes _____ No   Have high cholesterol

_____ Yes _____ No   Smoke more than a pack of cigarettes a day

_____ Yes _____ No   Am over 60 years of age and not accustomed to vigorous exercise

_____ Yes _____ No   Have bone or joint problems that would interfere with or be aggravated by exercise

_____ Yes _____ No   Have two or more of the following (check which ones):

  a. Family history of premature coronary heart disease
  b. Obesity
  c. Type A behavior with stressful occupation and/or lifestyle
  d. Diabetes

_____ Yes _____ No   Have a medical condition not mentioned here that might need special attention in an exercise program

_____ Yes _____ No   Taking medication for a cardiorespiratory problem

desired behavior changes. There are also a number of questions indicating a need for education (ED) in terms of exercise, nutrition, alcohol, smoking, or stress management. This information will be useful for the program director in deciding what workshops and educational materials should be offered to the participants.

KEY POINT.   Individuals who have moderate risk of CHD, conditions that might be affected by exercise, or borderline fitness scores should participate in a supervised program, receive education about their problems, and know what to do in emergencies. Exercise leaders who have unevaluated individuals in a group program should include some screening as part of the class.

CHANGE OF HEALTH/FITNESS STATUS

This chapter has dealt with the initial screenings and the resulting decisions concerning appropriate fitness programs. The HFI needs to understand that persons who are in exercise programs may have health/fitness changes that require a change in their program. One of the purposes of periodic testing is to determine whether persons should be reassigned to different programs. It will be common for individuals to make improvements that will safely allow additional exercise options as part of their fitness programs. In other cases, negative changes occur that need your attention. For example, if an individual in an unsupervised program develops symptoms during exercise, he or she should be referred to a physician, retested, or placed in the supervised program, depending on the severity of the problem.

There are reasons to _discontinue_ an exercise program, including severe psychological, medical, or drug- or alcohol-abuse problems that are not responding to therapy, or problems that are aggravated by activity [adapted from (4)].

There are other reasons to _temporarily defer_ exercise, including excessive heat, humidity, or pollution; sunburn; overindulgence in food, alcohol, stimulating beverages, or drugs such as decongestants, bronchodilators, atropine; dehydration; or anything that causes unusual discomfort with exercise. Exercise should be deferred with major changes in resting blood pressure, or emotional problems [adapted from (2, 4)].

SUMMARY

The HFI should support regular medical examinations, health screening, and low-intensity exercise for the public. One of the responsibilities of a fitness program is to help persons evaluate current health status. This information can be used to refer potential participants to appropriate professionals, low- or moderate-intensity exercise programs, or additional testing. The health status form and suggested fitness-test items presented in this chapter help you identify characteristics needing medical referral. This information helps distinguish conditions and risk factors suggesting a supervised, versus an unsupervised, exercise program. Conditions needing special attention, extra caution, and unique activities are listed. Finally, additional education is needed for fitness participants who are at higher risk for developing serious health problems.

CASE STUDIES FOR ANALYSIS

2.1 You are teaching an exercise-to-music class open to the public. Everyone in the class answered no to all the questions on the checklist for walk-in, moderate-intensity exercisers, except for one obese woman who answered that she got breathless after mild exercise. When you talk to her, it is obvious that she does not know her blood pressure or cholesterol levels. She has never done any fitness or sport activities and cannot climb a flight of stairs or walk two blocks without getting out of breath. She has been reading about the importance of exercise and decided that she should become active. What advice would you give her? (See Appendix A.)

2.2 An African-American male letter-carrier for the post office, aged 42, has just signed up for the fitness program. He appears to be a little nervous. According to his HSQ, he can engage in unsupervised exercise. You are checking his resting HR and BP prior to a GXT and get HR = 110 and BP = 180/86. What would you do? (See Appendix A.)

REFERENCES

1. American College of Sports Medicine (1991)
2. American Heart Association Joint National Committee (1987)
3. American Heart Association National Cholesterol Education Program (1988)
4. Painter and Haskell (1988)
5. Pollock and Wilmore (1990)
6. Sharkey (1990)
7. Shephard (1988)

See the Bibliography at the end of the book for a complete source listing.

Part II

Scientific Foundations

Chapter 3

Exercise Physiology

OBJECTIVES

The reader will be able to:

- Describe the structure of skeletal muscle, the sliding-filament theory of muscle contraction, and the power, speed, endurance, and metabolism of the different types of muscle fibers
- Describe tension development in terms of twitch, summation, and tetanus, and describe the role of recruitment of muscle fiber types in exercise of increasing intensities
- Indicate the methods by which muscle produces energy aerobically and anaerobically, and evaluate the importance of each type of energy production in fitness and sport activities
- Describe the various fuels for muscle work, and the effect of exercise intensity and duration on the respiratory exchange ratio
- Describe how the ventilatory threshold and the lactate threshold are indicators of fitness, as well as predictors of performance in endurance events
- Describe the blood pressure responses to changes in posture, static (isometric) exercise, weight lifting, and dynamic endurance exercise
- List the physiological adaptations of muscle structure, energy metabolism, and the cardiorespiratory responses at rest, during submaximal exercise, and during maximal exercise, following an endurance training program
- Describe the changes in each of the following variables to a graded exercise test taken to a subject's maximum: $\dot{V}O_2$, blood lactate, pulmonary ventilation, respiratory rate, tidal volume, cardiac output, heart rate, stroke volume, arteriovenous oxygen difference, systolic and diastolic blood pressures
- Describe the effect of an endurance training program on each of the variables identified in the preceding objective
- Describe the role of the trained-state of skeletal muscle in the heart-rate response to submaximal exercise, and relate this to the specificity of training
- Discuss the effect of stopping or reducing training on $\dot{V}O_2$max
- Describe the various mechanisms of heat loss, and the role of each in (a) submaximal exercise conducted in an environment that is increasing in temperature, and (b) a comfortable environment in which the intensity of exercise increases
- Describe the effect of altitude and carbon monoxide on $\dot{V}O_2$max
- Describe how males and females differ in their cardiovascular response to graded exercise

Terms

The reader will be able to define or describe:

A band	Arterioles
Actin	Autonomic nervous system
Actomyosin	Baroreceptors
Aerobic	Beta-adrenergic receptors
Anaerobic	Conduction
Anaerobic threshold	Convection

Creatine phosphate
Cross bridge
Diabetes
Double product
Ejection fraction
End diastolic volume
Epinephrine
Evaporation
Glycolysis
Hyperventilation
Hypoglycemia
H zone
I band
Insulin
Lactate threshold
Maximal aerobic power
Maximal oxygen uptake
Mitochondria
Muscle fiber
Myofibril
Myosin
Norepinephrine
Oxygen consumption
Oxygen debt
Oxygen deficit
Parasympathetic nervous system

Pulmonary ventilation
Radiation
Rate–pressure product
Relative humidity
Respiratory exchange ratio
Respiratory quotient
Sarcomeres
Sarcoplasmic reticulum
Saturation pressure
Sliding-filament theory
Steady-state oxygen requirement
Summation
Sweating
Sympathetic nervous system
Tetanus
Transverse tubules
Tropomyosin
Troponin
Twitch
Type I (slow oxidative) fibers
Type IIa (fast oxidative glycolytic) fibers
Type IIb (fast glycolytic) fibers
Ventilatory threshold
$\dot{V}O_2$max
Water vapor pressure gradient
Z line

The Health Fitness Instructor needs to know basic aspects of exercise physiology in order to prescribe appropriate activities, deal with weight loss concerns, and explain to participants what happens as a result of training or when exercise is done in a hot and humid environment. This chapter can't possibly cover the extensive detail found in an exercise physiology text; instead we summarize major topics and, where possible, apply the discussion to exercise testing and exercise prescription. We refer the interested reader to the exercise physiology texts on the Suggested Readings list at the end of this chapter.

MUSCLE STRUCTURE AND FUNCTION

Exercise means movement, and movement requires muscle action. To discuss human physiology related to exercise and endurance training, we must start with skeletal muscle, the tissue that converts the chemical energy of adenosine triphosphate (ATP) to mechanical work. How does a muscle do this? We will begin with a presentation of the structure of skeletal muscle.

Figure 3.1 shows the structure of skeletal muscle, from the intact muscle to the smallest functional unit. A **muscle fiber** is a cylindrical cell that has repeating light and dark bands, giving it the name *striated muscle*. The striations are due to a more basic structural component called the **myofibril**, which runs the length of the muscle. Each myofibril is composed of a long series of **sarcomeres**, the fundamental unit of muscle contraction. Figure 3.1 shows the sarcomere to be composed of the thick filament **myosin** and the thin filament **actin**, and is bounded by connective tissue called the **Z line** (54).

An enlargement of two sarcomeres in Figure 3.2 shows the **A band, I band** , and **H zone**, and the changes that take place when the sarcomere goes from the resting state to the contracted state. The I band is composed of actin and is bisected by the Z line, and the A band is composed of myosin and actin. According to the **sliding-filament theory** of muscle contraction, the thin filaments slide over the thick filaments, pulling the Z lines toward the center of the sarcomere. In this way the entire muscle shortens, but the contractile proteins do not change size. How does the muscle release the energy in ATP to make this happen?

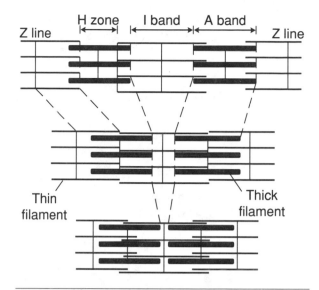

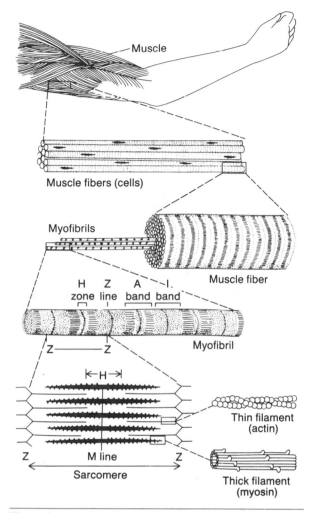

Figure 3.2 Changes in filament alignment and banding pattern in a myofibril during shortening. *Note.* From *Human Physiology* (3rd ed.) (p. 216) by A.J. Vander, J.H. Sherman, and D.S. Luciano, 1980, New York: McGraw Hill. Copyright 1980 by McGraw Hill. Reprinted by permisison.

- the cross bridge moves and pulls actin toward the center of the sarcomere; and
- ATP binds to and releases the cross bridge from actin to start the process over again.

If all of the components needed for muscle contraction are present, why aren't the cross bridges always moving and the muscle always in the state of contraction? At rest there are two proteins associated with actin that block the interaction of myosin with actin: **troponin**, which has the capacity to bind calcium, and **tropomyosin**. Figure 3.4 shows that when a muscle is depolarized (excited) by a motor nerve, the action potential spreads over the surface of the muscle fiber and enters the fiber through special channels called **transverse tubules**. Once inside the muscle fiber, this wave of depolarization spreads over the **sarcoplasmic reticulum** (SR), a membrane that surrounds the myofibril, and calcium is released from the SR into the sarcoplasm. When the calcium binds with troponin, the tropomyosin aligns the binding site on actin so the myosin cross bridge can interact with it. The formation of **actomyosin** releases the energy, the cross bridge that is bound to actin moves, and the sarcomere shortens. This sequence is repeated as long as there is calcium present and the muscle has ATP to replace what is used. Muscle relaxation is achieved when the calcium is pumped back into the sarcoplasmic reticulum and troponin and tropomyosin can again block the interaction of actin and myosin (54).

Figure 3.1 Levels of fibrillar organization within a skeletal muscle. *Note.* From *Human Physiology* (3rd ed.) (p. 212) by A.J. Vander, J.H. Sherman, and D.S. Luciano, 1980, New York: McGraw Hill. Copyright 1980 by McGraw Hill. Reprinted by permission.

If ATP is the energy supply, then an ATPase (an enzyme) must exist in muscle to split ATP and release the potential energy contained within its structure. The ATPase is found in an extension of the thick myosin filament, the **cross bridge**, which also possesses the ability to bind to actin. Figure 3.3 shows the interaction of ATP, the cross bridge, and actin that leads to the shortening of the sarcomere (54).

KEY POINT. Muscle contraction occurs when

- ATP is split to form a high-energy myosin-ATP cross bridge;
- the myosin-ATP cross bridge binds to actin and energy is released;

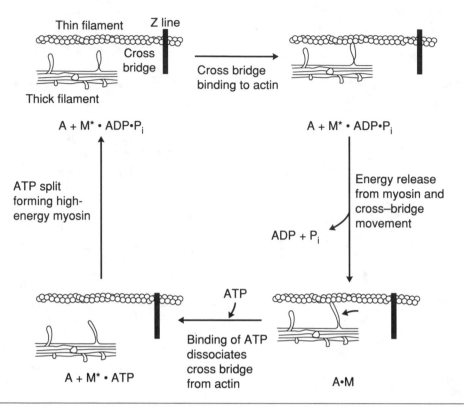

Figure 3.3 Chemical and mechanical changes during the four stages of a single cross-bridge cycle. Start reading the figure at the lower left. *Note.* From *Human Physiology* (4th ed.) (p. 263) by A.J. Vander, J.H. Sherman, and D.S. Luciano, 1985, New York: McGraw Hill. Copyright 1985 by McGraw Hill. Reprinted by permission.

The muscle needs ATP for cross-bridge movement, to pump the calcium back to the SR, and for the maintenance of the resting membrane potential that allows the muscle to be depolarized. Where does this ATP come from?

RELATIONSHIP OF ENERGY AND WORK

Several kinds of energy exist in biological systems: electrical energy in nerves and muscles; chemical energy in the synthesis of molecules; mechanical energy in the contraction of a muscle to move an object; and thermal energy, derived from all of these processes, that helps to maintain body temperature. The ultimate source of the energy for biological systems is the sun. The radiant energy from the sun is captured by plants and used to convert simple atoms and molecules into carbohydrates, fats, and proteins. The sun's energy is trapped within the chemical bonds of these food molecules.

For the cells to use this energy, the foodstuffs must be broken down in a manner that conserves most of the energy contained in the bonds of the carbohydrates, fats, and proteins. In addition, the final product must

be in a form that can be used by the cell. As mentioned above, cells use ATP as the primary energy source for biological work, whether electrical, mechanical, or chemical. ATP is a molecule that has three phosphates linked together by high-energy bonds. When the bond between the phosphates is broken, energy is released and may be used by the cell. At this point the ATP has been reduced to a lower energy state: adenosine diphosphate (ADP) and inorganic phosphate (Pi).

$$ATP \rightarrow ADP + Pi + \text{energy for work}$$

When a muscle is doing work, ATP is constantly being broken down to ADP and Pi. The ATP must be replaced as fast as it is being used if the cell is to continue to work. The muscle cell has a great capacity to replace ATP under a wide variety of circumstances, from a short, quick dash to a marathon. Edington and Edgerton (13) devised a logical approach to this topic of supplying energy for muscle contraction. They divided the energy sources into immediate, short-term, and long-term sources of ATP.

Immediate Sources of Energy

The very limited amount of ATP stored in a muscle might meet the energy demands of a maximal effort

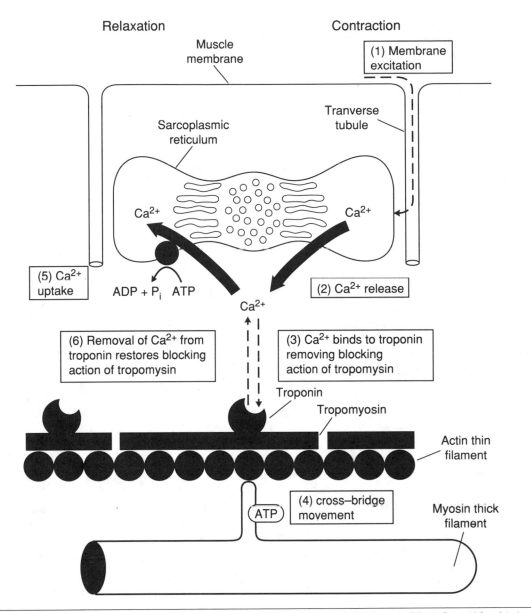

Figure 3.4 Role of calcium in muscle excitation-contraction coupling. *Note.* From *Human Physiology* (4th ed.) (p. 268) by A.J. Vander, J.H. Sherman, and D.S. Luciano, 1985, New York: McGraw Hill. Copyright 1985 by McGraw Hill. Reprinted by permission.

lasting about 1 s. **Creatine phosphate** (CP), another high-energy phosphate molecule stored in the muscle, is the most important immediate source of energy. CP can donate its phosphate (and the energy therein) to ADP to make ATP, allowing the muscle to continue working.

$$CP + ADP \rightarrow ATP + C$$

This reaction takes place as fast as the muscle forms ADP. Unfortunately, the CP store in muscle lasts only 3 to 5 s when the muscle is working maximally. This process does not require oxygen and is one of the **anaerobic** (without oxygen) mechanisms for producing ATP. CP would be the primary source of ATP during

a shot put, a vertical jump, or the first seconds of a sprint.

Short-Term Sources of Energy

As the muscle store of CP decreases, the cell begins to break down muscle glycogen (the muscle glucose store) to produce ATP at a very high rate. This process is called **glycolysis**, and it does not require oxygen (it is anaerobic).

Muscle glycogen → glucose → 2 lactic acid + 3 ATP

Glycolysis allows the muscle to continue doing intense

work, but only for a limited period of time. An end product of glycolysis is lactic acid; as exercise continues, lactic acid accumulates in the muscle cells and the blood. This accumulation of acid in the muscle slows down the rate at which the glycogen can be broken down and may actually interfere with the mechanism involved in muscle contraction. Supplying ATP via glycolysis has its obvious shortcomings, but it does allow a person to run at high rates of speed for short distances. This short-term source of energy is of primary importance in events involving maximal work lasting 2 to 3 min.

Long-Term Sources of Energy

The long-term source of energy involves the production of ATP from a variety of fuels, but this method requires the utilization of oxygen (it is **aerobic**). The primary fuels include muscle glycogen, blood glucose, plasma free fatty acids, and intramuscular fats. These molecules are broken down so they can transfer the energy contained in their chemical bonds to a site in the cell where ATP is synthesized. Most of these reactions occur in the **mitochondria** of the cell, where oxygen is used.

Carbohydrates and fats + O_2 → mitochondria → ATP

ATP production from this source is slower than from the immediate and short-term sources of energy, and during submaximal work it may be 2 or 3 min before the ATP needs of the cell are completely met by this aerobic process. One reason for this lag is the time it takes for the heart to increase the delivery of oxygen-enriched blood to the muscles at the rate needed to meet the ATP demands of the muscle. The aerobic production of ATP is the primary means of supplying energy to the muscle in maximal work lasting more than 2 to 3 min, and for all types of submaximal work.

KEY POINTS.

- ATP is supplied at a high rate by the anaerobic processes: creatine phosphate breakdown and glycolysis.
- ATP is supplied during prolonged exercise by the aerobic metabolism of carbohydrates and fats in the mitochondria of the muscle.

Interaction of Exercise Intensity, Duration, and Energy Production

The proportion of energy coming from the anaerobic sources (immediate and short-term) is very much influ-

enced by the intensity and duration of the activity. Figure 3.5 shows that during an all-out activity lasting less than 1 min (e.g., a 400-m dash), the muscles obtain most of the ATP from anaerobic sources. In a 2- to 3-min maximal effort, approximately 50% of the energy comes from anaerobic sources and 50% comes from aerobic sources; in a 10-min *maximal* effort, the anaerobic component drops to 15%. Thus the anaerobic component is considerably less than 15% in a typical *submaximal* training session.

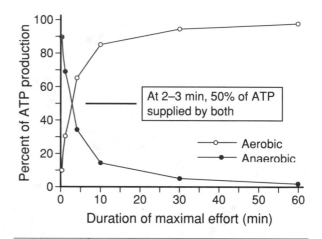

Figure 3.5   Percent contribution to total energy supply during maximal work of various durations. Adapted from Powers and Howley (1990).

Muscle Fiber Types and Performance

Muscle fibers vary in their abilities to produce ATP by the mechanisms described. Some muscle fibers contract quickly and have an innate capacity to produce great amounts of force, but they fatigue quickly. These muscle fibers produce most of their ATP by creatine phosphate breakdown and glycolysis, and are termed **fast glycolytic** (FG), or **Type IIb, fibers**. Other muscle fibers contract slowly and produce only small amounts of force, but they have great resistance to fatigue. These fibers produce most of their ATP aerobically in the mitochondria and are called **slow oxidative** (SO), or **Type I, fibers**. They have many mitochondria and a relatively large number of capillaries helping to deliver oxygen to the mitochondria. Lastly, there is a fiber with a combination of the Type I and Type IIb characteristics. It is a fast-contracting muscle fiber that produces a great force when stimulated, but it possesses a resistance to fatigue because of its large number of mitochondria and capillaries. These fibers are called **fast oxidative glycolytic** (FOG), or **Type IIa**, fibers.

KEY POINT.   Muscle fibers differ in speed of contraction, force, and resistance to fatigue:

- Type I—slow oxidative (SO): slow, low force, fatigue resistant
- Type IIa—fast oxidative glycolytic (FOG): fast, high force, fatigue resistant
- Type IIb—fast glycolytic (FG): fast twitch, high force, fatiguable

Genetics, Gender, and Training

In the average male and female, about 52% of the muscle fibers are Type I, with the fast-twitch fibers divided into 33% Type IIa and 13% Type IIb (47, 49). However, there is great variation in the distribution of fiber types in the population. On the basis of studies comparing identical to fraternal twins, the distribution of fast and slow fibers seems to be genetically fixed. Consequently, fast-twitch fibers *cannot* be converted to slow-twitch fibers, and vice versa. On the other hand, the capacity of the muscle fiber to produce ATP aerobically (its oxidative capacity) seems to be easily altered by endurance training. In fact, in some elite endurance athletes Type IIb fibers can't be found; they have been converted to the oxidative version, Type IIa (47). The increase in mitochondria and capillaries in endurance-trained muscles allows an individual to meet ATP demands via aerobic processes, with less glycogen depletion and lactate formation (25).

Tension (Force) Development

The tension or force generated by a muscle depends on more than the fiber type. When a single threshold-level stimulus excites a muscle fiber, a single, low-tension **twitch** results, a brief contraction followed by relaxation. If the frequency of stimulation is increased, the muscle fiber can't relax between stimuli, and the tension of one contraction is added on to the previous one. This is called **summation**. A further increase in the frequency of stimulation results in the contractions fusing together into a smooth, sustained, high-tension contraction called **tetanus**. However, force of contraction is dependent on more than frequency of stimulation; it is dependent also on the degree to which the muscle fibers contract simultaneously (synchronous firing) and the number of muscle fibers recruited. This latter factor is the most important.

Fiber-Type Recruitment

Figure 3.6 shows the order of recruitment of the different muscle fiber types as the intensity of exercise increases. The order is from the most to the least oxidative, from the slowest fiber to the fastest (45).

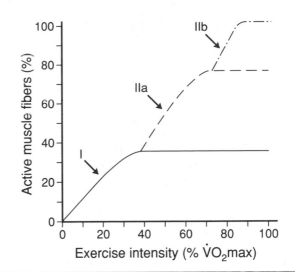

Figure 3.6 Order of muscle fiber type recruitment in exercise of increasing intensity. *Note.* From D.G. Sale, "Influence of Exercise & Training on Motor Unit Activation." In *Exercise and Sport Sciences Reviews*, Volume 15, edited by K.B. Pandolf, PhD. Copyright © 1987 American College of Sports Medicine. Adapted with permission of Macmillan Publishing Company.

Consequently, at higher work rates when the Type IIb fibers are being recruited, there is a greater chance of producing lactic acid. Although chronic light (<40% $\dot{V}O_2$max) exercise recruits and causes a training effect in only the Type I fibers, exercise beyond 70% $\dot{V}O_2$max involves all the fiber types. This has important implications in the specificity of training and the potential for transferring training effects from one activity to another. Obviously, if you don't use a muscle fiber, it can't become "trained."

METABOLIC, CARDIOVASCULAR, AND RESPIRATORY RESPONSES TO EXERCISE

A primary task of the HFI is to recommend physical activities that increase or maintain cardiorespiratory function. Activities that demand the production of energy (ATP) by aerobic mechanisms automatically cause the circulatory and respiratory systems to deliver oxygen to the muscle to meet the demand. The selected aerobic activities must be strenuous enough to challenge the cardiorespiratory systems to cause the systems to improve. This crucial link between aerobic activities and cardiorespiratory function provides the basis for much of exercise programming. The following sections present a summary of selected metabolic, cardiovascular, and respiratory responses to submaximal work and to a graded exercise test taken to maximum.

We will begin with a discussion of how oxygen uptake is measured.

Measurement of Oxygen Uptake

How does oxygen get to the mitochondria? Oxygen enters the lungs when a person inhales; it then diffuses from the alveoli of the lungs into the blood. Oxygen is bound to hemoglobin in the red blood cells, and the heart delivers the oxygen-enriched blood to the muscles. Oxygen then diffuses into the muscle cells to the mitochondria, where it is used (consumed) in the production of ATP. How is oxygen consumption measured during exercise?

Oxygen consumption ($\dot{V}O_2$) is measured by subtracting the volume of oxygen exhaled from the volume of oxygen inhaled.

$$(\dot{V}O_2) = \text{volume } O_2 \text{ inhaled} - \text{volume } O_2 \text{ exhaled}$$

In general, the subject breathes through a special valve that allows room air (containing 20.93% O_2 and 0.03% CO_2) to be inhaled into the lungs while directing exhaled air to a meterological balloon or Douglas bag (see Figure 3.7). A volume meter measures the liters of air inhaled per minute, which is called the **pulmonary ventilation**. The exhaled air contained in the meterological balloon is analyzed for its oxygen and carbon dioxide content, and the oxygen consumption (uptake) is calculated by simply multiplying the volume of air breathed by the percentage of oxygen extracted. Oxygen extraction is the percentage of oxygen extracted from the inhaled air, the difference between the 20.93% O_2 in room air and the percent O_2 in the meterological balloon.

The following example indicates the general steps used to calculate $\dot{V}O_2$—the exact procedure is in Appendix B.

$$\dot{V}O_2 = \text{ventilation (L} \cdot \text{min}^{-1}) \cdot$$

$$O_2 \text{ extraction (\%)}$$

If ventilation = 60 L $\cdot$ min^{-1}, and exhaled O_2 = 16.93%, then

$$\dot{V}O_2 = 60 \text{ L} \cdot \text{min}^{-1} \cdot (20.93\% \ O_2 -$$

$$16.93\% \ O_2)$$

$$= 60 \text{ L} \cdot \text{min}^{-1} \cdot 4.0\%$$

$$= 2.4 \text{ L} \cdot \text{min}^{-1}$$

Carbon dioxide (CO_2) is produced in the mitochondria, diffuses out of the muscle into the venous blood,

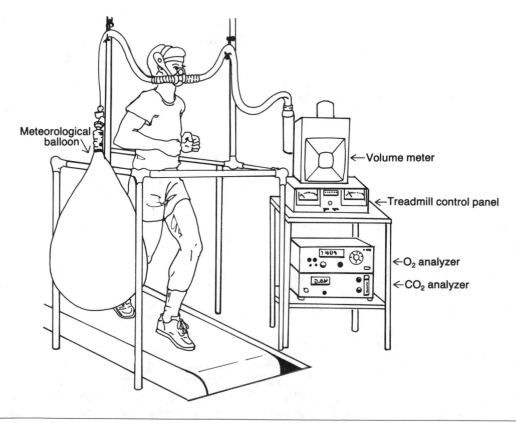

Figure 3.7 Conventional equipment involved in the measurement of oxygen uptake.

is carried back to the lungs where it diffuses into the alveoli, and is exhaled into the meterological balloon. Carbon dioxide production ($\dot{V}CO_2$) can be calculated as described for the $\dot{V}O_2$.

If ventilation $= 60\ L \cdot min^{-1}$, and exhaled $CO_2 = 3.03\%$, then

$$\dot{V}CO_2 = 60\ L \cdot min^{-1} \cdot (3.03\%\ CO_2 -$$

$$0.03\%\ CO_2)$$

$$= 60\ L \cdot min^{-1} \cdot 3.0\%$$

$$= 1.8\ L \cdot min^{-1}$$

The ratio of CO_2 production ($\dot{V}CO_2$) to oxygen consumption ($\dot{V}O_2$) at the cell is called the **respiratory quotient** (RQ). Because the measurements of $\dot{V}CO_2$ and $\dot{V}O_2$ are made at the mouth rather than at the tissue, this ratio is called the **respiratory exchange ratio** (R). R is an important measure in that it can tell us what type of fuel is being used during exercise.

$$R = \dot{V}CO_2 \div \dot{V}O_2$$

Using the values already calculated,

$$R = 1.8\ L \cdot min^{-1} \div 2.4\ L \cdot min^{-1} = 0.75$$

Fuel Utilization During Exercise

In general, protein contributes less than 5% to total energy production during exercise, and for our discussion it will be ignored (40). This leaves carbohydrate (muscle glycogen, and blood glucose, which is derived from liver glycogen) and fat (adipose tissue and intramuscular fat) as the primary fuels for exercise. The

ability of the respiratory exchange ratio to provide good information about the metabolism of fats and carbohydrates during exercise is due to the following observations about the metabolism of fats and glucose.

When R = 1.0, 100% of the energy is derived from carbohydrates, 0% from fat; when R = 0.7, it is the reverse. When R = 0.85, approximately 50% of the energy is derived from carbohydrates and 50% from fat. For the measurement to be correct, the subject must be in a steady state. If lactic acid is increasing in the blood, the plasma bicarbonate (HCO_3) buffer store will react with the acid (H^+) and produce CO_2, which will be exhaled as we are stimulated to hyperventilate:

$$H^+ + HCO_3^- \rightarrow H_2O + CO_2$$

This CO_2 is not the result of the aerobic metabolism of carbohydrate and fat, and when the CO_2 is exhaled it will result in an overestimation of the true value of R. During strenuous work when Type IIb fibers are recruited, lactic acid will be produced, driving R over 1.0.

Effect of Exercise Intensity

Figure 3.8 shows the changes in R during progressive work up to $\dot{V}O_2$max. In the progressive test, R increases at about 40% to 50% $\dot{V}O_2$max, indicating that Type IIa fibers are being recruited and carbohydrates are becoming a more important fuel source. This has an adaptive advantage—the muscle obtains about 6% more energy from each liter of O_2 when carbohydrates are used (5 kcal $\cdot$ L^{-1}) compared to when fat is used (4.7 kcal $\cdot$ L^{-1}). The primary carbohydrate used in exercise is muscle glycogen, with blood glucose contributing about 10% to 15% to the total energy supply. The

---

Respiratory Exchange Ratios for Carbohydrate and Fat

For glucose:

$$C_6H_{12}O_6 + 6\ O_2 \rightarrow 6\ CO_2 + 6\ H_2O + energy$$

$$R = \frac{6\ CO_2}{6\ O_2} = 1.0$$

For palmitate (a fatty acid):

$$C_{16}H_{32}O_2 + 23\ O_2 \rightarrow 16\ CO_2 + 16\ H_2O + energy$$

$$R = \frac{16\ CO_2}{23\ O_2} = 0.7$$

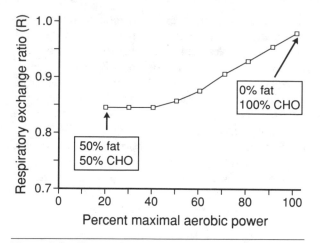

Figure 3.8 Changes in the respiratory exchange ratio with increasing exercise intensity. Adapted from Åstrand and Rodahl (1986).

higher the intensity of exercise, the greater the rate at which muscle glycogen is used; and in sustained heavy exercise (>75% $\dot{V}O_2$max), inadequate muscle glycogen results in premature fatigue (6).

Effect of Exercise Duration

Figure 3.9 shows the change in R during a 90-min test at 60% to 70% of the subject's $\dot{V}O_2$max (41). R decreases over time, indicating a greater reliance on fat

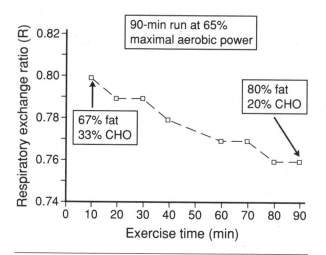

Figure 3.9 Changes in the respiratory exchange ratio during prolonged steady-state exercise. Data from Powers, Riley, and Howley (1980).

as a fuel. The fats are derived from both intramuscular fat stores and adipose tissue, which releases free fatty acids into the blood to be carried to the muscle. This increased use of fat spares the remaining carbohydrate stores and extends the time to exhaustion.

Hormones and Fuel Mobilization

Plasma glucose and free fatty acids used during exercise must be replaced with that stored in the liver and adipose tissue, respectively. A wide variety of hormones are involved in the mobilization of fuels, but special attention will be focused on **insulin**. Insulin secretion from the pancreas increases immediately following a meal to help store nutrients in the liver and adipose tissue. Without adequate insulin, the plasma glucose concentration would increase, because glucose would not be removed by the cells at the correct rate. You know this condition as **diabetes**. The fact that insulin is needed to take glucose into cells might suggest that you need more insulin during exercise because the muscle cells are using more glucose as fuel. However, that is not the case. During exercise the muscle membrane becomes more permeable to glucose, and less insulin is needed. This has important consequences for the diabetic, who may have to reduce the amount of insulin injected before certain types of exercise (see chapter 13). The plasma insulin concentration decreases during exercise; such a change favors the mobilization, not storage, of fuel. If insulin secretion increased during exercise, glucose would be removed from the plasma so fast that **hypoglycemia**, a low blood-glucose condition, would result.

Effect of Diet and Training

The type of fuel used during exercise is dependent on diet. It has been clearly demonstrated that a high-carbohydrate diet increases the muscle glycogen content and extends the time to exhaustion, compared to an average diet (28). Further, the capacity of the muscle to increase its glycogen store is increased if strenuous exercise is performed prior to eating the high-carbohydrate diet (28, 51).

The increase in the number of mitochondria in the muscle accompanying endurance training results in an increased capacity of the muscle to use fat as a fuel and an increased ability to process the available carbohydrate aerobically. This results in a sparing of the carbohydrate store and a reduction in lactate production, both of which favorably influence performance (25).

Transition From Rest to Steady-State Work

Some readers might mistakenly assume from the discussion of the immediate, short- and long-term sources of energy that these various sources of ATP are used in distinct activities and do not work together to allow a person to make the transition from rest to exercise. If an individual were to step onto a treadmill with the belt moving at a velocity of 200 m • min^{-1} (7.5 mi • hr^{-1}), the ATP requirement would increase from the low level needed to stand alongside the treadmill to the new level of ATP required by the muscles to run at 200 m • min^{-1}. This change in the ATP supply to the muscle must take place in the first step onto the treadmill. Failure to do so results in the individual going off the back of the treadmill. What energy sources supply ATP during the first minutes of work?

Oxygen Uptake

The cardiovascular and respiratory systems cannot instantaneously increase the delivery of oxygen to the muscles to completely meet the ATP demands by aerobic processes. In the interval between the time a person steps onto the treadmill and the time his or her cardiovascular and respiratory systems deliver the correct amount of oxygen, the immediate and short-term sources of energy supply the needed ATP. The volume of oxygen "missing" in the first few minutes of work is the **oxygen deficit** (Figure 3.10). Creatine phosphate supplies some of the needed ATP, and the anaerobic breakdown of glycogen to lactic acid provides the rest until the oxidative mechanisms come into play. When the oxygen uptake levels off during submaximal work, the oxygen uptake value is said to represent the **steady-state oxygen requirement** for the activity. At this point the ATP need of the cell is being met by the production of ATP with oxygen in the mitochondria of the muscle on a "pay as you go" basis.

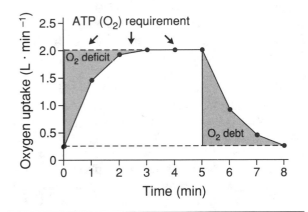

Figure 3.10 Oxygen deficit and oxygen debt (repayment) during a 5-minute run on a treadmill.

When the individual stops running and steps off the treadmill, the ATP need of the muscles that were involved in the activity drops suddenly back toward the resting value. The oxygen uptake decreases quickly at first and then more gradually approaches the resting

value. This elevated oxygen uptake in recovery from exercise is called the oxygen repayment, or **oxygen debt** (Figure 3.10). In part, the extra oxygen is being used to make additional ATP to bring the CP store of the muscle back to normal (remember that it was depleted somewhat at the onset of work). The remainder of the "extra" oxygen taken in during recovery from exercise is used to pay the ATP requirement for the higher heart rate and breathing during recovery (compared to rest). A small part of the oxygen repayment is used by the liver to convert a portion of the lactic acid produced at the onset of work into glucose (40).

If an individual reaches the steady-state oxygen requirement earlier during the first minutes of work, she or he incurs a smaller oxygen deficit. This results in less CP depletion and the production of less lactic acid. Endurance training speeds up the kinetics of oxygen transport; that is, it decreases the time needed to reach a steady state of oxygen uptake. People in poor condition, as well as people with cardiovascular or pulmonary disease, take longer to reach the steady-state oxygen requirement. As a result, they incur a larger oxygen deficit and must produce more ATP by the immediate and short-term sources of energy at the onset of work (20, 39).

Heart Rate and Pulmonary Ventilation

This link between the cardiorespiratory responses to work and the time it takes to reach the steady-state oxygen requirement should be no surprise. Figure 3.11 shows the typical heart-rate and pulmonary-ventilation responses to a submaximal run test. The shape of the curve in each case resembles the curve for oxygen uptake described earlier.

Additionally, the muscle has something to do with the lag in the oxygen-uptake response at the onset of work. An untrained muscle has relatively few mito-

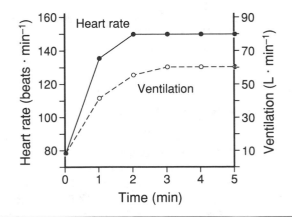

Figure 3.11 Heart-rate and pulmonary-ventilation responses during a 5-minute run on a treadmill.

chondria available to produce ATP aerobically and also has relatively few capillaries per muscle fiber to bring the oxygen-enriched arterial blood to those mitochondria. Following an endurance-training program, both of these factors increase, so the muscle can produce more ATP aerobically at the onset of work. The result is a reduction in lactic acid production and a lowering of the blood lactic acid concentration for a fixed submaximal work rate following an endurance-training program (20, 25, 39).

GRADED EXERCISE TEST

A clear link exists between oxygen consumption and cardiorespiratory fitness, because oxygen delivery to tissue is dependent on lung and heart function. One of the most common tests used to evaluate cardiorespiratory function is a graded exercise test (GXT) in which the subject exercises at progressively increasing work rates until maximum work tolerance is reached. During the test the subject may be monitored for cardiovascular variables (ECG, heart rate, blood pressure), respiratory variables (pulmonary ventilation, respiratory frequency), and metabolic variables (oxygen uptake, blood lactic acid level). The manner in which an individual responds to each stage of the GXT gives important information about cardiorespiratory function.

Oxygen Uptake and Maximal Aerobic Power

Oxygen uptake, measured as described earlier, is expressed per kilogram of body weight to facilitate comparisons between people and for the same person over time. The $\dot{V}O_2$ value in liters per minute is simply multiplied by 1,000 to convert the $\dot{V}O_2$ to ml $\cdot$ min^{-1}; that value is divided by the subject's body weight in kilograms to yield a value expressed in milliliters per kilogram per minute.

$$\dot{V}O_2 = 2.4\,L \cdot min^{-1} \cdot \frac{1,000\,ml}{L}$$

$$= 2,400\,ml \cdot min^{-1}$$

For a 60-kg subject,

$$2,400\,ml \cdot min^{-1} \div 60\,kg = 40\,ml \cdot kg^{-1} \cdot min^{-1}$$

Figure 3.12 shows a GXT conducted on a treadmill where the speed is constant (3 mi $\cdot$ hr^{-1}) and the grade changes 3% every 3 min. With each stage of a GXT the oxygen uptake increases to meet the ATP demand of the work rate. At each stage of the GXT the subject incurs a small oxygen deficit as the cardiovascular system tries to adjust to the new demand placed on it by the increased work rate.

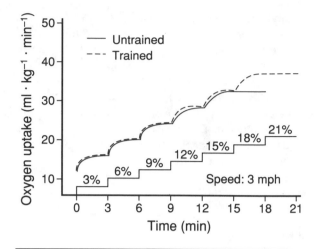

Figure 3.12 Oxygen uptake responses to a graded exercise test. Data adapted from *Nutrition, Weight Control, and Exercise* (p. 52) by F.I. Katch and W.D. McArdle, 1977, Boston: Houghton Mifflin.

It has been shown that apparently healthy individuals reach the steady-state requirement by 1.5 min or so of each stage of the test up to moderately heavy work (37, 38). Those who have low cardiorespiratory fitness or who possess cardiovascular and pulmonary diseases may not be able to reach the expected values in the same amount of time and might incur larger oxygen deficits with each stage of the test. The oxygen uptake measured at various stages of the test on these latter subjects would be lower than expected, because they could not reach the expected steady-state demands of the test at each stage.

Toward the end of a GXT, a point is reached at which the work rate changes (i.e., the grade on the treadmill is increased) but the oxygen uptake does not. In effect, the limits of the cardiovascular system to transport oxygen to the muscle have been reached. This point is called **maximal aerobic power,** or **maximal oxygen uptake ($\dot{V}O_2$max).** A complete leveling-off in the oxygen consumption is not seen in all cases, because it requires the subject to work one stage past the actual point at which $\dot{V}O_2$max is reached. This requires the subjects to be highly motivated. The "plateau" in oxygen uptake is judged against the criteria of less than 150 ml $\cdot$ min^{-1} or 2.1 ml $\cdot$ kg^{-1} $\cdot$ min^{-1} increase in $\dot{V}O_2$ from one stage to the next (53). Other criteria for having achieved $\dot{V}O_2$max include an R > 1.15 (29) and a blood lactate concentration greater than 8 mmol $\cdot$ L^{-1}, about 8 times the resting value (1). Participation in a 10- to 20-week endurance-training program causes an increase in $\dot{V}O_2$max. If this trained person were to retake the GXT, the oxygen-uptake response would be as shown by the dashed line in Figure 3.12. The subject reaches the steady state sooner at light to moderate work rates, and goes one stage further into the test, at which time the greater $\dot{V}O_2$max is measured.

Maximal aerobic power is the greatest rate at which the human body (primarily muscle) can produce ATP aerobically. It is also the upper limit at which the cardiovascular system can deliver oxygen-enriched blood to the muscles. Thus maximal aerobic power is not only a good index of cardiorespiratory fitness, it is also a good predictor of performance capability in aerobic events such as distance running, cycling, cross-country skiing, and swimming. In the apparently healthy person, maximal aerobic power is usually understood as the quantitative limit at which the cardiovascular system can deliver oxygen to tissues. This usual interpretation must be tempered by the mode of exercise (test type) used to impose the work rate on the subject.

Test Type

For the average person, the highest value for maximal aerobic power is measured when the subject completes a GXT involving uphill running. A GXT conducted at a walking speed usually results in a $\dot{V}O_2$max value 4% to 6% below the graded running value, and a test on a cycle ergometer may yield a value 10% to 12% lower than the graded running value (15, 35, 36). Lastly, if a subject works to exhaustion using an arm ergometer, then the highest oxygen-uptake value is less than 70% of that measured with the legs (18). Knowledge of these variations in maximal aerobic power is helpful in making recommendations about the intensity of different exercises needed to achieve target heart rate (THR). At any given rate, most physiological responses (heart rate, blood pressure, and blood lactic acid) are higher for arm work than for leg work (18, 50). Maximal aerobic power is influenced by more than the type of test used in its measurement. Other factors include endurance training, heredity, gender, age, altitude, and cardiovascular and pulmonary disease.

Training and Heredity

Typically, endurance-training programs increase $\dot{V}O_2$max 5% to 25%, with the magnitude of the change depending primarily on the initial level of fitness. A person with a low $\dot{V}O_2$max makes the largest percentage change as a result of a training program. Eventually a point is reached where further training does not increase $\dot{V}O_2$max. It has been demonstrated that approximately 40% of the extremely high values of maximal aerobic power found in elite cross-country skiers and distance runners are related to a genetic predisposition for having a superior cardiovascular system (3). Because typical endurance-training programs may increase $\dot{V}O_2$max by only 20% or so, it is unrealistic to expect a person with a $\dot{V}O_2$max of 40 ml • kg^{-1} • min^{-1} to increase the value to 80 ml • kg^{-1} • min^{-1}, a value measured in some elite cross-country skiers and distance runners (46). On the other hand, those who do severe interval training can achieve gains of 44% in $\dot{V}O_2$max (21).

Gender and Age

Women have $\dot{V}O_2$max values about 15% lower than men's; that difference exists across ages 20 to 60 years. The 15% difference between men and women is an average difference, and a considerable overlap in $\dot{V}O_2$max values exists in these populations (2). The aging effect indicates a gradual but systematic 1%-per-year reduction in $\dot{V}O_2$max in most people. Given that the average person becomes heavier and more sedentary with age, the decrease in $\dot{V}O_2$max may be as much a reflection of these changes as a specific aging effect. In fact, recent evidence indicates that individuals who remain active and maintain their body weight show little change in $\dot{V}O_2$max over the years (30, 31, 32).

Altitude and Pollution

Figure 3.13 shows that $\dot{V}O_2$max decreases with increasing altitude. At 7,400 ft (2,300 m) $\dot{V}O_2$max is only 88% of the sea-level value. This decrease in $\dot{V}O_2$max is due primarily to the reduction in the arterial oxygen content that occurs as the oxygen pressure decreases with increasing altitude. With the lower arterial oxygen content at altitude, the heart must pump more blood per minute to meet the oxygen needs of any task. As a result,

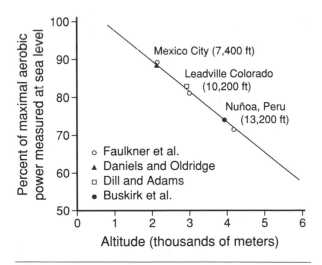

Figure 3.13 Changes in maximal aerobic power with increasing altitude. The sea-level value for maximal aerobic power is set to 100%. *Note.* From ''Effects of Altitude on Physical Performance'' by E.T. Howley. In *Encyclopedia of Physical Education, Fitness and Sports: Training, Environment, Nutrition and Fitness* (p. 180) by G.A. Stull and T.K. Cureton (Eds.), 1980, Reston, VA: AAHPERD. Copyright 1980 by AAHPERD. Reprinted by permission.

the heart-rate response is higher at *submaximal* intensities when performed at higher altitudes (27).

Carbon monoxide, produced from the burning of fossil fuel as well as from cigarette smoke, binds readily to hemoglobin and can decrease oxygen transport to muscles. The critical concentration of carbon monoxide in blood needed to decrease $\dot{V}O_2$max is 4.3%. After that, there is approximately a 1% decrease in $\dot{V}O_2$max for every 1% increase in the carbon monoxide concentration in blood (43).

Cardiovascular and Pulmonary Diseases

Pulmonary and cardiovascular diseases decrease $\dot{V}O_2$max by diminishing the delivery of oxygen from the air to the blood and reducing the capacity of the heart to deliver blood to the muscles. These patients have some of the lowest $\dot{V}O_2$max (functional capacity) values measured, but they also experience the largest percentage changes in $\dot{V}O_2$max in endurance-training programs. Table 3.1 shows common values for $\dot{V}O_2$max in a variety of populations (2, 17).

Table 3.1   Maximal Aerobic Power Measured in Healthy and Diseased Populations

	$\dot{V}O_2$max ($ml \cdot kg^{-1} \cdot min^{-1}$)	
Population	Men	Women
Cross-country skiing	82	66
Distance runners	79	62
College students	45	38
Middle-aged adults	35	30
Postmyocardial infarction patients	22	18
Severe pulmonary-diseased patients	13	13

Note. Data compiled from Åstrand and Rodahl (1986), Fox, Bowers, and Foss (1988), and the Fort Sanders Cardiac Rehabilitation Program.

Blood Lactic Acid

Lactic acid produced by a muscle is released into the blood. Figure 3.14 shows that during a GXT, blood lactate concentration changes little or not at all at the lower work rates; the lactate is metabolized as fast as it is produced (4). As the stages of the GXT continue to increase, a point is reached at which the blood lactate concentration suddenly increases. The work rate at which the lactate concentration suddenly increases is called the **lactate threshold**. It should not be called the **anaerobic threshold** because several conditions other

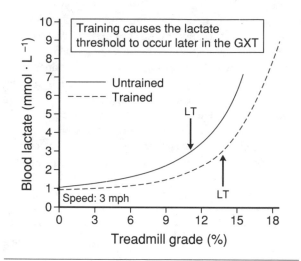

Figure 3.14   Changes in the blood lactic acid (lactate) concentration during a graded exercise test. LT indicates lactate threshold. Based on data from "Effect of Training on Circulatory Response to Exercise" by B. Ekblom, P.O. Åstrand, B. Saltin, J. Stenberg, and B. Wallstrom, 1968, *Journal of Applied Physiology,* 24.

than an oxygen lack (hypoxia) at the muscle cell can result in lactate production and release into the blood. An endurance-training program causes an increase in the mitochondria number of the trained muscles, allowing the aerobic metabolism of carbohydrates and the use of more fat as fuel. As a result, when the subject takes the GXT again, less lactate is produced and the lactate threshold is shifted to the right as shown in Figure 3.14. The lactate threshold is a good indicator of endurance performance and has been used to predict performance in marathon races (52).

Heart Rate

Figure 3.15 shows that once the heart rate reaches about 110 beats $\cdot$ min^{-1}, it increases linearly with each work rate in a GXT until the maximal heart rate is reached. Estimates of maximal heart rate are usually obtained by the formula 220 minus age, recognizing that the maximal heart rate decreases with increased age. When using this formula, however, it must be remembered that maximal heart rate varies considerably at any age. The maximal heart rate at the age of 30 might be calculated to be 190 beats $\cdot$ min^{-1}, but the range (expressed as plus or minus 3 standard deviations) is from 157 to 223. The dashed line on the graph shows the influence of a training program on the subject's heart-rate response at the same work rates. The lower heart rate at submaximal work rates is a beneficial effect because it decreases the oxygen needed by the heart muscle. Maximal heart rate shows no change or is slightly reduced as a result of an endurance-training program.

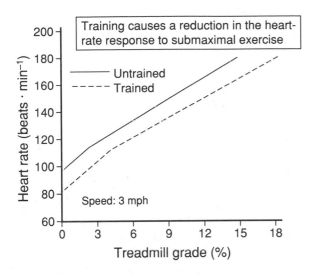

Figure 3.15 The heart-rate response to a graded exercise test. Based on data from "Effect of Training on Circulatory Response to Exercise" by B. Ekblom, P.O. Åstrand, B. Saltin, J. Stenberg, and B. Wallstrom, 1968, *Journal of Applied Physiology*, 24.

Stroke Volume

The volume of blood pumped by the heart per beat (ml•beat^{-1}) is called the stroke volume. Figure 3.16 shows the stroke volume response to a GXT. Stroke volume increases in the early stages of the GXT until

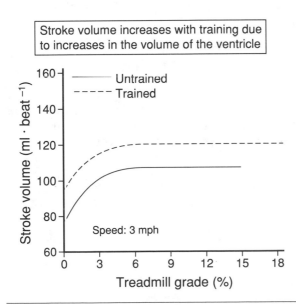

Figure 3.16 The stroke volume response to a graded exercise test. Based on data from "Effect of Training on Circulatory Response to Exercise" by B. Ekblom, P.O. Åstrand, B. Saltin, J. Stenberg, and B. Wallstrom, 1968, *Journal of Applied Physiology*, 24.

about 40% $\dot{V}O_2$max and then levels off. Consequently, the heart rate is the sole factor responsible for the increased flow of blood from the heart to the working muscles after a work rate equal to 40% of maximal aerobic power is reached. This is what makes the heart rate a good indicator of the metabolic rate during exercise. One of the primary effects of an endurance-training program is an increase in stroke volume at rest and during work (see Figure 3.16); this is due, in part, to an increase in the volume of the ventricle, without any change in ventricle-wall thickness (14). This increases the **end diastolic volume**, the volume of blood in the heart just before contraction. So, even if the same fraction of blood in the ventricle is pumped per beat (**ejection fraction**) following endurance training, the heart pumps more blood *per minute* at the same heart rate.

Cardiac Output

Cardiac output (liters per minute) is the volume of blood pumped by the heart per minute and is calculated by multiplying the heart rate (beats•min^{-1}) by the stroke volume (ml•beat^{-1}).

$$\text{Cardiac output} = \text{heart rate} \cdot \text{stroke volume}$$
$$= 60 \text{ beats•min}^{-1} \cdot 80 \text{ ml•beat}^{-1}$$
$$= 4,800 \text{ ml•min}^{-1} \text{ or } 4.8 \text{ L•min}^{-1}$$

Figure 3.17 shows cardiac output to increase linearly with work rate. Generally, the cardiac-output response to light and moderate work is not affected by an endurance-training program. What is changed is the manner in which the cardiac output is achieved, with a lower heart rate and a higher stroke volume (see Figures 3.15 and 3.16).

The maximal cardiac output (highest value reached in a GXT) is the most important cardiovascular variable determining maximal aerobic power, because the oxygen-enriched blood (carrying about 0.2 L O_2 per liter of blood) must be delivered to the muscle for the mitochondria to use. If a person's maximal cardiac output is 10 L•min^{-1}, only 2 L O_2 would leave the heart per minute for the tissues (i.e., 0.2 L O_2 per liter of blood times a cardiac output of 10 L•min^{-1}, thus 10 • 0.2 = 2). A person with a maximal cardiac output of 30 L•min^{-1} would deliver 6 L O_2 per minute to the tissues. One of the effects of an endurance-training program is an increase in the maximal cardiac output and thus the delivery of oxygen to muscles (see Figure 3.17). This increase in maximal cardiac output is matched by an increase in the capillary number in the muscle to allow the blood to move slowly enough through the muscle to maintain the time needed for oxygen to diffuse from the blood to the mitochondria (47). The increase in maximal cardiac

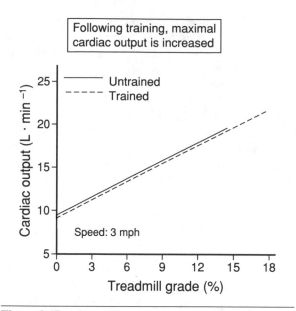

Following training, maximal cardiac output is increased

Speed: 3 mph

Untrained
Trained

Figure 3.17 The cardiac-output response to a graded exercise test. Based on data from "Effect of Training on Circulatory Response to Exercise" by B. Ekblom, P.O. Åstrand, B. Saltin, J. Stenberg, and B. Wallstrom, 1968, *Journal of Applied Physiology*, 24.

output explains 50% of the increase in maximal oxygen uptake that occurs in previously sedentary subjects who engage in endurance-training programs (44).

In the normal population the major variable influencing the maximal cardiac output is the stroke volume. Differences in maximal cardiac output and maximal aerobic power that exist between females and males, between trained and untrained individuals, and between the world-class endurance athlete and the average person can be explained to a large degree on the basis of differences in maximal stroke volume. This is shown clearly on Table 3.2, where $\dot{V}O_2$max varies by a factor of 3 among three distinct groups, whereas maximal heart rate is almost the same for all three groups. This clearly shows that maximal stroke volume is the primary factor related to $\dot{V}O_2$max.

KEY POINTS. Following an endurance-training program,

- heart rate is lower, and stroke volume is higher at rest and during submaximal work; and
- maximal cardiac output is increased, due to an increase in maximal stroke volume, with no change or a slight decrease in maximal heart rate.

What causes the increase in heart rate and stroke volume during exercise to cause the increase in cardiac output? The heart rate is under the control of the **parasympathetic** and **sympathetic** branches of the **autonomic nervous system**. At the onset of exercise, there is a decrease in the activity of the parasympathetic (vagus) nerve to the sinoatrial (SA) node of the heart, and the heart rate speeds up. Simultaneously, there is an increase in sympathetic nervous system activity, mediated through the direct release of **norepinephrine** at the SA node and the release of **epinephrine** from the adrenal medulla into the blood. These catecholamines, epinephrine and norepinephrine, bind to **beta- (ß-) adrenergic receptors** on cells of the SA node and cause intracellular changes that speed up the heart rate. Stroke volume is increased, in part due to the increased force of contraction of the ventricle caused by these catecholamines. In cardiac patients, or those with high blood pressure, a physician may prescribe drugs called beta-blockers (ß-blockers) that block the interaction of the ß-adrenergic receptor with the catecholamines. This reduces cardiac output, resulting in less work of the heart and a lower blood pressure. Chapter 15 spells out the details associated with medications and exercise.

Oxygen Extraction

Two factors determine the oxygen uptake at any time: the volume of blood delivered to the tissues per minute (cardiac output) and the volume of oxygen extracted from each liter of blood. Oxygen extraction is calcu-

Table 3.2   Maximal Values of $\dot{V}O_2$, Heart Rate, Stroke Volume, and (a-$\bar{v}$) Oxygen Difference in 3 Groups Having Very Low, Normal, and High Maximal $\dot{V}O_2$

Group	Max $\dot{V}O_2$ (L · min⁻¹)	=	Heart rate (beats · min⁻¹)	x	Stroke volume (ml)	x	(a-$\bar{v}$) Oxygen difference (ml · L⁻¹)
Mitral stenosis	1.60	=	190	x	50	x	170
Sedentary	3.20	=	200	x	100	x	160
Athlete	5.20	=	190	x	160	x	170

Note. From L. Rowell, "Circulation," *Medicine and Science in Sports*, **1**, pp. 15-22, 1969, © by the American College of Sports Medicine.

lated by subtracting the oxygen content of mixed venous blood (as it returns to the heart) from the oxygen content of the arterial blood. This is called the arteriovenous oxygen difference, or the $(a-\bar{v})O_2$ difference.

$$\dot{V}O_2 = \text{cardiac output} \cdot (a-\bar{v})O_2 \text{ difference}$$

At rest:

cardiac output $= 5 \text{ L blood} \cdot \text{min}^{-1}$,

arterial O_2 content $= 200 \text{ ml } O_2 \text{ per liter of blood}$

$(\text{ml } O_2 \cdot L^{-1})$,

mixed venous O_2 content $= 150 \text{ ml } O_2 \cdot L^{-1}$

$\dot{V}O_2 = (5 \text{ L blood} \cdot \text{min}^{-1}) \cdot (200 \text{ ml } O_2 \cdot L^{-1}$

$- 150 \text{ ml } O_2 \cdot L^{-1})$

$\dot{V}O_2 = 250 \text{ ml} \cdot \text{min}^{-1}$

The $(a-\bar{v})O_2$ difference is a measure of the ability of the muscle tissues to extract oxygen, and it increases with exercise intensity as shown in Figure 3.18. The ability of a tissue to extract oxygen is a function of the capillary-to-muscle-fiber ratio, the number of mitochondria in the muscle fiber, and the activity of the oxidative enzymes in the mitochondria. Endurance-training programs increase all of these factors, leading

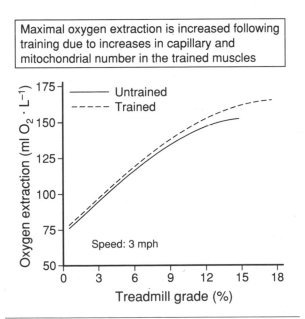

Figure 3.18 The changes in oxygen extraction (difference between the oxygen content of arterial blood and the mixed venous blood in the right heart) during a graded exercise test. Based on data from "Effect of Training on Circulatory Response to Exercise" by B. Ekblom, P.O. Åstrand, B. Saltin, J. Stenberg, and B. Wallstrom, 1968, *Journal of Applied Physiology*, 24.

to an increase in the maximal capacity to extract oxygen in the last stage of the GXT (47). This increase in the $(a-\bar{v})O_2$ difference explains about 50% of the increase in $\dot{V}O_2$max that occurs with endurance-training programs in previously sedentary subjects (44).

Blood Pressure

Blood pressure is dependent on the balance between cardiac output and the resistance the blood vessels offer to blood flow (total peripheral resistance). The resistance to blood flow is altered by the constriction or dilation of blood vessels called **arterioles**.

KEY POINT.   Blood Pressure = Cardiac Output × Total Peripheral Resistance

---

Blood pressure is sensed by **baroreceptors** in the arch of the aorta and in the carotid arteries. If there is a change in blood pressure, signals from the baroreceptors go to the cardiovascular control center in the brain, which in turn alters cardiac output or the diameter of arterioles. For example, when a person who has been lying in the supine position suddenly stands, blood pools in the lower extremities, stroke volume falls, and with it, blood pressure. If blood pressure is not restored, blood flow to the brain will be reduced, and the person might faint. The baroreceptors monitor this fall in blood pressure, and the cardiovascular control center simultaneously increases the heart rate and reduces the diameter of the arterioles (to increase total peripheral resistance) to try to return blood pressure to normal values. During exercise, a dilation of arterioles occurs in the active muscle to increase blood flow and meet metabolic demands. This dilation is matched with a constriction of arterioles in the liver, kidneys, and gastrointestinal tract, and an increase in heart rate and stroke volume as already mentioned. These coordinated changes maintain blood pressure.

Blood pressure is monitored at each stage of a GXT. Figure 3.19 shows the changes in systolic and diastolic pressures with increasing work rates. Systolic pressure increases with each stage until maximum work tolerance is reached. At that point, systolic pressure might decrease. A fall in systolic pressure with an increase in work rate is used as one of the indicators of maximal cardiovascular function and can aid in determining the end point for a test. Diastolic blood pressure tends to remain the same or decrease during a GXT. An increase in diastolic blood pressure toward the end of the test is an indicator that a person's functional capacity has been reached. Endurance-training programs result

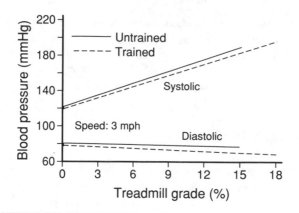

Figure 3.19 The systolic and diastolic blood pressure responses to a graded exercise test. Based on data from "Effect of Training on Circulatory Response to Exercise" by B. Ekblom, P.O. Åstrand, B. Saltin, J. Stenberg, and B. Wallstrom, 1968, *Journal of Applied Physiology*, 24.

in a reduction in the blood pressure responses at fixed submaximal work rates.

Two factors that determine the oxygen demand (work) of the heart during aerobic exercise are the heart rate and the systolic blood pressure. The product of these two variables is called the **rate–pressure product**, or the **double product**, and is proportional to the myocardial oxygen demand (i.e., the volume of oxygen needed by the heart muscle per minute to function properly). Factors that decrease the heart-rate and blood-pressure responses to work increase the chance that the coronary blood supply to the heart muscle will adequately meet the oxygen needs of the heart. Endurance

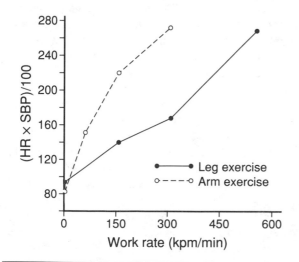

Figure 3.20 Rate–pressure product at rest and during arm and leg exercise. *Note.* From "A Comparison of the Response to Arm and Leg Work in Patients With Ischemic Heart Disease" by J. Schwade, C.G. Blomqvist, and W. Shapiro, 1977, *American Heart Journal*, **94**, p. 206. Copyright 1977 by Mosby-Year Book. Adapted by permission.

training decreases the heart-rate and blood-pressure responses to fixed submaximal work tasks and is seen as protective against any diminished blood supply (ischemia) to the myocardium. Drugs are also used to reduce the heart-rate and blood-pressure responses to try to reduce the work of the heart (see chapter 15).

Arm Versus Leg Work

When a person does the same rate of work with the arms as with the legs, the heart-rate and blood-pressure responses are considerably higher during the arm work. This is shown in Figure 3.20, in which the double product is plotted for various levels of arm and leg work. Given that the load on the heart and the potential for fatigue is greater for arm work, it is clear that an HFI should choose activities that use large muscle groups; this would result in lower heart-rate and blood-pressure responses, and in reduced perception of fatigue (18, 50).

Pulmonary Ventilation

Pulmonary ventilation is the volume of air inhaled or exhaled per minute and is calculated by multiplying the frequency (f) of breathing by the tidal volume (TV), the volume of air moved in one breath. For example,

$$\text{Ventilation (L} \cdot \text{min}^{-1}) = \text{TV (L} \cdot \text{breaths}^{-1}) \cdot$$
$$f \text{ (breaths} \cdot \text{min}^{-1})$$
$$30 \text{ L} \cdot \text{min}^{-1} = 1.5 \text{ L} \cdot \text{breaths}^{-1} \cdot$$
$$20 \text{ breaths} \cdot \text{min}^{-1}$$

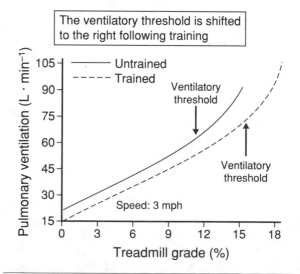

Figure 3.21 The pulmonary ventilation response to a graded exercise test. (The ventilatory threshold is shown with an arrow.)

Pulmonary ventilation increases linearly with work rate until 50% to 80% of $\dot{V}O_2$max, at which point a relative **hyperventilation** results (Figure 3.21). The inflection point in the pulmonary-ventilation response is called the **ventilatory threshold**. The ventilatory threshold has been used as a noninvasive indicator of the lactate threshold and as a predictor of performance (12, 42). The increase in pulmonary ventilation is mediated by changes in the frequency of breathing (from about 10 to 12 breaths$\cdot$min^{-1} at rest to 40 to 50 breaths$\cdot$min^{-1} during maximal work) and the tidal volume (from 0.5 L$\cdot$breath^{-1} at rest to 2 to 3 L$\cdot$breath^{-1} in maximal work). Endurance-training programs result in a lower pulmonary ventilation during submaximal work; the ventilatory threshold occurs later into the GXT. The maximal value for pulmonary ventilation tends to change in the direction of $\dot{V}O_2$max.

Effects of Endurance Training and Detraining

Various comments have been made about the effect of endurance training on various physiological responses to exercise. This section will try to show how some of the changes are interrelated.

- **Endurance training increases the number of mitochondria and capillaries in muscle, causing all active fibers to become more oxidative.** This effect is manifested by the increase in the Type IIa (FOG) fibers and a decrease in Type IIb fibers. These changes increase the endurance capacity of the muscle by using fat for a greater percentage of energy production, sparing the muscle glycogen store and reducing lactate production. This causes the lactate threshold to be shifted to the right, and performance times in distance races to improve.
- **Endurance training decreases the time it takes to achieve a steady state in submaximal exercise.** This results in a reduction in the oxygen deficit and less reliance on creatine phosphate and anaerobic glycolysis for energy.
- **Endurance training causes an increase in the volume of the ventricle, with no changes in ventricle-wall thickness.** This accommodates an increase in the end diastolic volume, such that more blood is pumped out per beat. This increase in stroke volume is accompanied by a decrease in heart rate during submaximal work, so the cardiac output remains the same. The oxygen needs of the tissues are met with less work of the heart.
- **Maximal aerobic power increases with endurance training, the increase being inversely related to the initial $\dot{V}O_2$max.** In formerly

sedentary individuals, about 50% of the increase in $\dot{V}O_2$max is due to an increase in maximal cardiac output, a change brought about by an increase in maximal stroke volume, given that maximal heart rate either remains the same or is decreased slightly. The other 50% of the increase in $\dot{V}O_2$max is due to an increase in oxygen extraction at the muscle, shown by an increase in the $(a-\bar{v})O_2$ difference. This occurs as a result of an increase in the number of capillaries in the trained muscle to allow the arterial blood to flow slowly enough for the oxygen to diffuse to the mitochondria.

Transfer of Training

The training effects that have been discussed are observed only when trained muscles are used in the exercise test. Although this may appear obvious for the decrease in blood lactate that is due, in part, to the increase in the mitochondria of the trained muscles, it is also the case for the changes that occur in the heart-rate response to submaximal work following the training program. Figure 3.22 shows the results of repeated submaximal exercise tests conducted on subjects who trained only one leg on a cycle ergometer for 13 days. The heart-rate response decreased as expected. At the end of the 13 days of training the untrained leg was now subjected to the same exercise test. The heart rate responded as if a training effect had not occurred. The point of this is to indicate that part of the reason the heart-rate response to submaximal exercise decreases as a result of the training program is due to signals coming back from the trained muscles (5, 44). This has important implications for training programs, in that being fit, and responding in a trained fashion (lower lactate, lower heart rate, more fat use, etc.), are related to doing the exercise with the muscle groups involved

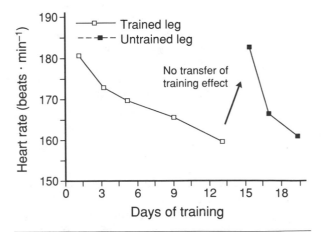

Figure 3.22 Lack of transfer of training effect. Data from Claytor (1985).

in the training. The probability of some carryover of the training effect to another activity is dependent on the degree to which the new activity uses the muscles that are already trained.

Detraining

How fast is a training effect lost? A number of investigations have explored this question by having subjects either reduce or completely cease training. Maximal oxygen uptake is usually used as the principal measure to evaluate changes due to detraining, but a subject's response to a submaximal work rate has also been used to track these changes over time.

Cessation of Training. The following study used subjects who had trained for 10 ± 3 years and agreed to cease training for 84 days (9). They were tested on days 12, 21, 56, and 84 of the detraining period. Figure 3.23 shows that $\dot{V}O_2$max decreased 7% within the first 12 days of detraining. {Remember that $\dot{V}O_2$max = Cardiac Output • $[(a-\bar{v})O_2$ diff].} The decrease in $\dot{V}O_2$max was due entirely to a decrease in maximal cardiac output, because the maximal oxygen extraction $[(a-\bar{v})O_2$ difference] was unchanged. In turn, the decrease in maximal cardiac output was due entirely to a decrease in maximal stroke volume, because maximal heart rate actually increased during the period of no training. A subsequent study showed that the reduced stroke volume was due to a reduction in plasma volume that occurred in the first 12 days of no training (7). In contrast, the decrease in $\dot{V}O_2$max that occurred between days 21 and 84 was due to a decrease in the oxygen extraction, because maximal cardiac output was unchanged (see Figure 3.23). This decrease in oxygen extraction appeared to be due to a reduction in the number of mitochondria in the muscle, given that the number of capillaries surrounding each muscle fiber was unchanged (10).

The same subjects also completed a standard (fixed work rate) submaximal exercise test during the 84 days of no training (8). Figure 3.24 shows that heart-rate and blood lactic acid responses to this work test increased throughout the period of detraining. The higher responses are related to the fact that the same work rate required a greater percentage of $\dot{V}O_2$max, because the latter variable was decreasing throughout training. However, the magnitude of change in heart-rate and blood lactic acid responses to this submaximal work bout make them very sensitive indicators of the training state of an individual.

Reduced Training. To evaluate the effect of a reduction in training, Hickson and colleagues (22, 23, 24) first trained subjects for 10 weeks to cause an increase in $\dot{V}O_2$max. The training program was conducted 40 min per day, 6 days per week. Three days involved running at near maximum intensity for 40 min; the

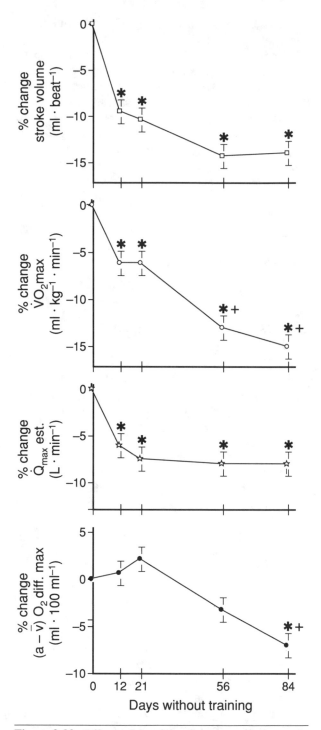

Figure 3.23 Effects of detraining upon percent changes in stroke volume during exercise, maximal O_2 uptake, or $\dot{V}O_2$max, maximal cardiac output, or $\dot{Q}_{max}$ est, and maximal arteriovenous O_2 difference, or $(a-\bar{v})O_2$ difference max. Original data from Coyle, E.F. et al. (1984). *Journal of Applied Physiology*, 57:1857-1864. Figure from Coyle, E.F. (1988). *Resource Manual for Guidelines for Graded Exercise Testing and Prescription.* Reprinted by permission.

other 3 days required six 5-min bouts at near-maximum intensity on a cycle ergometer, with a 2-min rest between work bouts. Subjects expended about 600 kcal

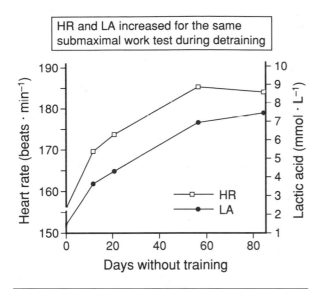

HR and LA increased for the same submaximal work test during detraining

Figure 3.24 Changes in the heart-rate and blood lactic acid concentration responses to a standard exercise test taken during 84 days of detraining. Adapted from Coyle et al. (1985).

per day of exercise, or 3,600 kcal per week. At the end of this 10-week training program the subjects were divided into groups that trained at either a one-third or a two-third reduction in the previous frequency (4 and 2 days per week), duration (26 and 13 min per day), or intensity (a one-third or two-thirds reduction in work done or distance run per 40-min session). Data collected on the maximal treadmill tests showed that the reduction in duration from 40 to 26 or 13 min, or a reduction in frequency from 6 to 4 or 2 days per week, did not affect $\dot{V}O_2$max. In contrast, $\dot{V}O_2$max was clearly decreased when the intensity of training was reduced by either one third or two thirds. What is interesting is that the subjects were able to maintain $\dot{V}O_2$max when the total exercise done per week was reduced from 3,600 kcal to 1,200 kcal in the two-thirds reduced frequency and duration treatments, but were not able to maintain $\dot{V}O_2$max when the intensity was reduced, even though the subjects were still expending about 1,200 kcal per week. This points to the importance of the exercise intensity in maintaining $\dot{V}O_2$max, and confirms that it takes less exercise to maintain $\dot{V}O_2$max than to achieve the level.

CARDIOVASCULAR RESPONSES TO EXERCISE FOR FEMALES AND MALES

Generally, little or no difference exists between boys and girls in $\dot{V}O_2$max or in their cardiovascular responses to submaximal exercise. During puberty, dif-

ferences between girls and boys appear and are related to the female's higher percent body fat, lower hemoglobin, and smaller heart size relative to body weight (2). These latter factors also affect a woman's cardiovascular responses to submaximal work. For example, if an 80-kg male were walking on a 10% grade on a treadmill at 3 mi•hr^{-1}, the $\dot{V}O_2$ would be 2.07 L•min^{-1}, or 25.9 ml•kg^{-1}•min^{-1}. The heart rate might be 140 beats• min^{-1} for this person. If he had to now carry a backpack weighing 15 kg, the $\dot{V}O_2$ expressed per kg would not change (25.9 ml•kg^{-1}•min^{-1}), but the total oxygen requirement would increase 389 ml•min^{-1} (i.e., 15 kg • 25.9 ml•kg^{-1}•min^{-1}) to carry the load. His heart rate would obviously be higher with this load than without, even thought the $\dot{V}O_2$ expressed per kilogram of body weight is the same. In like manner, performance in the 12-min run test to evaluate maximal aerobic power was decreased by 89 m when body weight was experimentally increased to simulate a 5% gain in body fat (11). When a postpubescent female walks on a treadmill at a given grade and speed, her heart rate is higher than a comparable male's heart rate because of the additional fat weight she carries. The lower hemoglobin and smaller relative heart size also cause the heart rate to be higher at the same oxygen uptake expressed per unit of body weight.

The differences between males and females in the cardiovascular response to submaximal work becomes more exaggerated when work is done on a cycle ergometer where a given work rate demands the same $\dot{V}O_2$ in liters per minute, independent of size, gender, or training. The average woman has less hemoglobin and a smaller heart volume compared to the average male. To deliver the same volume of oxygen to the muscles, the woman must have a higher heart rate to compensate for the smaller stroke volume and must have a slightly higher cardiac output to compensate for the lower hemoglobin concentration (2). These differences between women and men in the cardiovascular responses to cycle ergometry are shown in Figure 3.25.

CARDIOVASCULAR RESPONSES TO ISOMETRIC EXERCISE AND WEIGHT LIFTING

Most endurance exercise programs use dynamic activities involving large muscle masses to place loads on the cardiorespiratory system. The previous summary of the physiological responses to a GXT indicates the rather proportional nature of the cardiovascular load to the exercise intensity. But this is not necessarily the case for activities that fall into the strength-training category, in which a person can have a disproportionately high

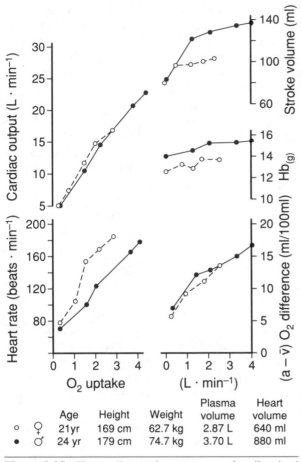

Figure 3.25 The cardiovascular responses of well-trained men and women to cycle ergometry exercise. From *Textbook of Work Physiology* (p. 198) by P.O. Åstrand and K. Rodahl, 1977, New York: McGraw-Hill. Reprinted by permission.

		Age	Height	Weight	Plasma volume	Heart volume
o	♀	21yr	169 cm	62.7 kg	2.87 L	640 ml
●	♂	24 yr	179 cm	74.7 kg	3.70 L	880 ml

cardiovascular load relative to the exercise intensity. In the previous discussion of cardiovascular responses to a GXT, there was a progressive rise in the heart-rate and systolic blood-pressure responses with each stage of the test. Figure 3.26 shows the heart-rate and blood-pressure response to an isometric exercise test (sustained handgrip) at only 30% maximal voluntary contraction strength, and to a treadmill test using two exercise intensities. The most impressive change during the sustained handgrip is in blood pressure; the systolic and diastolic pressures increase over time, and the magnitude of the systolic pressure exceeds 220 mmHg. This kind of exercise places an additional load on the heart and is not recommended for strength-training programs for older adults or people with heart disease (33).

Dynamic, heavy-resistance exercises can also cause extreme blood-pressure responses. Figure 3.27 shows the peak blood-pressure response achieved during exercises done at 95% to 100% of the maximum weight that could be lifted one time (1 RM). Note that both systolic and diastolic blood pressures are elevated, with average

values exceeding 300/200 mmHg for the two-leg leg press done to failure. The elevation in pressure was believed to be due to the compression of the arteries by the muscles, a reflex response due to the "static" component associated with near-maximal dynamic lifts, and the Valsalva maneuver, which can cause, independently, an elevation of blood pressure (34). Another study reported peak values of about 190/140 mmHg for exercises of 50%, 70%, and 80% of 1 RM done to fatigue in novice and untrained lifters. Body builders responded with lower pressures, indicating a cardiovascular adaptation to weight training (16).

TEMPERATURE REGULATION

Under resting conditions the body's core temperature is 37 °C, and there is a balance between heat production and heat loss. Heat production mechanisms include the basal metabolic rate, shivering, work, and exercise. When exercise is done, the mechanical efficiency is about 20% or less, which means that 80% or more of the energy production ($\dot{V}O_2$) is converted to heat. For example, if you are working on a cycle ergometer at a rate requiring a $\dot{V}O_2$ of 2.0 L•min^{-1}, your energy production is about 10 kcal•min^{-1}. At 20% efficiency, 2 kcal•min^{-1} goes to do work, and 8 kcal•min^{-1} is converted to heat that the body has to deal with. If this added heat is not lost, the core temperature might quickly rise to dangerous levels. How does the body lose heat?

Heat-Loss Mechanisms

Heat is lost from the body by four processes. In **radiation**, heat is transferred from the surface of one object to the surface of another, with no physical contact between the objects. Heat loss depends on the temperature gradient, that is, the temperature difference between the surfaces of the objects. When a person is seated at rest in a comfortable environment (21 to 22 °C), about 60% of body heat is lost through radiation to cooler objects. **Conduction** is the transfer of heat from one object to another by direct contact and, like radiation, is dependent on a temperature gradient. When we sit on cold marble benches, we lose heat from our bodies by conduction. **Convection** is a special case of conduction in which heat is transferred to air (or water) molecules, which become lighter and rise away from the body to be replaced by cold air (or water). Heat loss can be increased by increasing the movement of the air (or water) over the surface of the body. It should be clear that all of these heat-loss mechanisms can be heat-

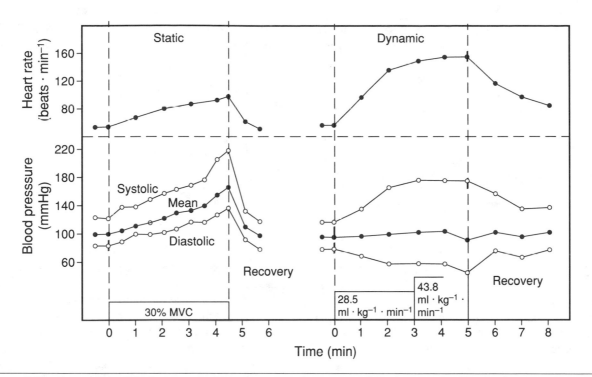

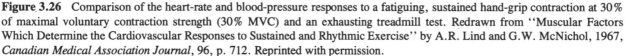

Figure 3.26 Comparison of the heart-rate and blood-pressure responses to a fatiguing, sustained hand-grip contraction at 30% of maximal voluntary contraction strength (30% MVC) and an exhausting treadmill test. Redrawn from ''Muscular Factors Which Determine the Cardiovascular Responses to Sustained and Rhythmic Exercise'' by A.R. Lind and G.W. McNichol, 1967, *Canadian Medical Association Journal*, 96, p. 712. Reprinted with permission.

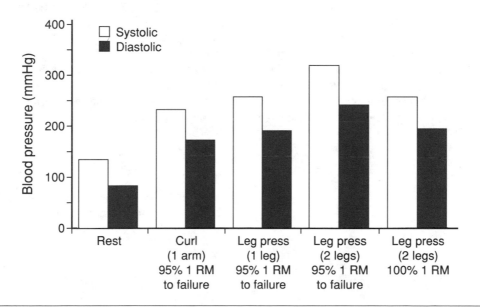

Figure 3.27 Blood-pressure responses during weight lifting. (RM = repetition maximum.) Data from MacDougall, Tuxen, Sale, Moroz, and Sutton (1985).

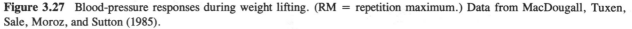

gain mechanisms. We gain heat from the sun by radiation across 93 million miles of space, and we gain heat from water in a hot tub by conduction because the water temperature is greater than skin temperature. Heat gained from the environment is added to that generated by exercise and puts an additional strain on heat-loss mechanisms.

The final heat-loss mechanism is the evaporation of sweat. **Sweating** is the process of producing a watery solution over the surface of the body. **Evaporation** is the process in which liquid water molecules are converted to a gas. This conversion requires about 580 kcal of heat per liter of sweat evaporated. The heat for this comes from the body, and thus, the body is cooled. At rest, about 25% of heat loss is due to evaporation, but during exercise it becomes the primary mechanism for heat loss.

Evaporation is dependent upon the **water vapor pressure gradient** between the skin and the air and is not directly dependent upon temperature. The water vapor pressure of the air is dependent on the **relative humidity** and the **saturation pressure** at that air temperature. For example, the relative humidity can be 90% in winter, but because the saturation pressure of cold air is low, on such a day the water vapor pressure of the air is also low, and you can see water vapor rising from your body following exercise. However, in warm temperatures the relative humidity is a good indicator of the water vapor pressure of the air. If the water vapor pressure of the air is too high, sweat will not evaporate, and sweat that does not evaporate does not cool the body (40).

Body Temperature Response to Exercise

Figure 3.28 shows that during exercise in a comfortable environment the core temperature increases to a level proportional to the relative intensity (%$\dot{V}O_2$max) of the exercise and then levels off (48). The gain in body heat that occurs early in exercise triggers the heat-loss mechanisms discussed in the preceding section, and after 10 to 20 minutes heat loss equals heat production, and the

core temperature remains steady (19). What are the most important heat-loss mechanisms during exercise?

Heat Loss During Exercise

Exercise intensity and environmental temperature have major impacts on which heat-loss mechanism is primarily responsible for maintaining the core temperature during exercise.

Exercise of Increasing Intensity

When a subject participates in a series of progressively more difficult exercise tests in an environment that allows heat loss by all the mechanisms we've just mentioned, the contribution that convection and radiation make to overall heat loss is modest (Figure 3.29). This is due to the fact that the temperature gradient between the skin and the room is not altered much during exercise, and consequently the rate of heat loss is relatively constant. To compensate for this, evaporation picks up when heat loss by convection and radiation levels off, and it is responsible for most of the heat loss in heavy exercise.

Exercise in High Environmental Temperatures

If a subject performs steady-state exercise in an environment in which the temperature is increasing, the role that evaporation plays becomes more important. Figure 3.30 shows that as environmental temperature increases, the gradient for heat loss by convection and radiation decreases, and with it, the rate of heat loss by these processes also decreases. As a result, evaporation must compensate to maintain core temperature.

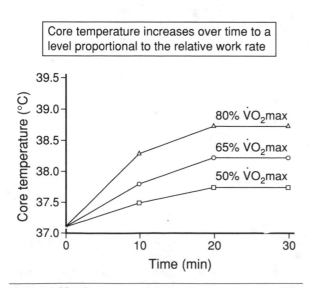

Figure 3.28 Core temperature response to exercise. Data from Saltin and Hermansen (1966).

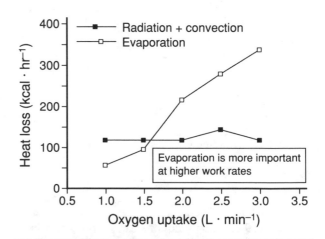

Figure 3.29 Importance of evaporation as a heat loss mechanism as exercise intensity increases. Based on figure on p. 595 in Åstrand and Rodahl (1986).

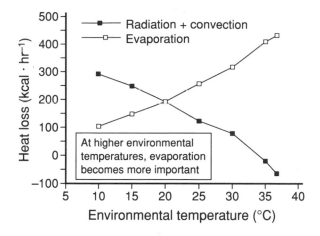

Figure 3.30 Importance of evaporation as a heat loss mechanism during exercise as environmental temperature increases. Based on figure on p. 598 in Åstrand and Rodahl (1986).

An important insight to be gained from these figures is that in strenuous exercise or hot environments, evaporation is the most important process for losing heat and maintaining body temperature in the safe range. It should be no surprise, then, that factors that affect sweat production (such as dehydration) or that interfere with the evaporation of sweat (such as impermeable clothing) are causes for concern. Chapter 13 provides the specifics on how to deal with heat and humidity when prescribing exercise, and chapter 16 provides important information on preventing and treating heat-related disorders.

Training, Acclimatization, and Evaporative Heat Loss

Training in a hot and humid environment for as little as 7 to 12 days results in specific adaptations that lead to improved heat tolerance, and as a result the subject's body temperature is lower during submaximal exercise (19). These adaptations include

- an increase in plasma volume,
- an earlier onset of sweating,
- a higher sweat rate,
- a reduction in salt loss in sweat, and
- a reduced skin blood flow.

SUMMARY

Muscles use ATP to develop tension; ATP must be supplied as fast as it is used, or else fatigue will occur. Muscles can supply ATP from stored energy sources (CP), anaerobic metabolism of carbohydrates (glycoly-

sis), and through the oxidation of carbohydrates and fats in the mitochondria. Muscle fiber types vary in their speed of contraction, force development, and resistance to fatigue. Three fiber types have been identified: Type I (slow twitch, low force, fatigue resistant), Type IIa (fast twitch, high force, fatigue resistant), and Type IIb (fast twitch, high force, fatiguable). The lag in the circulatory and ventilatory responses at the onset of submaximal exercise necessitates the use of anaerobic sources of ATP. In 2 to 3 min, the oxygen uptake meets the ATP demands of the muscles. During a GXT the oxygen uptake increases with each grade until the functional capacity of the cardiovascular system to deliver oxygen has been reached. This increased oxygen delivery is directly related to increases in heart rate, cardiac output, pulmonary ventilation, and extraction of oxygen from the arterial blood. Endurance training causes an increase in maximal cardiac output and oxygen extraction, resulting in an increase in maximal oxygen uptake. Heart rate, ventilation, lactate production, and blood pressure are lower at the same submaximal work rates following a training program. Cessation of long-term training results in an immediate decrease in $\dot{V}O_2$max due to a decrease in maximal stroke volume, with the long-term decrease due to a reduction in oxygen extraction. A reduction in the duration or frequency of training has minimal effect on $\dot{V}O_2$max as long as the intensity is maintained at very high levels. Women respond to submaximal exercise with a higher heart rate, due to a lower stroke volume, with an additional compensation in cardiac output made for the lower hemoglobin concentration. Dynamic exercise done with small muscle groups, isometric exercise, and weight lifting result in large increases in blood pressure in contrast to dynamic work done at moderate work rates. Body temperature is maintained at higher levels during exercise, proportional to the exercise intensity. The primary mechanism for heat loss during heavy exercise, or when exercise is done in a hot environment, is the evaporation of sweat.

REFERENCES

1. Åstrand (1952)
2. Åstrand and Rodahl (1977, 1986)
3. Bouchard, Lesage, Lortie, Simoneau, Hamel, Boulay, Perusse, Theriault, and Leblank. (1986)
4. Brooks (1985)
5. Claytor (1985)
6. Costill (1988)
7. Coyle, Hemmert, and Coggan (1986)
8. Coyle, Martin, Bloomfield, Lowry, and Holloszy (1985)

9. Coyle, Martin, Sinacore, Joyner, Hagberg, and Holloszy (1984)
10. Coyle (1988)
11. Cureton, Sparling, Evans, Johnson, Kong, and Purvis (1978)
12. Davis (1985)
13. Edington and Edgerton (1976)
14. Ekblom, Åstrand, Saltin, Stenberg, and Wallstrom (1968)
15. Faulkner (1971)
16. Fleck and Dean (1987)
17. Fox, Bowers, and Foss (1988)
18. Franklin (1985)
19. Gisolfi and Wenger (1984)
20. Hickson, Bomze, and Holloszy (1978)
21. Hickson, Bomze, and Holloszy (1977)
22. Hickson, Foster, Pollock, Galassi, and Rich (1985)
23. Hickson, Kanakis, Davis, Moore, and Rich (1982)
24. Hickson and Rosenkoetter (1981)
25. Holloszy and Coyle (1984)
26. Holmgren (1967)
27. Howley (1980)
28. Hultman (1967)
29. Issekutz, Birkhead, and Rodahl (1962)
30. Kasch, Boyer, Van Camp, Verity, and Wallace (1990)
31. Kasch, Wallace, and Van Camp (1985)
32. Kasch, Wallace, Van Camp, and Verity (1988)
33. Lind and McNicol (1967)
34. MacDougall, Tuxen, Sale, Moroz, and Sutton (1985)
35. McArdle, Katch, and Pechar (1973)
36. McArdle and Magel (1970)
37. Montoye, Ayen, Nagle, and Howley (1986)
38. Nagle, Balke, Baptista, Alleyia, and Howley (1971)
39. Powers, Dodd, and Beadle (1985)
40. Powers and Howley (1990)
41. Powers, Riley, and Howley (1980)
42. Powers, Dodd, Deason, Byrd, and McKnight (1983)
43. Raven (1974)
44. Rowell (1986)
45. Sale (1987)
46. Saltin (1969)
47. Saltin and Gollnick (1983)
48. Saltin and Hermansen (1966)
49. Saltin, Henriksson, Nygaard, Anderson, and Janssen (1977)
50. Schwade, Blomqvist, and Shapiro (1977)
51. Sherman (1983)
52. Tanaka and Matsuura (1984)
53. Taylor, Buskirk, and Henschel (1955)
54. Vander, Sherman, and Luciano (1985)

SUGGESTED READINGS

Åstrand and Rodahl (1986)
Brooks and Fahey (1987)
Fox, Bowers, and Foss (1988)
Lamb (1984)
McArdle, Katch, and Katch (1991)
Noble (1986)
Powers and Howley (1990)

See the Bibliography at the end of the book for a complete source listing.

Chapter 4

Anatomy and Biomechanics

Jean Lewis

OBJECTIVES

The reader will be able to:

- Describe the four classifications of bones by shape, and give an example of each type
- Describe the general structure of long bones
- Describe the process of ossification of long bones
- Identify the major bones of the skeletal system
- Distinguish between synarthrodial, amphiarthrodial, and diarthrodial joints, both structurally and functionally
- Identify the structures of a diarthrodial joint
- List the factors that determine range and direction of motion
- List and demonstrate the movements possible at each joint
- Describe forces that can cause joint movement
- Describe forces that can resist movement caused by another force
- Describe the gross structure of a muscle
- Explain the differences between concentric, eccentric, and isometric muscle contractions
- Identify the type of muscle contraction during slow movements
- Describe the phases of a ballistic movement
- List the major muscles in each muscle group
- List the major actions and joint(s) of involvement of the following muscles: trapezius, serratus anterior, deltoid, pectoralis major, latissimus dorsi, biceps brachii, brachialis, triceps brachii, flexor and extensor carpi radialis and ulnaris, rectus abdominus, external oblique, erector spinae, gluteus maximus, gluteus medias, iliopsoas, rectus femoris, the three vasti muscles, the three hamstring muscles, tibialis anterior, soleus, gastrocnemius
- Cite specific errors that occur during exercise movements
- Analyze locomotion, throwing, cycling, jumping, and swimming for the movements and muscle involvement
- Describe the three factors that determine stability
- Identify the interrelationships between line of gravity, base of support, balance, and stability, and describe the practical applications of these interrelationships during physical activity
- Describe torque
- Describe how an exerciser can change body segment positions to alter the resistive torque
- Describe how the mechanical principles of rotational inertia and angular momentum have application to movement
- Demonstrate the ability to recognize common error in body alignment and movement mechanics

TERMS

The reader will be able to define or describe:

Abduction	Isometric contraction
Adduction	Joint cavity
Agonist	Lateral rotation
Amphiarthrodial joint	Ligaments
Angular momentum	Medial rotation
Antagonist	Menisci
Aponeurosis	Motor unit
Articular capsule	Muscle group
Articular cartilage	Ossification
Ballistic movement	Perimysium
Bursae	Periosteum
Cartilaginous joints	Prime mover
Concentric contraction	Recruitment
Diaphysis	Resistance arm
Diarthrodial joint	Resistance force
Eccentric contraction	Rotation
Epimysium	Rotational inertia
Epiphyseal plates	Stability
Epiphyses	Summation
Extension	Synarthrodial joints
Fasciculi	Synovial joints
Flexion	Synovial membrane
Force arm	Torque
Hyperextension	Transfer of angular momentum

A knowledge of the bones, joints, and muscles; an understanding of the involvement of muscle forces and other forces; and the ability to apply biomechanical principles to human movement are essential for the health fitness instructor. With this knowledge and understanding the instructor will be better equipped to lead and direct physical activity in a safe manner for the participants that will lead to better exercise benefits. This knowledge will also help the instructor earn the respect of clients, who will view the instructor as a professional in the field, rather than a technician.

SKELETAL ANATOMY

Most of the 200 distinct bones in the human skeleton are involved in human movement. Their high mineral component gives them rigidity; the protein component makes them resistant to tension. The two types of bone tissue are (a) compact tissue, which is the dense, hard, outer layer of bone, and (b) spongy, or cancellous tissue, which has a latticelike structure to allow greater structural strength along the lines of stress at a reduced weight. Bones are often divided into four classifications according to their shapes—long, short, flat, and irregu-

lar. (In chapter 18, we describe computer software that will help you learn the human skeleton.)

Long Bones

The long bones, found in the limbs and digits, serve primarily as levers for movement. Each long bone consists of the **diaphysis**, or shaft, which is made up of thick, compact bone around the hollow medullary cavity; the expanded ends, or **epiphyses**, composed of spongy bone with a thin outer layer of compact bone; the **articular cartilage**, a thin layer of hyaline cartilage covering the articulating surfaces (the surfaces of a bone that meet or come into contact with another bone to form a joint) that provides a friction-free surface and helps absorb shock; and the **periosteum**, a fibrous membrane covering the entire bone except where the articular cartilage is present that serves as an attachment site for many muscles. (See Figure 4.1.)

KEY POINT.   The structures of a long bone include

- the diaphysis, or shaft;
- the epiphyses, or expanded ends;

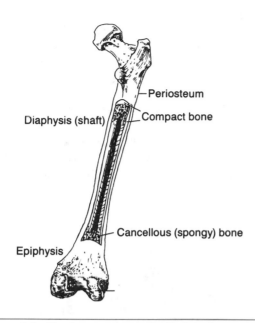

Figure 4.1 The femur, an example of a long bone.

- periosteum, which covers the bone except at the articulating surfaces; and
- articular cartilage at the articulating surfaces.

Short Bones

The tarsals (ankle) and carpals (wrist) are the short bones. Their cubic shapes and composition (spongy bone with a thin outside layer of compact bone) give greater strength but decrease movement potential.

Flat Bones

The flat bones, such as the ribs, ilia, and scapulae, serve primarily as broad sites for muscle attachments and, in the case of the ribs and ilia, to enclose cavities and protect internal organs. These bones are also spongy and covered with a thin layer of compact bone.

Irregular Bones

The ischium, pubis, and vertebrae are irregular shaped bones that serve special purposes such as protecting internal parts and supporting the body.

Ossification of Bones

The skeleton begins as a cartilaginous structure, which is gradually replaced by bone (**ossification**). This process

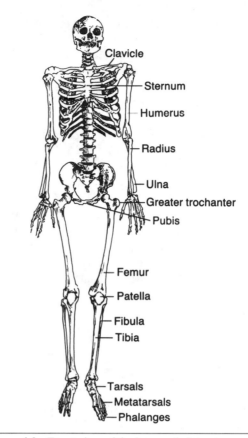

Figure 4.2 Front view of the human skeleton.

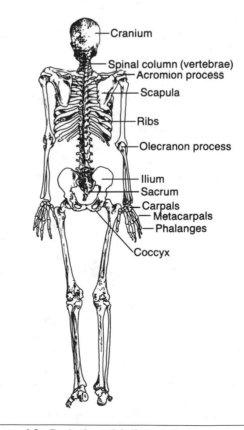

Figure 4.3 Back view of the human skeleton.

begins at the diaphysis of long bones (in centers of ossification) and spreads toward the epiphyses. The **epiphyseal plates** between the diaphyses and epiphyses are the growth areas where the cartilage is replaced by bone; bone growth in length and width continues until the epiphyseal plates are completely ossified. During growth, additional cartilage is laid down to eventually be replaced by bone. When no further cartilage is produced, and the cartilage present is replaced by bone, growth ceases. Other secondary centers of ossification develop in the epiphyses and in some bony protuberances, such as the tibial tuberosity and the articular condyles of the humerus. Short bones have one center of ossification. Dates of closure vary. Although bone fusion at some centers of ossification may occur by puberty or earlier, most of the long bones do not have complete ossification until the late teens. Premature closing, which results in a shorter bone length, can be caused by trauma, abnormal stresses, malnutrition, and drugs.

KEY POINT. Ossification is the development of bone. Generally, bone growth is completed by the late teens.

JOINTS

Joints, the places where bones meet or articulate, are often classified according to the amount of movement that can take place at those sites. The classifications are synarthrodial, amphiarthrodial, and diarthrodial joints.

The **synarthrodial joints** are the immovable joints. The bones merge into each other and are bound together by fibrous tissue that is continuous with the periosteum. The sutures, or the lines of junction, of the cranial bones are prime examples of this type of joint.

The **amphiarthrodial**, or **cartilaginous**, **joints** allow only slight movement in all directions. Usually a fibrocartilage disk separates the bones, and movement can occur only by deformation of the disk. Examples of these joints are found in the tibiofibular joints and the sacroiliac joints, and between the bodies of the vertebrae. **Ligaments**, which are tough, fibrous bands of connective tissue, connect the bones to each other.

Diarthrodial, or **synovial**, **joints** (Figure 4.4) are freely movable joints that allow a variety of movement direction and range; therefore, most of the joint movements during physical activity occur at diarthrodial joints. Strong and fairly inelastic ligaments, along with connective and muscle tissue that crosses the joint, are responsible for maintaining the integrity of the joint.

Diarthrodial joints have distinct physical characteristics that also differentiate them from the other types of joints. The articulating surfaces of the bones are covered by articular cartilage, a type of hyaline cartilage that reduces friction and acts somewhat as a shock absorber. Each joint is enclosed by an **articular capsule**, a ligamentous structure which may be fairly thin in spots or thick enough to be considered separate ligaments. The **synovial membrane**, which secretes synovial fluid into the **joint cavity** to bathe the joint, lines the inner surface of the capsule.

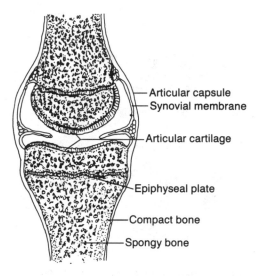

- Articular capsule
- Synovial membrane
- Articular cartilage
- Epiphyseal plate
- Compact bone
- Spongy bone

Figure 4.4 A synovial joint.

Normally, the joint cavity is small and therefore contains little synovial fluid, but an injury to the joint can result in an increased secretion of synovial fluid and swelling. Some diarthrodial joints, such as the sternoclavicular, distal radioulnar, and knee joints, also have a partial or complete fibrocartilage disk between the bones to aid in the absorption of shock and, in the case of the knee, to give greater stability to the joint. The partial, semilunar-shaped disks between the femur and tibia at the knee are called **menisci**.

To reduce frictional rubbing that occurs as the lengths of tendons change during muscle contraction, tendons are often surrounded by tendinous sheaths—cylindrical, tunnel-like sacs lined with synovial membrane. For example, the two proximal tendons of the biceps brachii muscle pass through these tunnels in the bicipital groove of the humerus. **Bursae**, or sacs of synovial fluid that lie between muscles, tendons, and/or bones, also reduce friction between the tissues and act as shock absorbers. Many bursae are found around the shoulder, elbow, hip, and knee. Bursitis, or the inflammation of a bursa, can be caused by repeated friction or mechanical irritation, or as a result of inflammatory or degenerative conditions of tendons.

KEY POINT.   The types of joints are

- synarthrodial, which do not allow movement;
- amphiarthrodial, which allow only slight movement; and
- diarthrodial, or synovial, joints, which are characterized functionally by their wide range of movement and structurally by the presence of articular cartilage, an articular capsule, synovial membrane, and synovial fluid within the joint cavity.

Factors That Determine Direction and Range of Motion

Most of the movement at a joint is rotary in nature—the bone moves around a fixed axis, the joint. The structures of the bones at and near their articulating ends largely determines both the direction and the range of movement. Ball-and-socket joints, which are found at the hip and shoulder, allow a wide range of movement in all directions; but a hinge joint, such as the elbow joint, restricts both direction and range of movement, because bone impinges on bone. The length of the ligaments, and to a lesser extent their elasticity, are also factors in range of movement. For example, the ilio-femoral ligament at the anterior hip joint is a strong but short ligament that prohibits much hip hyperextension. A third factor in range of movement, and the one that can be changed by appropriate exercise, is elasticity, or the ability of tendinous tissue to stretch and return to normal length. This elasticity is determined by the amount and type of physical activity an individual engages in.

KEY POINT.   The potential range and direction of motion is related to

- the shape of the articulating ends of the bones,
- the length of ligaments, and
- the elasticity of connective tissue.

Description of Joint Movements

Specific terminology is used to describe the direction of movement at the different joints. Although different terminology may be used for specific joints, **flexion** in general is anterior or posterior movement from the anatomical position that brings two bones together; **extension** is the return from flexion; **hyperextension**, the continuation of extension past the anatomical position. **Abduction** is the movement of a bone laterally from the anatomical position away from the trunk; **adduction**, the return back toward the anatomical position. **Rotation** occurs when the bone spins around so that its surface faces a different direction.

Shoulder Girdle

This joint complex includes the articulations between the sternum and clavicle and between the clavicle and scapula. Rotary joint movement occurs at those articulations, but the movement terms *elevation, depression, abduction, adduction,* and *upward* and *downward rotation* describe the resulting movements of the scapulae. (See Figure 4.5.) Abduction, adduction, and scapular elevation and depression can all occur without shoulder

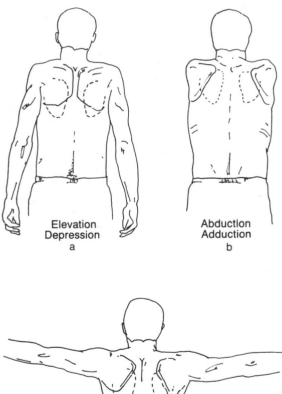

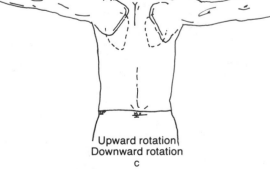

Figure 4.5   Movement of the scapula.

joint movement but may enhance it. Upward and downward rotation occur only when the humerus is moved upward and downward. If the scapulae cannot rotate upward, the arms cannot be elevated sideways above the horizon.

Shoulder Joint

Because of its ball-and-socket structure, the shoulder joint can have movement in all directions—flexion, extension, hyperextension, abduction, adduction, **lateral** and **medial rotation**, and circumduction, which is the circular movement of the arm. Horizontal abduction and horizontal adduction are movements of the arm parallel to the ground. (See Figure 4.6.)

Scapula movements can enhance shoulder-joint movements. As the arm flexes or horizontally flexes, scapula abduction can move the hand out farther in front. Scapula adduction can allow the arm to move back more during hyperextension and horizontal extension. Elevation of the

scapula can allow the hand to reach higher. Medial rotation may be accompanied by scapula abduction; lateral rotation, by scapula adduction.

Elbow Joint

Sometimes referred to as the humeroulnar joint for the bones involved in elbow-joint movement, the elbow joint allows only flexion and extension because of its bony arrangement. (See Figure 4.7.) The ability of some individuals to hyperextend the elbow joint is due to the shape of the articulating surfaces.

Radioulnar Joints

Pronation and supination are the movements of the radius around the ulna in the lower arm. (See Figure 4.8.) Although the wrist is not involved in these movements, the position of the radioulnar joints can be identified by the direction the palm of the hand is facing. When the

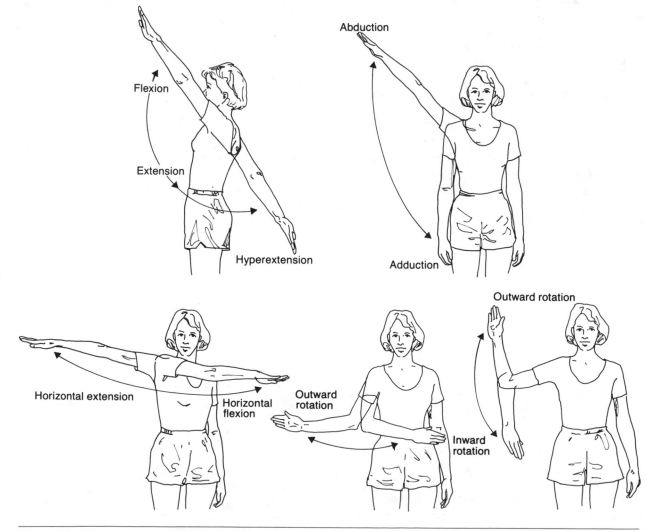

Figure 4.6 Movement of the shoulder joint.

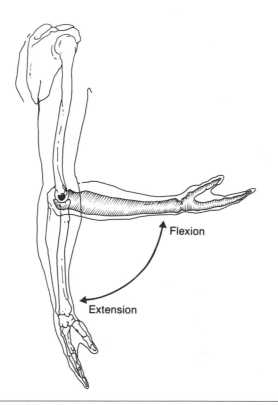

Figure 4.7   Movement of the elbow joint.

arms are hanging down alongside the trunk, the palm faces forward in the supinated position and toward the back in the pronated position. In the supinated position, the radius and ulnar are parallel to each other; in the pronated position, the radius lies across and on top of the ulna. Pronation combined with shoulder-joint medial rotation, and supination with shoulder-joint lateral rotation, moves the hand around even farther.

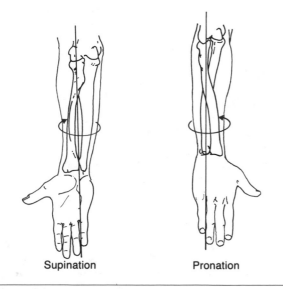

Supination   Pronation

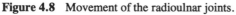

Figure 4.8   Movement of the radioulnar joints.

Wrist Joint

Movement at the wrist joint can occur in two planes of direction—flexion, extension, and hyperextension, and abduction (sometimes referred to as radial flexion) and adduction (ulnar flexion). (See Figure 4.9.)

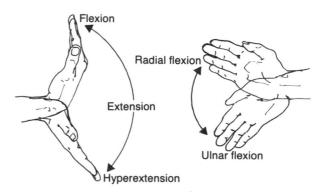

Figure 4.9   Movement of the wrist joint.

Metatarsophalangeal and Interphalangeal Joints

The second through the fifth metacarpophalangeal and all of the metatarsophalangeal (MP) joints allow flexion and extension, and abduction and adduction. The MP joint of the thumb allows only flexion and extension, but it is the only digit that also allows movement at the carpometacarpal joint (which gives the thumb its movement ability). All the interphalangeal (IP) joints of the fingers and toes have only flexion and extension.

Vertebral Column

Movements of the trunk—flexion, extension, hyperextension, lateral flexion, and rotation—occur at all the joints of the vertebral column. (See Figure 4.10.) It is possible to have movement at only one section; for example, the cervical vertebrae can show only hyperextension.

Lumbosacral Joint—Pelvis

The tilts of the pelvis (see Figure 4.11) occur mainly at the joint formed by the fifth lumbar vertebra and the pelvis. The reference point for the direction of the tilts is the iliac crest. As the crest moves forward and down, the pelvis is going toward a forward, or anterior, pelvic tilt; as the crest rotates toward the back, the pelvis has a backward, or posterior, tilt.

The anterior pelvic tilt is usually accompanied by a hyperextension of the lumbar vertebrae; a backward tilt by a flattening out of the lumbar vertebrae.

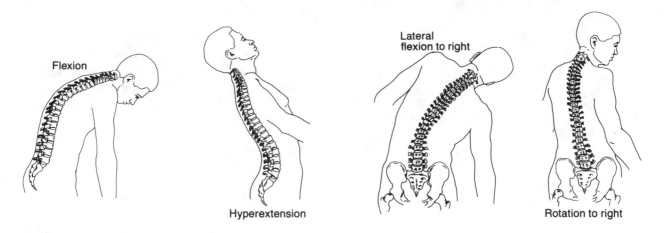

Figure 4.10 Movement of the vertebral column.

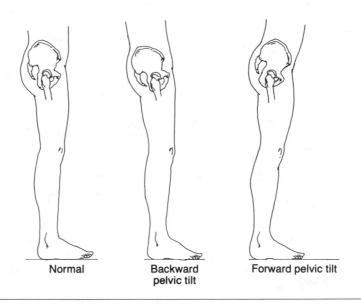

Figure 4.11 Movement of the lumbosacral joint.

Hip Joint

The hip joint structure is similar to the shoulder joint, a ball-and-socket arrangement, and the same movements are possible. (See Figure 4.12.) Because of the deepness of the socket and the tightness of the ligaments at the hip joint, range of motion at this joint, especially for hyperextension, is less than at the shoulder joint. True hip abduction is also limited to about 45° by bony impingement. The leg can be lifted higher only by rotating the hip laterally.

Knee Joint

Flexion and extension are the major movements. (See Figure 4.13.) When the knee is in a flexed position, a limited amount of rotation, abduction, and adduction is possible.

Ankle Joint

Also called the talocrural joint, the ankle is limited to movement in one plane only. Plantar flexion is still sometimes referred to as extension; dorsiflexion, as flexion. (See Figure 4.14.)

Intertarsal Joints

The sideways movements of the foot occur between the different tarsal joints in the foot. (See Figure 4.15.) Inversion can be considered a combination of pronation

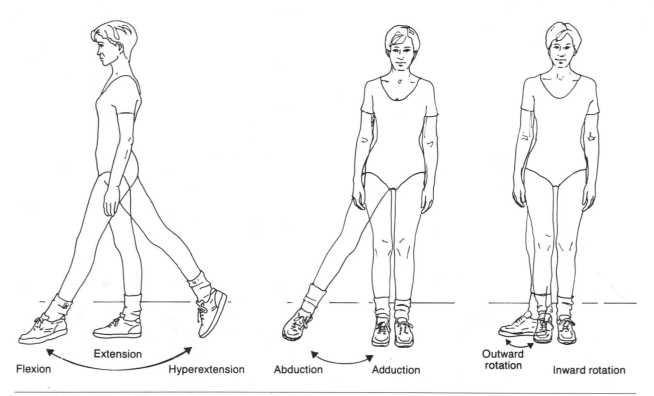

Figure 4.12   Movement of the hip joint.

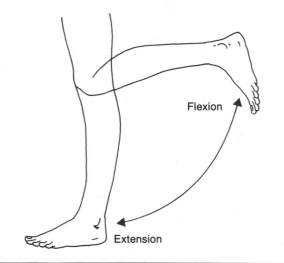

Flexion

Extension

Figure 4.13   Movement of the knee joint.

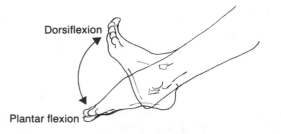

Dorsiflexion

Plantar flexion

Figure 4.14   Movement of the ankle joint.

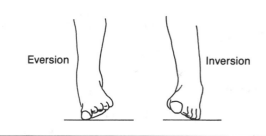

Eversion

Inversion

Figure 4.15   Movement of the intertarsal joints.

and adduction; eversion, a combination of supination and abduction.

Table 4.1 lists the possible movements at each joint.

Forces Related to Joint Movement

Several forces can act on the bones, forces that can cause, resist, or even prevent movement.

Forces That Cause Movement

Joint movement is primarily caused by either muscular contraction or gravitational pull, although other forces, such as another person pushing or pulling on a body part, may also cause joint movement. Whether or not muscle contraction will cause the movement depends

Table 4.1   Joint Movements

Joint	Movements
Shoulder girdle	Elevation, depression; abduction, adduction; upward rotation; downward rotation
Shoulder joint	Flexion, extension, hyperextension; abduction, adduction; medial rotation, lateral rotation; horizontal flexion, horizontal extension
Elbow joint	Flexion, extension
Radioulnar joint	Pronation, supination
Wrist joint	Flexion, extension, hyperextension; radial flexion, ulnar flexion
Vertebral column	Flexion, extension, hyperextension; lateral flexion; rotation
Lumbosacral joint	Forward pelvic tilt, backward pelvic tilt
Hip joint	Flexion, extension, hyperextension; abduction, adduction; medial rotation, lateral rotation
Knee joint	Flexion, extension
Ankle joint	Plantar flexion, dorsiflexion
Intertarsal joint	Eversion, inversion

upon the force of that contraction and the amount of resistance from the other forces.

Forces That Resist Movement Caused by Another Force

The same forces that can cause movement can also act to resist movement. Joint movement caused by gravity can be resisted or decelerated by muscle contraction. Gravity always resists movement occurring in the direction away from the earth. Other forces that can resist movement include internal tissue restriction, hydraulic or air pressure devices on resistance-training equipment, and water.

KEY POINT.   Forces that can both cause and resist joint movements are

- muscle contraction and
- gravity.

VOLUNTARY (SKELETAL) MUSCLE

A muscle consists of thousands of muscle fibers (e.g., the brachioradialis has approximately 130,000 fibers; the gastrocnemius has over 1 million) and connective tissue. Each fiber is enclosed by the connective tissue endomysium. The **fasciculi**, or bundles of fibers grouped together, are surrounded by the **perimysium**, and the entire muscle is enclosed by the **epimysium**. Each muscle is attached either to the bone itself, to the periosteum of the bone, or to deep, thick fascia by tendons and the perimysium and epimysium connective tissues. The sizes and the shapes of the tendons vary and depend upon their functions and the shape of the muscle itself. Some tendons (e.g., the hamstring muscle tendons found at the sides of the posterior knee and the Achilles tendon) are obvious and significant parts of the entire muscle length, but other muscles, such as the supraspinatus and infraspinatus, seem to lie directly on the bone with no observable tendon. Many of the distal attachments that are usually found on the bone that shows the greater movement have a more defined tendinous structure than the proximal attachments. Broad and flat tendons, such as the proximal tendinous sheath of the latissimus dorsi, are called **aponeuroses**. Refer to Figures 4.16 and 4.17 for anterior and posterior views of surface muscles. Other muscles lie under the surface muscles.

Muscle Contraction

Each muscle fiber is innervated by a branch of a motor neuron. The functional organization, or **motor unit**, consists of a single motor neuron and its branches and all the muscle fibers innervated by that motor neuron. With a sufficiently strong stimulus, each muscle fiber within that motor unit contracts maximally; muscular tension increases as a result of the stimulation of more motor units (**recruitment**) or an increased rate of stimulation (**summation**). A muscle that has as its primary purpose a strength or power movement (as does the gastrocnemius) rather than a delicate movement, has a large number of muscle fibers and also has many muscle fibers per motor unit. When a muscle develops tension, or contracts, it tends to shorten toward the middle, pulling on all of its bony attachments. Whether or not the bone(s) of attachment move as a result of that contraction depends upon the amount of the force of the contraction and the resistance to that movement from other forces.

Concentric Contraction

A **concentric contraction** occurs when a muscle contracts forcibly enough to actually shorten. This shortening pulls the bones of attachment closer to each other, causing movement at the joint. Figure 4.18 illustrates elbow flexion against gravity as a result of a concentric contraction—the muscles responsible for the flexion are able to contract with sufficient force to shorten, which

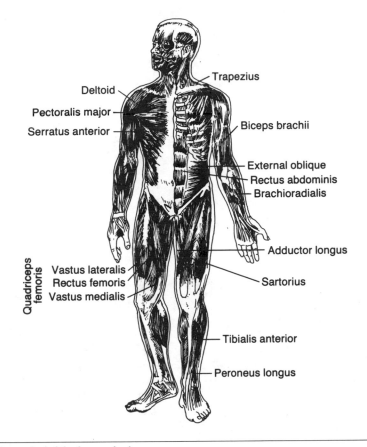

Deltoid
Pectoralis major
Serratus anterior
Trapezius
Biceps brachii
External oblique
Rectus abdominis
Brachioradialis
Adductor longus
Quadriceps femoris
Vastus lateralis
Rectus femoris
Vastus medialis
Sartorius
Tibialis anterior
Peroneus longus

Figure 4.16   Front view of muscles of the human body.

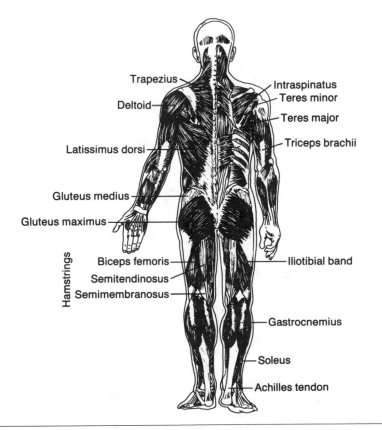

Trapezius
Deltoid
Latissimus dorsi
Gluteus medius
Gluteus maximus
Hamstrings
Biceps femoris
Semitendinosus
Semimembranosus
Intraspinatus
Teres minor
Teres major
Triceps brachii
Iliotibial band
Gastrocnemius
Soleus
Achilles tendon

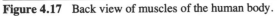

Figure 4.17   Back view of muscles of the human body.

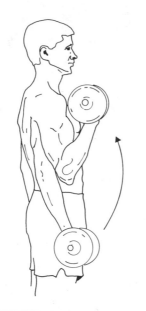

Figure 4.18   Concentric contraction by elbow flexors.

pulls the lower arm toward the humerus. Although the pull is on all bones of attachment, usually only the bone farthest from the trunk (e.g., a limb) will move. To stand up from a semisquat position, there must be extension at the hip joints and knee joints, but gravity is resisting that extension. The muscles must develop sufficient force to overcome the gravitational force; if sufficient force is developed, the muscle will shorten in a concentric contraction, pulling on the bones to cause extension. Resistance training with free weights uses gravitational pull as the resistance; the use of pulleys changes the direction of the gravitation pull, offering resistance to movement in other directions. Although gravity is not a factor in water, the water itself resists movement in all directions.

To exercise muscles by using gravity as the resisting force, the movements must be done in the direction opposite the pull of gravity—away from the earth. Arm abduction from a standing position is a movement opposite the pull of gravity, so a concentric contraction is required by the muscles that will pull the humerus into the abducted position. Movements such as shoulder horizontal flexion and extension (see Fig. 4.6) executed from a standing position occur parallel to the ground and therefore are not resisted by gravity—internal tissue friction is the only resistance, but concentric contraction by the muscles responsible for these movements is still necessary. During these movements, gravity is still trying to draw the arm toward the earth, but it is not interfering with the horizontal movement. To perform horizontal flexion and extension against the resistance of gravity, the performer must get into a position in which the movements are away from the pull of gravity. Lying prone (for horizontal extension) or supine (for

horizontal flexion) on a bench or floor, or flexing the trunk at the hip (horizontal extension), will result in those shoulder movements being against gravity.

A concentric contraction is also necessary for a rapid movement, regardless of the direction of another force. When an external force could cause the desired movement without any muscular contraction, but too slowly, concentric contractions produce the desired speed. An example of this is seen in the arm movements during the second count of a jumping jack, when the arms adduct from their abducted position—gravity would adduct the arms, but concentrically contracting muscles cause the movement to occur much more quickly.

A muscle that is very effective in causing a certain joint movement is a **prime mover**, or **agonist**. Assistant movers are muscles that are not as effective for the same movement. For example, the peroneus longus and brevis are prime movers for eversion of the intertarsal joints, but they can offer only a little assistance in plantar flexion of the ankle joint. During a concentric contraction, muscles that act opposite to the muscles causing the concentric contraction, the **antagonist** muscles, are basically passive and lengthen as the agonists shorten in contraction. For example, for elbow flexion to occur against the pull of gravity, the muscles responsible for elbow flexion are contracting concentrically; the antagonists, or the muscles responsible for elbow extension, relax and lengthen passively during the movement. However, in some fitness activities, such as aerobic dance, the antagonist muscles can be contracted to offer more resistance to the concentrically contracting muscles.

KEY POINT.   A concentric contraction, which results in a shortening of the muscle and therefore a pulling on the bones of attachment, is necessary if joint movement is to be

- in a direction opposite another force, such as gravity, and
- rapid, regardless of the direction of any other forces.

Eccentric Contraction

An **eccentric contraction** occurs when a muscle generates tension that is not great enough to cause movement but instead acts as a brake to control the speed of movement caused by another force. (See Figure 4.19.) The muscle exerts force, but its length increases. Arm abduction requires a concentric contraction of muscles; gravity will adduct the arm back down to the side. To adduct the arm more slowly than gravity, the same muscles that contracted concentrically to abduct the arm

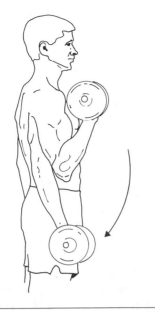

Figure 4.19 Eccentric contraction by elbow flexors.

now contract eccentrically to control the speed of the adduction caused by gravity. Eccentric contractions may also occur when a muscle's maximum effort still is not great enough to overcome the opposing force; movement will be caused by that force in spite of the maximally contracting muscle, which is still lengthening. Muscles antagonist to the eccentrically contracting muscles passively shorten during the movement.

KEY POINT.   An eccentric contraction, which results in a lengthening of the muscle, controls the velocity of movement caused by another force.

Ballistic Movements and Muscle Contraction

A **ballistic**, or fast, **movement** occurs when resistance is insignificant, as in throwing a ball, and requires a burst of concentric contractions to initiate the movement. Once movement has begun, the muscles that contracted to cause the movement basically shut down; any further contraction slows the movement. Other muscles actively guide the movement in the appropriate direction. Eccentric contractions of muscles that are antagonist, or opposite, to the muscles that initiated the movement decelerate and eventually stop the movement. For example, one of the most important movements in the actual throwing motion is medial rotation of the shoulder joint. The muscles responsible for medial rotation concentrically contract quickly to begin the throwing motion; after the ball is released, the muscles responsible for lateral rotation contract eccentrically to slow and eventually stop the movement; this is the follow-through. The reverse is true for the windup, or prepara-

tion for the actual throw. All of this occurs in an exceedingly short period of time.

KEY POINT.   A ballistic movement is a rapid movement that includes

- concentric contraction of the agonist muscles to initiate movement,
- "coasting," in which there is minimal muscle activity, and
- eccentric contraction of the antagonist muscles to decelerate the movement.

Isometric Contraction

During an **isometric**, or static, **contraction**, the muscle exerts a force that counteracts an opposing force. The muscle length does not change, so no movement occurs, and that joint position is maintained. The contractile part of the muscle shortens, but the elastic connective tissue lengthens proportionately; no overall change in the entire muscle length occurs. Holding the arm in an abducted position or maintaining a semisquat position requires an isometric contraction—just enough muscle force to counteract the pull of gravity, resulting in no movement. The effort involved in trying to move an immovable object is another example of isometric contractions; although the amount of muscular force can be maximal, no joint movement will occur. (See Figure 4.20.)

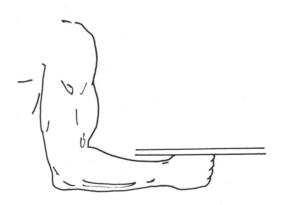

Figure 4.20 Isometric contraction by elbow flexors.

Quad sets, a rehabilitation exercise in which the knee extensor muscles are contracted with the knee already in the extended position, provide another example of a static contraction. A backward pelvic tilt desired during some exercises is maintained by isometric contraction by the abdominal muscles after they have contracted concentrically to tilt the pelvis backward.

Roles of Muscles

As has been mentioned in the discussion of muscular contractions, muscles can act in several ways and have several functions. They can cause movement (concentric contraction), decelerate movement caused by another force (eccentric contraction), or prevent movement (isometric contraction). Muscles may also contract isometrically to stabilize or prevent an undesirable body-segment movement. For example, during a push-up exercise, gravity tends to cause hyperextension of the vertebral column and hip joint. Isometric contraction of the abdominal muscles prevents this sagging—these muscles stabilize the trunk in its proper position. Another role of a muscle is to counteract an undesirable action caused by the concentric contraction of another muscle. The concentric contraction of most muscles causes more than one movement at the same joint, or movement at more than one joint. If only one of those movements is intended, another muscle would contract to prevent the undesirable movement. For example, concentric contraction of the upper trapezius fibers would cause elevation and some adduction of the scapula. If only adduction were desired, the lower trapezius fibers, which cause depression and adduction, contract to neutralize the undesirable elevation. In this example, the different fibers of the trapezius are neutralizing the unwanted action and also helping the desired action. The biceps brachii muscle causes elbow flexion and radioulnar supination; for only flexion to occur with biceps brachii contraction, the pronator teres also contracts to counteract the supination. Muscles also act to guide movements initiated or caused by other muscles. During activities against a great resistance, such as lifting free weights, muscles are contracting to help maintain balance or proper direction of the movement. After muscle force has initiated a ballistic movement, other muscles can help guide the movement in the proper direction.

KEY POINT.   The major roles of the muscles are to

- cause movement (concentric contraction) regardless of an opposing force,
- decelerate or control the speed of movement (eccentric contraction) caused by another force, and
- prevent movement (isometric contraction).

Muscle Groups

A **muscle group** includes all of the muscles that cause the same movement at the same joint. The group is named for the joint where the movement takes place and the common movement that is caused by the concentric contraction of those muscles. The elbow flexors, for example, is a muscle group composed of the specific muscles responsible for flexion at the elbow joint when the muscles contract concentrically. Table 4.2 lists the muscles that are prime (and assistant) movers of the muscle groups. Note that a movement being observed at a joint does not necessarily involve the muscle group for the movement that is occurring. The muscle group responsible for the opposite action may be contracting eccentrically to control the movement. For example, the elbow flexor muscle group exerts force to flex the elbow joint during the elbow curl exercise. To return to the starting position, the pull of gravity extends the joint to the original position, but the elbow flexor muscle group is still exerting force to control the speed of that movement with eccentric contractions. To maintain the elbow in a flexed position requires an isometric contraction by those same elbow flexors.

Specific muscles that cause more than one action at a joint or cause movement at more than one joint belong to more than one muscle group. For example, the flexor carpi ulnaris muscle belongs in both the wrist flexor and wrist adductor muscle groups. The biceps brachii is part of the elbow flexor and radioulnar supinator muscle groups. Table 4.2 lists the specific muscles in each muscle group.

KEY POINT.   A muscle group includes all the muscles that cause a specific movement at a specific joint.

COMMON EXERCISE ERRORS AND HINTS FOR EXERCISING MUSCLE GROUPS

Many of the errors in exercising and movement result from a lack of knowledge rather than a lack of muscular strength or coordination. By applying basic knowledge, an exerciser can perform better and more safely.

Shoulder-Girdle and Shoulder-Joint Complex

Movement can be enhanced and more muscles involved if a deliberate effort is made to incorporate shoulder-girdle

Table 4.2   Muscles That Are Prime Movers (and Assistant Movers)

Joint	Prime Movers (Assistant Movers)
Shoulder girdle	Abductors—serratus anterior, pectoralis minor Adductors—middle fibers of trapezius, rhomboids (upper and lower fibers of trapezius) Upward rotators—upper and lower fibers of trapezius; serratus anterior Downward rotators—rhomboids, pectoralis minor Elevators—levator scapulae, upper fibers of trapezius, rhomboids Depressors—lower fibers of trapezius, pectoralis minor
Shoulder joint	Flexors—anterior deltoid, clavicular portion of pectoralis major (short head of biceps brachii) Extensors—sternal portion of pectoralis major, latissimus dorsi, teres major (posterior deltoid, long head of triceps brachii, infraspinatus/teres minor) Hyperextensors—latissimus dorsi, teres major (posterior deltoid, infraspinatus, teres minor) Abductors—middle deltoid, supraspinatus (anterior deltoid, long head of biceps brachii) Adductors—latissimus dorsi, teres major, sternal portion of pectoralis major (short head of biceps brachii, long head of triceps brachii) Lateral rotators—*infraspinatus, *teres minor (posterior deltoid) Medial rotators—pectoralis major, *subscapularis, latissimus dorsi, teres major (anterior deltoid, *supraspinatus) Horizontal flexors—both portions of pectoralis major, anterior deltoid Horizontal extensors—latissimus dorsi, teres major, infraspinatus, teres minor, posterior deltoid
Elbow joint	Flexors—brachialis, biceps brachii, brachioradialis (pronator teres, flexor carpi ulnaris and radialis) Extensors—triceps brachii (anconeus, extensor carpi ulnaris and radialis)
Radioulnar joint	Pronators—pronator quadratus, pronator teres, brachioradialis Supinators—supinator, biceps brachii, brachioradialis
Wrist joint	Flexors—flexor carpi ulnaris, flexor carpi radialis (flexor digitorum superficialis and profundus) Extensors and hyperextensors—extensor carpi ulnaris, extensor carpi radialis longus and brevis (extensor digitorum) Abductors (radial flexors)—flexor carpi radialis, extensor carpi radialis longus and brevis (extensor pollicis) Adductors (ulnar flexors)—flexor carpi ulnaris, extensor carpi ulnaris
Lumbosacral joint	Forward pelvic tilters—iliopsoas (rectus femoris) Backward pelvic tilters—rectus abdominus, internal oblique (external oblique, gluteus maximus)
Spinal column (thoracic and lumbar areas)	Flexors—rectus abdominus, external oblique, internal oblique Extensors and hyperextensors—erector spinae group Rotators—internal oblique, external oblique, erector spinae, rotatores, multifidus Lateral flexors—internal oblique, external oblique, quadratus lumborum, multifidus, rotatores (erector spinae group)
Hip joint	Flexors—iliopsoas, pectineus, rectus femoris (sartorius, tensor fascia latae, gracilis, adductor longus and brevis) Extensors and hyperextensors—gluteus maximus, biceps femoris, semitendinosus, semimembranosus Abductors—gluteus medius (tensors fascia latae, iliopsoas, sartorius) Adductors—adductor brevis, adductor longus, gracilis, pectineus (adductor magnus) Lateral rotators—gluteus maximus, the six deep lateral rotator muscles (iliopsoas, sartorius) Medial rotators—gluteus minimus, gluteus medius (tensor fascia latae, pectineus)
Knee joint	Flexors—biceps femoris, semimembranosus, semitendinosus (sartorius, gracilis, gastronemius, plantaris) Extensors—rectus femoris, vastus medialis, vastus lateralis, vastus intermedius
Ankle joint	Plantar flexors—gastrocnemius, soleus (peroneus longus, peroneus brevis, tibialis posterior, flexor digitorum, flexor hallucis longus) Dorsiflexors—tibialis anterior, extensor digitorum longus, peroneus tertius (extensor hallucis longus)
Intertarsal joint	Inverters—tibialis anterior, tibialis posterior (extensor and flexor hallucis longus, flexor digitorum longus) Everters—extensor digitorum longus, peroneus brevis, peroneus longus, peroneus tertius

*Rotator cuff muscles.

movements with shoulder-joint movements. For instance, optimal involvement of these muscles can be achieved in the following exercises and movements.

- **Forward reaching.** Flexion can be accompanied by scapula abduction if the exerciser reaches the fingertips as far forward as possible.
- **Push-up.** At the completion of a push-up, the scapulae can be abducted to raise the chest a little bit more off the floor.
- **Overhead reaching.** Normally, there is some scapulae elevation when the arm is overhead. A conscious effort to reach as high as possible will involve the scapulae elevators more; conversely, a deliberate attempt to keep the shoulders low for a "long neck" look requires concentric contraction by the scapulae depressors.
- **Sideward arm reaching.** During shoulder-joint horizontal extension in movement or exercise, the arm can be moved farther back with scapula adduction.

Elbow and Radioulnar Joints

The position of the radioulnar joints, that is, whether the arm is supinated or pronated, does not affect the involvement of the elbow-joint muscles. Flexion against a resistance requires contraction of the flexor muscles. However, the degree to which muscles are used is affected by supination and pronation—a good point to remember when instructing participants how to do **curls.** Normally, flexion with the radioulnar joint in a pronated position is a weaker movement, because the biceps brachii muscle cannot contract as strongly as when the radioulnar joints are in a supinated position. (The distal tendon of the biceps brachii muscle is wrapped around the radius somewhat in the pronated position, which diminishes its force of pull.) The brachialis muscle, though, is not affected by the radioulnar joint position, because it is attached to the ulna, which is the nonmoving bone in radioulnar joint movements. Further, the brachioradialis muscle can contract with more force when the radioulnar joint is in a semi-pronated, semisupinated position. None of the extensor muscles is affected by the radioulnar joint positions, so supination or pronation would not affect **triceps presses.**

Wrist Joint

The wrist muscles during flexion and extension exercises are affected by the position of the radioulnar joints. When the elbow is in a flexed position, gravity can act as a resistance for wrist flexion when the radioulnar joints are in the supinated position and resistance for extension when the radioulnar joints are in the pronated position. Remind exercise participants that how they twist their lower arms will affect which muscles are strengthened during these exercises.

Vertebral Column and Lumbosacral Joints

Neither neck hyperextension nor hyperflexion is desirable. The same pairs of muscles that flex and extend can be strengthened or stretched, one side at a time, by cervical lateral flexion and rotation. The instructor should ask participants to **tilt** or **turn** the head from side to side rather than to bend the neck forward or back.

Many exercises require appropriate positioning of the lumbosacral joint and lumbar vertebrae, and contractions by the abdominal muscles for either movement or stabilization. A **curl-up** or **crunch** exercise should begin with a backward pelvic tilt that is maintained throughout the curl and return movement. If there is any indication that this backward pelvic tilt cannot be maintained, or if the exerciser feels tightness or an ache in the lumbar area, that exercise should be stopped. If the problem is inadequate strength to maintain the backward tilt position, the exercise should be modified to one that requires less abdominal muscle strength, one that the exerciser has sufficient abdominal strength to do correctly.

A full curl-up, in which the exerciser comes up to a sitting position, requires hip flexion by the hip flexor muscles during the last stages of the exercise. Initially, the abdominal muscles contract concentrically to tilt the pelvis backward and then to flex the vertebral column. Once the flexion is achieved, these muscles contract isometrically to keep the pelvis tilted backward and the trunk in a flexed position. There is a "sticking point" that can be felt by the exerciser during a full curl-up. This occurs when the trunk flexion is complete and the hip flexors begin to bring the trunk to an upright position. Doing partial curl-ups or crunches will help eliminate the role of the hip flexors.

The exercise called **leg lifts** is considered to be an abdominal exercise, but inadequate instruction is often given as to how to perform it correctly. The legs are lifted off the floor and held up by concentric and then isometric contraction of the hip flexors. Some of the hip flexor muscles also pull the lumbosacral joint into a forward-tilted position. It is the role of the abdominal muscles to prevent that forward tilt and to maintain a flattened lumbar spine and posterior pelvic tilt. The backward pelvic tilt should precede the hip flexion; and, as in the case of the curl-up exercise, if the proper tilt cannot be maintained, the exercise should not be done in that fashion.

There is also a tendency for the pelvis to tilt forward during **overhead arm movements** from a standing position. This can be prevented by keeping the arms in front of the ears and by flexing the knees somewhat.

When weights are lifted from a supine position, as in the **bench press**, there is a tendency to hyperextend the lumbar spine and tilt the pelvis forward. Although this can allow the exerciser to lift a somewhat heavier weight, it does not increase the work of the arm muscles, and it puts the lower back into a compromising position. Bench presses are best done with the hips and knees in a flexed position and feet on the bench or a bench extension. Upright presses are best done seated with the back supported.

Hip Joint

A common error during **side-lying leg raises** to exercise the hip abductor muscles is the attempt to move the foot as high as possible. Because the range of motion for true abduction is limited (about 45°), the exerciser often rotates the top leg laterally, which allows the foot to go higher. However, this rotation changes the muscle involvement more to the hip flexor muscles. To exercise the primary abductor muscles, the leg should not be rotated; the toes should face forward, not up. Turning the feet out comes from lateral rotation of the hips; there should be no attempt to rotate the knee or the ankle joints.

In **backward leg movements**, hyperextension is limited primarily by the tightness of the hip ligaments. A leg can appear to be more hyperextended if it is accompanied by a forward pelvic tilt. The exerciser should be cautioned to keep the pelvis in its proper position, even though some apparent hyperextension is lost.

A common exercise position is standing with feet shoulder-width apart. Often the exerciser has the feet turned somewhat outward (from hip lateral rotation). There is nothing gained from this foot position, and it is potentially dangerous. During any **squatting** or **standing** movement, the knee should be directly over the foot to prevent strain to the lateral and medial knee ligaments. Although the knee can be kept over the foot even in the toed-out position during a squat, some individuals have a tendency to let the knees move toward the inside of the feet. It is easier to determine whether the knee position is a correct one when the feet are parallel to each other. During the squat, the exerciser should be able to see the big toe on each foot.

Knee Joint

Hyperflexion can strain and stretch knee ligaments and put pressure on the menisci; therefore, *a full squat*, especially with additional weights, should not be attempted, nor should *sitting on the lower legs*. During any **lunging** movements or **forward-back stride** positions in which the front knee is in a flexed position, the knee should be over or in back of the foot, not in front. Any knee position that puts a twisting pressure on the knee-joint structures should also be avoided. The *hurdler position*, in which, from a sitting position, one leg is stretched out in front of the body and the other leg is out to the side and back with a flexed knee, should be avoided.

MUSCLE GROUP INVOLVEMENT IN SELECTED ACTIVITIES

Human movement is caused or controlled by muscle forces. The following sections briefly analyze the involvement of muscle groups in some common physical activities.

Walking, Jogging, Running

Jogging can be looked at as a modification of walking; and running, as a fast jog. The different phases and the muscle-group involvement in walking, jogging, and running are similar, but more forceful muscle contractions are needed to increase speed. The three basic phases are the pushoff, the recovery of the pushoff leg, and the landing.

Pushoff

The pushoff is accomplished by the concentric contraction of the hip hyperextensors, the talocrural plantar flexors, and, to a lesser extent, the foot metatarsophalangeal flexors. (See the back leg in Figure 4.21.) Because the knee is almost in the extended position at pushoff, little work is done by the knee extensors to help propel the body forward. The gluteus maximus muscle may assume a greater role in the hip hyperextension as speed increases. Medial rotation takes place at the hip joint, but because the foot is fixed on the ground, this movement is seen at the pelvis.

Recovery

At the beginning of the recovery phase, the hip flexors contract concentrically to begin the forward leg swing.

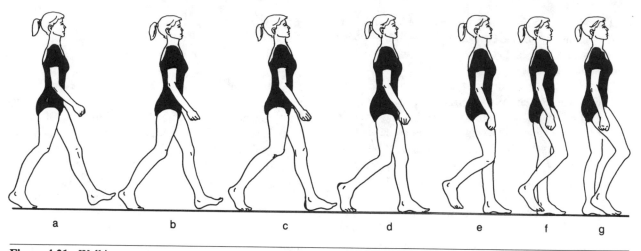

Figure 4.21 Walking movements.

This is basically a ballistic movement, so the momentum initiated by the hip flexors continues the motion. The knee flexors bend the knee at the beginning of hip flexion; the extensors initiate the straightening of the knee; the flexors then work eccentrically to control this knee extension at the end of the recovery phase. The talocrural joint is dorsiflexed to clear the foot from the ground and prepare for the landing. (See the recovery leg in frames d through g in Figure 4.21.) Running speed is a product of stride length and stride frequency. To increase both factors in running, the hip is flexed to a greater extent and with a much greater velocity. (See Figure 4.22, the recovery leg.)

Landing

Just prior to landing, the hip extensors contract eccentrically to decelerate the forward leg swing. On contact, the knee extensors contract eccentrically to cushion the impact. The heel should touch the ground first, during walking and jogging; as running speed increases, the ball of the foot or the entire foot may make contact. During the landing phase in walking, the talocrural dorsiflexors contract eccentrically to control the speed of movement of the ball of the foot to the ground.

The arm swing requires shoulder flexion and extension to hyperextension. As speed increases, the swing becomes more vigorous, and there is more elbow flexion. For the greatest efficiency, the arms should move in an anterior/posterior direction. To increase the upper limb muscle involvement, a walker can exaggerate the flexion and extension movements or can abduct and adduct or horizontal flex and extend the shoulder joint.

Walking or running up an incline elicits a greater force of contraction from the gluteus maximus muscle

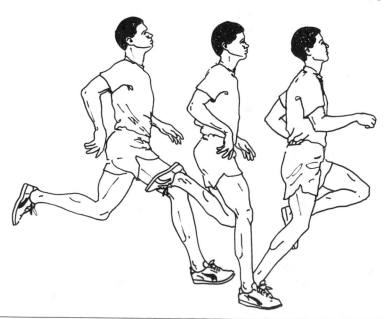

Figure 4.22 Running movements.

at the hip and from the knee extensors. The talocrural dorsiflexors are more active immediately before landing to position the talocrural joint to conform with the angle of the incline. Because the talocrural joint is in a more dorsiflexed position, the plantar flexors begin contracting during pushoff from a more stretched position. For these reasons, hill climbing requires greater flexibility in the plantar flexors, especially the soleus muscle, and greater strength in the dorsiflexors. There is also more eccentric contraction by the knee extensors during landing in downhill than in uphill running. As a result, these muscle groups are more apt to become fatigued and be sore afterward.

Jogging in place requires the talocrural plantar flexors to propel the body upward; they work more than any of the other lower extremity muscle groups. The knee extensors are primarily active in eccentric contraction to cushion the landing. At the landing during walking and jogging, the heel is the first part of the foot to make contact with the surface, but in jogging in place, the ball of the foot touches first. The plantar flexors therefore are also active during the landing, contracting eccentrically to control the speed and amount of dorsiflexion. It is better to have sufficient dorsiflexion so the heel briefly touches the ground rather than to always stay up on the toes, which can put quite a strain on the plantar flexors. There can be additional muscle involvement with the execution of movements with the leg immediately after pushoff and before the foot lands again—hip flexion with flexed or extended knee, hip hyperextension with flexed or extended knee, hip abduction/adduction, hip lateral rotation along with hip and knee flexion that brings the foot to the front of the trunk, and medial rotation with knee flexion that brings the foot posteriorly and to the side of the trunk.

KEY POINT.   The major muscle groups involved during locomotion are

- in the pushoff—hip hyperextensors and talocrural plantarflexors;
- in the recovery—hip and knee flexors, and talocrural dorsiflexors; and
- in the landing—knee extensors (eccentric) and talocrural plantarflexors (eccentric).

Cycling

The main force in cycling comes from the hip and knee extensor muscles during the downward push. With toe clips, the rider can use the hip and talocrural dorsiflexors to help return the pedal to the up position, if she or he makes a conscious effort to do so.

KEY POINT.   The major muscle groups involved in cycling are

- hip extensors and
- knee extensors.

Jumping

The hip and knee extensors, followed by the talocrural plantar flexors, forcibly contract to propel the body upward. The lean of the trunk primarily determines the angle of takeoff. The trunk extends, and the arms flex from a hyperextended position just before the leg action. If the reach height is important, the scapula elevates. During the landing, the hip and knee extensors and the talocrural plantar flexors contract eccentrically.

KEY POINT.   The major muscle groups involved in jumping are

- hip extensors,
- knee extensors, and
- talocrural plantarflexors.

Overarm Throwing

There are three phases in throwing: the windup, or preparation; the execution, or actual throw; and the followthrough, or recovery. (See Figure 4.23.)

Windup

In preparation for throwing, there is a weight shift to the back foot, a medial rotation of the back leg (because the leg is fixed to the ground, rotation is seen at the pelvis), trunk rotation and some lateral flexion and hyperextension, shoulder lateral rotation, some horizontal extension of the throwing arm accompanied by the adduction of the scapula, flexion of the elbow, and hyperextension of the wrist. The movements of the throwing arm are all ballistic. The lateral rotation at the shoulder is remarkably fast and powerful. Toward the end of the windup, the medial rotators begin to eccentrically contract to decelerate the rotation in preparation for the actual throw. (See Figure 4.23.)

Execution

The weight shift forward is the initial movement in the throwing pattern. This is accomplished by the hip abductors and hyperextensors, the talocrural plantar flexors,

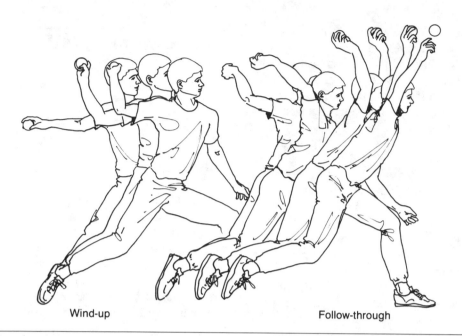

Wind-up   Follow-through

Figure 4.23 Throwing movements.

and the intertarsal evertors of the back leg. The front hip laterally rotates. The trunk then laterally flexes in the direction opposite that of the windup, and rotates, beginning at the lumbar area and continuing through the thoracic vertebrae, and then flexes. There is a forcible medial rotation of the shoulder, along with scapula abduction. Although there is some horizontal flexion, most of the force of the shoulder in an overhand throw comes from this medial rotation. The elbow extends, and the wrist moves toward flexion. Depending upon the desired spin on the ball, the radioulnar pronators and the wrist abductors or adductors may also be involved. (See Figure 4.23.)

Follow-Through

Because the actions at the shoulder and elbow joints are vigorous ballistic movements, the shoulder lateral rotators and horizontal extensors contract eccentrically to decelerate the movements; the elbow flexors contract eccentrically to prevent elbow hyperextension. (See Figure 4.23.)

KEY POINT. The major muscle groups involved in throwing, which requires both rapid concentric and rapid eccentric contractions, are

- shoulder-joint medial and lateral rotators (eccentric and concentric),
- elbow flexors (eccentric) and extensors (concentric), and
- trunk flexors and rotators.

Swimming and Exercise in Water

Swimming is a unique activity because the water medium offers resistance to movements of submerged body parts in all directions and at all speeds. Exercises or movements performed in water demand concentric contractions. Gravity is not a factor in water, so less stress is put on the weight-bearing joints. In stroke swimming, the following muscle groups and muscle location areas are primarily active during the propulsion phase:

Stroke	Muscle Group
Front crawl	Shoulder-girdle downward rotators and adductors, shoulder-joint extensors, hip flexors and extensors
Back crawl	Shoulder-girdle downward rotators and abductors, anterior shoulder-joint muscles, hip flexors and extensors
Side stroke	Leading arm: shoulder-girdle abductors, anterior shoulder-joint muscles; trailing arm: shoulder-girdle adductors, posterior shoulder muscles, hip flexors and extensors
Breast stroke	Shoulder-girdle adductors, posterior shoulder muscles, hip abductors and adductors

KEY POINT. All movements of limbs submerged in water require concentric contractions.

Lifting and Carrying Objects

The weight to be lifted from the ground should be located close to the lifter's spread feet; the lifter squats, keeping the trunk as erect as possible. The actual lifting should be accomplished by leg rather than spine or arm action. Proper lifting is begun by moving the trunk to a position as perpendicular to the floor as possible and then tilting the pelvis backward; the knee extensors along with the hip extensors then contract concentrically. (See Figure 4.24.) Insufficient leg strength can result in an incorrect lifting technique. The weight should be carried close to the body, with the trunk assuming a position that allows the line of gravity to fall well within the area of the base. The trunk lateral flexors are more active when the weight is carried on one side; the extensors are more active when the weight is in front of the body; and when the weight is carried across the top of the back, as in backpacking, the abdominals are more active.

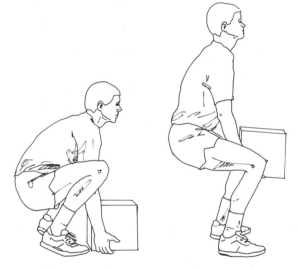

Figure 4.24   Lifting technique.

KEY POINT.   The steps in proper lifting are

- place the feet close to the weight,
- move the vertebral column to an upright position perpendicular to the floor,
- tilt the pelvis backward, and
- extend the hips and knees.

BASIC MECHANICAL CONCEPTS RELATED TO HUMAN MOVEMENT

Knowledge of the laws and principles of mechanics is also important to the understanding of human move-

ment. Some of these basic but important concepts are described below.

Stability

For an individual to maintain balance, his or her line of gravity must fall within the area of the base of support. In Figure 4.25, frame (a) illustrates the area of the base of support in a standing position with feet together; frame (b), with feet apart and forward and back.

Stability, or the ease with which balance can be maintained, is proportional to the distance from the line of gravity to the outer limits of the base that is farthest from a potentially upsetting force. Figure 4.26 compares more stable positions with less stable positions. A wide base of support usually, but not necessarily, insures greater stability. From a feet-apart position, if one leans so that the line of gravity falls directly over a foot, and a pushing force is applied from the opposite side, there is less stability than if the feet were together but with the line of gravity falling over the edge of the foot closer to the applied force.

The degree of stability is indirectly proportional to the height of the center of gravity above the base; the lower the center of gravity above the base, the greater the force needed to upset the stability. The degree of stability is also directly proportional to the weight of the body. With all other factors being equal, a heavy person is more stable than a lighter one.

KEY POINT.   Stability in humans is

- directly proportional to the distance of the line of gravity from the limits of the base,
- indirectly proportional to the height of the center of gravity above the base, and
- directly proportional to the weight of the body.

Stability may be increased by moving the feet apart to widen the base of support and by flexing the knees and hips to lower the center of gravity. During standing exercises that require some degree of balance, stability can also be aided by having a nearby object such as a wall or chair to hold or push against if necessary. Many exercises can also be executed from a sitting position. To help maintain stability against a potentially upsetting force, the weight should be shifted toward that force. When locomotion is going to occur, a position close to instability is attained by shifting the line of gravity closer to the outer limits of the base (which is the area of the pushoff foot) in the direction of the intended movement (see Figure 4.26). During locomotion, as the line of gravity moves outside the limits of the base, a

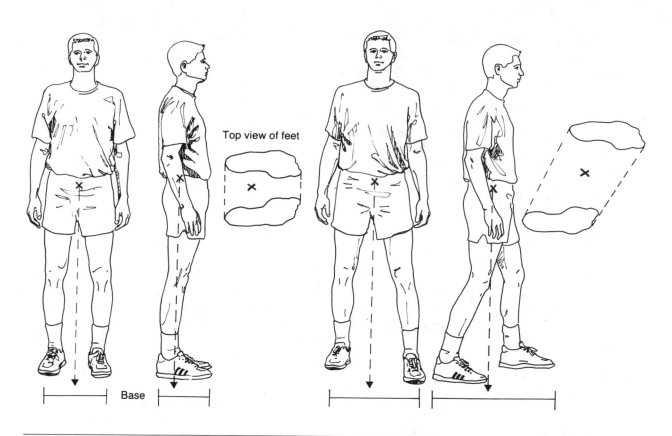

Top view of feet

Base

Figure 4.25   Areas of bases of support.

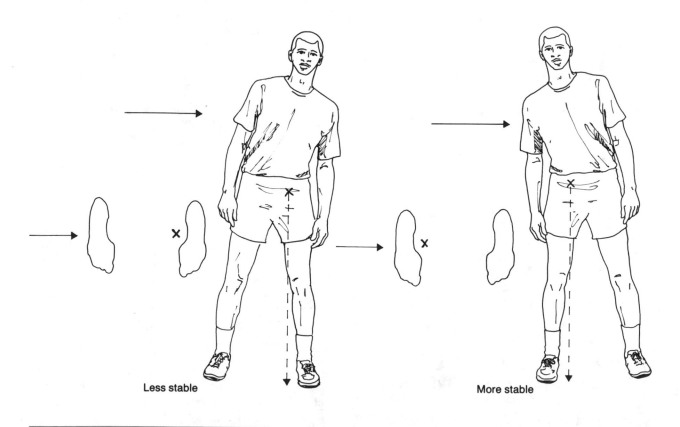

Less stable

More stable

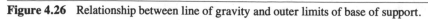

Figure 4.26   Relationship between line of gravity and outer limits of base of support.

new base is established when the other foot lands, and stability is maintained. If something prevents the foot from establishing a new base, stability is lost.

Torque

The effect produced when a force causes rotation is called **torque** (T). It is the product of the magnitude of the force (F) and the **force arm** (FA), which is the perpendicular distance from the axis to the direction of the application of that force. Algebraically, torque can be expressed as $T = F \times FA$. When two opposing forces are acting to produce rotation in opposite directions, one of the forces is often designated as the **resistance force** (R); its force arm, the **resistance arm** (RA). When considering the torque produced by sufficient muscle force to cause movement against gravity or some other external force, F and FA are designated for the muscle, R and RA for the gravitational or other opposing force.

KEY POINT.   Torque can be expressed algebraically as $T = F \times FA$, for the torque that produces the movement, or $T = R \times RA$, for the torque that is opposing the movement.

Application to Muscle Contraction

Muscle contraction can be considered the force; the FA is the perpendicular distance from the joint (axis) to the

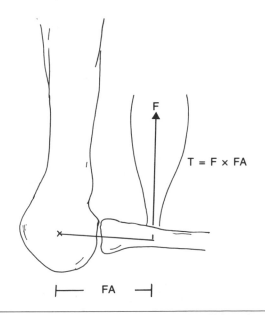

Figure 4.27   Force (F) and force arm (FA) of biceps brachii muscle.

direction of the force from its point of application (where the muscle attaches to the bone). Figure 4.27 illustrates the direction of pull of the biceps brachii muscle on the radius; the force arm is the perpendicular distance from the elbow joint to this line of force. If the muscle insertion were closer to the joint, the same force would produce less torque because of the shorter force arm; to produce the same torque, more muscle force must be produced.

Torque is also affected by joint position. Figure 4.28 again shows the direction of pull by the biceps brachii, but with the elbow in a less flexed position. This results in a shorter force arm, so the same muscle force produces less torque.

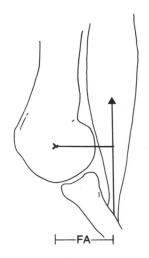

Figure 4.28   Effect of a less flexed position of the elbow joint on the force arm of the biceps brachii.

Torque Resulting From Other Forces

The force from gravitational pull will be treated as a resistance force. The resistive force produced by gravity pulling on a body part is the mass of the object; the resistance arm is the perpendicular distance from the axis of rotation to the point of the object that represents its center of gravity. Figure 4.29 illustrates the torque produced as a result of gravity acting on the arm. The torque opposing limb movements can be increased by adding weight to increase both the magnitude of force and the length of the resistance arm, or by adjusting the weight further from the axis. The resistance arm of a force applied by someone pushing or pulling on a limb is the perpendicular distance from the axis to the point of application of the push or pull.

For muscle contraction to cause movement of a bone, the muscle force must produce a torque greater than the opposing or resistance torque; the muscle contraction is concentric. A greater resistance torque results in

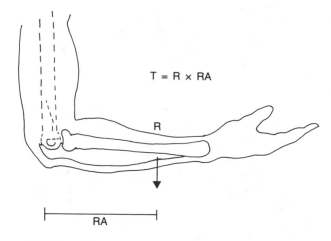

Figure 4.29 Resistance (R) and resistance arm (RA) of lower arm.

movement, and the muscle contracts eccentrically. Technically, it can be argued that the muscle force during an eccentric contraction should be considered the resistance, and the external force causing the movement, the force. When the muscular torque equals the resistance torque, no movement occurs; the muscle is contracting isometrically.

KEY POINTS.

- A concentric contraction produces a torque that is greater than the resistive torque.
- An eccentric contraction produces a torque that is less than the opposing torque.
- An isometric contraction produces a torque that is the same as the opposing torque.

Application to Exercising

Knowledge of torques can be applied to individualize exercises. The amount of muscular contraction necessary during the exercise can be modified to fit an individual's needs by altering the amount of resistance and/or the resistance arm to change the resistive torque. For example, resistance torque can be increased with the use of external weights, which would therefore require stronger muscle contractions. The resistance torque can also be changed by altering the position of the body parts. The modifications shown in Figure 4.30 that can be made by the exerciser to reduce the necessary muscle force include not using the weight, to reduce both the resistive force and the resistance arm, and flexing the elbow to reduce the length of the resistance arm.

The arm position during a curl-up exercise determines the length of the resistance arm and therefore the

amount of resistance torque against which the abdominal muscles have to work. Arms may be held at the sides of the body to bring the upper body mass closer to the axes of rotation to reduce the necessary muscle force; arms can be put overhead with hands on the scapulae to increase the resistive torque, therefore increasing the required muscle force. It is important to realize that modifications to lessen the resistance torque do not necessarily make the exercise "easy" for all individuals. If an exerciser with a lower strength level finds the resistive torque too great to overcome for a sufficient number of repetitions, the limb positions can be altered to reduce the torque against which the muscles have to work, but this individual is still working as hard as a stronger individual who did not have to reduce the resistive torque.

KEY POINT.   The torque that resists limb movements can be altered by

- increasing or decreasing the amount of the resistive force, and

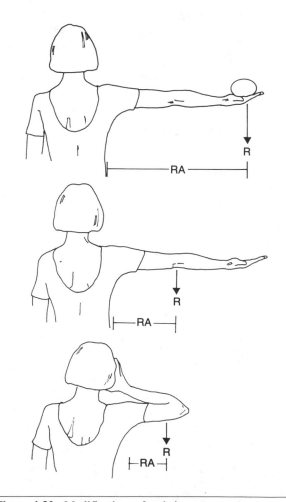

Figure 4.30 Modifications of resistive torque.

- changing the position of the resistive force relative to the joint to change the resistance arm.

Rotational Inertia

Rotational inertia (also referred to as the moment of inertia), or the reluctance of a body segment or segments to rotate around an axis or a joint, is dependent upon the body's mass and the distribution of that mass around the joint. A leg, for example, has more rotational inertia than an arm, not only because of its heavier mass but also because its mass is concentrated a greater distance away from its axis. A softball bat held by its fat end has less rotational inertia than if it were grasped in the usual manner.

Application to Exercising

The rotational inertia possessed by body segments before or during movement is dependent on the mass of the segments, which cannot be changed, and the distribution of the mass around the joints, which can be manipulated and result in a change of the rotational inertia. For example, an arm with elbow, wrist, and fingers extended has a greater rotational inertia than an arm with elbow, wrist, and fingers flexed; a leg with extended knee and ankle has more inertia than if the knee were flexed and the ankle dorsiflexed. The amount of muscular force necessary to cause rapid limb movement is proportional to the rotational inertia of the limb to be moved. During jogging, in which speed of running is not a factor, the knee of the recovery leg is flexed to reduce the leg's rotational inertia around the hip joint. Less muscular force is needed to swing the recovery leg forward, thus the possibility of local fatigue of the hip flexor muscles is reduced. In sprinting, the quicker the recovery leg is brought forward, the faster the running speed. Powerful contractions of the hip flexors, along with a greater knee flexion, results in the recovery leg coming through sooner, which results in increased speed. Another example of rapid movement to which this principle can be applied is in jumping jacks. Keeping the elbow flexed reduces the rotational inertia. This results in either the reduction of the amount of muscle force by the shoulder abductor and adductor muscle groups to maintain a certain cadence, or, if maximum muscle force is still applied, faster movements.

KEY POINT. Rotational inertia during fast limb movements can be decreased by moving the mass of the limb closer to the axis or joints.

Angular Momentum

Angular momentum, or the quantity of angular motion, is expressed as the product of the rotational inertia, which is determined by both the mass of the moving part and the distribution of the mass around the joints, and the angular velocity. A moving body part possesses angular momentum; the faster it is moving and the greater its rotational inertia, the greater the angular momentum. The amount of force necessary to change angular momentum is proportional to the amount of the momentum.

Application to Exercising

This concept can be applied to ballistic limb movements during exercise. A fast-moving body segment is decelerated by eccentric muscle contractions; the faster the movement, the greater the mass, or the greater the desired deceleration, the greater the muscle force that must be applied. Care must be taken when rapid ballistic limb movements, especially with added weights, are performed. A large amount of momentum may be generated, and considerable muscle strength may be required to decelerate and eventually stop the movement.

Transfer of Momentum

Transfer of angular momentum from one body segment to another can be achieved by stabilizing the initial moving body part at a joint, which will result in angular movement of another body part. For example, in performing a curl-up exercise for the trunk flexors, a flinging forward of the arms from an overhead position or of the elbows from alongside the head results in a transfer of their momentum to the trunk. This decreases the amount of muscular contraction needed by the trunk flexors, which may or may not be desired. A jump with a turn in the air can be better achieved if the arms are swung forcibly across the body in the intended direction of the spin just before takeoff.

KEY POINTS.

- The amount of angular momentum is dependent upon the rotational inertia and angular velocity of a moving body segment.
- The amount of eccentric force necessary to decelerate the angular velocity of a body segment is proportional to the amount of angular momentum of the body segment.
- Angular momentum can be transferred from one body segment to another.

COMMON MECHANICAL ERRORS DURING LOCOMOTION, THROWING, AND STRIKING

Success in activities depends in part on the proper execution of movements. Some of the more common errors that violate the laws of mechanics to some degree are discussed in the next sections.

Locomotion

Some beginning joggers have a tendency to run "stiff legged," or with insufficient knee flexion of the recovery leg. This results in a greater rotational inertia of the leg; the hip flexor muscles exert more force than if the knee were more flexed to bring the mass of the leg closer to the hip axis.

Another potential problem is direction of the arm and leg movements. All movements should be executed in the anterior and posterior directions. Swinging the hands across the trunk rotates the upper trunk; in reaction, the lower trunk rotates in the opposite direction. There also may be a tendency for hip medial rotation of the recovery leg; this swings the recovery foot to the outside. The touchdown foot should land in a forward–backward direction and not pointed to the outside. Sometimes runners are not aware of this, and a suggestion for them to "toe in" somewhat when landing will result in the correct foot alignment.

Some joggers and runners propel themselves too high off the ground during the airborne phase; this results in a shorter stride length. Although the length of time the body is airborne may be the same as when running with less loft, less horizontal distance is covered.

Overstriding, in which the line of gravity from the runner's center of gravity falls in front of the touchdown foot, will decelerate the running speed. No propulsion force against the ground for forward movement can take place until the line of gravity is over the foot. Understriding, in which the line of gravity falls well in back of the foot at touchdown, results in a shorter period of time during which the propulsion muscles can work.

Throwing and Striking

A ball is thrown for accuracy, speed, or distance, which depends in part on the speed of the ball when it leaves the hand. The speed of the ball in the hand just before release is the speed of the ball immediately after it leaves the hand. The more joints that can be involved in the throwing motions, the greater the speed of the ball when it is released. Proper throwing and striking techniques are the same for females and males. Many throwing problems, such as pushing the ball rather than throwing it, that result in low velocity stem from a lack of sufficient trunk rotation or from poor timing of this rotation and the shoulder-joint movements. The thrower should rotate the trunk and hips during the windup so that the pelvis is sideways to the intended direction of the throw and the shoulders rotated even more to the back. As the hips and then the different sections of the spinal column rotate back to begin the execution of the throw, the arm lags behind. This sets up for a whiplike action of the arm and an adequate length of time for the important medial rotation. Without this trunk rotation, there is inadequate arm rotation, resulting in a pushing motion during the throw. The vertebral column also has to rotate in a wavelike fashion, with the thoracic vertebrae being the last to rotate.

The same sequence of motion applies to striking events, such as tennis and badminton stroking and softball batting. A common fault in learning how to serve a tennis ball or smash a birdie is insufficient trunk rotation. It is easier to hit an object without trunk rotation, but the impact of the racket on the projectile will not be as great. In batting, a common error is the lack of timing between the different body segment movements. The hip, trunk, and arm movements follow one another so the bat is moving with great velocity upon contact with the ball. Beginners often stop one motion before beginning the next.

SUMMARY

Knowledge of the structure and function of muscles, bones, and joints is essential to understanding human movement. The lengths and shapes of the bones, the amounts of movement possible at a joint, the lengths and elasticity of the ligaments and tendons, and the types of muscle contractions all influence the rate and range of possible movement. While developing tension, muscles can shorten and cause movement (concentric contraction), lengthen and resist movement caused by other forces (eccentric contraction), or remain the same length to stabilize a body segment (isometric contraction). Information is given about the muscle groups involved in selected activities and about some common errors during exercise, along with some suggestions for exercising muscle groups. The basic mechanical concepts of stability, torque, rotational inertia, and angular momentum, as applied to human movement, are also summarized. Finally, some common mechanical errors in locomotion, throwing, and striking are discussed.

CASE STUDIES FOR ANALYSIS

4.1 You are supervising the resistance training area when you hear a lot of clanging noise coming from the seated leg press area. You discover that the exerciser at that machine is not controlling descent of the weights. You suggest that he slowly let the weights return rather than just letting them drop. He asks you for the reason for the suggestion—he doesn't see any benefit in a controlled return other than it is not as noisy. What do you tell him? (See Appendix A.)

4.2 You've told David that he should do two kinds of wall stretches—one keeping the knees extended to stretch the gastrocnemius muscles and another flexing at the knees to stretch the soleus muscles. He wants to know why just one of those won't stretch both of those calf muscles. How do you explain the need for two stretches? (See Appendix A.)

SUGGESTED READINGS

Adrian and Cooper (1989)
Barham (1978)
Basmajian and MacConaill (1977)
Brancazio (1984)
Broer and Zernicke (1979)
Cooper and Glassow (1982)
Gowitzke and Milner (1988)
Gray (1966)
Hay and Reid (1982)
Hinson (1981)
Jensen, Schultz, and Bangerter (1983)
Kreighbaum and Barthels (1990)
Logan and McKinney (1982)
Luttgens and Well (1982)
O'Connell and Gardner (1972)
Rasch and Burke (1986)
Thompson (1988)

See the Bibliography at the end of the book for a complete source listing.

Chapter 5

Measurement and Evaluation

OBJECTIVES

The reader will be able to:
- Describe components and types of validity
- Describe ways to improve accuracy of test scores
- Describe calibration of equipment
- Describe ways to interpret fitness test scores
- Describe use of tests in a fitness program

TERMS

The reader will be able to define or describe:

Calibration	Objectivity
Construct validity	Predictive validity
Content validity	Reliability
Criterion validity	Standard deviation
Error	True score

Fitness programs combine knowledge from several areas of the exercise sciences. Other chapters present information based on exercise physiology, biomechanics, and exercise psychology. This chapter summarizes aspects of measurement and evaluation that are related to fitness testing. Chapter 18 evaluates computer software related to fitness testing.

VALIDITY

The most important question to raise about a test is that of validity: Does the test measure the characteristic I'm interested in evaluating? The two key components of validity are consistency and relevance. Consistency includes the **reliability** of the test results as well as the **objectivity** of the testers. If the test is repeated without a change in the fitness of the person being tested and the same results are obtained, it is reliable. If different persons administer or score the test, and they obtain the same results, the test reflects objectivity.

Although a test could be reliable and objective and still not be valid, tests that are unreliable or lack objectivity cannot be valid. After the consistency of the test is assured, there are three major ways to determine whether the test measures what it is supposed to measure: content, criterion, and construct validity. **Content validity** indicates that the test seems to be good based on logic, expert testimony, and widespread use. **Criterion validity** involves having an externally valid criterion for the test. For example, underwater weighing serves as the criterion measure for validating skinfold assessment of body fatness. With **predictive validity**, the criterion is measured at some point in the future. For example, risk factors for coronary heart disease (CHD) have been validated with a criterion that is measured in the future (i.e., actual development of CHD). **Construct validity** is provided by showing that a test responds in the ways one would expect based on theoretical understanding of that characteristic. For example, step tests have some validity because those who are physically active score better than inactive people.

KEY POINT. The most important question to ask about a test is whether it measures the characteristics you are interested in. To do so, a test must

- give consistent results (reliability), even with different testers (objectivity), and

- have evidence that it is related to the selected characteristic (validity) in terms of expert opinion, comparison with good tests of the same variable, and theoretical support.

The fitness tests recommended in this book have been shown to be reliable and objective when carefully administered by trained professionals. Maximal oxygen uptake and percent-fat estimation by underwater weighing are considered valid tests (and are often used as the "gold standards" for cardiorespiratory fitness and relative leanness, respectively). They have been recommended and used by experts in numerous research investigations and fitness programs (content validity). The field tests recommended in chapters 7, 9, and 10 also have *content* validity in that they are recommended and used by fitness experts. In addition, the endurance run and skinfold fat tests have *criterion* validity in that they are highly related (correlated) with maximal oxygen uptake and underwater weighing, respectively (1). There is some *construct* validity for all of the tests, in that they have been shown to be related to other tests of the same variable, they improve with the type of physical conditioning thought to improve the characteristic, and performance on these tests changes with changes in training states.

KEY POINT.   There are valid fitness tests for cardio-respiratory function (maximal oxygen uptake, endur-

ance run of at least 1 mi); relative leanness (underwater weighing, skinfolds); strength and endurance (curl-ups, modified pull-ups); and flexibility (sit and reach).

TIPS FOR INCREASING THE ACCURACY OF TESTING

An observed test score includes the individual's **true score** plus **error**. The error can result from the testing environment, the equipment, normal variation of the person, and the tester. There are a number of things that fitness leaders can do to obtain more accurate results (i.e., less error) from testing. These include

- properly preparing the person to be tested,
- organizing the testing session, and
- attending to details.

Preparation of the Subject

The best test results are found with persons who understand what test procedures are going to be used, have practiced any unusual or novel aspects of the test, have complied with pretest instructions in terms of rest, food, drink, drugs, and exercise, and who are physically and mentally prepared to take the test. See the

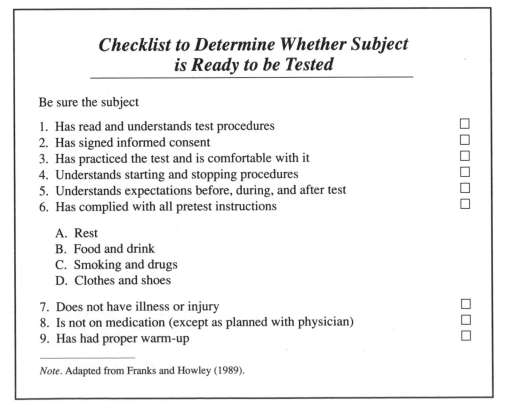

Checklist to Determine Whether Subject is Ready to be Tested

Be sure the subject

1. Has read and understands test procedures ☐
2. Has signed informed consent ☐
3. Has practiced the test and is comfortable with it ☐
4. Understands starting and stopping procedures ☐
5. Understands expectations before, during, and after test ☐
6. Has complied with all pretest instructions ☐

    A. Rest
    B. Food and drink
    C. Smoking and drugs
    D. Clothes and shoes

7. Does not have illness or injury ☐
8. Is not on medication (except as planned with physician) ☐
9. Has had proper warm-up ☐

Note. Adapted from Franks and Howley (1989).

Checklist to Determine Whether Subject is Ready to be Tested.

Organization

Preparation of the subject is part of organizing the test session. In addition to the items listed in the preceding section, the fitness tester will want to ensure that everything is ready to test persons accurately and efficiently (see the Checklist for Fitness Tester form).

Attention to Details

The most fundamental thing a tester can do to improve the accuracy of the testing situation is to pay close attention to all the details (such as those listed in the preced-

ing checklists). Preparation of the subject, organization of the testing situation, and precision of data collection can be accurately completed only when the tester attends to each aspect of the test protocol.

KEY POINT.   Accuracy of testing can be improved by careful preparation of the person to be tested and having the tester be precise in an organized testing session.

INTERPRETING TEST SCORES

What does a body weight of 180 lb reflect? It may mean this: The person really weighs 183, she or he just lost

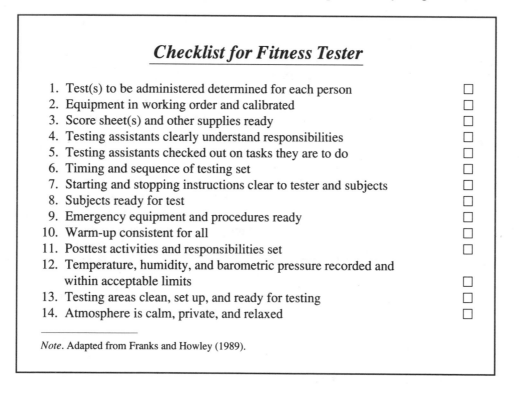

Checklist for Fitness Tester

1. Test(s) to be administered determined for each person ☐
2. Equipment in working order and calibrated ☐
3. Score sheet(s) and other supplies ready ☐
4. Testing assistants clearly understand responsibilities ☐
5. Testing assistants checked out on tasks they are to do ☐
6. Timing and sequence of testing set ☐
7. Starting and stopping instructions clear to tester and subjects ☐
8. Subjects ready for test ☐
9. Emergency equipment and procedures ready ☐
10. Warm-up consistent for all ☐
11. Posttest activities and responsibilities set ☐
12. Temperature, humidity, and barometric pressure recorded and within acceptable limits ☐
13. Testing areas clean, set up, and ready for testing ☐
14. Atmosphere is calm, private, and relaxed ☐

Note. Adapted from Franks and Howley (1989).

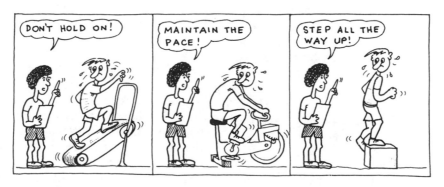

Figure 5.1 Tips for testers.

1 lb of water weight in a workout, the scales weigh 3 lb light, and we have misread the scale 1 lb heavy, resulting in:

$$183 - 1 - 3 + 1 = 180$$

Any observed test result includes true score plus error. The error may be caused by equipment, environment, psychological factors, inconsistency of the subject, or the tester. Some of the error may be *constant* (which can be corrected with a constant) or *random* (which cannot be predicted or corrected). In the body-weight example, the scale error could have been corrected by adding 3 lb to the weight, but the tester error cannot be predicted, in that it might be light one time and heavy the next. **One reason several trials are taken for a test is based on the assumption that the random errors will average out;** thus if you were to take the average of three body weights, it would reduce the effect of random error.

One way to deal with variability is to use the **standard deviation** from the mean. The mean is the average. So if a large number of 20-year-old women were tested, one might find that the mean maximal heart rate was 200 beats•min^{-1}. If you looked at each individual's maximal heart rate, you would find a large number that had maximal heart rates within a few beats of 200. You would find a few women who had maximal heart rates several beats above or below 200. In the case of maximal heart rate, the standard deviation is about 11 beats •min^{-1} for different ages (10). In a normal distribution, standard deviation includes a set percentage of people:

- Mean plus and minus 1 standard deviation = 68% of group
- Mean plus and minus 2 standard deviations = 95% of group
- Mean plus and minus 3 standard deviations = 99+% of group

In the example of maximal heart rate, you would expect to find 68% of 20-year-old women with maximal heart rates between 189 and 211, and 95% between 178 and 221; and almost all 20-year-old women would have a maximal heart rate between 167 and 233.

Two conclusions can be drawn from the variability of fitness tests. The first one is that when carefully used, fitness tests can give *accurate* estimates of fitness components. The second one is that the fitness test results are *approximations* of the fitness components. Thus we can differentiate among cardiorespiratory fitness (CRF) levels of 14, 9, and 6 METs (see chapter 8), but would not be able to pinpoint differences between 8.6 and 9.4 METs.

KEY POINT.　Test scores include the true score, constant error, and random error. The standard deviation

from the mean can be used to describe variability. Fitness tests can provide good *approximations* of fitness levels.

HOW TO EXPLAIN TEST SCORES TO INDIVIDUALS

You can help participants evaluate their fitness test scores by doing the following (2, 5).

- Emphasize health status rather than comparison with others.
- Emphasize change rather than current status.
- Provide specific recommendations based on the test data and your understanding of the individual.

Criterion Health Status

One common approach is to compare the fitness participant with persons of the same gender and similar age (e.g., "On the 1.5-mi-run test, you were better than 60% of the people your age and sex"). Although individuals may ask for this type of feedback, it is probably the least useful in terms of fitness. Much of the individual comparison with others is based on heredity and early experience. There are limits to how much change can be made even with a great deal of effort. It is unfortunate that many people in fitness programs try to use the "performance" model of being number one. The emphasis should not be on who can run the fastest or who has the lowest cholesterol, but rather on helping all people understand and try to obtain and maintain healthy levels of cardiorespiratory fitness, body composition, and low-back function. Thus, in the first testing session, the feedback should be based on whether or not people meet desirable health standards rather than what percentage of the population they could "beat" on a test. This is the approach we have used in this book.

We have set fitness standards for persons based on what is needed for good health. For example, we would like all women to have from 16% to 25% fat, and children and men, from 7% to 18% (see chapter 7). It doesn't matter what percentage of the population currently is in that range. What does matter is that if persons have less fat than the lower limit of the range, they have health risks associated with having too little fat, and if they have more fat than the upper limit of the range, their risks of developing (or making worse) major health problems increases. The fitness leader should encourage all participants to try to reach and maintain the health standards for cardiorespiratory fitness, body composition, and low-back function. Health standards for field tests (see chapters 7, 9, and 10 for details of the tests) for different ages are provided on the Fitness Test Standards form. Standards for maximal oxygen uptake are included in chapter 9. Although it is common for persons to perform at lower levels on fitness tests as they get older, it is not healthy to decrease CRF, gain fat, or reduce midtrunk flexibility and abdominal muscle endurance. Therefore, we expect performance times (e.g., time needed to win a 10K race) to decrease, but the minimal fitness standards are the same for adults of all ages. It should be noted that more research is needed to be able to refine these standards—thus these may need to be modified as we find out more about the relationship between test scores and positive health.

Improvement

The most important question for a fitness participant is *not* what her or his status is at this moment in life, but rather what it will be 6 months, 2 years, or 20 years from now. Thus, one deals with the person's status compared with health standards and helps the individual set reasonable, desirable, and achievable goals for the next testing period.

Specific Fitness Goals

Another way that test results can be used is to help individuals meet specific goals. It may be that the health standards are not appropriate or reasonable for an individual. For example, the mile-run standards cannot be used for people who are swimming for their fitness workouts or for individuals in wheelchairs. However, individual goals for covering a certain distance in the water or in a wheelchair can be established. Or the fitness leader may want to set subgoals for an individual who is very unfit. For example, it would be discouraging to discuss mile-run standards for a person who can only walk a quarter of a mile without stopping. The initial goal for that person may be to work up to being able to walk a mile without stopping. As indicated in chapter 12, it is important to set goals and subgoals to help people begin and continue healthy behaviors.

Healthy Behaviors

Fitness and lifestyle behaviors (such as getting adequate exercise, nutrition, and rest; avoiding substance abuse; coping with stress) and fitness test scores are related. However, the fitness leader should *emphasize* the fitness *behaviors*. It is more important to have people begin and continue regular physical activity than to reach a certain level on a graded exercise test. It is more im-

portant to have people eating properly than to have a certain percent body fat. By emphasizing healthy behaviors, one can recognize people for their efforts, and in the long run this will be the best way to improve their fitness test scores. An overemphasis on test scores can discourage some participants.

KEY POINT. Individuals should be recognized and rewarded for healthy behaviors, improving in fitness status, achieving specific fitness goals, and maintaining a healthy fitness status in each component of physical fitness.

FEEDBACK

The health standards and emphasis on improvement and healthy behaviors provide the basis for the feedback given to individual participants. Another factor to consider is the individual's own nature and likes. The key to feedback is to provide the best recommendations concerning activities (type, total work, intensity, frequency, etc.) that would be healthy, helpful, and interesting to this individual (thus providing motivation for participants to continue). Assistance is especially important early in the fitness program.

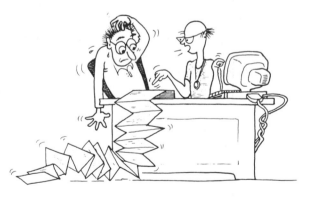

Figure 5.2 Feedback on fitness test results.

PROGRAM REVISION

Analysis of test scores from different fitness classes can assist in deciding what revisions need to be made. How many people drop out of various classes? What kinds of aerobic, body fatness, and low-back function changes are being made? How many injuries are related to the various classes? The answers to such questions help you to evaluate, revise, and improve your fitness programs. You might consider your programs to be improving rather than

Fitness Test Standards

Test item	Age (years)					
	6-9	10-12	13-15	16-30	31-50	51-70

Mile run (min)

Males						
Good	14	12	11	10	10	10
Borderline	16	14	13	12	12	12
Needs work	≥ 18	≥ 16	≥ 15	≥ 14	≥ 14	≥ 14
Females						
Good	14	12	13	12	12	12
Borderline	16	14	15	14	14	14
Needs work	≥ 18	≥ 16	≥ 17	≥ 16	≥ 16	≥ 16

Percent fat (%)

Males						
Good	7-18	7-18	7-18	7-18	7-18	7-18
Borderline	22	22	22	22	22	22
Needs work	< 5	< 5	< 5	< 5	< 5	< 5
	> 25	> 25	> 25	> 25	> 25	> 25
Females						
Good	7-18	7-18	16-25	16-25	16-25	16-25
Borderline	22	22	27	27	27	27
Needs work	< 5	< 5	< 14	< 14	< 14	< 14
	> 25	> 25	> 30	> 30	> 30	> 30

Curl-ups (#)

Good	≥ 20	≥ 25	≥ 30	≥ 35	≥ 35	≥ 35
Borderline	12	15	22	25	25	25
Needs work	≤ 5	≤ 10	≤ 13	≤ 15	≤ 15	≤ 15

Sit and reach (in.)[a]

Good	12	12	12	12	12	12
Borderline	8	8	8	8	8	8
Needs work	≤ 6	≤ 6	≤ 6	≤ 6	≤ 6	≤ 6

Mod. pull-ups (#)

Good	≥ 10	≥ 12	≥ 15	≥ 15	≥ 15	≥ 15
Borderline	6	8	10	10	10	10
Needs work	≤ 2	≤ 4	≤ 5	≤ 5	≤ 5	≤ 5

Note. Adapted from *YMCA Youth Fitness Test Manual* (pp. 42-47) by B.D. Franks, 1989, Champaign, IL: Human Kinetics. Copyright 1989 by National Council of Young Men's Christian Associations of the United States of America. Adapted by permission.

aThe feet touch the base of the box at 9 in.—a score of 9 indicates the person can touch his or her feet.

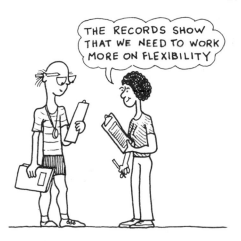

Figure 5.3 Modification of fitness program.

as having reached "perfection." This improvement can result from program evaluation.

Another use of test scores is to help educate the public and to get positive attention for your program. What percentage of the participants stay with the program long enough to make important fitness gains? What is the total amount of fat lost by participants in 1 year? How many miles have the participants run during the year? Careful testing, record keeping, and analysis can provide helpful information about your program to the public.

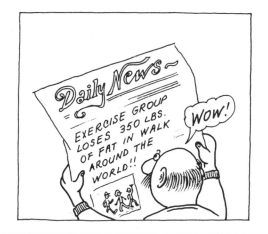

Figure 5.4 Publicity.

KEY POINT.   Fitness scores, along with individuals' interests, can help modify exercise recommendations for participants. The testing results from all the participants can provide the basis for evaluation and modification of the fitness center's program.

CALIBRATION OF EQUIPMENT

To calibrate is to check the accuracy of a measuring device by comparing it with a known standard and adjusting it to provide an accurate reading. This section deals with the **calibration** of equipment used in exercise testing. However, it should not be viewed as a replacement for the specific procedures recommended by the equipment manufacturer (8).

Treadmill

The treadmill's speed and grade settings must be calibrated because they determine physiological demand and are crucial in estimating cardiorespiratory fitness.

Speed Calibration

An easy way to calibrate the speed on any treadmill is to measure the length of the belt and count the number of belt revolutions in a certain time period. The specific steps are these (8):

1. Measure exact length of the belt in meters, and record the value.
2. Place a small piece of tape near the edge of the belt surface.
3. Turn on the treadmill to a given speed using the speed control.
4. Count 20 revolutions of the belt while tracking time with a stopwatch. Start your watch as the tape first moves past the fixed point, beginning your counting with "zero."
5. Convert the number of revolutions to revolutions per minute. For example, if the belt made 20 complete revolutions in 35 s:

$$35 \text{ s} \div 60 \text{ s} \cdot \text{min}^{-1} = .583 \text{ min}$$

So,

$$20 \text{ rev} \div .583 \text{ min} = 34.3 \text{ rev} \cdot \text{min}^{-1}$$

6. Multiply the calculated revolutions per minute (step 5) times the belt length (step 1). This will give you the belt speed in meters per minute. For example, if the belt length is 5.025 m:

$$34.3 \text{ rev} \cdot \text{min}^{-1} \cdot 5.025 \text{ m} \cdot \text{rev}^{-1}$$

$$= 172.35 \text{ m} \cdot \text{min}^{-1}$$

7. To convert meters per minute to miles per hour $(\text{mi} \cdot \text{hr}^{-1})$, divide the answer in step 6 by 26.8 $(\text{m} \cdot \text{min}^{-1}) \cdot (\text{mi} \cdot \text{hr}^{-1})^{-1}$:

$$172.35 \text{ m} \cdot \text{min}^{-1} \div 26.8 \,([\text{m} \cdot \text{min}^{-1}]$$

$$\cdot [\text{mi} \cdot \text{hr}^{-1}]^{-1})$$

$$= 6.43 \text{ mi} \cdot \text{hr}^{-1}$$

8. The value obtained in step 7 is the actual treadmill speed in miles per hour. If the speed indicator does not agree with this value, adjust the dial to the proper reading. Check your instruction manual for the location of the speed adjustment.
9. Repeat for a number of different speeds to assure accuracy across the speeds used in test protocols.

Elevation Calibration

Treadmill manuals describe how to calibrate the grade using a simple carpenter's level and a square edge. This calibration procedure consists of three steps.

1. Use a carpenter's level to make sure that the treadmill is level, and check the zero setting on the grade meter under these conditions (with the treadmill electronics turned on). If the meter does not read zero, follow instructions to make the adjustment (usually by using the small screw on the face of the dial).
2. Elevate the treadmill so that the percent-grade dial reads approximately 20%. Measure the exact incline of the treadmill as shown in Figure 5.5. When the level's bubble is exactly in the center of the tube, the rise measurement is obtained.
3. Calculate the grade as the rise over the "run" (tangent θ), and adjust the treadmill meter to read that exact grade. For example, if the rise were 4.5 in. to the run's 22.5 in., the fractional grade would be

$$\text{Grade} = \text{tangent } \theta$$

$$= \text{rise} \div \text{run}$$

$$= 4.5 \text{ in.} \div 22.5 \text{ in.}$$

$$= 0.20$$

$$= 20\%$$

This rise-over-run method is a typical engineering method for calculating grade, giving the tangent of the angle (the opposite side divided by the horizontal distance, as shown in Figure 5.5). Although the sine of the angle (opposite side divided by the hypotenuse) provides the most accurate setting of grade, Table 5.1 shows that the tangent value is a good approximation of the sine value for grades less than 20%, or 12°. However, the rise-over-run method can also be used for calibrating steep grades. One would obtain the tangent

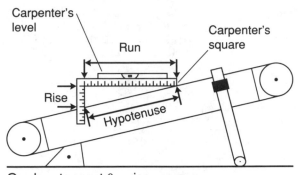

Grade = tangent θ = rise ÷ run
Grade = sine θ = rise ÷ hypotenuse

Figure 5.5 Calibration of grade by tangent method (rise ÷ run) with carpenter's square and level. *Note.* From "The Exercise Testing Laboratory" by E.T. Howley. In *Resource Manual for Guidelines for Exercise Testing and Prescription* (p. 409) by S.N. Blair, P. Painter, R.R. Pate, L.K. Smith, and C.B. Taylor (Eds.), 1988, Philadelphia: Lea & Febiger. Copyright 1988 by Lea & Febiger. Reprinted by permission.

value as described above and simply look across Table 5.1 to obtain the correct sine value to set on the treadmill dial. For example, if the rise-over-run method yielded 0.268, or 26.8% (tangent), the "correct" set-

Table 5.1   Table of Natural Sines and Tangents

Degrees	Sine	% Grade	Tangent	% Grade
0	0.0000	0.0	0.0000	0.0
1	0.0175	1.7	0.0175	1.7
2	0.0349	3.5	0.0349	3.5
3	0.0523	5.2	0.0524	5.2
4	0.0698	7.0	0.0699	7.0
5	0.0872	8.7	0.0875	8.7
6	0.1045	10.4	0.1051	10.5
7	0.1219	12.2	0.1228	12.3
8	0.1392	13.9	0.1405	14.0
9	0.1564	15.6	0.1584	15.8
10	0.1736	17.4	0.1763	17.6
11	0.1908	19.1	0.1944	19.4
12	0.2079	20.8	0.2126	21.3
13	0.2250	22.5	0.2309	23.1
14	0.2419	24.2	0.2493	24.9
15	0.2588	25.9	0.2679	26.8
20	0.3420	34.2	0.3640	36.4
25	0.4067	40.7	0.4452	44.5

Note. From "The Exercise Testing Laboratory" by E.T. Howley. In *Resource Manual for Guidelines for Exercise Testing and Prescription* (p. 410) by S.N. Blair, P. Painter, R.R. Pate, L.K. Smith, and C.B. Taylor (Eds.), 1988, Philadelphia: Lea & Febiger. Copyright 1988 by Lea & Febiger. Reprinted by Permission.

ting would be 25.9% (sine). The latter value is set on the grade dial of the treadmill.

Cycle Ergometer

The cycle ergometer must be calibrated on a routine basis to assure that the work rate is accurate. The work rate on the cycle ergometer is varied by altering either the pedal rate or the load on the wheel. Work is equal to force times the distance through which the force acts: $W = F \times d$. The kilopond (kp) is a common unit used to express force, *not* the kilogram, which is a unit of mass. The kilopond is defined as the force acting on a mass of 1 kg at the normal acceleration of gravity.

On a mechanically braked cycle ergometer, the force (kp) is moved through a distance (meters), so work is expressed in kpm. Because work is accomplished over some period of time (minutes), the activity is referred to as a *work rate* or *power output* (kpm•min^{-1}), not a workload. On the Monark cycle ergometer, a point on the rim of the wheel travels 6 m per pedal revolution, so at 50 rev•min^{-1} the wheel travels 300 m•min^{-1} [i.e., (6 m•rev^{-1}) • (50 rev•min^{-1}) = 300 m•min^{-1}]. If a force of 1 kp were hanging from that wheel, the work rate, or power output, would be 300 kpm•min^{-1} [i.e., 1 kp •(300 m•min^{-1}) = 300 kpm•min^{-1}]. From these simple calculations you can see the importance of maintaining a correct pedal rate during the test—if the subject were pedaling at 60 rev•min^{-1}, the work rate would actually be 20% higher (360 vs. 300 kpm•min^{-1}) than it appears to be. The force setting (resistance on the wheel) must also be carefully set and checked, because it tends to drift as the test progresses. However, it is crucial that the force (resistance) values on the scale be correct. The following six steps outline the procedures for calibrating the Monark cycle ergometer scale (3).

1. Using a carpenter's level, adjust a table to ensure that it is *level*, and put the ergometer on it.
2. Disconnect the "belt" at the spring.
3. Adjust the set screw on the front of the bike against which the force scale rests so that the vertical mark on the pendulum weight is matched with "0" KP on the weight scale. The pendulum must be free-swinging. Lock the adjustment screw.
4. Suspend a 0.5-kg weight from the spring so that no contact is made with the flywheel, and see if the pendulum moves to the 0.5-kp mark. If it doesn't, place tape over the scale, and make a mark in line with the pendulum.
5. Systematically add weight (0.5 kg at a time) to the spring. The pendulum mark should match the

weight-scale mark for each weight. If the marks do not match, put tape over the marks and numbers on the weight scale, and label the taped scale appropriately. Note: Be sure to calibrate the ergometer through the range of values to be used in your tests.
6. Reassemble the cycle ergometer.

Sphygmomanometer

A sphygmomanometer is a blood-pressure measurement system composed of an inflatable rubber bladder, an instrument to indicate the applied pressure, an inflation bulb to create pressure, and an adjustable valve to deflate the system. The cuff and the measuring instrument are the most crucial in terms of measurement accuracy. The width of the cuff should be about 20% wider than the diameter of the limb to which it is applied, and when inflated, the bladder should not cause a bulging or displacement. If the bladder is too wide,

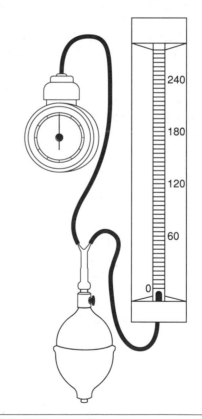

Figure 5.6 Calibration of aneroid manometer with mercury manometer. *Note.* Reproduced with permission. "Recommendations for Human Blood Pressure Determination by Sphygmomanometers," 1987. Copyright American Heart Association. Article by E.D. Frohlich, C. Grim, D.R. Labarthe, M.H. Maxwell, D. Perloff, and W.H. Weidman. *Circulation*, **77**, pp. 501A-514A.

blood pressure will be underestimated; if too narrow, pressure will be overestimated. Consequently, bladder size (length × width) varies with the type of cuff: child (21.5 × 10 cm), adult (24 × 12.5 cm), and large adult (33 or 42 × 15 cm).

The pressure-measuring device, the manometer, can be a mercury or an aneroid type. The mercury type is the standard, and its calibration is easily maintained. The mercury column should rise and fall smoothly, form a clear meniscus, and read zero when the bladder is deflated. If the mercury sticks in the tube, remove the cap and swab out the inside. If it is very dirty, the tube should be removed and cleaned (with detergent, a water rinse, and alcohol for drying). If the mercury column falls below zero, add mercury to bring the meniscus exactly to the zero mark (4, 7, 8).

The aneroid gauge uses a metal bellows assembly that expands when pressure is applied, and the expansion moves the pointer on the indicator dial. A spring attached to the pointer moves the pointer downscale to zero when the bladder is deflated. This gauge should be calibrated at least once every 6 months at a variety of settings, using the mercury column just described. A simple Y tube is used to connect the two systems together (see Figure 5.6). Readings should be taken with pressure falling to simulate the readings during an actual measurement (8).

KEY POINT.   Testing equipment should be carefully selected and calibrated.

SUMMARY

Validity of fitness tests includes ensuring consistency in tests and testers and checking content, criterion, and construct validity. The accuracy of testing can be enhanced by paying attention to the details of preparation of the subject and organization of the testing situation. Interpretation of test scores should emphasize criterion health status, improvement, and specific feedback based on the results and the individual's nature. The fitness behaviors should be emphasized in helping indi-

viduals enhance their positive health. Fitness-test evaluation can help the individual assess his or her health status by comparing current test results with desired health standards. Fitness programs can benefit from analysis of test results in terms of needed revisions and public relations. The calibration of equipment is an important part of obtaining accurate results. Details of calibration for the treadmill, cycle ergometer, and blood pressure equipment are included.

REFERENCES

1. American Alliance for Health, Physical Education, Recreation and Dance (1984)
2. American Alliance for Health, Physical Education, Recreation and Dance (1988)
3. Åstrand (n.d.)
4. Baum (1961)
5. Franks (1989)
6. Franks and Howley (1989)
7. Frohlich et al. (1987)
8. Howley (1988)
9. Kirkendall, Feinleib, Freis, and Mark (1980)
10. Londeree and Moeschberger (1982)
11. Quinton Instruments Instruction Manual (1970)

SUGGESTED READINGS

American College of Sports Medicine (1991)
Åstrand and Rodahl (1970)
Baumgartner and Jackson (1987)
Blair et al. (1989)
Franks and Deutsch (1973)
Hanson (1988)
Paffenbarger, Hyde, and Wing (1990)
Safrit (1986)
Thompson (1988)

See the Bibliography at the end of the book for a complete source listing.

Part III

Physical Fitness

Chapter 6

Nutrition

Wendy J. Bubb

OBJECTIVES

The reader will be able to:
- List six essential nutrients and describe the roles of each
- Identify the functions of fat and water-soluble vitamins and discuss the potential risk of toxicity with oversupplementation
- Compare the macrominerals and microminerals
- List the common dietary sources of calcium and iron, and indicate the populations at risk for, and the potential consequences to health of, inadequate intake
- Discuss guidelines for caloric intake for an individual desiring to lose or gain weight
- List the Basic Four Food Groups and indicate the suggested number of daily servings and foods for each
- Discuss the inappropriate use of diet pills, protein powder, liquid protein diets, and other nutritional supplements
- Describe the contraindications to very low-calorie diets and the proper role of medical supervision in caloric-restriction programs of various levels
- Demonstrate familiarity with the dietary guidelines recommended by the U.S. Department of Health and Human Services relative to carbohydrate, saturated and unsaturated fat, protein, cholesterol, and salt
- Compare and contrast the Recommended Dietary Allowances (RDAs) and the U.S. Recommended Daily Allowances (U.S. RDAs)
- Describe various methods used to assess dietary habits
- Describe the effects of diet and exercise on the lipoprotein profile
- Explain the concept of energy balance as it relates to weight control
- Describe the myths and consequences associated with inappropriate weight-loss methods such as saunas, vibrating belts, body wraps, and sweat suits
- Describe appropriate weekly weight-loss goals
- Demonstrate familiarity with the exchange lists of the American Dietetic Association, the dietary recommendations of the American Heart Association, and the ACSM position on proper and improper weight-loss programs

TERMS

The reader will be able to define or describe:

Amino acids
Basic Four Food Groups
Dietary exchange lists
Fat-soluble vitamin
Fiber
High-density lipoprotein (HDL)

Iron-deficiency anemia
Low-density lipoprotein (LDL)
Macromineral
Micromineral
Monosaccharide
Nutrient density

Osteoporosis
Polysaccharide
Recommended Dietary Allowances (RDAs)
Saturated fat
Unsaturated fat

U.S. Recommended Daily Allowances
(U.S. RDAs)
Very low-density lipoprotein (VLDL)
Water-soluble vitamin

Clear evidence shows that diet and nutrition are of considerable importance to positive health. Daily dietary habits can influence the risk of developing heart disease, stroke, high blood pressure, and one of America's leading health problems, obesity, which is linked to an increase in the incidence of diabetes (3).

A healthy diet depends not on any single nutrient or group of nutrients; rather, the overall structure of the diet is important. Individual foods are not nutritionally complete. A basic nutritional principle is to consume a wide variety of foods containing complementary patterns of nutrients. This is the premise behind structuring the diet according to the Basic Four Food Groups discussed in a later section. Foods are placed in a particular group because the foods in that group tend to contain the same nutrients. Thus, by choosing foods from all four of the basic groups, the nutritional needs of the body are easily met.

BASIC FOODS AND FUNCTIONS

More than 50 known nutrients are needed by the body. The nutrients are divided into carbohydrates, fats, proteins, vitamins, minerals, and water. This section discusses each of these basic nutrients, including their functions and food sources. Where appropriate, their roles as energy sources during exercise are addressed.

Carbohydrates

Carbohydrates are commonly referred to as sugars or starches. Sugars are **monosaccharides** such as glucose, galactose, and fructose. Vegetables, fruits, grains, and refined sugars are sources of glucose. Fruits and sugars also provide fructose. Galactose is primarily supplied by milk products. Three or more molecules of monosaccharides form a **polysaccharide**, or starch. Vegetable foods such as potatoes, beans, corn, and peas contain polysaccharides, as do various grains used in breads, cereals, pastries, and spaghetti. The recommendation for the current U.S. diet is to increase carbohydrate consumption to 55% to 60% of the total caloric intake, while deriving less from refined sugar and more

from complex carbohydrates including vegetables, fruits, cereals, and breads.

Carbohydrates are a primary source for the production of ATP. This includes blood glucose, which is used by all tissues in the body and is the exclusive energy source for the central nervous system. In addition, liver and muscle tissues store excess carbohydrates in the form of many glucose molecules linked together to form large glycogen molecules. One g of carbohydrate provides 4 kcal of energy.

Dietary **fiber** is a type of complex carbohydrate that cannot be digested by the body. It passes through the digestive tract, providing bulk and aiding in elimination of the stool. Although the recommended daily fiber intake is 25 to 50 g, the average American consumes only 10 to 20 g per day. Fiber can be classified into two categories. Water-insoluble fiber acts primarily in the large intestine to absorb water and produce soft stools that move through the digestive system more quickly. Examples are cellulose, hemicellulose, and lignin. Dietary sources of insoluble fiber are whole-grain products, especially bran. Water-soluble fiber is contained in pectin or gum. Dietary sources are citrus fruits and apples.

Dietary fiber has been linked to the prevention of certain diseases. Water-insoluble fiber may play a role in preventing irritable-bowel syndrome, a condition affecting the lining of the intestines, and diverticular disease, or outpouchings in weak areas of the large intestine. A diet high in water-soluble fiber may protect against colon cancer and elevated cholesterol levels. Adequate fiber intake in the diet can be assured by eating more fruits and vegetables, especially raw, more whole-grain products, and fewer processed foods (9).

KEY POINT. Complex carbohydrates are good sources of dietary fiber, which has been linked to the prevention of certain diseases.

Fats

Fats found in the body are classified as simple fats, compound fats, and derived fats. These are also referred to, respectively, as triglycerides, phospholipids, and cholesterol. Triglycerides, consisting of a glycerol and three fatty-acid molecules, represent more than 90% of the fat stored in the body. Fatty acids differ in the number of carbon atoms they contain and the degree of saturation of the carbon atoms in the fatty-acid chain with hydrogen. Free fatty acids are saturated when the carbon atoms are saturated with hydrogen atoms, and unsaturated when the carbon atoms are not saturated with hydrogen atoms. Fats with large amounts of **saturated fats** are solid at room temperature and come primarily from animal sources. Beef, pork, lamb, shellfish, and many dairy products contain high levels of saturated fats. Vegetable sources of saturated fat include palm oil, coconut oil, and cocoa butter. **Unsaturated fats**, which are liquid at room temperature, are vegetable oils such as canola, corn, cottonseed, peanut, and soybean oils. Recommendations for dietary fat include a reduction in the number of calories from fat to no more than 30%, with 10% or fewer calories coming from saturated fat. The compound fats, particularly lipoproteins, and derived fats such as cholesterol are discussed in the section dealing with diet, exercise, and lipids.

Because they are stored in large quantities in adipose tissue and muscle tissue throughout the body, triglycerides represent a large potential energy store. In addition, they are a concentrated source of energy; 1 g of fat contains 9 kcal, more than twice the energy provided by carbohydrates and proteins. Besides their energy-supplying functions, fats protect vital organs against trauma and insulate during cold exposure. Dietary fats also transport the fat-soluble vitamins A, D, E, and K throughout the body.

KEY POINT.   Saturated and unsaturated dietary fats provide the same amount of energy.

Proteins

Protein is constructed from separate subunits, called **amino acids**, arranged in various chemical and physical configurations. Of the 22 different amino acids required by the body, 8 are considered indispensable, or essential, because of the body's inability to synthesize them—they must be provided in the daily dietary intake. Dietary proteins vary in amino acid composition and in their provision of the indispensable amino acids for protein synthesis. Animal proteins such as meat, fish, poultry, milk, and eggs are high-quality proteins because they contain all 8 indispensable amino acids. Because they lack certain amino acids, plant sources are lower in quality. The protein requirement can be met

on a vegetarian diet, but combinations of foods must be carefully planned, because indispensable amino acids must be consumed together to be synthesized together into proteins.

The daily protein requirement is 0.8 to 0.9 g of protein per kilogram of body weight. For children, this value increases to approximately 3 g per kilogram of body weight. Contrary to popular belief, protein is the least important nutrient as an energy source at rest or during exercise. Its key value is to furnish the chemical building blocks for bodily structures. Under resting conditions, protein metabolism equals 3.1 g$\cdot$hr^{-1} and supplies approximately 17% of the body's energy needs. During exercise, the rate of protein metabolism remains at 3.1 g$\cdot$hr^{-1}. Because the metabolic rate is elevated by a factor of 10 or more above the resting level during exercise, protein constitutes less than 2% of the energy for muscular work. Thus carbohydrates and fats are the primary fuels of concern during exercise. One g of protein contains 4.0 kcal of energy (see Powers and Howley).

KEY POINT.   The daily protein requirement is 0.8 to 0.9 g per kilogram of body weight.

Research has demonstrated that protein requirements do not increase with activity, either for energy needs or for increased muscle mass. Like excess calories from any nutrient, additional protein calories are converted to and stored as fat, primarily in adipose tissue. A commonly held myth is that athletes involved in strength programs and growing athletes have special requirements for supplemental protein. The excess calories typically consumed by these individuals should meet any additional protein needs. An intake of 1 g of protein per kilogram of body weight provides a sufficient margin of safety for any increase in body mass that occurs in adult athletes (2).

KEY POINT.

   1 g carbohydrate → 4 kcal
   1 g fat → 9 kcal
   1 g protein → 4.0 kcal

Vitamins

Vitamins as a group of nutrients have attracted considerable attention. The importance of these organic substances has long been known. Contrary to popular opinion, however, they provide no calories and therefore cannot increase a person's level of energy. Because the body generally cannot manufacture vitamins, they are required in the diet though in very small amounts (i.e., milligram or microgram quantities).

The 14 known vitamins are classified as water soluble or fat soluble. Daily intake of the four **fat-soluble vitamins**, A, D, E, and K, is not essential, because they can be stored in the fat tissues of the body. The **water-soluble vitamins** include eight B-complex vitamins and vitamin C. Because excess water-soluble vitamins are not stored in the body, adequate daily consumption is essential. Excess water-soluble vitamins are eventually eliminated via urine or sweat.

Some people have only marginal nutrient intake, and vitamin supplementation is justified for them. Likewise, vitamins are correctly prescribed for pregnant women and infants. Although in the normal population a daily multivitamin is no reason for alarm, such supplementation is not a suitable remedy for poor dietary habits. The potentially dangerous megadosing of vitamins is strongly discouraged. Taking too many vitamins may pose serious health hazards and is economically unjustified. Because the body can store fat-soluble vitamins, megadoses of these can lead to conditions of hypervitaminosis with potential severe consequences, including liver and kidney damage. Studies have also indicated that excess water-soluble vitamins, once thought to be safe, also pose dangers when ingested in large amounts (2).

Vitamins have various functions; most are involved in regulating the metabolic reactions whereby energy is released from carbohydrates, fats, and proteins. Generally they serve as coenzymes by assisting enzymes in carrying out their functions. Table 6.1 summarizes the primary functions and dietary sources, and gives the requirements, for each of the vitamins.

Table 6.1 Vitamins and Their Functions

Vitamin	Function	Sources	Daily adult requirement[a]	
			Men	Women
Thiamin (B-1)	Functions as part of a coenzyme to aid utilization of energy	Whole grains, nuts, lean pork	1.5 mg[b]	1.1 mg
Riboflavin (B-2)	Involved in energy metabolism as part of a coenzyme	Milk, yogurt, cheese	1.7 mg	1.3 mg
Niacin	Facilitates energy production in cells	Lean meat, fish, poultry, grains	19.0 mg	15.0 mg
Vitamin B-6	Absorbs and metabolizes protein; aids in red blood cell formation	Lean meat, vegetables, whole grains	2.0 mg	1.6 mg
Pantothenic acid	Aids in metabolism of carbohydrate, fat, and protein	Whole-grain cereals, bread, dark green vegetables	4-7 mg	4-7 mg
Folic acid	Functions as coenzyme in synthesis of nucleic acids and protein	Green vegetables, beans, whole-wheat products	200 µg	180 µg
Vitamin B-12	Involved in synthesis of nucleic acids, red blood cell formation	Only in animal foods, not plant foods	2 µg	2 µg
Biotin	Coenzyme in synthesis of fatty acids and glycogen formation	Egg yolk, dark green vegetables	30-100 µg	30-100 µg
C	Intracellular maintenance of bone, capillaries, and teeth	Citrus fruits, green peppers, tomatoes	60 mg	60 mg
A	Functions in visual processes; formation and maintenance of skin and mucous membranes	Carrots, sweet potatoes, margarine, butter, liver	1,000 µg	800 µg[c]
D	Aids in growth and formation of bones and teeth; promotes calcium absorption	Eggs, tuna, liver, fortified milk	5 µg	5 µg
E	Protects polyunsaturated fats; prevents cell membrane damage	Vegetable oils, whole-grain cereal and bread, green leafy vegetables	10 mg	8 mg
K	Important in blood clotting	Green leafy vegetables, peas, potatoes	80 µg	65 µg

Note. From Franks and Howley (1989).

[a]Values are for adults 25 to 50 years of age. The requirements vary for children and pregnant or lactating women. See Appendix C.

[b]mg = milligram, µg = microgram, IU = international unit.

[c]µg vitamin A requirements are expressed in microgram of Retinol equivalents.

KEY POINT. Vitamins are classified as fat soluble (A, D, E, and K) or water soluble (C and B-complex).

Minerals

Minerals are inorganic compounds that are found in miniscule quantities in the body and that carry out a wide range of functions. Major minerals, or **macrominerals**, include calcium, potassium, magnesium, sulfur, sodium, and chloride. Iron, iodine, copper, zinc, fluorine, selenium, manganese, molybdenum, and chromium compose the trace minerals, or **microminerals**. The key functions of minerals are as enzyme components in cellular metabolism. Table 6.2 lists the functions, sources, and daily requirements for minerals.

The daily requirement of essential minerals can usu-

ally be met through the foods a person eats; supplementation is generally not necessary. Exceptions to this may include calcium among the macrominerals and iron and zinc from the microminerals. Inadequate iron in the diet may lead to **iron-deficiency anemia**, the most common nutritional deficiency in the U.S. American women of childbearing age, infants, young children, and adolescents are most likely to suffer. It has also been observed in athletes, especially long-distance runners, in a condition called sports anemia. The requirements for iron for adult men and women are 10 $mg \cdot day^{-1}$ and 15 $mg \cdot day^{-1}$, respectively (5). Although the actual requirements are only about 1/10 this amount, dietary iron is poorly absorbed by the body. Therefore, dietary intake must exceed the actual need. The average American woman consumes only 10 to 12 mg of iron per day. Its absorption is tripled if iron is consumed with vitamin C. Good dietary sources of iron include beans, peas,

Table 6.2 Minerals and Their Functions

Mineral	Function	Sources	Daily adult requirement[a] Men	Women
		MAJOR MINERALS		
Calcium	Bones, teeth, blood clotting, nerve and muscle function	Milk, sardines, dark green vegetables, nuts	800 mg	800 mg
Chloride	Nerve and muscle function, water balance (with sodium)	Table salt	750 mg	750 mg[b]
Magnesium	Bone growth; nerve, muscle, and enzyme function	Nuts, seafood, whole grains, leafy green vegetables	350 mg	280 mg
Phosphorus	Bone, teeth, energy transfer	Meats, poultry, seafood, eggs, milk, beans	800 mg	800 mg
Potassium	Nerve and muscle function	Fresh vegetables, bananas, citrus fruits, milk, meats, fish	2000 mg	2000 mg[b]
Sodium	Nerve and muscle function, water balance	Table salt	500 mg	500 mg[b]
		TRACE MINERALS		
Chromium	Glucose metabolism	Meats, liver, whole grains, dried beans	.05-.2 mg	.05-.2 mg
Copper	Enzyme function, energy production	Meats, seafood, nuts, grains	1.5-3 mg	1.5-3 mg
Fluoride	Bone and teeth growth	Drinking water, fish, milk	1.5-4 mg	1.5-4 mg
Iodine	Thyroid hormone formation	Iodized salt, seafood	150 µg	150 µg
Iron	O_2 transport in red blood cells; enzyme function	Red met, liver, eggs, beans, leafy vegetables, shell fish	10 mg	15 mg
Manganese	Enzyme function	Whole grains, nuts, fruits, vegetables	2.5-5 mg	2.5-5 mg
Molybdenum	Energy metabolism in cells	Whole grains, organ meats, peas, beans	.075-.25 mg	.075-.25 mg
Selenium	Works with vitamin E	Meat, fish, whole grains, eggs	70 µg	55 µg
Zinc	Part of enzymes, growth	Meat, shellfish, yeast, whole grains	15 mg	12 mg

Note. From Franks and Howley (1989). Adapted from Christian and Greger (1985) and Williams (1988).

[a]Values are for adults 25 to 50 years of age. Requirements vary for children and pregnant or lactating women. See Appendix C.

[b]Minimum requirements for healthy persons. See Appendix C.

green leafy vegetables, whole grains, and organ meats such as heart, liver, and kidney.

Calcium is important for the growth and maintenance of the teeth and bones. With insufficient calcium in the diet, calcium will be drawn from the bones to meet the needs of the body. Over a period of time, the bones will become more porous, and bone mass will be decreased, a condition known as **osteoporosis**. The RDA for calcium is 1,200 mg through age 24, and 800 mg thereafter, but approximately half of American women consume less than 500 mg each day, with 25% consuming less than 300 mg each day. If there is inadequate calcium in the diet, calcium supplementation is generally recommended to prevent osteoporosis.

KEY POINT. Two minerals commonly deficient in women are iron and calcium, leading to iron-deficiency anemia and osteoporosis, respectively.

Water

Although it contains no calories and does not contribute any nutrients to the diet, water is necessary for life. It serves as a transport mechanism for nutrients, gases, and waste products. It is also involved in heat-regulating functions of the body.

DIETARY GOALS AND EVALUATION OF DIETARY INTAKE

Beginning in the 1970s, Americans became increasingly interested in nutrition, partly as a result of scientific research linking America's leading ills to poor nutritional habits. An evaluation by the Senate Select Committee on Nutrition and Human Needs indicated that the typical U.S. diet contains too much fat (particularly saturated fat), too much refined sugar, and too many calories. Most dietary protein comes from animal sources and is rich in fat and cholesterol. Based on this evaluation, the committee made some general recommendations to ease nutrition-related diseases, including heart disease, stroke, and obesity. Accepting the initiative from the Senate committee, other agencies such as the U.S. Departments of Agriculture and Health, Education, and Welfare have made similar recommendations. Figure 6.1 presents the recommended goals. See also the Recommended Dietary Goals and Recommended Dietary Changes lists.

These guidelines are clearly shaping America's nutritional behavior. Recent data gathered by the National

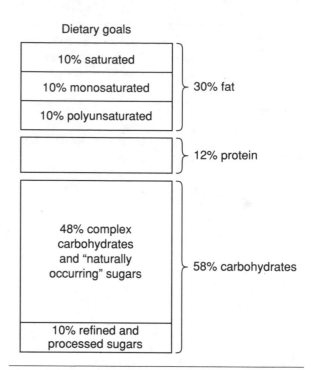

Figure 6.1 Dietary goals for the United States. (Percentages represent portions of total caloric intake.) From Senate Select Committee on Nutrition and Human Needs. Used with permission.

Institutes of Health, and the Agricultural Research Services of the United States Department of Agriculture, indicate that some progress has been made in attaining the goals since they were first set in 1977. Data from 1985 indicated that fat constitutes 35% of the typical U.S. diet, and that 13% of that fat is saturated. These figures are down from 42% and 16%, respectively, in 1977. There has been a corresponding increase in the consumption of complex carbohydrates during this same time period. Remember that what is important is the overall structure of the diet, rather than an underemphasis or overemphasis on certain food items. This means that variety in selection should be emphasized as the easiest and most realistic way to achieve the dietary recommendations. Likewise, a gradual change in a person's eating habits is preferred over immediate drastic changes that may lead to resentment and poor adherence.

KEY POINT. The typical American diet is characterized by too much saturated fat, too much refined sugar, and too many calories.

Recommended Dietary Allowances

The **Recommended Dietary Allowances**, or **RDAs** (Appendix C), established by the National Research

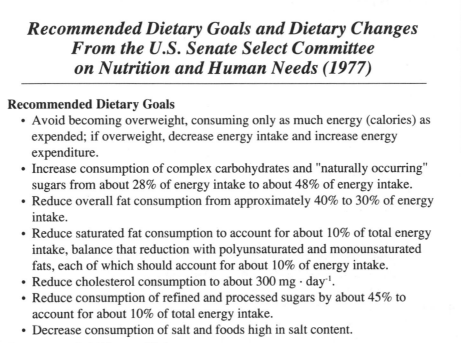

Recommended Dietary Goals and Dietary Changes From the U.S. Senate Select Committee on Nutrition and Human Needs (1977)

Recommended Dietary Goals
- Avoid becoming overweight, consuming only as much energy (calories) as expended; if overweight, decrease energy intake and increase energy expenditure.
- Increase consumption of complex carbohydrates and "naturally occurring" sugars from about 28% of energy intake to about 48% of energy intake.
- Reduce overall fat consumption from approximately 40% to 30% of energy intake.
- Reduce saturated fat consumption to account for about 10% of total energy intake, balance that reduction with polyunsaturated and monounsaturated fats, each of which should account for about 10% of energy intake.
- Reduce cholesterol consumption to about 300 mg · day^{-1}.
- Reduce consumption of refined and processed sugars by about 45% to account for about 10% of total energy intake.
- Decrease consumption of salt and foods high in salt content.

Recommended Dietary Changes
- Increase consumption of fruits, vegetables, and whole grains.
- Decrease consumption of animal fat, and substitute poultry and fish, which decrease saturated fat.
- Decrease consumption of foods high in total fat, and particularly replace saturated with polyunsaturated fat.
- Except for young children, substitute lowfat and nonfat milk for whole milk, and substitute lowfat dairy products for high-fat products.
- Decrease consumption of butterfat, eggs, and other high-cholesterol sources.
- Decrease consumption of refined and other processed sugars and foods high in such sugars.
- Decrease consumption of salt and foods high in salt content.

Council of the National Academy of Sciences, are the levels of intake of essential nutrients considered to be adequate to meet the needs of almost all healthy people. The RDAs are to be applied to population groups and should not be confused with requirements for a specific individual. They are designed to meet the needs of 98% of the population. They represent acceptable nutrient intake for nearly all healthy people and are generous levels for most people. The RDAs are established by estimating average population requirements and variability for each nutrient. This number is then increased to meet the needs of 90% of the population, followed by an additional increase in the allowance to counter inefficient nutrient utilization such as poor absorption or inadequate conversion of a precursor to an active form. Therefore, to meet the needs of those individuals with the highest requirements, the RDAs exceed what

most people require. For ease of application, the RDAs are recommended as daily allowances. There is no cause for alarm, though, if a person's diet is below one day and above the next day, because mechanisms exist to compensate for previous deficiencies. Averaging intakes over a period of several days to a week is acceptable.

In addition to those nutrients for which the RDA has been established, some nutrients are listed as estimated safe and adequate daily dietary intakes. The levels for these nutrients, which are listed in Appendix C, are based on less complete data than the RDA and are presented as ranges. They serve as useful guides and represent the best available knowledge.

Of the approximately 50 known nutrients, the RDAs have been determined for some, and estimated safe and adequate intake ranges have been identified for others.

Some nutrients, however, are known to be required but have no established allowances. It is therefore assumed that attempts to achieve the recommended dietary allowances are based on a wide variety of food selections. A varied diet that meets the requirements of known nutrients also likely satisfies the requirements of those nutrients for which no allowance has been established.

U.S. Recommended Daily Allowances

The **U.S. Recommended Daily Allowances (U.S. RDAs)** were developed by the Food and Drug Administration to be used for nutritional labeling. The 26 age and gender categories of the RDA have been condensed into four groups: infants, children under 4 years of age, males and females over 4 years old, and pregnant and lactating women. For several reasons, the U.S. RDAs on food labels exceed the requirements of most people. In addition to the added amounts included in the RDAs, the U.S. RDAs for males and females over 4 years of age are based on the highest RDAs (i.e., those for teenage boys).

The nutritional guidelines discussed are designed to serve as useful guides in food selection. Nevertheless, meal planning should not become a mathematical frustration. A variety of enjoyable foods is the most important factor in meal planning, because unappealing foods that are not eaten have no nutritional value. Several methods are available to aid the nutritionally conscious person in meeting the suggested dietary standards. Perhaps the best known of these is the **Basic Four Food Groups**, which is a convenient grouping of foods based on similar nutrient content. Foods are placed into one of four groups:

1. **Meat, fish, and poultry**
2. **Milk and milk products**
3. **Bread and cereal**
4. **Fruits and vegetables**

Examples of foods in each category are given in One Serving Equivalents in the Four Food Groups Plan.

Adequate nutrition is based on combining specified numbers of servings of foods chosen from each group to receive all of the required nutrients (Table 6.3). Even diets that meet the requirements of the Basic Four Food Groups are frequently deficient in vitamins E and B-6, magnesium, zinc, and iron. The following modifications of the Basic Four are recommended to compensate for these common deficiencies.

- The meat group should be met using low-fat meats and protein from vegetable sources.
- Foods high in saturated fat, salt, and refined sugar should be strongly discouraged.

Table 6.3   The Basic Four Food Groups Plan

| Food group | Daily servings | | | Main nutrients |
	Child	Teen	Adult	
Milk	3	4	2	Vitamin D Calcium Riboflavin Protein
Meat	2	2	2	Protein Calcium Iron Thiamin Riboflavin
Fruits and vegetables	4	4	4	Vitamin A Vitamin C Carbohydrate
Bread and cereal	4	4	4	Carbohydrate Thiamin Iron Niacin

- Cooking methods should limit excess fat, salt, and sugar.
- People should be encouraged to meet the daily requirement by using foods containing less than 2% fat.
- Selections from the bread and cereal group should include whole-grain products.
- Selections from the fruits and vegetables group should include daily servings of a dark-green vegetable and a source rich in vitamin C (6).

Dietary Exchange Lists

Dietary exchange lists are another popular dietary management system. Although they were first developed for diabetics, their use has been extended, through the combined efforts of the American Diabetes Association and the American Dietetic Association, to others who require a more structured dietary regimen, particularly for weight management. The exchange lists consist of six groups of foods that have been classed together because of similar caloric content and similar percentages of carbohydrate, fat, and protein. Therefore, foods within a group may be exchanged for any other food in the same group. Table 6.4 shows the six exchange groups. Appendix D lists the foods that constitute an exchange for each of the groups. The dietary exchange lists are particularly useful for weight control programs, because total daily caloric intake can be determined by the number of exchanges within each

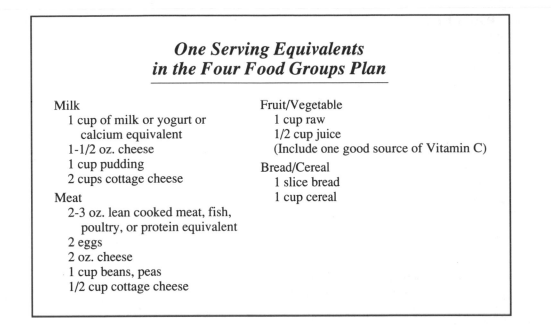

One Serving Equivalents in the Four Food Groups Plan

Milk
    1 cup of milk or yogurt or
       calcium equivalent
    1-1/2 oz. cheese
    1 cup pudding
    2 cups cottage cheese

Meat
    2-3 oz. lean cooked meat, fish,
      poultry, or protein equivalent
    2 eggs
    2 oz. cheese
    1 cup beans, peas
    1/2 cup cottage cheese

Fruit/Vegetable
    1 cup raw
    1/2 cup juice
    (Include one good source of Vitamin C)

Bread/Cereal
    1 slice bread
    1 cup cereal

group. The exchange groups also allow selection of foods based on personal preference, while still assuring adequate nutrient content. See the 1,800-Calorie Diet Utilizing the Food-Exchange System.

Another new concept in nutrition education is **nutrient density**. The nutrient density of a food measures the amount of proteins, carbohydrates, fats, vitamins, and minerals per 100 kcal of the food. Low-nutrient-density foods, foods rich in calories containing a low level of essential nutrients, should be discouraged, particularly for people on caloric-restrictive diets. As calories are restricted, the nutrient density of foods should be higher to assure that the person will receive all of the required nutrients. Nutrient Densities of Typical Lunches compares the nutrient density of three different lunch selections.

KEY POINT.   A person's dietary intake may be evaluated based on the Recommended Dietary Allowances, the Basic Four Food Groups, dietary exchange lists, and nutrient density.

Success in changing a person's dietary habits depends on determining what is eaten, how it is prepared, and how much is eaten. A simple dietary history should be taken before making specific recommendations. The Suggested Questions for a Dietary History provide insight into how a person's lifestyle affects his or her dietary choices.

In addition to a diet history, a food record should be completed in which the food eaten throughout the day is recorded. To insure an accurate assessment of dietary habits, individuals must be encouraged to meticulously record everything that is eaten, preferably for 7 consecutive days. If this is not possible, an alternative is to record food intake on 2 weekdays and 1 weekend day. Because many people have significantly different eating patterns on Saturdays and Sundays than on other days of the week, the food record must include sampling from a weekend. It is not uncommon for individuals to become more aware of their food habits while recording dietary intakes, and as a result of this awareness they make changes in food habits. Thus, participants should be instructed to maintain usual eating habits during the recording period, and to provide as much information as possible regarding the nature of the foods, how they were prepared, and how much was eaten. Showing pictures or models of food portions will assist in providing accurate estimates of the amounts of food eaten. Individuals should be instructed to report only the amount eaten or drunk, not the amount served, and to also estimate and record what was sampled or tasted during food preparation. The caloric content of each food is found in available tables, and the total daily caloric intake is determined. Inexpensive calorie-counting guides that list most foods are available; many guides list foods according to commercial brand names.

Studies show that many factors besides food influence eating behavior. Included among these are certain places, life events, and emotions. Recording the time of eating, mood, degree of hunger, associated activity, and place of eating with types and quantities of foods eaten provides additional information that may be valuable in restructuring a person's eating habits. See the Suggested Dietary Recall Form. Chapter 12 deals more specifically with behavioral modification of dietary habits.

Table 6.4   The Dietary Exchange Groups of the American Diabetes Association[a]

Group	Serving size	Similar foods	Carbohydrate (g)	Protein (g)	Fat (g)	Energy (kcal)
Milk (skim)	1 cup	1 cup skim milk 1 cup yogurt from skim milk	12	8	Trace	90
Vegetable	1/2 cup	String beans Greens Carrots Beets	5	2	0	25
Fruit	1 serving	1/2 small banana 1 small apple 1/2 grapefruit 1/2 cup orange juice	15	0	0	60
Bread (starch)	1 slice	3/4 cup ready-to-eat cereal 1/2 cup beans 1/3 cup corn 1 small potato	15	3	Trace	80
Meat (lean)	1 oz	1 oz chicken meat, without skin 1 oz fish 1/4 cup canned tuna, or salmon 1 oz low-fat cheese (< 5% butterfat)	0	7	3	55
Fat	1 tsp	1 tsp margarine 1 tsp oil 1 tbsp salad dressing 1 strip crisp bacon	0	0	5	45

[a]Appendix D is a more complete list of foods in each exchange.

Note. The Exchange Lists are the basis of a meal planning system designed by a committee of the American Diabetes Association and The American Dietetic Association. While designed primarily for people with diabetes and others who must follow special diets, the Exchange Lists are based on principles of good nutrition that apply to everyone. Copyright © 1989 by American Diabetes Association, The American Dietetic Association.

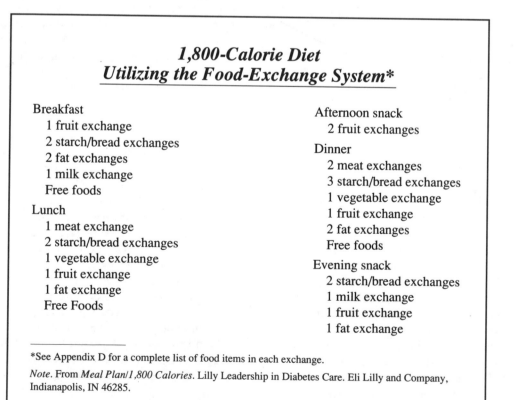

1,800-Calorie Diet
*Utilizing the Food-Exchange System**

Breakfast
  1 fruit exchange
  2 starch/bread exchanges
  2 fat exchanges
  1 milk exchange
  Free foods

Lunch
  1 meat exchange
  2 starch/bread exchanges
  1 vegetable exchange
  1 fruit exchange
  1 fat exchange
  Free Foods

Afternoon snack
  2 fruit exchanges

Dinner
  2 meat exchanges
  3 starch/bread exchanges
  1 vegetable exchange
  1 fruit exchange
  2 fat exchanges
  Free foods

Evening snack
  2 starch/bread exchanges
  1 milk exchange
  1 fruit exchange
  1 fat exchange

*See Appendix D for a complete list of food items in each exchange.

Note. From *Meal Plan/1,800 Calories.* Lilly Leadership in Diabetes Care. Eli Lilly and Company, Indianapolis, IN 46285.

Nutrient Densities of Typical Lunches

Chicken*	Ham/cheese	Cheeseburger

Chicken sandwich:
2 oz. chicken breast
2 slices whole wheat bread
1 Tbsp. mayonnaise
2 slices tomato
Celery & carrot sticks—3 each
Strawberries—1/2 cup fresh strawberries
    1 Tbsp. sugar
Vanilla wafers—two
Skim milk (1 glass)
	Ham & cheese sandwich:
	1 slice boiled ham
	1 slice American cheese
	2 slices rye bread
	1 Tbsp. margarine
	1 tsp. mustard
	Tossed salad:
	1 cup tossed greens (lettuce)
	2 Tbsp. French dressing
	Strawberry sundae:
	1/4 cup fresh strawberries
	1 Tbsp. sugar
	1/2 pint ice cream
	Coffee
		Cheeseburger:
		1 hamburger patty (4 oz.)
		1 slice American cheese
		1 enriched roll
		2 slices tomato
		French-fried potatoes—
		    10 strips
		Coleslaw—1/2 cup
		Apple pie a la mode—
		    1/6 pie
		1/2 cup ice cream
		Cola

	Chicken	Ham/cheese	Cheeseburger
Total Calories	545	870	1480

Nutrients per 100 calories

	Chicken	Ham/cheese	Cheeseburger
Protein (g)	6.3	2.7	3.3
Vitamin A (IU)	430	195	95
Vitamin C (mg)	13.0	3.2	3.4
Thiamine (mg)	0.062	0.328	0.029
Riboflavin (mg)	0.122	0.543	0.049
Niacin (mg)	1.73	0.23	1.37
Calcium (mg)	75	52	27
Iron (mg)	0.60	0.34	0.47
Protein (g)	6.3	2.7	3.3
Fat, total (g)	3.1	6.1	5.1
[including saturated fat]	[0.6]	[2.1]	[1.7]
Carbohydrate (g)	12.3	9.2	10.4

Note. Adapted from "Choosing Foods for Health" by G.A. Leveille and A. Dean, 1979. In D.T. Mason and H. Guthrie (Eds.), *The Medicine Called Nutrition* (p. 25), Englewood Cliffs, NJ: Best Foods. Reprinted by permission of Mazola Nutrition/Health Information Service (Mazola corn oil).

*Note nutrient advantages of this meal with fewer calories.

In addition to total caloric intake, the information gathered from daily food records can be used to assess the general overall nutritional value of a person's diet. The amount of fat, protein, and carbohydrate, and the vitamin and mineral content of each item, can also be determined from the available food lists. The percentage of total calories from fat, protein, and carbohydrate can be calculated; this provides useful information relative to the dietary guidelines for Americans. The Dietary Composition Form provides a means to record this information. The foods eaten each day can also be evaluated on the basis of meeting the recommended number of servings from each of the Basic Four Food Groups. A suggested format for this purpose is shown in the Three-Day Record for the Four Food Groups.

Another useful tool in dietary evaluation and coun-

Suggested Questions for a Dietary History

1. How often do you eat?
2. Do you enjoy eating?
3. Do you eat only when you are hungry, or do you eat according to a time schedule?
4. At what time do you eat meals? Snacks?
5. What foods do you eat most often?
6. What are your favorite snacks?
7. What are some of your least favorite foods?
8. How long does it take you to eat a meal?
9. Would you estimate that you eat more or less than most other people?
10. Do you follow, or have you recently followed, any special diet plan? If so, describe it.
11. Do you take vitamin supplements?
12. Describe your use of fats and oils.
13. Do you add salt to foods during cooking? At the table?
14. What kinds of meat and dairy products do you normally eat?
15. How are most of your foods prepared?
16. How long has your weight been about what it is now?
17. Who usually cooks the food if you eat at home?
18. How often do you eat out? For what meals?

Note. Adapted from "Choosing Foods for Health" by G.A. Leveille and A. Dean, 1979. In D.T. Mason and H. Guthrie (Eds.), *The Medicine Called Nutrition* (p. 25), Englewood Cliffs, NJ: Best Foods. Reprinted by permission of Mazola Nutrition/Health Information Service (Mazola corn oil).

---

seling is a computer-assisted analysis of food intake. A person's daily caloric intake can be evaluated based on the RDAs for essential vitamins, minerals, carbohydrates, fats, and proteins. Total daily cholesterol and sodium intake are also frequently assessed. In addition to the quantitative information supplied, some marketed programs assess the input relative to recommended levels of nutrients for age, gender, and activity level, and offer specific individual recommendations to increase or decrease levels of certain nutrients or calories. With increasing numbers of dietary analysis programs available, identifying and evaluating programs may be time consuming and frustrating. Some software programs are effective, but some may be more a hindrance than a help. Chapter 18 evaluates these computer programs and can be used by HFIs to select software programs that are most appropriate to the intended use and their particular needs.

GUIDELINES FOR WEIGHT CONTROL

Millions of people are involved in weight-reduction programs. In the United States, over $100 million are spent annually on weight reduction. In spite of this, there has been no nationwide decrease in obesity. As many as 90% of all individuals who lose weight regain it within 1 year. With large numbers of men and women reporting that they are trying to lose weight, an obvious need exists for guidelines to properly control weight.

In *Proper and Improper Weight-Loss Programs*, the American College of Sports Medicine (1) made specific recommendations for a desirable weight-loss program. **A desirable weight-loss program is one that**

- **provides a caloric intake not lower than 1,200 kcal·day^{-1} for normal adults, to meet nutritional needs;**
- **includes food acceptable to the dieter based on sociocultural background, usual habits, taste, cost, and ease of acquisition and preparation;**
- **provides a negative caloric balance not to exceed 500 to 1,000 kcal·day^{-1}, to result in maximal weight loss of 2 lb·week^{-1};**
- **includes behavioral-modification techniques to identify and eliminate poor nutritional habits; and**
- **includes an endurance exercise program of at least 3 days·week^{-1}, 20 to 30 min in duration, at a minimum intensity of 60% of maximal heart rate.**

Suggested Dietary Recall Form

	Time	Food	Amount	Calories	Where are you?	Who is with you?	What are you doing?	How do you feel?
Day 1								
Breakfast								
Lunch								
Dinner								
Day 2								
Breakfast								
Lunch								
Dinner								
Day 3								
Breakfast								
Lunch								
Dinner								

Note. Adapted from Nutrition, Weight Control, and Exercise (p. 164) by F.I. Katch and W.D. McArdle, 1977, Boston: Houghton Mifflin Co. And from Slim Chance in a Fat World: Behavioral Control of Obesity by R.B. Stuart and B. Davies, 1971. Champaign, IL: Research Press. Copyright 1977 by Houghton Mifflin Company and copyright 1971 by Research Press. Adapted by permission.

Dietary Composition Form

Food	Amount	Calories	Protein g	Fat g	Saturated fat g	Cholesterol mg	Carbohydrate g	Calcium mg	Iron mg	Sodium mg	Vitamin A IU	Thiamin mg	Riboflavin mg	Niacin mg	Vitamin C mg

Totals

RDA

% RDA

% total calories

Instructions:
1. Multiply the number of fat, protein, and carbohydrate grams by 9 kcal · g^{-1}, 4.0 kcal · g^{-1}, and 4 kcal · g^{-1}, respectively.
2. Divide the number of fat calories by the total daily calories to determine the percentage of your diet composed of fat. Repeat for carbohydrate and protein.
3. Compare to Dietary Goals for the United States.

Three-Day Record for the Four Food Groups

Instructions
1. By referring to your record of food intake, determine for each day the actual number of servings you had in each food group, and record this in the appropriate box below. If you ate no servings in a food group, record a zero.
2. The Vegetables and Fruits Group is divided into three categories. Treat each of these separately. If you ate more than one serving of food high in vitamin A or vitamin C, record just one serving for that vitamin, and count the servings above one in the additional group.
3. Total the number of servings in each food group for the 3 days, and record this in the appropriate box.
4. Divide this by the number given, which represents the recommended minimum servings of that group for 3 days.
5. Multiply the above results by 100 to find the percentage, and record it in the appropriate box.

Food groups	Rec. min. daily servings	1st day	2nd day	3rd day	Total	Divide by	Average daily percentage
1. Meat group	2					6	
2. Vegetable and fruit group	A–1					3	
	C–1					3	
	additional—2					6	
3. Milk group	2					6	
4. Bread and cereal group	4					12	

With these guidelines in mind, a tool similar to the Weight-Loss Diet Evaluation Checklist can be used to evaluate weight-reduction diets.

Many individuals successfully lose weight by decreasing caloric intake and increasing energy expenditure through exercise. Unfortunately, after they have achieved their desired weight-loss goals, most of these individuals regain the weight they had lost. This is because most weight-control programs do not result in permanent lifestyle changes.

Caloric deficits can be created by decreasing food intake, increasing energy expenditure, or preferably combining these two. Two points should be emphasized in counseling individuals for weight control.

1. No single method of weight control can be recommended for all people. The necessity of structuring the program to the individual cannot be overemphasized.
2. One of the most important goals should be to reeducate a person's dietary and exercise habits, resulting in lifestyle patterns that can be continued indefinitely.

Commercial Diets and Fad Diets

The public is bombarded with a barrage of commercial and fad diets, dietetic foods, appetite suppressants, and exercise devices aimed at quick and easy weight loss. Unfortunately, much of this is medically unsound, potentially dangerous, ineffective, and expensive. We cannot discuss every type of fad and crash diet available here, but they tend to have certain characteristics in

---

Weight-Loss Diet Evaluation Checklist

The following checklist can be used to evaluate weight-loss diets. A *no* answer to any of the questions indicates an inadequate weight-reduction plan. Does your weight-reduction plan

	Yes	No
1. Aim for a weight loss of 1-2 lb per week?	☐	☐
2. Provide at least 1,200 kcal per day?	☐	☐
3. Recommend a regular endurance exercise program?	☐	☐
4. Provide a balance of foods from all four food groups?	☐	☐
5. Provide for variety to prevent boredom?	☐	☐
6. Establish eating and exercise habits that can be maintained the rest of your life?	☐	☐
7. Conform to your personal lifestyle?	☐	☐
8. Work without pills, drugs, or other gadgets?	☐	☐

---

common. The person searching for a proper weight-reduction plan can also be alerted to claims and gimmicks that seem to characterize many improper weight-loss programs. The series of claims presented in the Unsafe Claims Checklist can be used to identify ineffective or potentially dangerous weight-loss diets. Following is a brief description of broad types of fad diets, including their proposed mechanisms of action and possible harmful effects. All of these dietary regimens have the disadvantage of not being long-lasting plans. No provision is made for long-term maintenance of weight loss.

High-protein diets require almost exclusive consumption of protein and large amounts of water. They are based on the theory that because protein is a complex molecule, its digestion expends extra calories. It has been claimed that as much as 20% to 30% of the food energy from protein is expended for its digestion. This value is probably not that high, but even if it were, weight loss would likely be no greater than 0.5 lb per week. This small potential weight loss must be weighed against the increased risk of ketone bodies (from increased fat metabolism) in the blood and urine, and the accompanying health hazards of this condition, includ-

---

Unsafe Claims Checklist

Improper weight-control programs frequently make the following claims. A *yes* answer to any question indicates a questionable practice. Does your weight-control program

	Yes	No
1. Claim that calories do not count?	☐	☐
2. Guarantee spot reduction and sudden weight loss?	☐	☐
3. Promise cure for disease through diet and say that most disease is because of faulty diet?	☐	☐
4. Recommend drastic changes in a person's eating habits?	☐	☐
5. Not recommend an exercise program?	☐	☐
6. Guarantee quick, easy weight loss and success for everyone?	☐	☐
7. Recommend extreme amounts of certain nutrients or the elimination of certain nutrients?	☐	☐
8. Use spectacular advertising claims including testimonials to back up its claims?	☐	☐
9. Recommend that everyone take vitamins or health foods and claim that natural vitamins are better than synthetic ones?	☐	☐

ing kidney stones, calcium loss, and danger to an unborn child. Furthermore, because most high-protein foods are also high in saturated fats and cholesterol, blood cholesterol levels may become elevated.

Low-carbohydrate diets drastically reduce, without completely eliminating, carbohydrates from the diet. Many of these diets are not nutritionally sound and recommend that carbohydrates in the form of complex sugars be eliminated. This leads to decreased caloric intake and weight loss. Much of the weight loss is likely to be water, especially initially, as the body's carbohydrate stores are diminished.

High-fat diets aim at eating foods high in fat while consuming little or no carbohydrates. Their promoters claim that this leads to the mobilization and utilization of fat as fuel. In addition, the promoters claim that the urination of ketone bodies, a potential energy source, permits consumption of large numbers of calories while still losing weight. The dangers associated with ketosis and diets high in saturated fats have already been discussed. Diarrhea, fatigue, dehydration, and hypotension are frequently associated with these diets. The diets can be further criticized because no evidence exists to suggest, as is claimed, that weight loss can occur without a caloric deficit.

Besides being nutritionally unbalanced, diets consisting of one or two foods, such as grapefruit, eggs, or bananas, have as their greatest disadvantage their failure to bring about a permanent change in a person's eating habits. They can be initially effective for weight loss, but monotony soon dictates a return to previous eating patterns, and weight is frequently regained.

Recent years have seen the advent of medically supervised very low-calorie diet (VLCD) programs. These diets, which are designed to produce large and rapid weight loss without loss of lean body mass, consist of 400 to 800 kcal·day^{-1}, including 45 to 100 g of high-quality protein. They typically come as a powder that is mixed with water and consumed three to five times per day. Vitamin and mineral supplementation, and consumption of a minimum of 2 L of fluids, are required each day. The diets are usually followed for 12 to 16 weeks, followed by introduction to solid food over a 3- to 6-week period. The average weight loss is approximately 3.5 lb per week for females, and 4.5 lb per week for males. The aggressive marketing and public attraction to these diets have raised concern within the medical community (10).

VLCD programs can be administered with minimal risk by physicians who are trained in their use, including training in body composition, cardiac function during severe caloric restriction, and energy metabolism. In certain qualified patients, the programs can be effective at reducing multiple and life-threatening cardiovascular risk factors and achieving weight-loss goals.

Patients should be carefully selected; they should be restricted to those who are at least 30% fat and 40 lb overweight, in whom a medical examination and electrocardiogram have ruled out contraindications. In these patients, acceptable levels of lean body mass will be retained, and the risk of cardiovascular complications is minimized. Weekly medical examinations and biweekly assessment of electrolyte levels are recommended. Inclusion of regular exercise in the overall plan is also critical for minimizing loss of lean body mass while maximizing loss of adipose tissue. It is widely accepted that VLCDs decrease metabolic rate in their users. This leads to reduced energy expenditure and energy requirements, and could further complicate the difficulty of attempting to lose weight. Regular exercise should also be recommended to offset the reduced metabolic rate. Proper treatment of severe obesity requires a multidisciplinary approach, including the availability of a physician, a dietician, a behavioral psychologist, and an exercise professional. Modification of lifestyle and exercise habits should be emphasized.

The increased risk of complications with the improper use of VLCDs has led to legitimate concerns when they are used (1) without medical supervision, (2) by the mildly obese, and (3) by untrained physicians. Perhaps the greatest danger is for the unsupervised dieter who self-prescribes a VLCD by decreasing caloric intake to less than 800 kcal·day^{-1}, or who misuses commercial powdered diets by using them as their only nutritional and caloric source. Without medical supervision, complications such as dehydration and electrolyte imbalances go unnoticed, creating potentially serious complications. Dangerous cardiac arrhythmias may occur during the period of caloric restriction and may also be induced by abrupt feeding following severe caloric restriction (10).

Because the safety of VLCDs has been demonstrated only in severely obese individuals, concern is raised over their use in the mildly obese, in whom more lean body mass will be lost. This could precipitate cardiac abnormalities and damage other organs. Large decreases in lean body mass will also decrease metabolic rate, leading to reduced energy expenditure and energy requirements. The frequently observed plateau, or slowing of weight loss, may be due to the reduced energy expenditure, which may further contribute to difficulty maintaining weight loss.

Diet Medications and Appliances

A variety of diet medications are available both as over-the-counter drugs and by prescription. Many of these preparations serve as appetite suppressants and are effective for only 1 to 6 weeks for most individuals. These may lead to physical or psychological dependence, nervousness, irritability, and depression (8).

- *Diuretics* cause temporary weight loss by eliminating water. Side effects include dehydration, nausea, and vomiting.
- *Laxatives* speed the passage of food through the intestinal tract to decrease nutrient absorption of foods before they are eliminated as waste products. The loss of calories by this method is minimal, and any potential weight loss is far outweighed by possible health hazards from long-term laxative use.
- *Rubber or plastic suits* worn during exercise are effective for losing water weight, but they serve no useful purpose in fat reduction. During exercise the body must continually release heat from metabolism. The evaporation of sweat from the body is important in removing heat from the body. Rubber or plastic suits prevent sweat from reaching the air to be evaporated and are therefore very dangerous, particularly when the temperature and relative humidity are higher.
- *Elastic or inflatable belts* are advertised as increasing the temperature around the waistline and "melting" away fat. The falsity of this claim is obvious, because no caloric deficit is created. In some cases, the belts may result in a temporary decrease in waist size, but this is caused by compression of tissues and abdominal strengthening exercises that are included in the instructions.
- *Sauna baths* result in temporary weight loss that is only water loss. When liquids are consumed, water is replenished and the weight loss is regained.
- *Vibrators and massagers* are frequently promoted as effective weight-loss mechanisms. These may be effective muscle relaxants, but claims that they "break-up" fat are unfounded; only energy expended by the body, not by machines, can contribute to caloric deficits.

DIET, EXERCISE, AND LIPIDS

There is a strong relationship between the risk of heart disease and dietary levels of triglycerides and cholesterol. Although the mechanism of this relationship is not entirely clear, the communication of its existence to the public had led to significant dietary changes. The American public today consumes less saturated fat and cholesterol and more unsaturated fat than previously. Cholesterol is present in the body and serves many important functions; it is a component of cell membrane and nerve fibers, and is required for the production of steroid hormones, bile acids, and vitamin D. In addition

to that which is ingested (mostly in egg yolks, red meats, and whole-milk products), the body synthesizes approximately 1,000 mg of cholesterol each day. In fact, on the average, 65% to 70% of the cholesterol in the body is produced by the body itself. The biosynthesis of cholesterol occurs in nearly all cell types, but the liver and small intestine mucosa are the primary organs that produce cholesterol.

Triglycerides and cholesterol do not circulate freely in the plasma. They are carried in the bloodstream, bound to a protein, forming a lipoprotein. The partitioning of cholesterol into its lipoprotein fractions is of great importance. The total cholesterol level represents the cholesterol contained in different lipoproteins, namely, **very low-density lipoproteins (VLDL), low-density lipoproteins (LDL)**, and **high-density lipoproteins (HDL)**. The distribution of cholesterol among these various lipoproteins may be a more powerful predictor of heart disease than simply the total blood cholesterol level. The plasma total cholesterol is only weakly related to coronary artery disease risk, and the ratio of HDL to LDL, or HDL to total cholesterol may be the best lipid index (Table 6.5). The total cholesterol/HDL ratio is frequently used diagnostically. For example, two individuals may each have a blood cholesterol level of 240 mg$\cdot$dl^{-1}. If one of them has an HDL level of 80 mg$\cdot$dl^{-1}, the total cholesterol/HDL ratio is 3.00, which represents average risk. On the other hand, if the other person has an HDL level of 25 mg$\cdot$dl^{-1}, her or his total cholesterol/HDL index is 10.4. This is more than 2 times the average risk. LDL and VLDL encourage cholesterol to remain in the circu-

Table 6.5   Predicting Coronary Heart Disease Risk Based on LDL/HDL Ratio or Total Cholesterol/HDL Ratio

Risk	LDL/HDL	Total cholesterol/HDL
	WOMEN	
Below average	1.47	3.27
Average	3.22	4.44
2 x average	5.03	7.05
3 x average	6.14	11.04
	MEN	
Below average	1.00	3.43
Average	3.55	4.97
2 x average	6.25	9.55
3 x average	7.99	23.39

Note. From "Nutrition and Atherosclerosis" by W.B. Kannel, 1979. In D.T. Mason and H. Guthrie (Eds.), *The Medicine Called Nutrition* (p. 37). Englewood Cliffs, NJ: Best Foods. Copyright 1979 by Best Foods. Printed with permission of Mazola Nutrition/Health Information Service.

lation network by transporting it throughout the body to the cells, including the smooth muscle layers of the arterial walls, which frequently leads to narrowing of the arteries. The portion of total cholesterol in LDL is the primary atherogenic component of total blood cholesterol. HDL apparently serves as a cholesterol scavenger by removing cholesterol from the periphery, including arterial walls, and returning it to the liver where it can be excreted as bile. HDL may also interfere with the binding of LDL to the cell membrane. Because of the contrasting roles of these types of lipoproteins, HDL is frequently referred to as the "good" kind of cholesterol.

Epidemiological data and longitudinal studies indicate that the risk of coronary artery disease (CAD) is positively correlated with LDL levels and inversely related to the plasma HDL concentration. In fact, an inverse HDL–CAD relationship persists even after adjusting for the major CAD risk factors. The low incidence of CAD among people with high levels of HDL has led to the suggestion that HDL is an independent risk-lowering factor (4).

KEY POINT. A strong relationship exists between blood lipid levels and the risk of coronary heart disease. The ratio of LDL to HDL and of total cholesterol to HDL are useful indexes.

Understandably, there has been considerable interest in factors that appear to enhance HDL levels. Although not in complete agreement, results of studies relating HDL concentrations to physical activity and dietary factors show a somewhat consistent pattern. Regular physical activity is associated with decreased plasma triglycerides, VLDL, and LDL, and increased levels of HDL. Also, total blood cholesterol sometimes, but not always, falls. In addition, high HDL levels are strongly related to lower plasma triglyceride levels, decreased smoking, and loss of body weight.

Dietary manipulation can significantly influence the body's rate of cholesterol synthesis. With very little dietary cholesterol consumption, enough cholesterol is manufactured to maintain body functions. If the amount of cholesterol from food increases, the body responds with compensatory mechanisms, including reduced cholesterol synthesis and increased cholesterol excretion. The efficacy of these compensatory mechanisms varies among individuals. In some individuals they are not effective and instead lead to elevations in blood cholesterol levels. In people prone to tissue deposition of cholesterol, the risk of atherosclerosis may be enhanced.

The extent to which diet affects the total cholesterol to HDL ratio remains unclear. Studies comparing runners, joggers, and sedentary people indicate that HDL differences are associated more with total distance run than with dietary factors. The results of research studies have served as a reassurance that measures to prevent CHD do not adversely affect the blood lipid profile. If anything, conventional preventive measures are related to increased levels of HDL cholesterol. Until further investigations differentiate and clarify the causality of these factors, increased physical activity, weight reduction, smoking cessation, and a fat-controlled diet can be recommended to positively influence HDL levels and presumably decrease a person's risk of heart disease (4).

SUMMARY

Proper nutrition is important in reducing the risks associated with hypertension, stroke, obesity, and diabetes. Basic nutrients include proteins, carbohydrates, fats, vitamins, minerals, and water. Dietary goals recommend that the total caloric intake be divided among fat (30%), protein (12%), and carbohydrate (58%). Vitamins are essential for good health, but an excess will not increase health; in fact, large quantities of vitamins can be harmful. The use of extreme diets, drugs, and appliances to lose body fat usually produces only a temporary reduction in water weight. Diet and exercise interact to favorably influence the blood lipid profile by lowering total cholesterol and raising the HDL cholesterol.

REFERENCES

1. American College of Sports Medicine (1983)
2. American Dietetic Association (1987)
3. American Heart Association Committee Report (1982)
4. Caspersen and Heath (1988)
5. Food and Nutrition Board (1989)
6. King, Cohenour, Corruccini, and Schneeman (1978)
7. National Dairy Council (1989)
8. The fad-free diet (1985, July/Aug.)
9. U.S. Senate Select Committee on Nutrition and Human Needs (1977)
10. Wadden, Van Itallie, and Blackburn (1990)

SUGGESTED READINGS

American Heart Association (1987a)
Franks and Howley (1989)

Kannel (1979)
Powers and Howley (1990)
Stuart and Davies (1971)

See the Bibliography at the end of the book for a complete source
listing.

Chapter 7

Relative Leanness

Wendy J. Bubb

OBJECTIVES

The reader will be able to:

- State the rationale for determining body composition
- Discuss the relationship between body composition and health
- Demonstrate various techniques of assessing body composition and discuss advantages and disadvantages of each
- Calculate fat weight, fat-free weight, and body weight at a specific percent body fat, given current weight and percent fat
- Describe the health implications of variation in body-fat distribution patterns and the significance of waist-to-hip ratios
- Discuss how knowledge of an individual's overall health status and cardiac risk profile should be used in determining a recommended body weight
- Locate the common sites for measurement of skinfold thickness for estimation of body composition
- Describe appropriate weekly weight-loss goals
- Explain the set-point theory of weight control
- Distinguish between android-type and gynoid-type obesity
- Discuss the proper use of height/weight tables
- Calculate relative weight, and indicate values for overweight and obesity
- Calculate body mass index and indicate its relationship to the risk of cardiovascular and metabolic diseases
- Discuss the physiological effects of diet plus exercise, diet alone, and exercise alone as methods for modifying body composition
- Discuss the contribution of postexercise energy expenditure to total energy expenditure and weight control
- Describe anorexia nervosa and bulimia, and discuss factors contributing to their development
- Distinguish between isocaloric, negative caloric, and positive caloric balance, and describe their long-term consequences for weight control
- Describe the contribution of resting metabolic rate (RMR) to total energy expenditure, and describe factors that influence the RMR

TERMS

The reader will be able to define or describe:

Adipose tissue

Android-type obesity

Anorexia nervosa

Basal metabolic rate (BMR)

Bioelectric impedance

Body mass index (BMI)

Bulimia

Calorie

Gynoid-type obesity

Hydrostatic weighing

Isocaloric balance

Kilocalorie (kcal)

Lean body mass
Negative caloric balance
Overfat
Overweight
Positive caloric balance
Postexercise energy expenditure

Regional fat distribution
Relative weight (RW)
Residual volume
Resting metabolic rate (RMR)
Set-point theory
Waist-to-hip ratio

Obesity is a significant public health problem. It affects a large proportion of the population and adversely affects health and longevity. It either is a cause of or is correlated with health problems such as diabetes, coronary heart disease, and hypertension, disturbance of normal functions of the body including ventilation and excessive wear of joints, and such psychological effects as depression, withdrawal, poor self-concept, and self-pity (13). Overfat individuals are subjected to negative comments by peers and might not be selected for teams, jobs, and projects. Many agree that reducing the incidence of obesity would advance public health.

Our society is tremendously preoccupied with obesity. Physicians and their afflicted patients engage in frustrating efforts to correct it. Data from a 1985 National Health Interview Survey (19) indicated that 45% of females and 27% of males were trying to lose weight. Weight reduction is a multibillion-dollar industry; programs specifically aimed at weight management have spread rapidly in recent years. Nevertheless, obesity persists in our society.

BODY COMPOSITION

Body weight consists of many components, the relative proportions of which vary among individuals. Total body weight, which includes bone, muscle, fat, blood, and viscera, is conveniently divided into the lean body mass and fat mass. **Lean body mass** is the weight of all body tissue except fat. Body fat is stored in various organs of the body, such as the heart, liver, lungs, and brain. In addition, body fat is retained in **adipose tissue**, including the fat surrounding various internal organs as well as the subcutaneous layer of fat just beneath the skin. Some body fat is essential as an energy store, for protection of internal organs, as a component of nerves and cell membranes, and as insulation against heat loss. Essential body fat is 3% to 5% and 11% to 14% of the total body weight for adult males and females, respectively. These values represent the lower limits of body fat necessary to maintain good health.

The amount and sites of fat deposition vary among individuals and between sexes. The larger quantities of fat in females presumably relates to childbearing functions. Patterns of fat deposition are genetically unique to each individual. The hormone estrogen dictates fat deposition in the thighs, buttocks, and breasts in women. Men have minimal fat in these areas because they have lower levels of estrogen. A man is more likely to have fat in his back, lower abdomen, and at the top of his iliac crest.

The difference between being **overweight** and being **overfat** is an important distinction. Overweight is frequently defined as 10% in excess of the midpoint of the normal body weight range in the Metropolitan Life Insurance tables. Unfortunately, this does not consider the amount of body fat. Regarding relative leanness for positive health, the percentage of a person's body weight that is body fat is far more meaningful. Women and men are obese if they possess greater than 32% and 25% body fat, respectively. Body fatness is addressed more fully in the next section.

Recent studies suggest that not only percent fat but also **regional fat distribution** must be considered. Excess fat in the abdominal region is associated with greater risk of cardiovascular disease and a greater incidence of Type II (non–insulin dependent) diabetes. In determining regional body-fatness distribution, measurements should also be made of the waist and hip circumferences. **Waist-to-hip** circumference **ratios** greater than 0.8 and 0.9 for women and men, respectively, have been associated with greater risk of hypertriglyceridemia, Type II diabetes, hyperinsulinemia, and hypertension (18). A preponderance of abdominal fat and a high waist-to-hip ratio are characteristic of **android-type obesity**. This type of obesity involves hypertrophy (increase in size of adipose cells). **Gynoid-type obesity** is characterized by greater fat deposition on the buttocks, hips, and thighs, a low waist-to-hip ratio, and hyperplasia (increase in number of fat cells).

KEY POINT.   Regional fat distribution is related to risk of cardiovascular disease and diabetes. A high waist-to-hip circumference ratio is associated with increased risk.

Research has shown that the number and size of fat cells in the body are also important criteria in the degree of fatness. In adults, fat loss or gain occurs because of a decrease or increase, respectively, in the size of fat cells, with no change in the number of fat cells. For children, however, obesity occurs when there is an increase in the number and the size of fat cells. This is also believed to be related to the difficulty obese children have in being cured of obesity. Some studies suggest that an overabundance of fat cells may cause regulatory or metabolic dysfunctions that make it difficult for a person with a large number of fat cells to lose weight and maintain weight loss.

The difficulty experienced by obese individuals attempting to maintain weight loss has been used to explain physiological attempts by the body to maintain body weight and body fatness within a certain range. This concept of a "natural weight" for each individual is known as the **set-point theory**. It is important to recognize that the set-point body weight is a theoretical concept and not an actual physiological mechanism. Booth (3) has proposed both physiological and cognitive models of the set-point concept. According to the physiological set-point model, the body-weight set point is regulated by the hypothalamus as it receives input regarding blood glucose levels, the amount of fat stored in fat cells, and body weight. Food intake is regulated (decreased or increased) based on this input so that the set-point body weight can be maintained. Although dieting doesn't affect the set point, exercise appears to have a lowering effect. The cognitive set-point model focuses on the effects of environmental and cognitive signals on body weight. Information received about appearance, body weight, clothing size, health, and so on leads to eating and physical-activity behaviors designed to bring body weight in line with the perceived ideal weight.

EVALUATION OF BODY FATNESS

An evaluation of body composition is essential prior to making specific recommendations about a person's need to lose or gain body weight.

Relative Weight

Frequently, recommendations for weight loss have been made on the basis of the standard-weight-for-height charts published by the Metropolitan Life Insurance Company (Table 7.1). These tables, which were derived from insurance company policyholders, indicate the body weights associated with the lowest mortality rate within each height and frame size category. It

Table 7.1   Metropolitan Height and Weight Tables for Men and Women Between the Ages of 25 and 59

Height[a]		Frame		
Feet	Inches	Small	Medium	Large
		MEN		
5	2	112-120	118-129	126-141
5	3	115-123	121-133	129-144
5	4	118-126	124-136	132-148
5	5	121-129	127-139	135-152
5	6	124-133	130-143	138-156
5	7	128-137	134-147	142-161
5	8	132-141	138-152	147-166
5	9	136-145	142-156	151-170
5	10	140-150	146-160	155-174
5	11	144-154	150-165	159-179
6	0	148-158	154-170	164-184
6	1	152-162	158-175	168-189
6	2	156-167	162-180	173-194
6	3	160-171	167-185	178-199
6	4	164-175	172-190	182-204
		WOMEN		
4	10	92-98	96-107	104-119
4	11	94-101	98-110	106-122
5	0	96-104	101-113	109-125
5	1	99-107	104-116	112-128
5	2	102-110	107-119	115-131
5	3	105-113	110-122	118-134
5	4	108-116	113-126	121-138
5	5	111-119	116-130	125-142
5	6	114-123	120-135	129-146
5	7	118-127	124-139	133-150
5	8	122-131	128-143	137-154
5	9	126-135	132-147	141-158
5	10	130-140	136-151	145-163
5	11	134-144	140-155	149-168
6	0	138-148	144-159	153-173

[a]With shoes with one-inch heels for men, two-inch heels for women.

Note. From Metropolitan Life Insurance Company. Reprinted by permission.

has generally been suggested that a person whose body weight is 10% above the midpoint range for a medium frame according to insurance company statistics is overweight; 20% above the average weight for height is classified as obesity. The height/weight tables are also frequently used to calculate a **relative weight (RW)**. A person's body weight is divided by the midpoint in the weight range given for her or his height and frame size. If a person's body weight equals the midpoint of the range, the RW equals 1.00. For example, a woman who is 5 ft 5 in. tall with a medium frame and weighs 135 lb has a relative weight of 1.10 (135 lb ÷ 123 lb). At 10% above normal, she would be classified as overweight. Unfortunately, definition of body frame size often becomes an arbitrary judgment. In addition, these tables fail to consider the relative amounts of muscle and fat tissue. Physically fit athletes frequently weigh more than the body weight considered average or desirable by these standards. By evaluating body composition, however, it may be determined that they actually have a relatively low percentage of body fat and do not need to reduce weight. Likewise, some individuals may be considered underweight according to height and weight standards but have a high percentage of body fat. In the "average" population, excess weight is generally fat weight. Thus for many people, "overweight" and "overfat" can be used interchangeably. Height and weight standards are not as precise as some of the others to be discussed, and people with small or large amounts of muscle may be misevaluated.

Body Mass Index (BMI)

Another expression of height and weight data used to characterize body fatness is the **body mass index (BMI)**: BMI = weight (kg) ÷ height^2 (m). For example, a man who is 178 cm tall and weighs 77 kg has a BMI of 26.6 kg/m^2 (77 ÷ 1.78^2). In the original Framingham Heart Study, significant positive relationships were observed between BMI and blood pressure, high serum triglyceride levels, high total cholesterol, low HDL-cholesterol levels, and glucose intolerance. A 26-year follow-up study of the subjects in the Framingham study supported the earlier findings by showing a significant association between high BMI and cardiovascular disease (7). For women, desirable BMI is 21 to 23 kg/m^2; for men it is 22 to 24 kg/m^2. The risk of cardiovascular disease increases sharply at a BMI of about 27.8 kg/m^2 for men and 27.3 kg/m^2 for women (1).

KEY POINT.   Body mass index (BMI) = weight (kg) ÷ height^2 (m). A high BMI is associated with greater risk of cardiovascular diseases and diabetes.

Recognizing what information is provided by scale weight, and how to properly interpret the information obtained, should lead to the proper utilization of scale weights. Several factors influence scale weight independent of adipose tissue loss. Scale weight can vary during the day as a result of eating, urinary and fecal elimination, and loss of sweat. Certain factors can cause temporary loss or retention of water. A low-carbohydrate diet, for example, may cause an immediate weight

loss due to water being released by the body. This apparent weight loss is temporary, and the body will return to its original weight when its carbohydrate store is restored. Diarrhea can result in temporary weight loss for the same reason. On the other hand, a high-carbohydrate diet or menstruation may lead to water retention and temporary weight gain. This does not reflect changes in adipose tissue stores.

When using weighing scales, the following guidelines are recommended:

- **Beam scales with nondetachable weights should be used. They should be calibrated to zero and permit reading to the nearest 0.25 lb.**
- **Weighing should be done prior to breakfast, after the bladder has been emptied.**
- **Clothing should be light, without shoes.**
- **Measurements should be accurately noted and recorded and compared with previous weight measurements to determine possible weight loss.**

The most accurate methods to determine body composition are by chemical analysis of human cadavers; however, this is of no use to the Health Fitness Instructor. Several indirect methods that are widely used by exercise specialists have been validated by the information obtained from these direct measurements. These include

- hydrostatic (underwater) weighing,
- measurement of skinfold thickness, and
- measurement of bioelectrical impedance.

Underwater Weighing

With the application of Archimedes' principle, percent body fat can be calculated from body density using **hydrostatic**, or underwater, **weighing**. Body density is equal to the ratio of body weight (mass) to body volume (weight ÷ volume); scales are used to measure weight (mass), and hydrostatic weighing is used to determine body volume. Because an object's loss of weight in water is equal to the weight of the volume of water that it displaces, body volume can be calculated as the difference between body weight in air and body weight measured during water submersion (i.e., body volume = weight in air − weight in water). Therefore

$$\text{Body density} = \frac{\text{body weight in air}}{\text{weight in air} - \text{weight in water}}$$

The greatest disadvantages of hydrostatic weighing are the time and equipment necessary to perform it. The essential equipment includes a special chair suspended from a balance scale that measures to the nearest 10 g, a weight belt, and a tank into which the subject is submerged. A swimming pool with the chair and scale suspended from a support at the side of the pool is a suitable alternative to the tank. In addition, for accurate measurements a closed-circuit dilution system is necessary to measure residual volume.

Body weight is determined in air with a balance scale, with the subject dressed in a lightweight swimming suit. The subject is then seated in the chair suspended from the scale and submerged beneath the water (Figure 7.1). In many equipment setups, a weight belt fitted around the waist prevents the subject from floating toward the surface. Prior to submersion, as much air as possible is expired from the lungs. This forced expiration is maintained for 5 to 10 s while the underwater weight is recorded. The underwater weight of the belt and the chair is determined beforehand and subtracted from the total underwater weight of the subject. With repeated weighing, subjects may learn to expel more air from the lungs. It is recommended that measurements be repeated until three trials are obtained to a range of 100 g or less (2). The scale pointer will tend to fluctuate during the measurement; therefore, weight should be recorded as the midpoint of the fluctuation.

Following a maximal expiration, some air, defined as the **residual volume**, remains in the lungs. Because this volume contributes to buoyancy, the total volume must be corrected for the residual lung volume prior to the actual calculation of body density. An error in determining the relatively large residual volume (1,000 to 1,500 ml) could seriously affect the accuracy and usefulness of the underwater weighing technique. Without measuring residual volume directly, an assumed average value for all subjects, or an estimated value based on height and weight, can be used. In addition, residual volume can be estimated as the vital capacity × 0.24 for males and vital capacity × 0.28 for females, although the relationship between these parameters is relatively low. Because the accuracy of the residual-volume measurement can seriously affect the validity of subsequent calculations of body density and thus body fat, the practice of either using an assumed average value for all subjects or predicting the residual volume from other parameters is questionable. For example, an error of 500 to 1,000 ml in the residual volume results in percent-fatness values that are inaccurate by 2.0% to 5.5% fat (13). The extra time and cost may not be justified for hydrostatic weighing if measurement of residual volume using standard dilution techniques is not possible. The temperature of the water

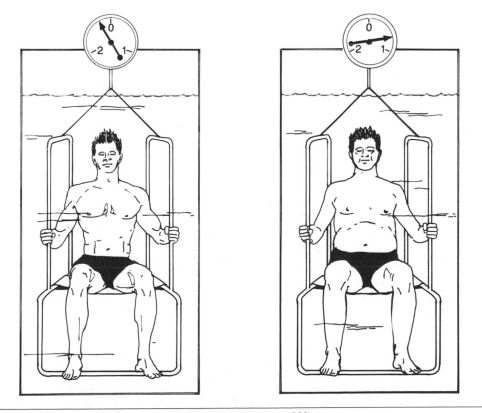

Figure 7.1 Underwater weighing. Adapted from Pollock and Wilmore (1990).

is recorded, and the volume is corrected for the density of the water at the recorded temperature. With these corrections, the body density equation becomes

Body density $(g \cdot cc^{-1})$

$$= \frac{\text{Weight in air}}{\dfrac{\text{weight in air} - \text{weight in water}}{\text{Density of water}} - \text{residual volume}}$$

The following example illustrates the use of these measurements in calculating body density:

Body weight	100 kg
Underwater weight	4.0 kg
Residual volume	1.0 L
Water density	0.9965 kg·L^{-1}

$$\text{Body density } (kg \cdot L^{-1}) = \frac{100 \text{ kg}}{\dfrac{100 \text{ kg} - 4 \text{ kg}}{0.9965 \text{ kg} \cdot L^{-1}} - 1.0 \text{ L}}$$

$$= 1.05 \text{ kg} \cdot L^{-1} \text{ or } 1.05 \text{ g} \cdot cc^{-1}$$

Equations presented later are used to calculate percent body fat (5, 17).

KEY POINT.   Hydrostatic, or underwater, weighing is the most accurate technique for determining body density, from which percent body fatness can be calculated. For greatest accuracy, the residual volume must be measured rather than estimated.

Skinfold Method

Determination of body composition by measuring the thickness of skinfolds has had the widest use, compared to the other techniques. The basis for measuring body fat in this way is that approximately 50% of the total fat content of the body is subcutaneous, or just beneath the skin. Measuring the thickness of a skinfold involves grasping a fold of skin and fat away from the underlying muscle. A skinfold caliper is used to measure the skinfold thickness to the nearest 0.5 mm. We recommend Harpenden calipers (Quinton Instrument Co., Seattle, WA) and Lange calipers (Cambridge Scientific Industries, Cambridge, MD), but other, less expensive calipers are suitable alternatives (for example, the Fat-O-Meter by Health Education Services Corp., Bensenville, IL; Fat Control, Inc., Towson, MD) except for research studies requiring greater precision.

The success of skinfold measurement depends on meticulous attention to detail in the techniques. Practice of the techniques should be extensive, and anatomical locations should be correct to establish test/retest reliability prior to performing the technique on a group of subjects. Although some suggest taking three consecutive measurements at a single site and using the middle score, a more objective technique is to measure different sites in succession, repeating the sequence two to three times without looking at the previous value. Average two or three measurements to determine skinfold thickness. If consecutive measurements are made at a given site before moving to another, the technique of measurement should be repeated completely, including locating the site and regrasping the skinfold. For test/retest reliability, where possible, the same test administrator should be used on subsequent testing periods. If more than one person is to be used for skinfold measurements, each person should be checked for objectivity against a standard (i.e., an experienced tester).

The most frequently measured skinfold sites are the triceps, subscapular, suprailiac, thigh, abdomen, calf, and chest. These are the specific anatomical locations:

Triceps—a fold parallel to the longitudinal axis of the upper arm measured at the midline halfway between the olecranon and acromion processes with the arm hanging freely at the side

Subscapular—an oblique fold measured just below the inferior angle of the scapula

Suprailiac—a slightly oblique fold that is lifted to follow the natural contour of the skinfold just above the iliac crest at the anterior axillary line

Thigh—a vertical fold in the anterior midline of the thigh, taken midway between the patella and the hip

Abdomen—a vertical fold measured 2 cm (1 in.) to the right of the umbilicus

Calf—a vertical fold measured on the medial aspect of the lower leg at the level of the greatest calf girth

Chest—a diagonal fold located one half of the distance between the anterior axillary line and the nipple, for men, and one third of the distance, for women

These sites are illustrated in Figure 7.2. The skinfold, which is grasped between the thumb and forefinger, includes two thicknesses of skin and subcutaneous fat, but no muscle. The caliper is placed 0.5 in. above or below the finger, midway between the crest and the base of the skinfold. All measurements are conventionally made on the right side of the standing subject's body.

The values obtained from skinfold measurements can be used in several ways. Values from several sites can be totaled to arrive at the sum of skinfolds. The sum of skinfolds can be used to rank-order individuals within a given group. This indicates a person's relative fatness compared to others in the group. The sum of skinfolds

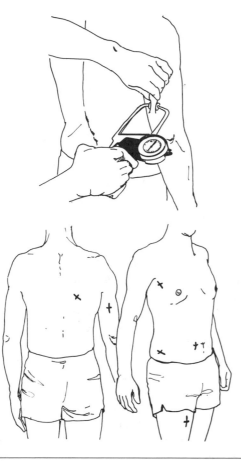

Figure 7.2 Skinfold sites used in the evaluation of body fatness.

can also be used to evaluate body fatness changes following dietary restriction or exercise conditioning programs. The use of the sum of skinfolds can be recommended as a guide toward achieving the goal of decreasing the total amount of body fat, independent of a fixed body-fat percentage. Using this approach, a person's sum of skinfolds is compared over time to assess relative changes in body fatness.

Skinfold measurements can also be used with mathematical equations to predict percent body fat. A word of caution is warranted regarding the more than 100 prediction equations available. These equations have been unequivocally proven to be more specific than general. That is, equations derived from one segment of the population do a poor job of predicting percent body fat when used on other populations. The equations are applicable only to groups similar in age and activity level to those from which the equations are derived. As might be expected, the equations are also gender specific. Most of the equations were formulated with data from average college-age men and women and, therefore, are best applied to these populations. The equation specificity points out the need for discriminat-

ing use of some of these equations for very fat or very thin individuals, athletic women and men, or individuals involved in strenuous weight-training programs.

The regression equations combine such variables as skinfold thickness, girth, height, and weight to most commonly predict body density, and less often predict percent body fat or lean body weight. Where body density is predicted, as in underwater weighing, percent body fat is computed with formulas such as the following:

$$\text{Percent fat} = \frac{495}{\text{density}} - 450$$

[See (17).]

$$\text{Percent fat} = \frac{4.570}{\text{density}} - 4.142 \cdot 100$$

[See (5).]

These equations are based on density values of 0.900 g•cc^{-1} and 1.100 g•cc^{-1} for fat tissue, and fat-free tissue, respectively. However, for certain populations the density of fat-free tissue is less than 1.100 g•cc^{-1}. For example, children and women, who have less bone mineral content per unit fat-free mass, have fat-free density values less than 1.100 g•cc^{-1}, whereas blacks have density values above 1.100 g•cc^{-1}. With consideration of these differences in the density of fat-free mass, **modifications of the Siri equation for specific populations** have been recommended:

Young women

$$\text{Percent fat} = \frac{509}{\text{density}} - 465$$

[See (11, 12).]

Children (ages 11 to 12)

$$\text{Percent fat} = \frac{530}{\text{density}} - 489$$

[See (11, 12).]

Blacks

$$\text{Percent fat} = \frac{437}{\text{density}} - 393$$

[See (15).]

Obviously, selection of the correct equation to determine body-fat values from body-density measures is crucial to the accurate application of these techniques for various populations.

Discussion of the various regression equations that have been derived for various populations is beyond the scope of this chapter. For the HFI, a convenient method to determine body density, especially with large numbers of subjects, is to use one of the recently developed generalized equations. These equations can be used with samples that vary greatly in age and body fatness. The obvious advantage of generalized equations is that one equation replaces several without compromising accuracy. The following **generalized equations** [from (9, 10)] are recommended for use by the HFI. Separate equations are provided for men and women to account for sex differences:

Men

Body density $= 1.10938 - 0.0008267(X_1)$
$$+ 0.0000016(X_1)^2 - 0.0002574(X_2)$$

X_1 = sum of chest, abdomen, and thigh skinfolds
X_2 = age in years

[See (9).]

Women

Body density $= 1.0994921 - 0.0009929(X_1)$
$$+ 0.0000023(X_1)^2 - 0.0001392(X_2)$$

X_1 = sum of triceps, suprailiac, and thigh skinfolds
X_2 = age in years

[See (10).]

Tables 7.2 and 7.3 are provided to expedite the calculation of percent body fat from these equations. Because the equations were developed on women and men 18 to 61 years of age, their use is not recommended for subjects outside this age range. Furthermore, larger than normal prediction errors can be expected with extremely obese and extremely thin individuals. Therefore, these equations should be used cautiously with such individuals. It is important to recognize the error inherent in estimating body-fat percentages from skinfold measurements. Using the above generalized equations, the standard error of the estimate ($\pm$ one standard deviation) is $\pm$ 3.6% and $\pm$ 3.9% for men and women, respectively. Thus, 68% ($\pm$ 1 SD) of all women who are estimated to have a body fatness of 23% will actually be between 19.1% and 26.9% fat.

Bioelectrical Impedance

Bioelectrical impedance has also been applied to body composition measurements. Due to the larger electrolyte content of lean tissue, the electrical conductivity of fat-free mass exceeds that of fat mass. The measurement technique involves using a small portable instrument and placing four electrodes on the skin to measure conductance of a very weak electrical current (Figure 7.3). The use of impedance-measuring devices is attractive because of their speed and ease of use, portability, lower expense, and reduction of intertester error, and the measurements can be applied to various ages and health states. There are, however, limitations to their accuracy due to variations in water balance, electrolyte levels, and skin temperature. Because total body water influences the fat-free mass, fluctuations in this component can adversely affect precision. For example, loss of body water will decrease impedance and lead to lower percent-fat values when no change has occurred in the fat mass. Recent studies have shown that the accuracy of body-fat measurements using bioelectrical impedance is no better than the skinfold technique (8, 16). Before widespread use of body-impedance measurements can be recommended, further research is needed from various populations on reliability and validity and on the identification and standardization of factors that affect whole-body impedance.

Calculation of Desirable Body Weight

Once it has been determined what percentage of a person's body weight is fat, simple calculations are used to arrive at a desirable body weight based on the present lean body weight. The steps are shown in Equations to Calculate Desirable Weight.

A range of desirable weights should be used to account for the measurement error associated with estimating body fatness. For example, a man with an initial body fatness of 23% may have 20% as an initial goal, followed by further reductions to 18% or lower to be classified in the fitness category. Furthermore, individ-

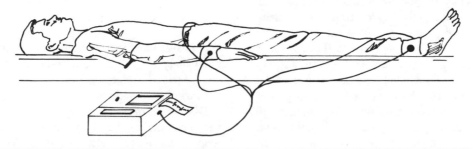

Figure 7.3 Impedance measuring device.

Table 7.2 Percent Body Fat[a] Estimation for Men from Age and the Sum of Chest, Abdominal, and Thigh Skinfolds

Sum of skinfolds (mm)	Age to the last year								
	Under 22	23 to 27	28 to 32	33 to 37	38 to 42	43 to 47	48 to 52	53 to 57	Over 57
8-10	1.3	1.8	2.3	2.9	3.4	3.9	4.5	5.0	5.5
11-13	2.2	2.8	3.3	3.9	4.4	4.9	5.5	6.0	6.5
14-16	3.2	3.8	4.3	4.8	5.4	5.9	6.4	7.0	7.5
17-19	4.2	4.7	5.3	5.8	6.3	6.9	7.4	8.0	8.5
20-22	5.1	5.7	6.2	6.8	7.3	7.9	8.4	8.9	9.5
23-25	6.1	6.6	7.2	7.7	8.3	8.8	9.4	9.9	10.5
26-28	7.0	7.6	8.1	8.7	9.2	9.8	10.3	10.9	11.4
29-31	8.0	8.5	9.1	9.6	10.2	10.7	11.3	11.8	12.4
32-34	8.9	9.4	10.0	10.5	11.1	11.6	12.2	12.8	13.3
35-37	9.8	10.4	10.9	11.5	12.0	12.6	13.1	13.7	14.3
38-40	10.7	11.3	11.8	12.4	12.9	13.5	14.1	14.6	15.2
41-43	11.6	12.2	12.7	13.3	13.8	14.4	15.0	15.5	16.1
44-46	12.5	13.1	13.6	14.2	14.7	15.3	15.9	16.4	17.0
47-49	13.4	13.9	14.5	15.1	15.6	16.2	16.8	17.3	17.9
50-52	14.3	14.8	15.4	15.9	16.5	17.1	17.6	18.2	18.8
53-55	15.1	15.7	16.2	16.8	17.4	17.9	18.5	19.1	19.7
56-58	16.0	16.5	17.1	17.7	18.2	18.8	19.4	20.0	20.5
59-61	16.9	17.4	17.9	18.5	19.1	19.7	20.2	20.8	21.4
62-64	17.6	18.2	18.8	19.4	19.9	20.5	21.1	21.7	22.2
65-67	18.5	19.0	19.6	20.2	20.8	21.3	21.9	22.5	23.1
68-70	19.3	19.9	20.4	21.0	21.6	22.2	22.7	23.3	23.9
71-73	20.1	20.7	21.2	21.8	22.4	23.0	23.6	24.1	24.7
74-76	20.9	21.5	22.0	22.6	23.2	23.8	24.4	25.0	25.5
77-79	21.7	22.2	22.8	23.4	24.0	24.6	25.2	25.8	26.3
80-82	22.4	23.0	23.6	24.2	24.8	25.4	25.9	26.5	27.1
83-85	23.2	23.8	24.4	25.0	25.5	26.1	26.7	27.3	27.9
86-88	24.0	24.5	25.1	25.7	26.3	26.9	27.5	28.1	28.7
89-91	24.7	25.3	25.9	26.5	27.1	27.6	28.2	28.8	29.4
92-94	25.4	26.0	26.6	27.2	27.8	28.4	29.0	29.6	30.2
95-97	26.1	26.7	27.3	27.9	28.5	29.1	29.7	30.3	30.9
98-100	26.9	27.4	28.0	28.6	29.2	29.8	30.4	31.0	31.6
101-103	27.5	28.1	28.7	29.3	29.9	30.5	31.1	31.7	32.3
104-106	28.2	28.8	29.4	30.0	30.6	31.2	31.8	32.4	33.0
107-109	28.9	29.5	30.1	30.7	31.3	31.9	32.5	33.1	33.7
110-112	29.6	30.2	30.8	31.4	32.0	32.6	33.2	33.8	34.4
113-115	30.2	30.8	31.4	32.0	32.6	33.2	33.8	34.5	35.1
116-118	30.9	31.5	32.1	32.7	33.3	33.9	34.5	35.1	35.7
119-121	31.5	32.1	32.7	33.3	33.9	34.5	35.1	35.7	36.4
122-124	32.1	32.7	33.3	33.9	34.5	35.1	35.8	36.4	37.0
125-127	32.7	33.3	33.9	34.5	35.1	35.8	36.4	37.0	37.6

Note. From "Measurement of Cardiorespiratory Fitness and Body Composition in a Clinical Setting" by M.L. Pollock, D.H. Schmidt, and A.S. Jackson, 1980, *Comprehensive Therapy*, **6**, pp. 12-27. Copyright 1980 by International Publishing Group. Adapted by permission.

[a]Percent fat calculated by the formula of Siri: percent fat = $[(4.95/D_b) - 4.5] \times 100$. Where D_b = body density.

uals should be reevaluated on these variables when they have reached the halfway points of their original goals.

Because so many factors influence body weight and body fatness, making specific recommendations about body fat is difficult. Desirable body weight likely varies from individual to individual. First, as implied in Table 7.4, different standards are applied for different purposes. An athlete, for example, should expect to maintain a lower fat percentage than an individual desiring fitness for positive health. Second, desirable body-fat

Table 7.3   Percent Body Fat[a] Estimation for Women from Age and Triceps, Suprailium, and Thigh Skinfolds

Sum of skinfolds (mm)	Age to the last year								
	Under 22	23 to 27	28 to 32	33 to 37	38 to 42	43 to 47	48 to 52	53 to 57	Over 57
23-25	9.7	9.9	10.2	10.4	10.7	10.9	11.2	11.4	11.7
26-28	11.0	11.2	11.5	11.7	12.0	12.3	12.5	12.7	13.0
29-31	12.3	12.5	12.8	13.0	13.3	13.5	13.8	14.0	14.3
32-34	13.6	13.8	14.0	14.3	14.5	14.8	15.0	15.3	15.5
35-37	14.8	15.0	15.3	15.5	15.8	16.0	16.3	16.5	16.8
38-40	16.0	16.3	16.5	16.7	17.0	17.2	17.5	17.7	18.0
41-43	17.2	17.4	17.7	17.9	18.2	18.4	18.7	18.9	19.2
44-46	18.3	18.6	18.8	19.1	19.3	19.6	19.8	20.1	20.3
47-49	19.5	19.7	20.0	20.2	20.5	20.7	21.0	21.2	21.5
50-52	20.6	20.8	21.1	21.3	21.6	21.8	22.1	22.3	22.6
53-55	21.7	21.9	22.1	22.4	22.6	22.9	23.1	23.4	23.6
56-58	22.7	23.0	23.2	23.4	23.7	23.9	24.2	24.4	24.7
59-61	23.7	24.0	24.2	24.5	24.7	25.0	25.2	25.5	25.7
62-64	24.7	25.0	25.2	25.5	25.7	26.0	26.2	26.4	26.7
65-67	25.7	25.9	26.2	26.4	26.7	26.9	27.2	27.4	27.7
68-70	26.6	26.9	27.1	27.4	27.6	27.9	28.1	28.4	28.6
71-73	27.5	27.8	28.0	28.3	28.5	28.8	29.0	29.3	29.5
74-76	28.4	28.7	28.9	29.2	29.4	29.7	29.9	30.2	30.4
77-79	29.3	29.5	29.8	30.0	30.3	30.5	30.8	31.0	31.3
80-82	30.1	30.4	30.6	30.9	31.1	31.4	31.6	31.9	32.1
83-85	30.9	31.2	31.4	31.7	31.9	32.2	32.4	32.7	32.9
86-88	31.7	32.0	32.2	32.5	32.7	32.9	33.2	33.4	33.7
89-91	32.5	32.7	33.0	33.2	33.5	33.7	33.9	34.2	34.4
92-94	33.2	33.4	33.7	33.9	34.2	34.4	34.7	34.9	35.2
95-97	33.9	34.1	34.4	34.6	34.9	35.1	35.4	35.6	35.9
98-100	34.6	34.8	35.1	35.3	35.5	35.8	36.0	36.3	36.5
101-103	35.3	35.4	35.7	35.9	36.2	36.4	36.7	36.9	37.2
104-106	35.8	36.1	36.3	36.6	36.8	37.1	37.3	37.5	37.8
107-109	36.4	36.7	36.9	37.1	37.4	37.6	37.9	38.1	38.4
110-112	37.0	37.2	37.5	37.7	38.0	38.2	38.5	38.7	38.9
113-115	37.5	37.8	38.0	38.2	38.5	38.7	39.0	39.2	39.5
116-118	38.0	38.3	38.5	38.8	39.0	39.3	39.5	39.7	40.0
119-121	38.5	38.7	39.0	39.2	39.5	39.7	40.0	40.2	40.5
122-124	39.0	39.2	39.4	39.7	39.9	40.2	30.4	40.7	40.9
125-127	39.4	39.6	39.9	40.1	40.4	40.6	40.9	41.1	41.4
128-130	39.8	40.0	40.3	40.5	40.8	41.0	41.3	41.5	41.8

Note. From "Measurement of Cardiorespiratory Fitness and Body Composition in a Clinical Setting" by M.L. Pollock, D.H. Schmidt, and A.S. Jackson, 1980, *Comprehensive Therapy*, **6**, pp. 12-27. Copyright 1980 by International Publishing Group. Adapted by permission.

[a]Percent fat calculated by the formula of Siri: percent fat = $[(4.95/D_b) - 4.5] \times 100$. Where D_b = body density.

percentages are presented as ranges in order to deal with the imprecision in all of the methods used to arrive at these percentages. Finally, as with high levels of serum cholesterol and blood pressure, health problems increase progressively as percent body fatness exceeds what is recommended. There is little question that health risks are greater for those with percent body fat in excess of 25% and 32% for males and females, respectively. However, there is reason to consider the values of 26% to 31% for females and 19% to 24% for males to represent a "gray area" of potential risk to which one should attend. It is recommended that women and men should maintain body-fat percentages of 16% to 25% and 12% to 18%, respectively. For people who have very high percentages of body fat, the first goal should be to achieve and maintain the values in the "gray area" and, with further evaluation, progress toward the lower values.

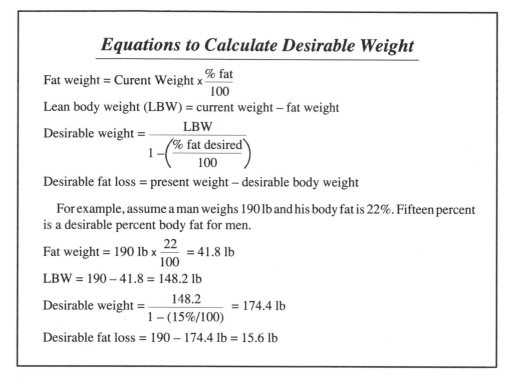

Equations to Calculate Desirable Weight

Fat weight = Curent Weight $\times \dfrac{\% \text{ fat}}{100}$

Lean body weight (LBW) = current weight − fat weight

Desirable weight = $\dfrac{\text{LBW}}{1 - \left(\dfrac{\% \text{ fat desired}}{100}\right)}$

Desirable fat loss = present weight − desirable body weight

For example, assume a man weighs 190 lb and his body fat is 22%. Fifteen percent is a desirable percent body fat for men.

Fat weight = 190 lb $\times \dfrac{22}{100}$ = 41.8 lb

LBW = 190 − 41.8 = 148.2 lb

Desirable weight = $\dfrac{148.2}{1 - (15\%/100)}$ = 174.4 lb

Desirable fat loss = 190 − 174.4 lb = 15.6 lb

Table 7.4 Body-Fat Norms Based on Percentage of Body Weight That is Fat

Classification	% Fat Women	% Fat Men
Essential fat	11.0-14.0	3.0-5.0
Athletes	12.0-22.0	5.0-13.0
Fitness	16.0-25.0	12.0-18.0
Potential risk	26.0-31.0	19.0-24.0
Obese	32.0 and higher	25.0 and higher

Note. Females before puberty use male scale. There is no health reason for increased body fat with age, thus the same standards are applied to all ages.

Adapted from Doxey GE, Fairbanks B, Housh TH, Johnson GO, Datch F, and Lohman T. Body composition roundtable: Part 1. Scientific considerations. *National Strength and Conditioning Association Journal* 9:14-15, 1987.

Societal pressures and media emphasis on the thin, model-type body may lead some individuals to become obsessed with body image, which may develop into the eating disorders **anorexia nervosa** and **bulimia**. Eating disorders are chronic, progressive, and potentially fatal. The problems are especially common in young women, although men are also affected. Anorexia nervosa usually begins as a normal weight-loss diet, but develops into a psychological disorder characterized by obsessive dieting and intense fear of becoming obese.

To stay thin, the anorexic skips meals, may go several days without food, and frequently exercises excessively. Anorexia is a serious psychological disorder requiring medical attention, because if it is not properly treated, death through starvation may ensue. Bulimia is characterized by episodes of binge-eating large quantities of food, followed by purging the food eaten using self-induced vomiting or laxatives. Binges occur most often during times of depression, anxiety, or loneliness. The most pervasive symptom of both eating disorders is denial that a problem exists or that help is needed. Early recognition and prompt treatment by trained medical personnel are the keys to successful treatment.

CALORIC BALANCE AND WEIGHT CONTROL

Caloric balance is the relationship between caloric intake and caloric expenditure (i.e., the number of calories taken in from food and drink compared to those expended by basal metabolism and voluntary activity). The energy-balance equation expresses this relationship mathematically as

Caloric intake = caloric expenditure

A **calorie** is a unit of energy defined as the amount of heat necessary to raise the temperature of 1 g of water 1 °C. In nutrition and exercise circles, the term *calorie* is frequently used for what is actually a **kilocalorie (kcal)**. A kilocalorie is the amount of heat needed to increase the temperature of 1 kg of water 1 °C. One kcal equals 1,000 cal.

Several terms have evolved to refer to the various relations that can exist between caloric intake and caloric expenditure. In **isocaloric balance**, caloric intake and caloric expenditure are equal. For example, if a person consumes an average of 2,500 kcal per day and expends 2,500 kcal per day, the energy equation is in balance; tissue mass neither increases or decreases.

When caloric intake exceeds caloric expenditure, a person is in **positive caloric balance**. For example, a caloric intake of 2,800 kcal per day while expending only 2,500 kcal per day leads to a positive 300-kcal balance per day. These 300 kcal that are not expended by the body are stored as adipose tissue, resulting in weight gain.

If energy expenditure exceeds caloric intake, a person is in **negative caloric balance**, and a caloric deficit exists. An example would be a person who consumes 2,500 kcal per day while expending 3,000 kcal. The 500-kcal caloric deficit leads to weight loss as the body primarily uses stored adipose tissue to meet its daily energy needs.

People in physical-activity and weight-reduction programs need to know that a balance must be achieved between the number of calories taken in and the number expended, to stay at the same weight. If more calories are consumed than expended, fat is stored in adipose tissue. One lb of adipose tissue equals 3,500 kcal. Thus, if 3,500 more kcal are eaten than are expended, 1 lb of adipose tissue is gained. Conversely, to lose 1 lb of body fat, a 3,500-kcal deficit must occur. A deficit of 500 kcal per day, therefore, leads to the loss of approximately 1 lb of adipose tissue in 1 week.

Negative caloric balance can be attained by decreasing caloric intake, increasing energy expenditure through exercise, or combining a decrease in caloric intake and increased participation in regular physical activity. As discussed in a subsequent section, a combination of restricted caloric intake and exercise is recommended. In any case, daily caloric deficit should not exceed 1,000 to 1,200 kcal per day. This results in a body-weight loss of approximately 2 lb per week.

KEY POINT.   A negative caloric balance of 3,500 kcal is required to lose 1 lb of adipose tissue. It is recommended that the caloric deficit be achieved through a combination of caloric restriction and increased physical activity.

Total caloric intake comes from the consumption of foods and drinks. The carbohydrates, fats, and proteins in these foods contain energy that is expressed in terms of kcal (see chapter 6).

Many factors affect a person's caloric intake at any particular time. Included among these are cultural and family influences. Some people react to various emotional states such as stress or depression by over- or undereating. Various physiological mechanisms may influence food intake. Hormonal or central nervous system regulatory mechanisms may be impaired, leading to overconsumption of food.

Resting Metabolic Rate

Total caloric expenditure, or the number of calories used by the body, is determined by basal metabolism and voluntary metabolism. Basal metabolism is the energy expended when the body is at rest. **Basal metabolic rate (BMR)** is usually measured in the morning after at least 8 hr of sleep and at least 12 hr after the last meal (i.e., in a postabsorptive state). Due to the difficulty of obtaining metabolic measurements in the basal state, the **resting metabolic rate (RMR)** is most commonly measured. The measurement is made 3 to 4 hr after the last meal and following a 30-min resting period on a day when there has been no vigorous physical activity. The RMR can be directly measured using calorimeters constructed for this purpose. However, for practical reasons, RMR is usually determined by indirect calorimetry. In this procedure, the amount of oxygen consumed and carbon dioxide produced is measured, with the person supine in a quiet, comfortable room. Oxygen consumption can be related to the number of calories expended in the resting state because approximately 5 kcal are produced per liter of oxygen consumed.

Resting metabolic rate is influenced by several factors; the primary determinant is body size. Specifically, RMR is in direct proportion to body surface area, which is related to height and weight. RMR decreases with age and is highest in a growing child. The decrease with advancing age may be because of muscle-tissue loss and an increase in percent body fat. When corrections are made for body size, women have lower RMRs than men; however, when expressed per unit of lean mass, RMRs for men and women are not different.

Voluntary metabolism is the energy required for muscle contraction and represents all of the energy expended by the body above the RMR. The number of calories expended by voluntary activity depends primarily on body weight and the amount of physical activity in which a person engages. Caloric expenditure is directly related to an individual's body weight. If two people, one weighing 100 lb and the other weighing 130 lb, jog 1 mi together, the heavier person will expend more energy. In addition, caloric expenditure is directly proportional to the amount of physical activity involved. Thus, the caloric cost of running or jogging is greater than for walking the same distance (see chapter 8).

Resting metabolic rate can be measured directly or indirectly, as already described. The limited size of calorimeters constructed to accommodate humans presents practical difficulty in determining the caloric cost of various physical activities. Therefore, the caloric expenditure of various physical activities is determined almost exclusively by indirect calorimetry. In this procedure, the oxygen consumed during various activities is measured. Like the RMR, oxygen consumption can be related to caloric expenditure because approximately 5 kcal are expended for each liter of oxygen consumed. The caloric cost of various activities is discussed in chapter 8.

Several convenient methods can be used to estimate a person's daily total caloric expenditure. Because the caloric costs of many activities have been determined, daily energy expenditure can be approximated by keeping a minute-by-minute daily activity record and finding the caloric cost of the activities. Adding together the cost of all activities provides an estimation of the total daily expenditure. This method of estimation is cumbersome, and precisely recording all activities in an entire day is difficult. Furthermore, as previously mentioned, caloric costs of activities depend on the amount of physical activity involved. For example, many of the available caloric-cost tables fail to indicate whether the reported cost of a given activity was determined at a leisurely or a fast pace.

Several equations estimate resting metabolic rate. The World Health Organization equations are listed in

Table 7.5   World Health Organization Equations for Estimating Resting Metabolic Rate (RMR)

Age	Equation for RMR (kcal/day)	SD
	MALES	
18-30	15.3 (kg)[a] + 679	151
30-60	11.6 (kg) + 879	164
> 60	13.5 (kg) + 487	148
	FEMALES	
18-30	14.7 (kg) + 496	121
30-60	8.7 (kg) + 829	108
> 60	10.5 (kg) + 596	108

[a](kg) = body weight in kilograms.

Report of a Joint FAO/WHO Expert Consultation. Energy and Protein Requirements. World Health Organization, 1985.

Table 7.5. Additional calories should be added to the estimated RMR, based on physical activity level. Depending on whether the person is sedentary or very active, 400 to 800 kcal may be added. For example, a 25-year-old female who weighs 55 kg has an estimated RMR of approximately 1,304 kcal·day[-1] [(14.7) (55 kg) + 496]. If she is moderately active, 600 kcal per day is added to account for voluntary activity. Thus, her total daily energy expenditure is estimated to be approximately 1,904 kcal·day[-1]. Based on the standard deviation for this estimate, 68% (± 1SD) of moderately active 55-kg women will have true values between 1,783 and 2,025 kcal·day[-1].

EXERCISE AND WEIGHT CONTROL

Many weight-control programs attend almost exclusively to reducing caloric intake, and they leave energy expenditure virtually unexplored. Although the value of exercise as an integral part of weight-loss programs has been repeatedly emphasized, the results of recent studies suggest that many adults do not follow the weight-loss guidelines of combining caloric restriction with exercise. In the 1985 National Health Interview Survey (19), only 58% of males and 57% of females increased their physical activity during a weight-loss program. Further, a 1987 Behavioral Risk Factor Surveillance System study of overweight men and women found that only 20.2% and 31.4%, respectively, combined caloric reduction and exercise in attempts to lose weight. Exercise provides a way to increase energy output relative to energy input, which may cause weight loss in itself or accelerate the effects of a reduction in caloric intake by dieting. If energy intake remains constant over time, an increase in energy expenditure can produce a negative energy balance and weight loss, regardless of the cause of excess accumulation of adipose tissue.

A common misconception is that exercise cannot create an effective caloric deficit because of its stimulatory effects on appetite. Actually, food intake is regulated by physical activity for nonsedentary individuals. Thus when activity increases, intake increases slightly. However, no change in body weight or body fat occurs. But very high levels of physical activity have a definite appetite-stimulating effect. For example, lumberjacks and marathon runners may consume more than 6,000 kcal per day. However, this increased caloric intake is required just to meet the body's daily energy output. This is evident from the fact that individuals engaged in physical labor and intense athletic training are characteristically quite lean, in spite of large caloric intakes. On the other hand, when there is no physical activity, the regulation of caloric intake is disrupted, and intake paradoxically increases. Sedentary individuals eat more, rather than less, and are heavier.

Regarding the acute effects of exercise on appetite, Epstein, Masek, and Marshall (6) found that decreased food intake followed prelunch exercise in previously sedentary obese children. The amount of exercise was inversely related to the decrease in caloric intake: The greatest decrease in intake was observed in children with the greatest increase in energy expenditure. One frequently overlooked benefit of a regular program of physical activity is its diversionary effects on caloric intake. In other words, while exercising, a person cannot be eating or snacking. The longer and more frequent the exercise, the greater the potential caloric deficit by decreasing eating.

Another frequently advanced argument against exercise as an effective weight-management tool is that relatively little energy is expended. For example, in jogging 1 mi, a 150-lb man expends only 100 kcal. At a cost of 3,500 kcal per pound of fat, if caloric intake remains constant, he must jog 35 mi to create a deficit equal to 1-lb fat loss. On a long-term basis, however, the situation is not as discouraging. If he jogs 2 mi per day, 5 days per week, he will lose approximately 1 lb of fat every 3.5 weeks. This is equivalent to 16 lb per year if caloric intake is not changed. With a concomitant slight decrease in intake, a weight loss can be substantially accelerated. Remember that a caloric deficit of 3,500 kcal results in a 1-lb fat loss, whether it occurs all at once or over a long period of time. Exercise should also be emphasized as an integral part of weight-management programs due to its positive relationship to maintenance of weight loss. Follow-up studies of individuals who are in weight-loss programs indicate that those who maintain their weight losses are those who exercise (18).

Individuals involved in weight-management programs should be encouraged to make exercise a regular part of their daily routine at home, work, or school by substituting physical work for patterns of inactivity. Chapter 12 deals with specific suggestions for increasing energy expenditure as a part of the regular daily routine. In addition, increased energy expenditure should be promoted during leisure time by using exercise programs. A major criterion for selection of an exercise for weight loss is total caloric expenditure. This choice, however, must be balanced against behavioral and physiological requirements. Long-duration exercise increases caloric expenditure, but it may also cause decreased adherence. For most people, social activities promote adherence more than solitary ones, and the activity chosen should not promote injuries that would limit further participation. A model exercise for weight control would, therefore, be aerobic in nature and lead to a large total energy expenditure (compared to calisthenics, for example). Exercise should be done with others, require minimal equipment, and should not have a high injury rate, and many people should be able to experience success in its participation. We recommend walking, swimming, and bicycling, because of the low-impact nature of these activities. Once the person can walk about 4 mi (or do the equivalent, for swimming or bicycling), she or he can progress to jogging or exercise-to-music programs (see chapter 14 for details).

Postexercise Energy Expenditure

An attractive idea, particularly to those interested in weight control, is that a single exercise bout may have a prolonged effect on RMR that could contribute to the total energy cost of the exercise. Although some studies report a rapid decline in metabolic rate following exercise, others report an increase in energy expenditure up to 24 hr postexercise for exercise of prolonged duration. The increase in **postexercise energy expenditure** has been reported to be linear with exercise intensity and duration. However, this is due to variations in total work accomplished during the exercise bout, rather than varying intensities and durations per se. Detecting small changes in RMR requires that before and after measurements be standardized, including adequate control of diet and physical activity prior to measurement of the baseline RMR. With appropriate controls, there will be few fluctuations in RMR, with day-to-day reproducibility. Individuals should not expect a significant calorigenic effect during recovery from exercise, unless the exercise is intense and of prolonged duration. For low- to moderately high-intensity exercise, the elevation is not of sufficient magnitude to contribute significantly to negative caloric balance in a weight-management program (4).

Spot Reduction

Many people think exercise that involves a certain area of the body actually reduces the amount of fat over that area. Unfortunately, this is not true. Genetic and hormonal factors control fat deposition to a large extent. Even with considerable energy expenditure, nothing guarantees that fat will be lost in the area exercised. This is not to imply that calisthenics and resistance exercises are of no value. They can increase strength and muscle tone, giving a slimming effect. In general, fat loss occurs first from the area of the body where it was last deposited.

INTERACTION OF DIET AND EXERCISE

One way the energy equation can be unbalanced to achieve weight reduction is to reduce caloric intake. For example, suppose a woman consumes an average of 2,650 kcal each day. If she reduces her caloric intake by 500 kcal per day to 2,150 kcal and maintains the same level of physical activity, she will lose approximately 1 lb of body fat per week. By maintaining this reduced intake she will lose approximately 4 lb per month, or 48 lb per year. However, a serious drawback to weight reduction by caloric restriction alone is apparent. Research has shown that significant amounts of the weight loss is lean body tissue with this method of weight control (21).

Exercise can also be used to produce a caloric deficit. To achieve the same daily 500-kcal deficit as above using exercise alone would require that a person do the equivalent of a 5-mi run or jog each day. Such a commitment is overwhelming for most people. Regarding body composition changes, it has been shown that regular exercise generally leads to the loss of body weight accompanied by a decrease in percent body fat. Lean body mass may increase or not change.

A more reasonable way to create a caloric deficit is through a combination of caloric restriction and exercise. For example, caloric intake can be decreased by 300 kcal per day and caloric expenditure can be increased by 200 kcal per day (the equivalent of a 2-mi run/jog). This leads to the same loss of approximately 1 lb per week. However, there is more fat loss with this method than with caloric restriction alone, and less than one half of the loss of lean muscle mass (21). Additional advantages are increased muscle tone and improved cardiovascular fitness.

Also consider the consequences of weight gain resulting from a positive caloric balance. If caloric intake exceeds caloric expenditure, and a person is engaging in a strenuous exercise program, weight gain is primarily in the form of muscle gain. Because of the hormone testosterone, men have more muscle-weight gain than women. On the other hand, if a person is not engaging in exercise, and caloric intake exceeds expenditure, then the weight gain is in the form of fat. If caloric consumption and expenditure are in balance, and a person engages in regular exercise, lean muscle mass increases and fat tissue correspondingly decreases.

Conversely, if a person is in caloric balance and decreases physical activity, lean muscle mass is lost and fat tissue increases.

SUMMARY

Excess body fat is a risk factor for heart disease and diabetes. The HFI must be able to estimate body fatness and predict an ideal weight consistent with optimal health. Underwater weighing, skinfold measurement, and bioelectrical impedance are being used for this purpose. For body weight to be maintained, caloric intake must equal caloric expenditure. Caloric intake can be estimated by dietary recall, and caloric expenditure can be predicted on the basis of body size, gender, and estimated activity level. A deficit of 3,500 kcal is needed to lose 1 lb of fat. A balanced program of exercise and dietary reduction, rather than diet alone, is recommended for weight loss.

CASE STUDIES FOR ANALYSIS

7.1 A large frame male is 6 ft 2 in. tall and weighs 220 lbs. His weight in water is 3.0 kg. The water density is .9965 kg•L^{-1}, and his residual volume is 900 ml.

Determine his relative weight (RW), and classify him according to his RW.

Determine his Body Mass Index (BMI) and indicate what this means with regard to his health.

Using the body fat values recommended for "fitness," calculate the following:

1) Fat weight
2) Lean body weight
3) Desirable weight (use upper value in the "fitness" range)
4) Desirable adipose tissue loss

If this subject decreases his average caloric intake to 2600 kcal per day, and increases his average daily expenditure to 3350 kcal per day, how long will it take for him to reach his desirable weight? (See Appendix A.)

7.2 A 175 lb female is 34% body fat and has waist and hip circumferences of 36 in. and 42 in., respectively. Based on her waist to hip ratio, what would you conclude about her relative risk of cardiovascular disease? (See Appendix A.)

REFERENCES

1. American College of Sports Medicine (1991)
2. Bonge and Donnelly (1989)
3. Booth (1980)
4. Brehm (1988)
5. Brozek, Grande, Anderson, and Keys (1963)
6. Epstein, Masek, and Marshall (1978)
7. Hubert (1983)
8. Jackson, Pollock, Graves, and Mahar (1988)
9. Jackson and Pollock (1978)
10. Jackson, Pollock, and Ward (1980)
11. Lohman (1985)
12. Lohman (1986)
13. Pollock and Wilmore (1990)
14. Schull (1990)
15. Schutte and Linkswiler (1984)
16. Segal, Gutin, Presta, Wang, and Van Itallie (1985)
17. Siri (1956)
18. Stunkard (1984)
19. U.S. Department of Health and Human Services (1985)
20. Van Itallie (1988)
21. Zuti and Golding (1976)

SUGGESTED READINGS

Doxey, Fairbanks, Housh, Johnson, Katch, and Lohman (1987)
Hubert, Feinleib, McNamara, and Castelli (1983)
World Health Organization (1985)

See the Bibliography at the end of the book for a complete source listing.

Chapter 8

Energy Costs of Activity

OBJECTIVES

The reader will be able to:

- Distinguish between direct and indirect calorimetry and between open and closed systems to measure oxygen consumption
- List the number of calories derived per liter of oxygen and per gram of carbohydrate, fat, and protein
- Express energy expenditure as $L \cdot min^{-1}$, $kcal \cdot min^{-1}$, $ml \cdot kg^{-1} \cdot min^{-1}$, METs, and $kcal \cdot kg^{-1} \cdot hr^{-1}$
- Estimate the energy cost of walking, jogging, cycle ergometry, and stepping
- Identify the approximate energy cost of recreational, sport, and work activities

TERMS

The reader will be able to define or describe:

Caloric equivalent of oxygen

Closed-circuit spirometry

Direct calorimetry

Indirect calorimetry

Open-circuit spirometry

Respiratory exchange ratio (R)

Respiratory quotient (RQ)

Health Fitness Instructors are usually concerned about the following two questions when they recommend specific physical activities to participants:

1. Are the activities appropriate, in terms of exercise intensity, to achieve the target heart rate? (see chapter 13), and
2. Is the combination of intensity and duration appropriate for achieving an energy expenditure goal to balance or exceed caloric intake? (see chapter 7).

To deal with these questions, the HFI should become familiar with the energy costs of various activities. The purpose of this chapter is to offer some basic information about how to estimate the energy requirement of various physical activities and to summarize the values associated with common recreational activities.

WAYS TO MEASURE ENERGY EXPENDITURE

Energy expenditure can be measured by direct and indirect calorimetry. **Direct calorimetry** requires that the person perform an activity within a specially constructed chamber that is insulated and has water flowing through its walls. The water is warmed by the heat given off by the subject, and heat production can be calculated by knowing the volume of water flowing through the chamber per minute and the change in the temperature of the water from entry to exit. For example, a person does bench-stepping exercise in the chamber at the rate of 30 $steps \cdot min^{-1}$ using a 20-cm bench. The water flows through the walls of the chamber at 20

$L \cdot min^{-1}$, and the increase in the temperature of the water from entry to exit is 0.5 °C. Because it takes approximately 1 kcal to raise the temperature of 1 L of water 1 °C, the following calculation yields the approximate energy expenditure.

$$\frac{20\,L}{min} \cdot \frac{1\,kcal}{°C} \cdot 0.5\,°C = \frac{10\,kcal}{min}$$

Additional heat is lost from the subject by evaporation of water from the skin and respiratory passages. This heat loss can be measured and added to that picked up by the water to yield the rate of energy produced by the subject for that task.

Indirect calorimetry estimates energy production by measuring oxygen consumption. This technique, already described in chapter 3, relies on certain constants to convert liters of oxygen consumption to kilocalories expended. The constants are derived from measurements made in a bomb calorimeter, a heavy metal chamber into which carbohydrate, fat, or protein can be placed with 100% oxygen under pressure. The chamber is immersed in a water bath, and the food stuff is oxidized to CO_2 and H_2O when an electric spark sets the process in motion. The heat given off warms the water; it has been determined that carbohydrates, fats, and proteins give off approximately 4, 9, and 5.6 kcal of heat per gram, respectively. However, because the nitrogen in protein cannot be completely oxidized in the body and is excreted as urea, the physiological value for protein is $4.0\ kcal \cdot g^{-1}$. Knowing how many liters of oxygen are required to oxidize carbohydrates, fats, and proteins makes it possible to calculate the number of kilocalories we obtain when we use 1 L of oxygen. This is called the **caloric equivalent of oxygen**. Values for carbohydrate, fat, and protein are listed in Table 8.1. The table shows that carbohydrates give more *energy per liter* of oxygen than fats (5.0 vs. $4.7\ kcal \cdot L^{-1}$), whereas fats give more *energy per gram* of substrate than carbohydrate (9 vs. $4\ kcal \cdot g^{-1}$). If a person is using a 50/50 mixture of carbohydrates and fats during exercise, the caloric equivalent is $4.85\ kcal \cdot L^{-1}$, halfway between the value of 4.7 for fat and 5.0 for carbohydrates (16). The ratio of the carbon dioxide produced to the oxygen consumed is the **respiratory quotient (RQ)**, or the **respiratory exchange ratio (R)** (see chapter 3).

Indirect calorimetry employs two techniques to measure oxygen consumption: **closed-circuit** and **open-circuit spirometry**. In the closed-circuit technique the subject usually breathes 100% oxygen from a spirometer; the exhaled air passes through a chemical to absorb the carbon dioxide. The decrease in the volume of oxygen contained in the spirometer is a measure of the oxygen consumption. Because the carbon dioxide is absorbed, one cannot calculate a respiratory quotient, so a caloric equivalent of $4.82\ kcal \cdot L^{-1}$ is used to indicate that a mixture of carbohydrates, fats, and proteins is used. This closed-circuit technique has been used extensively to measure the basal metabolic rate (16).

Table 8.1   The Caloric Density, Caloric Equivalent, and the Respiratory Quotient Associated With the Oxidation of Carbohydrate, Fat, and Protein

Measurement	Carbohydrate	Fat	Protein[a]
Caloric density (kcal/g)	4.0	9.0	4.0
Caloric equivalent of 1 L of O_2 (kcal/L)	5.0	4.7	4.5
Respiratory quotient	1.0	0.7	0.8

Note. Adapted from "Energy Metabolism" by L.K. Knoebel. In *Physiology* (5th edition) by E. Selkurt (Ed.), 1984, Boston: Little Brown & Co.

[a]Does not include the energy derived from the oxidation of nitrogen in the amino acids, because the body excretes this as urea.

The open-circuit technique for measuring oxygen consumption and carbon dioxide production is the most common indirect calorimetry technique. In this procedure, oxygen consumption is calculated by simply subtracting the volume of oxygen exhaled from the volume of oxygen inhaled. The difference is taken as the oxygen uptake or oxygen consumption (see chapter 3 for details). Carbon dioxide production is calculated in the same manner. This makes it possible to calculate the respiratory exchange ratio (R). One can then determine which substrate, fat or carbohydrate, provided the most energy during work, and also determine what value to use for the caloric equivalent of 1 L of oxygen in the calculation of energy expenditure (i.e., 5.0 $kcal \cdot L^{-1}$ for carbohydrates and 4.7 $kcal \cdot L^{-1}$ for fats).

KEY POINT.   Although fats provide more than twice as many kilocalories per gram than do carbohydrates, 9 vs. 4 $kcal \cdot gm^{-1}$, carbohydrates provide more kilocalories per liter of O_2 than do fats, 5.0 vs. 4.7 $kcal \cdot L^{-1}$.

WAYS TO EXPRESS ENERGY EXPENDITURE

The energy requirement for an activity is calculated on the basis of a subject's steady-state oxygen uptake ($\dot{V}O_2$) measured during an activity. Once the steady-state (leveling-off) oxygen uptake is reached, the energy (ATP) supplied to the muscles is derived from the aerobic metabolism of the various substrates. The measured oxygen uptake can then be used to express energy expenditure in different ways. The five most common expressions follow:

1. $\dot{V}O_2$ ($L \cdot min^{-1}$). The calculation of oxygen uptake (chapter 3 and Appendix B) yields a value expressed in liters of oxygen used per minute. For example, the following data were collected during a submaximal run on a treadmill on an 80-kg man: pulmonary ventilation = 60 $L \cdot min^{-1}$; expired O_2 = 16.93%.

$$\dot{V}O_2 (L \cdot min^{-1}) = 60 \, L \cdot min^{-1} \cdot (20.93\% \, O_2 - 16.93\% \, O_2)$$

$$= 2.4 \, L \cdot min^{-1}$$

2. $Kcal \cdot min^{-1}$. Oxygen uptake can be expressed in kilocalories used per minute. The caloric equivalent of 1 L of O_2 ranges from 4.7 kcal when fat is used as the sole fuel to 5.0 kcal when carbohydrate is used as the only fuel. For practical reasons, and with little loss in precision, 5 kcal per liter of O_2 is used to convert the oxygen uptake to kilocalories per minute. The total kilocalorie expenditure is calculated by multiplying the kilocalories expended per minute (kcals $\cdot min^{-1}$) by the duration of the activity in minutes. For example, if the 80-kg subject mentioned above runs on the treadmill for 30 min at a $\dot{V}O_2$ = 2.4 $L \cdot min^{-1}$, the total caloric expenditure can be calculated as follows.

$$\frac{2.4 \, L}{min} \cdot \frac{5 \, kcal}{L \, O_2} = \frac{12 \, kcal}{min}$$

$$\frac{12 \, kcal}{min} \cdot 30 \, min = 360 \, kcal$$

3. $\dot{V}O_2$ ($ml \cdot kg^{-1} \cdot min^{-1}$). If the measured oxygen uptake, expressed in liters per minute, is multiplied by 1,000 to yield milliliters per minute and then divided by the subject's body weight in kilograms, the value is expressed in ml O_2 per kilogram of body weight per minute, or $ml \cdot kg^{-1} \cdot min^{-1}$. This facilitates comparisons among people of different body sizes. For example, for the 80-kg subject with a $\dot{V}O_2$ = 2.4 $L \cdot min^{-1}$:

$$\frac{2.4 \, L}{min} \cdot \frac{1,000 \, ml}{L} \div 80 \, kg = (30 \, ml \cdot kg^{-1} \cdot min^{-1})$$

4. **METs.** The resting metabolic rate (oxygen uptake) is approximately 3.5 ml•kg^{-1}•min^{-1}. This is called 1 MET. Activities are expressed in terms of multiples of the MET unit. For example, using the values presented above,

$$30 \text{ ml•kg}^{-1}\text{•min}^{-1} \div 3.5 \text{ ml•kg}^{-1}\text{•min}^{-1} = 8.6 \text{ METs}$$

5. **Kcal•kg^{-1}•hr^{-1}.** The MET expression of energy expenditure carries a special bonus; the value also indicates the number of kilocalories the subject uses per kilogram of body weight per hour. In the example mentioned above, the subject is working at 8.6 METs, or about 30 ml•kg^{-1}•min^{-1}. When this value is multiplied by 60 min•hr^{-1}, it equals 1,800 ml•kg^{-1}•hr^{-1}, or 1.8 L•kg^{-1}•hr^{-1}. If the person is using a mixture of carbohydrates and fats as the fuel, then this oxygen consumption is multiplied by 4.85 kcal per L O$_2$ to give 8.7 kcal•kg^{-1}•hr^{-1}. The following steps show the detail.

$$8.6 \text{ METs} \cdot \frac{3.5 \text{ ml•kg}^{-1}\text{•min}^{-1}}{\text{MET}} = 30 \text{ ml•kg}^{-1}\text{•min}^{-1}$$

$$30 \text{ ml•kg}^{-1}\text{•min}^{-1} \cdot 60 \text{ min•hr}^{-1} = 1,800 \text{ ml•kg}^{-1}\text{•hr}^{-1} = 1.8 \text{ L•kg}^{-1}\text{•hr}^{-1}$$

$$1.8 \text{ L•kg}^{-1}\text{•hr}^{-1} \cdot 4.85 \text{ kcal•L O}_2^{-1} = 8.7 \text{ kcal•kg}^{-1}\text{•hr}^{-1}$$

FORMULAS FOR ESTIMATING THE ENERGY COST OF ACTIVITIES

In the mid-1970s the American College of Sports Medicine (ACSM) identified some simple formulas to estimate the steady-state energy requirement associated with common modes of activities used in graded exercise stress tests (GXTs): walking, stepping, running, and cycle ergometry (1). The oxygen uptake calculated from these formulas is an *estimate*, and a typical standard deviation associated with the actual *measured average* value is about 9% of the value (7). This normal variation in the energy cost of activities is important to remember when using these equations in prescribing exercise.

The ACSM formulas have been applied to GXTs to estimate functional capacity, or maximal aerobic power. This application has been shown to give reasonable estimates when the subjects are healthy and the rate at which the GXT progresses is slow enough to allow a steady-state oxygen uptake to be achieved at each stage (18, 19). When the increments in the stages of the GXT are large or the subject being tested is somewhat unfit, the subject's oxygen uptake will not keep pace with each stage of the test. In these cases the formulas overestimate the actual measured oxygen uptake (12). The fact that this overestimation is more likely to happen in diseased populations (e.g., cardiac) suggests that the GXTs used may be too aggressive. A test that progresses at a slower rate and allows the subject to reach the steady-state $\dot{V}O_2$ at each stage reduces the chance of an overestimation of functional capacity and still requires the subject to work at an appropriate metabolic rate to overload the system (see chapter 9). The previous information is presented to clarify the usefulness of the following equations. The formulas *estimate the steady-state energy requirements* for activities.

In the development of the ACSM equations, an attempt was made to use a true physiological oxygen-cost for each type of work. Each activity is broken down into the energy components. That is, in estimating the total oxygen cost of grade walking, add the net oxygen cost of the horizontal walk to the net oxygen cost of the vertical (grade) walk to the resting metabolic rate, which is taken to be 1 MET (3.5 ml•kg^{-1}•min^{-1}).

$$\text{Total O}_2 \text{ cost} = \text{net oxygen cost of activity} + 3.5 \text{ ml•kg}^{-1}\text{•min}^{-1}$$

Note that for the formulas to estimate the oxygen cost of the activity, the subject must follow instructions carefully (e.g., to not hold on to the treadmill railing; to maintain pedal cadence), and the work instruments (treadmill, cycle ergometer) must be calibrated so the settings are correct (see chapter 5).

ENERGY REQUIREMENTS OF COMMON ACTIVITIES

The following sections provide formulas to estimate the energy cost of walking, running, cycle ergometry, and stepping. These activities are common to cardiac rehabilitation and adult fitness programs. Examples are provided to show how the formulas are used in designing exercise programs.

Walking

On a Horizontal Surface

One of the most common activities used in an exercise program and in GXTs is walking. The following formula can be used to estimate the energy requirement between the walking speeds of 50 and 100 $m \cdot min^{-1}$ (1.9 to 3.7 $mi \cdot hr^{-1}$).

- **Multiply miles per hour by 26.8 to obtain meters per minute.**
- **Divide meters per minute by 26.8 to obtain miles per hour.**

Dill (9) showed that the net cost of walking 1 $m \cdot min^{-1}$ on a horizontal surface is 0.100 to 0.106 $ml \cdot kg^{-1} \cdot min^{-1}$. A value of 0.1 $ml \cdot kg^{-1} \cdot min^{-1}$ is used in the ACSM equations to simplify calculations without too much loss in precision. The equation for calculating the oxygen cost ($ml \cdot kg^{-1} \cdot min^{-1}$) of walking on a flat surface is

$$\dot{V}O_2 = 0.1\ ml \cdot kg^{-1} \cdot min^{-1} \text{ (horizontal velocity)} + 3.5\ ml \cdot kg^{-1} \cdot min^{-1}$$

QUESTION: What are the estimated steady-state $\dot{V}O_2$ and METs for a walking speed of 90 $m \cdot min^{-1}$ (3.4 $mi \cdot hr^{-1}$)?

ANSWER:

$$\dot{V}O_2 = 90\ m \cdot min^{-1} \cdot \frac{0.1\ ml \cdot kg^{-1} \cdot min^{-1}}{m \cdot min^{-1}} + 3.5\ ml \cdot kg^{-1} \cdot min^{-1}$$

$$\dot{V}O_2 = 9.0\ ml \cdot kg^{-1} \cdot min^{-1} + 3.5\ ml \cdot kg^{-1} \cdot min^{-1} = 12.5\ ml \cdot kg^{-1} \cdot min^{-1}$$

$$METs = 12.5\ ml \cdot kg^{-1} \cdot min^{-1} \div 3.5\ ml \cdot kg^{-1} \cdot min^{-1} = 3.6$$

The formulas can also be used to predict the level of activity required to elicit a specific energy expenditure.

QUESTION: An unfit participant is told to exercise at 11.5 $ml \cdot kg^{-1} \cdot min^{-1}$ to achieve the proper exercise intensity. What walking speed would you recommend?

ANSWER:

$$11.5\ ml \cdot kg^{-1} \cdot min^{-1} = ?\ m \cdot min^{-1} \cdot \frac{0.1\ ml \cdot kg^{-1} \cdot min^{-1}}{m \cdot min^{-1}} + 3.5\ ml \cdot kg^{-1} \cdot min^{-1}$$

Subtract 3.5 $ml \cdot kg^{-1} \cdot min^{-1}$ from 11.5 $ml \cdot kg^{-1} \cdot min^{-1}$ to obtain the *net O_2 cost* of the activity (8.0 $ml \cdot kg^{-1} \cdot min^{-1}$). The net cost is divided by 0.1 $ml \cdot kg^{-1} \cdot min^{-1}$ per $m \cdot min^{-1}$ to yield 80 $m \cdot min^{-1}$ (3 $mi \cdot hr^{-1}$):

$$8\ ml \cdot kg^{-1} \cdot min^{-1} = ?\ m \cdot min^{-1} \cdot \frac{0.1\ ml \cdot kg^{-1} \cdot min^{-1}}{m \cdot min^{-1}}$$

$$80 \text{ m} \cdot \text{min}^{-1} = 8 \text{ ml} \cdot \text{kg}^{-1} \cdot \text{min}^{-1} \div \frac{0.1 \text{ ml} \cdot \text{kg}^{-1} \cdot \text{min}^{-1}}{\text{m} \cdot \text{min}^{-1}}$$

$$3.0 \text{ mi} \cdot \text{hr}^{-1} = 80 \text{ m} \cdot \text{min}^{-1} \div \frac{26.8 \text{ m} \cdot \text{min}^{-1}}{\text{mi} \cdot \text{hr}^{-1}}$$

Up a Grade

The oxygen cost of grade walking is the sum of the oxygen cost of horizontal walking, the oxygen cost of the vertical component, and 3.5 ml·kg⁻¹·min⁻¹ for rest. Studies have shown that the oxygen cost of moving (walking or stepping) 1 m·min⁻¹ vertically is 1.8 ml·kg⁻¹·min⁻¹ [see (5, 20)]. The vertical velocity is calculated by multiplying the grade (expressed as a fraction) times the speed in meters per minute. A person walking at 80 m·min⁻¹ on a 10% grade is walking 8 m·min⁻¹ vertically (10% of 80 m·min⁻¹). The equation for calculating the oxygen cost (ml·kg⁻¹·min⁻¹) of walking on a grade is

$$\dot{V}O_2 = 0.1 \text{ ml} \cdot \text{kg}^{-1} \cdot \text{min}^{-1} \text{ (horizontal velocity)} +$$

$$1.8 \text{ ml} \cdot \text{kg}^{-1} \cdot \text{min}^{-1} \text{ (vertical velocity)} + 3.5 \text{ ml} \cdot \text{kg}^{-1} \cdot \text{min}^{-1}$$

QUESTION: What is the total oxygen cost of walking 90 m·min⁻¹ up a 12% grade?

ANSWER:

Horizontal component: Calculated as in preceding equation and equals 9 ml·kg⁻¹·min⁻¹

Vertical component:

$$\dot{V}O_2 = 0.12 \text{ (grade)} \cdot 90 \text{ m} \cdot \text{min}^{-1} \cdot \frac{1.8 \text{ ml} \cdot \text{kg}^{-1} \cdot \text{min}^{-1}}{\text{m} \cdot \text{min}^{-1}}$$

$$= 19.4 \text{ ml} \cdot \text{kg}^{-1} \cdot \text{min}^{-1}$$

$$\dot{V}O_2 \text{ (ml} \cdot \text{kg}^{-1} \cdot \text{min}^{-1}) = 9.0 \text{ (horizontal)} + 19.4 \text{ (vertical)} + 3.5 \text{ (rest)}$$

$$= 31.9 \text{ ml} \cdot \text{kg}^{-1} \cdot \text{min}^{-1}, \text{ or } 9.1 \text{ METs}$$

As indicated earlier, the formulas can be used to estimate the settings needed to elicit a specific oxygen uptake.

QUESTION: Set the treadmill grade to achieve an energy requirement of 6 METs (21.0 ml·kg⁻¹·min⁻¹) when walking at 60 m·min⁻¹.

ANSWER:

The net O_2 cost of the activity is equal to 21 minus 3.5, or 17.5 ml·kg⁻¹·min⁻¹.

$$\text{Horizontal component} = 60 \text{ m} \cdot \text{min}^{-1} \cdot \frac{0.1 \text{ ml} \cdot \text{kg}^{-1} \cdot \text{min}^{-1}}{\text{m} \cdot \text{min}^{-1}}$$

$$= 6.0 \text{ ml} \cdot \text{kg}^{-1} \cdot \text{min}^{-1}$$

$$\text{Vertical component} = 17.5 - 6.0 = 11.5 \text{ ml} \cdot \text{kg}^{-1} \cdot \text{min}^{-1}$$

$$11.5 \text{ ml} \cdot \text{kg}^{-1} \cdot \text{min}^{-1} = \text{fractional grade} \cdot 60 \text{ m} \cdot \text{min}^{-1} \cdot \frac{1.8 \text{ ml} \cdot \text{kg}^{-1} \cdot \text{min}^{-1}}{\text{m} \cdot \text{min}^{-1}}$$

$$11.5 \text{ ml} \cdot \text{kg}^{-1} \cdot \text{min}^{-1} = \text{fractional grade} \cdot 108 \text{ ml} \cdot \text{kg}^{-1} \cdot \text{min}^{-1}$$

$$\text{Fractional grade} = 11.5 \div 108 = 0.106 \cdot 100\% = 10.6\% \text{ grade}$$

At Different Speeds

The preceding formulas are useful within the range of walking speeds of 50 to 100 m•min^{-1} (1.9 to 3.7 mi•hr^{-1}); beyond that, the oxygen requirement for walking increases in a curvilinear manner (7). Because many people choose to walk at a fast speed rather than jog, knowledge of the energy requirements for walking at these higher speeds is useful in prescribing exercise. Values for the energy requirement for walking on the level and at various grades at these faster speeds (4.0 to 5.0 mi•hr^{-1}) are included in Table 8.2.

Table 8.2 Energy Requirement, in METs, for Walking at Various Speeds (mi · hr^{-1} or m · min^{-1}) and Grades (%)

	Miles per hour/Meters per minute						
% Grade	2.0/54	2.5/67	3.0/80	3.5/94	4.0/107	4.5/121	5.0/134
0	2.5	2.9	3.3	3.7	4.9	6.2	7.9
2	3.1	3.6	4.1	4.7	5.9	7.4	9.3
4	3.6	4.3	4.9	5.6	7.1	8.7	10.6
6	4.2	5.0	5.8	6.6	8.1	9.9	12.0
8	4.7	5.7	6.6	7.5	9.3	11.1	13.4
10	5.3	6.3	7.4	8.5	10.4	12.4	14.8
12	5.8	7.1	8.3	9.5	11.4	13.6	16.6
14	6.4	7.7	9.1	10.4	12.6	14.9	17.5
16	6.9	8.4	9.9	11.4	13.6	16.1	18.9
18	7.5	9.1	10.7	12.4	14.8	17.4	20.3
20	8.1	9.8	11.6	13.3	15.9	18.6	21.7
22	8.6	10.3	12.4	14.3	17.0	19.9	23.1
24	9.1	11.1	13.2	15.3	18.1	21.1	
26	9.7	11.9	14.0	16.2	19.2	22.3	
28	10.3	12.5	14.9	17.2	20.3	23.6	
30	10.8	13.2	15.7	18.2	21.4		

Note. Adapted from *Guidelines for Exercise Stress Testing and Prescription* (3rd edition, 1986) and W.J. Bubb, A.D. Martin, and E.T. Howley (1985).

One of the most common and useful ways the energy cost of walking can be expressed is in kilocalories per minute. In this way, the HFI can simply look up the speed of the walk in a table, identify the number of calories used per minute, and calculate the total energy expenditure, depending on the duration of the walk. Table 8.3 presents the energy cost (in kilocalories per minute) for walking at speeds of 2 to 5 mi•hr^{-1} and includes values for people of different body weights. It is no surprise that the energy cost of walking increases with the speed of the walk; however, the rate of increase is higher at the higher speeds. For example, when walking speed increases from 2 to 3 mi•hr^{-1} for a 170-lb participant, the energy cost increases from 3.2 to 4.2 kcal•min^{-1}. But going from 4 to 5 mi•hr^{-1} requires an increase from 6.3 to 10.2 kcal•min^{-1}. It is clear that the very sedentary individual can walk at slow speeds and achieve the desired exercise intensity, and the relatively fit individual can walk at high speeds at which the elevated energy requirement provides the necessary stimulus for a training effect. As a participant loses weight, the energy cost of walking at a certain speed decreases, because the energy cost is dependent on body weight. One can compensate by walking for a longer period of time or increasing the speed of the walk.

Jogging and Running

Jogging and running are common activities used in fitness programs for apparently healthy individuals. Using the ACSM equations it is possible to estimate the oxygen cost of these

Table 8.3 Energy Costs of Walking (kcal · min⁻¹)

| Body weight | | Miles per hour | | | | | | |
kg	lb	2.0	2.5	3.0	3.5	4.0	4.5	5.0
50.0	110	2.1	2.4	2.8	3.1	4.1	5.2	6.6
54.5	120	2.3	2.6	3.0	3.4	4.4	5.6	7.2
59.1	130	2.5	2.9	3.2	3.6	4.8	6.1	7.8
63.6	140	2.7	3.1	3.5	3.9	5.2	6.6	8.4
68.2	150	2.8	3.3	3.7	4.2	5.6	7.0	9.0
72.7	160	3.0	3.5	4.0	4.5	5.9	7.5	9.6
77.3	170	3.2	3.7	4.2	4.8	6.3	8.0	10.2
81.8	180	3.4	4.0	4.5	5.0	6.7	8.4	10.8
86.4	190	3.6	4.2	4.7	5.3	7.0	8.9	11.4
90.9	200	3.8	4.4	5.0	5.6	7.4	9.4	12.0
95.4	210	4.0	4.6	5.2	5.9	7.8	9.9	12.6
100.0	220	4.2	4.8	5.5	6.2	8.2	10.3	13.2

Note. Multiply value by the duration of the activity to obtain total calories expended.

activities for a broad range of speeds, generally from 130 to 350 $m \cdot min^{-1}$. However, the equations are also useful at speeds below 130 $m \cdot min^{-1}$ as long as the person is really jogging. The fact that a person can walk or jog at speeds below 130 $m \cdot min^{-1}$ complicates the issue. The O_2 cost of walking is less than that of jogging at slow speeds; however, at approximately 135 to 140 $m \cdot min^{-1}$, the oxygen cost of jogging and walking are about the same. Above this speed the oxygen cost of walking exceeds that of jogging (3).

On a Horizontal Surface

The net oxygen cost of jogging or running 1 $m \cdot min^{-1}$ on a horizontal surface is about twice that of walking, 0.2 $ml \cdot kg^{-1} \cdot min^{-1}$ per $m \cdot min^{-1}$ (5, 6, 17). Remember that the equation will, in general, yield a reasonable estimate of the oxygen cost of running for average individuals. It is well known that trained runners are more economical than the average person, and also that running economy varies within any specific group, trained or untrained (6, 8). The equation used to estimate the oxygen cost ($ml \cdot kg^{-1} \cdot min^{-1}$) of running is

$$\dot{V}O_2 = 0.2\ ml \cdot kg^{-1} \cdot min^{-1}\ (\text{horizontal velocity}) + 3.5\ ml \cdot kg^{-1} \cdot min^{-1}$$

QUESTION: What is the oxygen requirement for running a 10K race on a track in 60 min?

ANSWER:

$$10{,}000\ m \div 60\ min = 167\ m \cdot min^{-1}$$

$$\dot{V}O_2 = 167\ m \cdot min^{-1} \cdot \frac{0.2\ ml \cdot kg^{-1} \cdot min^{-1}}{m \cdot min^{-1}} + 3.5\ ml \cdot kg^{-1} \cdot min^{-1}$$

$$\dot{V}O_2 = 36.9\ ml \cdot kg^{-1} \cdot min^{-1},\ \text{or } 10.5\ \text{METs}$$

QUESTION: A 20-year-old female distance runner with a $\dot{V}O_2max$ of 50 $ml \cdot kg^{-1} \cdot min^{-1}$ wants to run intervals at 90% of $\dot{V}O_2max$. At what speed should she run on a track?

ANSWER:
90% of 50 = 45 $ml \cdot kg^{-1} \cdot min^{-1}$, and the net cost of the run is equal to 45 $ml \cdot kg^{-1} \cdot min^{-1}$ minus 3.5 $ml \cdot kg^{-1} \cdot min^{-1}$, or 41.5 $ml \cdot kg^{-1} \cdot min^{-1}$.

$$41.5 \text{ ml} \cdot \text{kg}^{-1} \cdot \text{min}^{-1} \div \frac{0.2 \text{ ml} \cdot \text{kg}^{-1} \cdot \text{min}^{-1}}{\text{m} \cdot \text{min}^{-1}} = 207 \text{ m} \cdot \text{min}^{-1}$$

$$1{,}610 \text{ m} \cdot \text{mi}^{-1} \div 207 \text{ m} \cdot \text{min}^{-1} = 7.78 \text{ min, or } 7{:}47\text{- (min:s) mi pace}$$

Up a Grade

There is not as much information about the oxygen cost of grade running as there is about the previous activities. But one thing is clear—the oxygen cost of running up a grade is about one half that of walking up a grade (17). Some of the vertical lift associated with running on a flat surface is used to accomplish some grade work during inclined running, lowering the net oxygen requirement for the vertical work. The oxygen cost of running 1 m·min^{-1} vertically is about 0.9 ml·kg^{-1}·min^{-1}. As in grade walking, the vertical velocity is calculated by multiplying the fractional grade times the horizontal velocity. The following equation is used for calculating the oxygen cost of grade running.

$$\dot{V}O_2 = 0.2 \text{ ml} \cdot \text{kg}^{-1} \cdot \text{min}^{-1} \text{ (horizontal velocity)} +$$

$$0.9 \text{ ml} \cdot \text{kg}^{-1} \cdot \text{min}^{-1} \text{ (vertical velocity)} + 3.5 \text{ ml} \cdot \text{kg}^{-1} \cdot \text{min}^{-1}$$

QUESTION: What is the oxygen cost of running 150 m·min^{-1} up a 10% grade?

ANSWER:
Horizontal component:

$$\dot{V}O_2 = 150 \text{ m} \cdot \text{min}^{-1} \cdot \frac{0.2 \text{ ml} \cdot \text{kg}^{-1} \cdot \text{min}^{-1}}{\text{m} \cdot \text{min}^{-1}} = 30 \text{ ml} \cdot \text{kg}^{-1} \cdot \text{min}^{-1}$$

Vertical component:

$$\dot{V}O_2 = 0.10 \text{ (fractional grade)} \cdot 150 \text{ m} \cdot \text{min}^{-1} \cdot \frac{0.9 \text{ ml} \cdot \text{kg}^{-1} \cdot \text{min}^{-1}}{\text{m} \cdot \text{min}^{-1}}$$

$$= 13.5 \text{ ml} \cdot \text{kg}^{-1} \cdot \text{min}^{-1}$$

$$\dot{V}O_2 = 30.0 \text{ (horizontal)} + 13.5 \text{ (vertical)} + 3.5 \text{ (rest)} = 47 \text{ ml} \cdot \text{kg}^{-1} \cdot \text{min}^{-1}$$

QUESTION: The oxygen cost of running 350 m·min^{-1} on the flat is about 73.5 ml·kg^{-1}·min^{-1}. What grade should be set on a treadmill for a speed of 300 m·min^{-1}, to achieve the same $\dot{V}O_2$?

ANSWER:
Horizontal component:

$$\dot{V}O_2 = 300 \text{ m} \cdot \text{min}^{-1} \cdot 0.2 \text{ ml} \cdot \text{kg}^{-1} \cdot \text{min}^{-1} \text{ per m} \cdot \text{min}^{-1} = 60 \text{ ml} \cdot \text{kg}^{-1} \cdot \text{min}^{-1}$$

Vertical component:

$$\text{Net } \dot{V}O_2 = 73.5 \text{ (total)} - 60 \text{ (horizontal)} - 3.5 \text{ (rest)} = 10.0 \text{ ml} \cdot \text{kg}^{-1} \cdot \text{min}^{-1}.$$

$$10 \text{ ml} \cdot \text{kg}^{-1} \cdot \text{min}^{-1} = \text{fractional grade} \cdot 300 \text{ m} \cdot \text{min}^{-1} \cdot \frac{0.9 \text{ ml} \cdot \text{kg}^{-1} \cdot \text{min}^{-1}}{\text{m} \cdot \text{min}^{-1}}$$

$$\text{Fractional grade} = 10 \text{ ml} \cdot \text{kg}^{-1} \cdot \text{min}^{-1} \div 270 \text{ ml} \cdot \text{kg}^{-1} \cdot \text{min}^{-1}$$

$$= .037 \text{ or } 3.7\% \text{ grade}$$

Table 8.4 summarizes the oxygen cost of running for level and graded running.

Table 8.4   Energy Requirement, in METs, for Jogging/Running at Various Speeds (mi · hr⁻¹ or m · min⁻¹) and Grades

	Miles per hour/Meters per minute							
% Grade	3/80	4/107	5/134	6/161	7/188	8/215	9/241	10/268
0	5.6	7.1	8.7	10.2	11.7	13.3	14.8	16.3
1	5.8	7.4	9.0	10.6	12.2	13.8	15.4	17.0
2	6.0	7.7	9.3	11.0	12.7	14.4	16.0	17.7
3	6.2	7.9	9.7	11.4	13.2	14.9	16.6	18.4
4	6.4	8.2	10.0	11.9	13.7	15.5	17.3	19.1
5	6.6	8.5	10.4	12.3	14.2	16.1	17.9	19.8
6	6.8	8.8	10.7	12.7	14.6	16.6	18.5	20.4
7	7.0	9.0	11.0	13.1	15.1	17.1	19.1	21.1
8	7.2	9.3	11.4	13.5	15.6	17.7	19.7	21.8
9	7.4	9.6	11.7	13.9	16.1	18.3	20.3	22.5
10	7.6	9.9	12.1	14.3	16.6	18.8	21.0	23.2

Note. Data from ACSM (1991).

At Different Speeds

In contrast to walking, the energy cost of jogging and running increases in a linear and predictable manner with increasing speed. Table 8.5 shows the caloric cost of running, in kilocalories per minute, for participants of different body weights. If we consider the 170-lb participant, the energy cost increases from 7.2 to 11.2 kcal•min⁻¹ when increasing speed from 3 to 5 mi•hr⁻¹; the increase is also 4 kcal•min⁻¹ when increasing the speed from 7 to 9 mi•hr⁻¹. As with walking, the energy cost is higher for heavier individuals.

Cycle Ergometry

Cycle ergometry exercise is common to a sport club, home, or rehabilitation program. Generally, energy expenditure is accomplished with less trauma to ankle, knee, and hip joints com-

Table 8.5   Energy Costs of Jogging and Running (kcal · min⁻¹)

Body weight		Miles per hour							
kg	lb	3.0	4.0	5.0	6.0	7.0	8.0	9.0	10.0
50.0	110	4.7	5.9	7.2	8.5	9.8	11.1	12.3	13.6
54.5	120	5.1	6.4	7.9	9.3	10.6	12.1	13.4	14.8
59.1	130	5.5	7.0	8.6	10.0	11.5	13.1	14.6	16.1
63.6	140	5.9	7.5	9.2	10.8	12.4	14.1	15.7	17.3
68.2	150	6.4	8.1	9.9	11.6	13.3	15.1	16.8	18.5
72.7	160	6.8	8.6	10.5	12.4	14.2	16.1	17.9	19.8
77.3	170	7.2	9.1	11.2	13.1	15.1	17.1	19.1	21.0
81.8	180	7.6	9.7	11.8	13.9	15.9	18.1	20.2	22.2
86.4	190	8.1	10.2	12.5	14.7	16.8	19.1	21.3	23.5
90.9	200	8.5	10.8	13.2	15.4	17.7	20.1	22.4	24.7
95.4	210	8.9	11.3	13.8	16.2	18.6	21.1	23.5	25.9
100.0	220	9.3	11.8	14.5	17.0	19.5	22.2	24.7	27.2

Note. Multiply value by the duration of the activity to obtain total calories expended.

pared to jogging. Cycle ergometers are used for conventional leg-exercise programs, but they are also adapted for arm exercise (by placing the ergometer on a table). The following sections describe how to estimate the energy costs of doing leg and arm cycle ergometry.

Legs

In the previous activities the individual was carrying his or her body weight, and the oxygen requirement was therefore proportional to body weight ($ml \cdot kg^{-1} \cdot min^{-1}$). This is not the case in cycle ergometry, in which an individual's body weight is supported by the cycle seat and the work rate is determined by the pedal rate and the resistance on the wheel. The oxygen requirement, in liters per minute, is *approximately* the same for people of different sizes for the same work rate. Thus, when a light person is doing the same work rate as a heavy person, the relative $\dot{V}O_2$ ($ml \cdot kg^{-1} \cdot min^{-1}$), or MET level, is higher for the lighter person.

The work rate is set on the simple, mechanically braked cycle ergometers by varying the force (weight, or load) on the wheel and the number of pedal revolutions per minute ($rev \cdot min^{-1}$). On the Monark cycle ergometer the wheel travels 6 m per pedal revolution; on the Tunturi ergometer the wheel travels only 3 m per revolution. Using the Monark ergometer as an example, a pedal rate of 50 $rev \cdot min^{-1}$ causes the wheel to travel a distance of 300 m (6 m per pedal revolution times 50 $rev \cdot min^{-1}$). If a 1-kilopond (kp) force (1-kg weight) were applied to the wheel, the work rate would be 300 kilopond meters per minute (300 $kpm \cdot min^{-1}$). Work rates are also expressed in watts (W), where 6.1 $kpm \cdot min^{-1}$ is equal to 1 W; the 300 $kpm \cdot min^{-1}$ work rate would be expressed as 50 W. The work rate can be doubled by changing the force from 1 kp to 2 kp or by changing the pedal rate from 50 to 100 $rev \cdot min^{-1}$. In contrast, some cycle ergometers are electrically controlled to deliver a specific work rate somewhat independent of pedal rate; as the pedal rate falls, the load on the wheel is proportionally increased.

The oxygen cost of doing 1 kpm of work is approximately 1.8 ml. During cycle ergometer exercise, some unmeasured "friction" work occurs in addition to the work rate that is set on the basis of pedal rate and force. This additional work requires about 10% of the oxygen required to do the measured work, so 0.2 $ml \cdot kpm^{-1}$ is added to the 1.8 $ml \cdot kpm^{-1}$ to get the net cost per kilopond meter of work on a cycle ergometer (2 $ml \cdot kpm^{-1}$). The oxygen cost of sitting on the cycle ergometer is approximately 300 $ml \cdot min^{-1}$ (2). The estimates from the following equation are reasonable for work rates between approximately 150 and 1,200 $kpm \cdot min^{-1}$ (see Table 8.6).

$$\dot{V}O_2 \ (ml \cdot min^{-1}) = \text{work rate} \ (kpm \cdot min^{-1}) \ (2 \ ml \ O^2 \cdot kpm^{-1}) + 300 \ ml \ O_2 \cdot min^{-1}$$

$$\dot{V}O_2 \ (ml \cdot min^{-1}) = \text{work rate} \ (W) \ (12 \ ml \ O_2 \cdot W^{-1}) + 300 \ ml \ O_2 \cdot min^{-1}$$

Table 8.6   Energy Expenditure, in METs, for Cycle Ergometry for Legs and Arms

Body weight		Work Rate ($kpm \cdot min^{-1}$ and watts)						
kg	lb	300/50	450/75	600/100	750/125	900/150	1050/175	1200/200
50	110	5.1 (6.9)	6.9 (9.4)	8.6 (12.0)	10.3 (—)	12.0 (—)	13.7 (—)	15.4 (—)
60	132	4.3 (5.7)	5.7 (7.8)	7.1 (10.0)	8.6 (12.1)	10.0 (—)	11.4 (—)	12.9 (—)
70	154	3.7 (4.9)	4.9 (6.7)	6.1 (8.6)	7.3 (10.4)	8.6 (12.2)	9.8 (—)	11.0 (—)
80	176	3.2 (4.3)	4.3 (5.9)	5.4 (7.5)	6.4 (9.1)	7.5 (10.7)	8.6 (12.3)	9.6 (—)
90	198	2.9 (3.8)	3.8 (5.2)	4.8 (6.7)	5.7 (8.1)	6.7 (9.5)	7.6 (10.9)	8.6 (12.3)
100	220	2.6 (3.4)	3.4 (4.7)	4.3 (6.0)	5.1 (7.3)	6.0 (8.6)	6.9 (9.9)	7.7 (11.1)

Note. Values in ( ) are for arm work. Adapted from *Guidelines for Exercise Stress Testing and Prescription* (4th ed.) (p. 299) by American College of Sports Medicine, 1991, Philadelphia: Lea and Febiger. Copyright 1991 by Lea and Febiger. And Franklin, Vanders, Wrisley, and Rubenfire (1983).

QUESTION: What is the oxygen cost of doing 600 kpm•min^{-1} (100 W) on a cycle ergometer for 50-kg and 100-kg subjects?

ANSWER:

$$\dot{V}O_2 = 600 \text{ kpm•min}^{-1} \cdot 2 \text{ ml } O_2\text{•kpm}^{-1} + 300 \text{ ml•min}^{-1}$$

$$\dot{V}O_2 = 1{,}500 \text{ ml•min}^{-1}, \text{ or } 1.5 \text{ L•min}^{-1}$$

For the 50-kg subject: $1{,}500 \text{ ml•min}^{-1} \div 50 \text{ kg} = 30 \text{ ml•kg}^{-1}\text{•min}^{-1}$, or 8.6 METs

For the 100-kg subject: $1{,}500 \text{ ml•min}^{-1} \div 100 \text{ kg} = 15 \text{ ml•kg}^{-1}\text{•min}^{-1}$, or 4.3 METs

In some exercise programs a participant might use a variety of pieces of exercise equipment to achieve a training effect, and might like to be able to set about the same intensity on each. In this regard, the formula for the cycle ergometer can be used to set the load to achieve a particular MET value on the cycle ergometer and bring it in balance with what is done during walking or jogging.

QUESTION: A 70-kg participant must work at 6 METs to match the intensity of his walking program. What force (load) should be set on a Monark cycle ergometer at a pedal rate of 50 rev•min^{-1}?

ANSWER:

$$6 \text{ METs} = 6 \,(3.5 \text{ ml•kg}^{-1}\text{•min}^{-1}) \cdot 70 \text{ kg} = 1{,}470 \text{ ml•min}^{-1}$$

$$\dot{V}O_2 = \text{kpm•min}^{-1} \cdot 2 \text{ ml } O_2\text{•kpm}^{-1} + 300 \text{ ml•min}^{-1}$$

$$\text{Net cost of cycling} = 1{,}470 - 300 = 1{,}170 \text{ ml•min}^{-1}$$

$$1{,}170 \text{ ml•min}^{-1} = ? \text{ kpm•min}^{-1} \cdot 2 \text{ ml•kpm}^{-1}$$

$$\text{Work rate (kpm•min}^{-1}) = 1{,}170 \div 2 = 585 \text{ kpm•min}^{-1}$$

$$585 \text{ kpm•min}^{-1} = (50 \text{ rev•min}^{-1} \cdot 6 \text{ m•rev}^{-1}) \cdot \text{force}$$

$$585 \text{ kpm•min}^{-1} = 300 \text{ m•min}^{-1} \cdot \text{force}$$

$$\text{Force} = 585 \text{ kpm•min}^{-1} \div 300 \text{ m•min}^{-1} = 1.95 \text{ kp}$$

Arms

A cycle ergometer can be used to exercise the arms and shoulder-girdle muscles by modifying the pedals and placing the cycle on a table. Arm ergometry is used on a limited basis as a GXT to evaluate cardiovascular function. It is used more generally as a routine exercise in rehabilitation programs (10).

Remember several factors when considering this type of exercise: (a) Functional capacity ($\dot{V}O_2$max) for the arms is only 70% of that measured with the legs in a normal healthy population, and less in an unfit, elderly, or diseased population; (b) the natural endurance of the muscles used in this work is less than that of the legs; (c) the HR and BP responses are higher for arm work compared to leg work at the same $\dot{V}O_2$; and (d) the oxygen cost of doing 1 kpm of work is about 50% higher (3 ml O_2•kpm^{-1}) for arm work because of the action's inefficiency (11). The formula for estimating the oxygen cost of arm work is

$$\dot{V}O_2 \text{ (ml•min}^{-1}) = \text{work rate (kpm•min}^{-1}) \,(3 \text{ ml } O_2\text{•kpm}^{-1}) + 300 \text{ ml•min}^{-1}$$

QUESTION: What is the oxygen requirement of doing 150 kpm•min^{-1} on an arm ergometer?

ANSWER:

$$\dot{V}O_2 = (150 \text{ kpm•min}^{-1}) \cdot (3 \text{ ml•kpm}^{-1}) + 300 \text{ ml•min}^{-1} = 750 \text{ ml•min}^{-1}$$

Stepping

One of the most useful and inexpensive forms of exercise is bench stepping. The activity is easily done at home and requires little or no equipment. The work rate is easily adjusted by simply increasing step height or cadence (number of lifts per minute).

The total oxygen cost of this exercise is the sum of the costs of (a) stepping up, (b) stepping down, and (c) moving back and forth on a level surface at the specified cadence. The oxygen cost of stepping up is $1.8 \text{ ml} \cdot \text{kg}^{-1} \cdot \text{min}^{-1}$ per $\text{m} \cdot \text{min}^{-1}$, as in walking (20). The oxygen cost of stepping down is a third of the cost of stepping up, therefore the oxygen cost of stepping up and down is 1.33 times the cost of stepping up. The number of meters moved up or down per minute is calculated by multiplying the number of lifts per minute by the height of the step (e.g., if the step height is 0.2 m (20 cm) and the cadence is 27 $\text{lifts} \cdot \text{min}^{-1}$, then the total lift or descent per minute is 27 times 0.2 m, or 5.4 $\text{m} \cdot \text{min}^{-1}$).

For step height

- **Multiply inches by 2.54 to obtain centimeters.**
- **Divide centimeters by 100 to obtain meters.**

The oxygen cost of stepping back and forth on a flat surface is proportional to the cadence. If the cadence is 15, the energy cost of moving back and forth at that rate is *about* 1.5 METs; if the cadence is 27, the energy requirement for moving back and forth on a flat surface is *about* 2.7 METs. In essence the oxygen cost of stepping back and forth on a flat surface can be estimated in METs by dividing the step rate by 10. Because 1 MET is $3.5 \text{ ml} \cdot \text{kg}^{-1} \cdot \text{min}^{-1}$, the oxygen cost of stepping back and forth can be estimated as 0.35 times the step rate (step rate $\cdot$ $0.35 \text{ ml} \cdot \text{kg}^{-1} \cdot \text{min}^{-1}$). The formula for estimating the energy requirement for stepping is

$$\dot{V}O_2 = (\text{step height in meters}) \, (\text{lifts} \cdot \text{min}^{-1}) \, (1.33) \, (1.8 \text{ ml} \cdot \text{kg}^{-1} \cdot \text{min}^{-1}) +$$

$$\text{step rate} \, (0.35 \text{ ml} \cdot \text{kg}^{-1} \cdot \text{min}^{-1})$$

QUESTION: What is the oxygen requirement for stepping at a rate of 20 $\text{lifts} \cdot \text{min}^{-1}$ on a 20-cm bench?

ANSWER:

$$\dot{V}O_2 = \frac{0.2 \text{ m}}{\text{lift}} \cdot \frac{20 \text{ lifts}}{\text{min}} \cdot 1.33 \cdot \frac{1.8 \text{ ml} \cdot \text{kg}^{-1} \cdot \text{min}^{-1}}{\text{m} \cdot \text{min}^{-1}} +$$

$$20 \, (0.35 \text{ ml} \cdot \text{kg}^{-1} \cdot \text{min}^{-1})$$

$$= 9.6 \text{ ml} \cdot \text{kg}^{-1} \cdot \text{min}^{-1} + 7.0 \text{ ml} \cdot \text{kg}^{-1} \cdot \text{min}^{-1}$$

$$= 16.6 \text{ ml} \cdot \text{kg}^{-1} \cdot \text{min}^{-1}, \text{ or } 4.7 \text{ METs}$$

Table 8.7 presents a summary of the energy requirements of stepping at different rates.

CALORIC COST OF WALKING AND RUNNING 1 MILE

In spite of the vast amount of information available regarding the costs of walking and running, a good deal of misunderstanding still exists. We hear claims that the energy cost of walking 1 mi is equal to that of running the same distance. In general, this is not the case (14). The formulas for estimating the energy cost of walking and running can be used to estimate the caloric cost of walking and running 1 mi, a piece of information that is useful in achieving energy expenditure goals.

Table 8.7   Energy Expenditure in METs During Stepping at Different Rates on Steps of Different Heights

Step height		Steps per minute			
cm	in.	12	18	24	30
0	0	1.2	1.8	2.4	3.0
4	1.6	1.5	2.3	3.1	3.8
8	3.2	1.9	2.8	3.7	4.6
12	4.7	2.2	3.3	4.4	5.5
16	6.3	2.5	3.8	5.0	6.3
20	7.9	2.8	4.3	5.7	7.1
24	9.4	3.2	4.8	6.3	7.9
28	11.0	3.5	5.2	7.0	8.7
32	12.6	3.8	5.7	7.7	9.6
36	14.2	4.1	6.2	8.3	10.4
40	15.8	4.5	6.7	9.0	11.2

Note. From *Guidelines for Graded Exercise Testing and Exercise Prescription*, ACSM, 1980, Philadelphia: Lea & Febiger. Copyright 1980 by Lea & Febiger. Reprinted with permission.

Walking

If a person walks at 3 mi•hr^{-1} (80 m•min^{-1}), 1 mi will be completed in 20 min. The caloric cost for walking 1 mi for a 70-kg person is

$$\dot{V}O_2 = 80 \text{ m•min}^{-1} \cdot 0.1 \text{ ml•kg}^{-1}\text{•min}^{-1} + 3.5 \text{ ml•kg}^{-1}\text{•min}^{-1}$$

$$\dot{V}O_2 = 11.5 \text{ ml•kg}^{-1}\text{•min}^{-1}$$

$$\dot{V}O_2 \text{ (ml•mi}^{-1}) = 11.5 \text{ ml•kg}^{-1}\text{•min}^{-1} \cdot 70 \text{ kg} \cdot 20 \text{ min•mi}^{-1} = 16{,}100 \text{ ml•mi}^{-1}$$

$$\dot{V}O_2 \text{ (L•min}^{-1}) = 16{,}100 \text{ ml•min}^{-1} \div 1{,}000 \text{ ml•L}^{-1} = 16.1 \text{ L•mi}^{-1}$$

At about 5.0 kcal per L O_2, the *gross caloric cost* per mi of walking is 80.5 kcal (5 kcal•L^{-1} • 16.1 L•mi^{-1}). The *net caloric cost* for the mile walk can be calculated by subtracting the oxygen cost of 20 min of rest from the gross cost of the 3 mi•hr^{-1} walk. For example, 20 min of rest times 70 kg times 3.5 ml•kg^{-1}•min^{-1} = 4,900 ml, or 4.9 L. Using 5 kcal•L^{-1}, this equals 24.5 kcal for 20 min of rest. The net cost of the mile walk is 80.5 kcal minus 24.5 kcal, or 56 kcal per mile.

Running

If the same 70-kg individual ran the mile at 6 mi•hr^{-1} (161 m•min^{-1}), the O_2 cost could be calculated by the following method.

$$\dot{V}O_2 = 161 \text{ m•min}^{-1} \cdot 0.2 \text{ ml•kg}^{-1}\text{•min}^{-1} + 3.5 \text{ ml•kg}^{-1}\text{•min}^{-1}$$

$$\dot{V}O_2 = 35.7 \text{ ml•kg}^{-1}\text{•min}^{-1}$$

$$\dot{V}O_2 \text{ (ml•mi}^{-1}) = 35.7 \text{ ml•kg}^{-1}\text{•min}^{-1} \cdot 70 \text{ kg} \cdot 10 \text{ min•mi}^{-1} = 25{,}000 \text{ ml•mi}^{-1}$$

$$\dot{V}O_2 \text{ (L•mi}^{-1}) = 25{,}000 \text{ ml•mi}^{-1} \div 1{,}000 \text{ ml•L}^{-1} = 25 \text{ L•mi}^{-1}$$

At about 5 kcal per L O$_2$, 125 kcal are used to jog or run 1 mi (5 kcal•L^{-1} • 25 L•mi^{-1}). The gross caloric cost per mile is about 50% higher for jogging than for walking (125 vs. 80 kcal). However, the net caloric cost of jogging or running 1 mi (kilocalories used above resting) is relatively independent of speed and is about twice that of walking. For example, when we subtract the caloric cost for 10 min of rest (12 kcal) from the gross caloric cost of the run (125 kcal), the net cost is 113 kcal, or twice that for the walk (56 kcal). Tables 8.8 and 8.9 list values for the net and gross caloric costs of walking and running 1 mi for a variety of body weights, with the values expressed in kilocalories per mile.

For weight control it is important to use the net cost of the activity, as it measures the energy used over and above that of sitting around. When moving at slow to moderate speeds (2 to 3.5 mi•hr^{-1}), the net cost of walking a mile is about half that of jogging or running the mile. This means that a person who jogs a mile at 3 mi•hr^{-1} will be working at a higher metabolic rate than someone who walks at the same speed, and of course the heart-rate response will be higher

Table 8.8   Gross and Net (Gross/Net) Cost in kcal · mi^{-1} for Walking

Body weight		Miles per hour						
kg	lb	2.0	2.5	3.0	3.5	4.0	4.5	5.0
50.0	110	64/39	58/39	54/39	53/39	60/48	68/57	79/69
54.5	120	69/42	63/42	59/42	57/42	66/52	75/63	86/75
59.1	130	75/45	68/45	64/45	62/45	71/57	81/68	93/81
63.6	140	80/49	73/49	69/49	67/49	77/61	87/73	100/88
68.2	150	87/52	79/52	74/52	72/52	82/65	93/78	108/94
72.7	160	92/56	84/56	79/56	76/56	88/70	100/84	115/100
77.3	170	98/59	90/59	84/59	81/59	93/74	106/89	122/107
81.8	180	104/63	95/63	89/63	86/63	99/78	112/94	129/113
86.4	190	110/66	100/66	94/66	91/66	104/83	118/99	136/119
90.9	200	115/70	105/70	99/70	95/70	110/87	124/104	144/125
95.4	210	121/73	111/73	104/73	100/73	115/92	131/110	151/132
100.0	220	127/77	116/77	109/77	105/77	121/96	137/115	158/138

Note. Multiply value by the number of miles walked to obtain the total (gross/net) calories expended.

Table 8.9   Gross and Net (Gross/Net) Cost in kcal · mi^{-1} for Jogging and Running

Body weight		Miles per hour						
kg	lb	3.0	4.0	5.0	6.0	7.0	8.0	9.0	10.0
50.0	110	93/77	89/77	86/77	84/77	84/77	83/77	82/77	81/77
54.5	120	101/83	97/83	94/83	92/83	92/83	90/83	89/83	89/83
59.1	130	110/90	105/90	102/90	100/90	99/90	98/90	97/90	96/90
63.6	140	118/97	113/97	110/97	108/97	107/97	106/97	104/97	104/97
68.2	150	127/104	121/104	118/104	115/104	114/104	113/104	112/104	111/104
72.7	160	135/111	129/111	125/111	123/111	122/111	121/111	119/111	119/111
77.3	170	144/118	137/118	133/118	131/118	130/118	128/118	127/118	126/118
81.8	180	152/125	146/125	141/125	138/125	137/125	136/125	134/125	133/125
86.4	190	161/132	154/132	149/132	146/132	145/132	143/132	141/132	141/132
90.9	200	169/139	162/139	157/139	154/139	153/139	151/139	149/139	148/139
95.4	210	177/146	170/146	165/146	161/146	160/146	158/146	156/146	155/146
100.0	220	186/153	178/153	173/153	169/153	168/153	166/153	164/153	163/153

Note. Multiply value by the number of miles jogged or run to obtain the total (gross/net) calories expended.

as well. Because many people walk at these slower speeds, it is important to remember that the net energy cost of the mile is half that of running. However, if we look at very high walking speeds (5 mi•hr^{-1}, or 1 mi in 12 min), we see that the net energy cost of walking 1 mi is only 10% less than that of running.

KEY POINT.   The net caloric cost of jogging or running a mile is twice that of walking a mile at moderate speeds.

Table 8.9 shows that the net cost of running a mile is independent of speed. It does not matter whether participants jog at 3 mi•hr^{-1} or run at 6 mi•hr^{-1}—the net caloric cost is the same. At 6 mi•hr^{-1} the individual will be expending energy at about twice the rate measured at 3 mi•hr^{-1}, but because the mile is finished in half the time, the net energy expenditure is about the same. Heart rate will, of course, be higher in the 6 mi•hr^{-1} run in order to deliver the oxygen to the muscles at the higher rate.

CALORIC COSTS OF OTHER ACTIVITIES

Many activities are available to you when you are designing a fitness program (see chapter 14). These include exercise to music, rope skipping, swimming, and games. Not surprisingly, the energy expenditure associated with these activities is difficult to predict when compared to walking or running, in which the energy cost between people is similar because of the natural movements associated with those activities. In contrast, many activities have variable energy costs, dependent on the skill level of the participants and the motivation they bring to the activity. This will be clear in the following examples. A summary of estimates of the energy requirements of some common aerobic activities is included.

Exercise to Music

Exercising to music is a good alternative to walking and running. The energy requirement depends on whether the session is high or low impact, done at a low, medium, or high intensity, and done with or without hand weights (22). A person who is starting out might simply walk through the movements, whereas an experienced person might go through the full range of motion with each step. Thus the energy costs of this activity vary considerably. Values might range from as low as 4 METs for someone walking through the routine to 10 METs for the experienced dancer working at a high intensity in either a low- or high-impact session (22). Remember that this activity often involves small muscle groups and includes some static (stabilizing) muscle contractions; as a result, HR response is higher for the same oxygen uptake measured in walking and running. Table 8.10 summarizes the caloric expenditure associated with exercise to music when done at low, moderate, and high intensities.

Rope Skipping

In walking and running, the energy requirement is proportional to the rate at which the person moves. But the energy requirement for rope skipping at only 60 to 80 turns per minute (about as slow as the rope can be turned) is about 9 METs. At 120 turns per minute the energy cost increases to only 11 METs (15). Consequently, rope skipping is not a graded activity as are walking and running. Secondly, the HR response is higher than expected from the oxygen cost of the activity. This, again, may be because a small muscle mass (lower leg) is the primary muscle group involved in the activity. In spite of this, rope skipping can be included as an

Table 8.10   Gross Energy Cost of Exercise to Music
(kcal · min⁻¹)

| Body weight | | Low | Moderate | High |
kg	lb	intensity	intensity	intensity
50.0	110	3.3	5.8	8.3
54.5	120	3.6	6.4	9.1
59.1	130	3.9	6.9	9.8
63.6	140	4.2	7.4	10.6
68.2	150	4.5	7.9	11.3
72.7	160	4.8	8.5	12.1
77.3	170	5.1	9.0	12.8
81.8	180	5.4	9.5	13.6
86.4	190	5.7	10.1	14.3
90.9	200	6.0	10.6	15.1
95.4	210	6.3	11.1	15.9
100.0	220	6.6	11.7	16.7

Note. Multiply value by the duration of the aerobic phase of the exercise-to-music class to obtain total calories expended.

effective *part* of a fitness program when done intermittently, using target heart rate (THR) as the guide (see chapter 13). However, rope skipping *should not* be used in the early part of a fitness program. Table 8.11 presents a summary of the energy costs of skipping rope at two speeds.

Swimming

Swimming is a preferred activity for many people because of the dynamic, large-muscle nature of the task and because little joint trauma is associated with it. The limitation is in finding a

Table 8.11   Gross Energy Cost of Rope Skipping
(kcal · min⁻¹)

| Body weight | | Slow skipping | Fast skipping |
kg	lb		
50.0	110	7.5	9.2
54.5	120	8.2	10.0
59.1	130	8.9	10.9
63.6	140	9.5	11.7
68.2	150	10.2	12.5
72.7	160	10.9	13.4
77.3	170	11.6	14.2
81.8	180	12.3	15.0
86.4	190	13.0	15.9
90.9	200	13.6	16.7
95.4	210	14.3	17.5
100.0	220	15.0	18.4

Note. Multiply value by the duration of the rope-skipping session to obtain total calories expended.

convenient facility that allows lap swimming and, of course, having enough skill to do the activity. The energy requirement depends on the velocity of movement and the stroke being used, but it is also influenced by the skill of the swimmer. A skilled swimmer requires less energy to move through the water, so that person has to swim a greater distance than an unskilled person to achieve the same caloric expenditure.

The energy cost of simply treading water can be as high as 1.5 L•min^{-1} (7.5 kcal•min^{-1}). Elite swimmers use this same number of kilocalories per minute to swim at 36 m•min^{-1}, whereas an unskilled swimmer might require twice that energy expenditure to maintain the same velocity. For elite swimmers, the front and back crawl are the most efficient, and the butterfly is the least efficient. The net caloric cost per mile of swimming has been estimated to be more than 400 kcal, or about 4 times that of running 1 mi and about 8 times that of walking 1 mi. However, the actual caloric cost per mile of swimming varies greatly, depending on skill and gender. Table 8.12 is a summary of the values presented by Holmer (13) for men and women.

Table 8.12   Caloric Cost Per Mile (kcal · mi^{-1}) of Swimming the Front Crawl for Men and Women by Skill Level

Skill level	Women	Men
Competitive	180	280
Skilled	260	360
Average	300	440
Unskilled	360	560
Poor	440	720

Note. Adapted from "Physiology of Swimming Man" by I. Holmer. In *Exercise and Sport Sciences Review*, 7, by R.S. Hutton and D.I. Miller (Eds.), 1979.

The HR response measured during swimming at a specific $\dot{V}O_2$ is lower than that measured during running at the same $\dot{V}O_2$. In fact, the maximal HR response is about 14 beats•min^{-1} lower for swimming. With this in mind, the THR range should be decreased when prescribing swimming activities.

Table 8.13 contains a summary of the measured energy requirements for a variety of physical activities. Please keep in mind that a range of values is presented for most activities and that in some cases the values are based on small sample sizes.

ESTIMATION OF ENERGY EXPENDITURE WITHOUT FORMULAS

The HFI selects activities that cause the fitness participant to exercise in the range of 60% to 80% of $\dot{V}O_2$max, the intensity needed to improve or maintain cardiorespiratory fitness. It should therefore be possible to estimate the energy expenditure for each individual on the basis of the subject's $\dot{V}O_2$max and the portion of the THR range at which the person is working. If a person has a functional capacity of 10 METs, energy expenditure can be estimated in the following way. Ten METs are equal to about 10 kcal•kg^{-1}•hr^{-1}. If a person is working at the bottom portion of the THR range, at about 60% $\dot{V}O_2$max, then the energy expenditure should be about 6 METs (60% of 10 METs). If the person weighs 70 kg, then 420 kcal are expended per hour

Table 8.13 Summary of Measured Energy Cost of Various Physical Activities

Activity	METs	kcal · kg⁻¹ · min⁻¹	kcal/hour 50 kg/110 lb	kcal/hour 70 kg/154 lb	kcal/hour 90 kg /198 lb
Archery	3-4	.050-.066	150-200	210-280	270-360
Backpacking	5-11	.083-.183	250-550	350-770	450-990
Badminton	4-9+	.066-.150	200-450	280-630	360-810
Basketball	3-12+	.050-.200	150-600	210-840	270-1080
Billiards	2.5	.042	125	175	225
Bowling	2-4	.033-.066	100-200	140-280	180-360
Boxing	8-13	.133-.216	400-650	560-910	720-1170
Canoeing, rowing, and kayaking	3-8	.050-.133	150-400	210-560	270-720
Cricket	4-7	.066-.117	200-350	280-490	360-630
Croquet	3.5	.058	175	245	315
Cycling	3-8+	.050-.133+	150-400+	210-560+	270-720+
Dancing—social/tap	3-7	.050-.117	150-350	210-490	270-630
aerobic	4-10	.066-.167	200-500	280-700	360-900
Fencing	6-10	.100-.167	300-500	420-700	540-900
Field hockey	8	.133	400	560	720
Fishing—from bank	2-4	.033-.066	100-200	140-280	180-360
wading	5-6	.083-.100	250-300	350-420	450-540
Football (touch)	6-10	.100-.167	300-500	420-700	540-900
Golf—power cart	2-3	.033-.050	100-150	140-210	180-270
pull/carry clubs	4-7	.066-.117	200-350	280-490	360-630
Handball	8-12	.133-.200	400-600	560-840	720-1080
Hiking	3-7	.050-.117	150-350	210-490	270-630
Horseback riding	3-8	.050-.133	150-400	210-560	270-720
Horseshoe pitching	2-3	.033-.050	100-150	140-210	180-270
Hunting (bow/gun) small game	3-7	.050-.117	150-350	210-490	270-630
Jogging (see Table 8.9)					
	5-10	.083-.167	250-500	350-700	450-900
Paddleball/racquetball	8-12	.133-.200	400-600	560-840	720-1080
Rope jumping	9-12	.150-.20	450-600	630-840	810-1080
Running (see Table 8.9)					
Sailing	2-5	.033-.083	100-250	140-350	180-450
Scuba diving	5-10	.083-.167	250-500	350-700	450-900
Shuffleboard	2-3	.033-.050	100-150	140-210	180-270
Skating (ice and roller)	5-8	.083-.133	250-400	350-560	450-720
Skiing (snow) downhill	5-8	.083-.133	250-400	350-560	450-720
cross-country	6-12	.100-.200	300-600	420-840	540-1080
Skiing (water)	5-7	.083-.117	250-350	350-490	450-630
Sledding, tobogganing	4-8	.066-.113	200-400	280-560	360-720
Snowshoeing	7-14	.117-.233	350-700	490-980	630-1260
Squash	8-12	.133-.200	400-600	560-840	720-1080
Soccer	5-12	.083-.200	250-600	350-840	450-1080
Swimming (see Table 8.12)					
Table tennis	3-5	.050-.083	150-250	210-350	270-450
Tennis	4-9	.066-.150	200-450	280-630	360-810
Volleyball (recreational)	3-6	.050-.100	150-300	210-420	270-540

Note. Adapted from *Guidelines for Graded Exercise Testing and Exercise Prescription* by American College of Sports Medicine, 1991, Philadelphia: Lea & Febiger. And from *Exercise Physiology* by W.D. McArdle, F.I. Katch, and V.L. Katch, 1986, Philadelphia: Lea & Febiger.

(70 kg • 6 kcal•kg^{-1}•hr^{-1}). A 30-min workout would require half this, or about 210 kcal. These simple calculations assume that the person is performing a large-muscle activity. Table 8.14 shows the estimated kilocalorie expenditure for a 30-min workout at 70% $\dot{V}O_2$max for a variety of fitness levels and body weights (21).

Table 8.14   Estimated Energy Expenditure for 30 Min of Exercise at 70% Functional Capacity ($\dot{V}O_2$max) for Persons of Various Body Weight (kg and lb)

$\dot{V}O_2$max METs (kcal · kg^{-1} · hr^{-1})	70% Max METs (kcal · kg^{-1} · hr^{-1})	Kcal/30 min		
		50 kg/ 110 lb	70 kg/ 154 lb	90 kg/ 198 lb
20	14.0	350	490	630
18	12.6	315	441	567
16	11.2	280	392	504
14	9.8	245	343	441
12	8.4	210	294	378
10	7.0	175	245	315
8	5.6	140	196	252
6	4.2	105	147	189

Note. Data from *Physiology of Fitness* by B.J. Sharkey, 1990, Champaign, IL: Human Kinetics.

ENVIRONMENTAL CONCERNS

Although changes in temperature, relative humidity, pollution, and altitude do not change the energy requirements for exercise, they do change the participant's response to the exercise bout. Remember that a person's HR response is the best indicator of the relative stress being experienced due to the interaction of exercise intensity, duration, and environmental factors. The participant should be instructed to cut back on the intensity of the activity when environmental factors drive the HR response. The duration of the activity can be increased to accommodate any energy expenditure goal.

SUMMARY

Energy expenditure is measured by direct and indirect calorimetry. Indirect calorimetry estimates energy expenditure by measuring oxygen consumption, knowing that 1 L of oxygen equals 4.7 to 5.0 kcal. Indirect calorimetry uses either a closed system, in which the subject breathes 100% oxygen from a spirometer, or an open system, in which the subject breathes room air. Energy expenditure is expressed in L O_2•min^{-1}, ml O_2•kg^{-1}•min^{-1}, METs, kcal•min^{-1}, and kcal•kg^{-1}•hr^{-1}. The ACSM has developed formulas for estimating the steady-state energy requirements of a variety of activities—walking, running, stepping, and cycle ergometry exercise. The net caloric cost of jogging (0.2 ml•kg^{-1}•min^{-1} per m•min^{-1}) is twice that of walking at moderate speeds (0.1 ml•kg^{-1}•min^{-1}). The oxygen cost of cycling is dependent on the work rate, not on body weight (which is supported by the seat). The oxygen cost of stepping is dependent on stepping rate and step height. The oxygen cost of exercise to music is about 4 METs at low intensities and 10 METs at high intensities. Rope skipping, even at 60 to 80 turns•min^{-1}, requires about 9 METs. The oxygen cost of swimming varies with skill, being lower for the more highly skilled, and with gender, with females requiring less energy expenditure to swim at the same speed. One can estimate energy expenditure during moderate exercise by taking 70% of the person's functional capacity, expressed in $kcal \cdot kg^{-1} \cdot hr^{-1}$, and multiplying by the person's body weight. A table showing the energy costs of common activities is presented.

REFERENCES

1. American College of Sports Medicine (1991)
2. Åstrand (n.d.)
3. Åstrand and Rodahl (1986)
4. Balke (1963)
5. Balke and Ware (1959)
6. Bransford and Howley (1977)
7. Bubb, Martin, and Howley (1985)
8. Daniels (1985)
9. Dill (1965)
10. Franklin (1985)
11. Franklin, Vanders, Wrisley, and Rubenfire (1983)
12. Haskell, Savin, Oldridge, and DeBisk (1982)
13. Holmer (1979)
14. Howley and Glover (1974)
15. Howley and Martin (1978)
16. Knoebel (1984)
17. Margaria, Cerretelli, Aghemo, and Sassi (1963)
18. Montoye, Ayen, Nagle, and Howley (1986)
19. Nagle, Balke, Baptista, Alleyia, and Howley (1971)
20. Nagle, Balke, and Naughton (1965)
21. Sharkey (1984)
22. Williford, Scharff-Olson, and Blessing (1989)

See the Bibliography at the end of the book for a complete source listing.

Chapter 9

Cardiorespiratory Fitness

OBJECTIVES

The reader will be able to:
- Describe the relationship of cardiorespiratory fitness (CRF) to health
- List reasons for CRF testing
- Present a logical sequence of testing
- Conduct walking and jogging field tests
- Conduct submaximal and maximal treadmill, cycle ergometer, and bench-step graded exercise tests (GXT)
- List variables measured during a GXT
- Describe procedures used prior to, during, and following testing

TERMS

The reader will be able to define or describe:

Bench stepping

Cycle ergometers

Diastolic blood pressure (DBP)

Functional capacity

Graded exercise test (GXT)

Heart rate (HR)

Informed consent

Maximal

Rating of perceived exertion (RPE)

Submaximal

Systolic blood pressure (SBP)

Treadmill

The usual introduction to cardiorespiratory fitness (CRF) delineates heart disease as the major cause of death and proceeds to describe the role of exercise in prevention and rehabilitation programs. However, it is more important to focus attention on a high level of CRF as a normal, lifelong goal that is needed to enjoy life. That alone merits the inclusion of CRF in any discussion about positive health. Cardiorespiratory fitness, also called cardiovascular, or aerobic, fitness, is a good measure of the heart's ability to pump oxygen-rich blood to the muscles. Although the terms *cardio-* (heart), *vascular* (blood vessels), *respiratory* (lungs and ventilation), and *aerobic* (working with oxygen) differ technically, they all reflect different aspects of this component of fitness. The person with a healthy heart can pump great volumes of blood with each beat and will have a high level of CRF. CRF values are expressed in the following ways:

- Liters of oxygen used by the body per minute ($L \cdot min^{-1}$)

- Milliliters of oxygen used per kilogram of body weight per minute ($ml \cdot kg^{-1} \cdot min^{-1}$)
- METs, multiples of resting metabolic rate, where $1 \text{ MET} = 3.5 \text{ ml} \cdot kg^{-1} \cdot min^{-1}$

A person with the ability to use $35 \text{ ml} \cdot kg^{-1} \cdot min^{-1}$ during maximal exercise is said to have a CRF equal to 10 METs ($35 \div 3.5 = 10$). Aerobic-training programs increase the heart's ability to pump blood, so it is no surprise that CRF improves as a result of such programs.

Chapter 3 described how CRF variables respond to acute exercise. Chapter 13 deals with the recommendation of activities for improvement of CRF. This chapter emphasizes the evaluation of CRF.

Historically, measurements of **heart rate (HR)**, blood pressure (BP), and the electrocardiogram (ECG) taken at rest were used to evaluate CRF. In addition, some static pulmonary function tests (e.g., vital capacity) were used to characterize respiratory function. However, it became clear that measurements made at rest told a physician little about the way a person's cardiorespiratory systems respond to physical activity. We are now familiar with the use of a graded exercise test (GXT) to evaluate HR, ECG, BP, ventilation, and oxygen-uptake responses during work.

REASONS FOR CARDIORESPIRATORY FITNESS TESTING

The results from cardiorespiratory fitness tests are used to write exercise recommendations and allow the HFI or physician to evaluate positive or negative changes in CRF as a result of physical conditioning, aging, illness, or inactivity. Given the recent increase in obesity and inactivity in children, there is good reason to include an evaluation of CRF throughout life, from early childhood to old age. This information can serve as a marker of where the individual stands relative to health-criterion test scores, and it will alert the individual to subtle changes in lifestyle that may compromise positive health. The nature of the tests and the level of monitoring should vary across the ages to reflect the type of information that is needed.

CRF testing depends on the purpose(s) of the test, the type of person to be evaluated, and the work tasks available. Reasons for testing include

- determining physiological responses at rest and during submaximal and/or maximal work,
- providing a basis for exercise programming,
- screening for coronary heart disease (CHD), and
- determining ability to perform a specific work task.

The choice of an appropriate test depends on several factors. People differ in age, fitness levels, known health problems, and risks of CHD. Also, financial considerations determine the amount of time that can be devoted to each individual and the type of work tasks available.

RISKS OF CRF TESTING

One point typically made about exercise tests or activities is the risk involved. For exercise testing (including postcardiac patients) there are about five incidents resulting in hospital treatment and one death per 10,000 tests. In terms of exercise-related death, there is about one per year for every 15,000 to 20,000 healthy persons. Because of the decreased risk of heart disease in

active or fit persons, the overall risk of a cardiovascular problem is greater for those who maintain sedentary habits (19, 31). This view is consistent with recent evidence that low levels of physical activity and CRF are directly related to a higher risk of heart disease and death (9, 27).

KEY POINT. Cardiorespiratory fitness is an important aspect of quality of life for healthy individuals. The ability to utilize oxygen during exercise is the basis for this fitness component.

SEQUENCE OF TESTING

A logical sequence for fitness testing (and activities) exists when people come to the same fitness center over a substantial period of time. This sequence progresses from the initial screening to fitness testing and programming, with opportunities for reviewing the program as fitness gains are made. (See Sequence of Testing and Activity Prescription.) For people who come in for fitness testing but do not have continuing involvement with the fitness center, the submaximal and maximal tests are usually a part of the same GXT protocol. Chapter 18 evaluates computer software that can assist the HFI in CRF testing.

Health History

Chapter 2 deals with procedures for determining current health status. This information can be used to determine appropriate testing protocol and activity recommendations. In addition, follow-up testing should be advised for people with symptoms of health problems. Referrals to other professionals might be warranted based on the person's history.

Screening

We recommended, in chapter 2, that individuals have regular medical examinations and health screening and engage in low-intensity exercise. Fitness programs need to determine whether or not the person needs medical permission to be in a fitness program involving moderate-intensity activities. People with CHD or other known major health problems *must have* medical supervision or clearance before any fitness testing or program beyond low-intensity exercise.

The ACSM has identified conditions where the risk

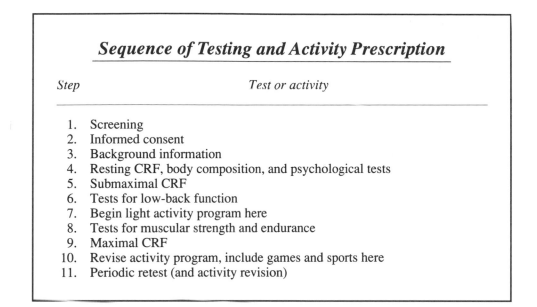

Sequence of Testing and Activity Prescription

Step	Test or activity
1.	Screening
2.	Informed consent
3.	Background information
4.	Resting CRF, body composition, and psychological tests
5.	Submaximal CRF
6.	Tests for low-back function
7.	Begin light activity program here
8.	Tests for muscular strength and endurance
9.	Maximal CRF
10.	Revise activity program, include games and sports here
11.	Periodic retest (and activity revision)

of testing outweighs the possible benefits (see Contraindications to Exercise Testing). Other conditions increase the risk of exercise testing—these persons should only be tested if the medical judgment is that the need for the test outweighs the potential risk.

Apparently healthy people who have no known major health problems or symptoms can be tested or begin the type of fitness program recommended in this book with minimal risk. Chapter 2 identifies the people who need medical clearance, a carefully supervised program, and educational information about health problems and behaviors.

Informed Consent

Fitness participants should be informed volunteers. The fitness program should clearly describe all of its procedures and the potential risks and benefits of the fitness tests and activities. The participants should understand that their individual data will be confidential and that any test or activity can be terminated at any time by the individual participant. A written **informed-consent** form should be signed by the participant after reading a description of the program and having all questions answered. A sample consent form is included in chapter 17.

Resting Measurements

Typical *resting* tests may include CRF measures (e.g., 12-lead ECG, BP, and blood chemistry profile) as well as other fitness variables, such as body composition and psychological traits. Evaluation of the ECG by a

physician determines whether any abnormalities require further medical attention. Those people with extreme BP or blood chemistry values (see chapter 2) should also be referred to their personal physicians.

Submaximal Tests to Estimate CRF

If the resting tests reflect normal values, then a submaximal test is administered. The **submaximal** test usually provides the HR and BP response to different intensities of work, from light up to a predetermined point (usually 85% of predicted maximum HR). This test can use a bench, cycle ergometer, or treadmill. Once again, if unusual responses to the submaximal test appear, then the person is referred for further medical tests. If the results appear normal, then an activity program is begun at intensities less than those reached on the test (e.g., a person goes to 85% of maximum HR on the test and starts the fitness program at 70%). After the person has become accustomed to regular exercise and appears to be adjusting to fitness activities, a maximal test can be administered.

Submaximal tests can also be used to estimate maximal functional capacity (maximal oxygen uptake) by extrapolating HR to a predicted maximum, then using the linear relationship between HR and oxygen uptake to estimate functional capacity. Although this estimated maximum is useful for evaluating a person's current status and prescribing or revising exercise, there is considerable error involved in the estimation. In addition to measuring submaximal CRF, measurements of flexibility and muscular strength and endurance (especially related to low-back function) are often included at this stage (see chapter 10).

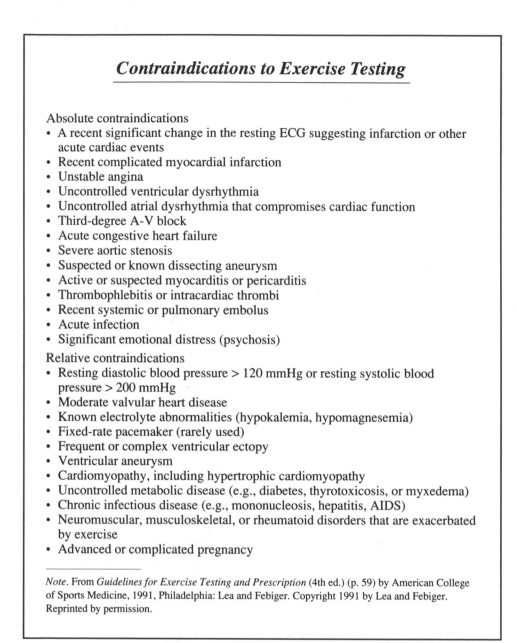

Contraindications to Exercise Testing

Absolute contraindications
- A recent significant change in the resting ECG suggesting infarction or other acute cardiac events
- Recent complicated myocardial infarction
- Unstable angina
- Uncontrolled ventricular dysrhythmia
- Uncontrolled atrial dysrhythmia that compromises cardiac function
- Third-degree A-V block
- Acute congestive heart failure
- Severe aortic stenosis
- Suspected or known dissecting aneurysm
- Active or suspected myocarditis or pericarditis
- Thrombophlebitis or intracardiac thrombi
- Recent systemic or pulmonary embolus
- Acute infection
- Significant emotional distress (psychosis)

Relative contraindications
- Resting diastolic blood pressure > 120 mmHg or resting systolic blood pressure > 200 mmHg
- Moderate valvular heart disease
- Known electrolyte abnormalities (hypokalemia, hypomagnesemia)
- Fixed-rate pacemaker (rarely used)
- Frequent or complex ventricular ectopy
- Ventricular aneurysm
- Cardiomyopathy, including hypertrophic cardiomyopathy
- Uncontrolled metabolic disease (e.g., diabetes, thyrotoxicosis, or myxedema)
- Chronic infectious disease (e.g., mononucleosis, hepatitis, AIDS)
- Neuromuscular, musculoskeletal, or rheumatoid disorders that are exacerbated by exercise
- Advanced or complicated pregnancy

Note. From *Guidelines for Exercise Testing and Prescription* (4th ed.) (p. 59) by American College of Sports Medicine, 1991, Philadelphia: Lea and Febiger. Copyright 1991 by Lea and Febiger. Reprinted by permission.

Maximal Tests to Estimate or Measure CRF

If no problems occur up to this point, a maximal test is administered. Two basic types of **maximal** tests are used to indicate CRF—laboratory tests involving the measurement of physiological responses (e.g., HR, BP) to increasing levels of work, and all-out endurance performance tests (e.g., time on a 1-mi run). The results of the maximal test can be used to revise the activity program. The use of the person's maximal functional capacity provides a new basis for selection of fitness activities. The person's measured maximal HR should now be used for determining target HR (instead of using the estimated maximal HR).

Program Modification

After a minimum level of fitness has been achieved, a wider variety of activities (e.g., games and sports) can be included in the fitness program. Finally, all of the tests should be retaken periodically to determine the progress being made and to revise the program in areas where the gains are not as great as desired.

FIELD TESTS

There are a variety of field tests that can be used to obtain an estimate of CRF. These are called "field tests'' because they require very little equipment, can be done just about anywhere, and use the simple activities of walking and running. Because these tests involve running or walking as fast as possible over a set distance, they are *not* recommended at the start of an exercise program. Instead, we recommend that participants complete the graduated walking program before taking the walking test, and the graduated jogging program before taking the running test. The walk/jog programs are found in chapter 14. The graduated nature of the fitness program allows participants to start at a low and safe level of activity and gradually improve. It is then appropriate to administer an endurance-run test to evaluate fitness status.

Field tests rely on the observation that for one to walk or run at high speeds over long distances, the heart must pump great volumes of oxygen to the muscles. It is in this way that the average speed maintained in these walk/run tests gives an estimate of CRF. The higher the CRF score, the greater the heart's capacity to transport oxygen. An endurance run of a set distance for time, or set time for distance, provides information about a person's CR endurance, as long as it is 1 mi or more. The advantages include its moderately high correlation to maximum oxygen uptake, the use of a natural activity, and the large numbers of participants that can be tested in a short period of time. The disadvantages of endurance running are that it is difficult to monitor physiological responses, that other factors affect the outcome (e.g., motivation), and that it cannot be used for graded or submaximal testing.

Walk Test

A 1-mi-walk test used to predict CRF was recently developed, with the focus on the older adult. **The following elements are needed for the walk test:**

- **A person to start and read the time from a stopwatch**
- **A partner with a watch (with a second hand) for each runner (perhaps with a sheet to mark off laps)**
- **Flat surface, marked off**
- **A stopwatch (with a spare ready)**
- **A scoresheet or scorecard**

In this test the individual walks as fast as possible on a measured track, and heart rate is measured at the end of the last quarter mile (see Steps in Administration of Mile Walk). The following equation is used to calculate $\dot{V}O_2$max ($ml \cdot kg^{-1} \cdot min^{-1}$):

$$\dot{V}O_2max = 132.853 - 0.0769 \text{ (weight)}$$
$$- 0.3877 \text{ (age)} + 6.315 \text{ (sex)}$$
$$- 3.2649 \text{ (time)} - 0.1565 \text{ (HR)}$$

where (weight) is body weight in pounds, (age) is in years, (sex) equals 0 for female and 1 for male, (time) is in minutes and hundredths of minutes, and (HR) is in $beats \cdot min^{-1}$. The formula was developed and validated on populations of females and males aged 30 to 69 years (see Kline et al., 1987).

QUESTION: What is the CRF of a 25-year-old, 170-lb male who walks the mile in 20 min and has an *immediate* postexercise heart rate of 140 $beats \cdot min^{-1}$?

ANSWER:

$$\dot{V}O_2max = 132.853 - 0.0769 \text{ (weight)} - 0.3877 \text{ (age)}$$
$$+ 6.315 \text{ (sex)} - 3.2649 \text{ (time)} - 0.1565 \text{ (HR)}$$
$$\dot{V}O_2max = 132.853 - 0.0769 \text{ (170)} - 0.3877 \text{ (25)}$$
$$+ 6.315 \text{ (1)} - 3.2649 \text{ (20.0)} - 0.1565 \text{ (140)}$$
$$\dot{V}O_2max = 29.2 \ ml \cdot kg^{-1} \cdot min^{-1}$$

To simplify the steps in using this 1-mi-walk test, Table 9.1 was generated on the basis of the above formula, for men weighing 170 lb and women weighing 125 lb. For each 15 lb beyond these weights, subtract about 1 $ml \cdot kg^{-1} \cdot min^{-1}$.

To use Table 9.1, find the part of the table for the individual's sex and age, then go across the top until you find the time (to the nearest minute) it took to walk a mile, and then go down that column until it intersects with the person's postexercise HR (listed on the left side). The number at which the mile time and postexercise HR meet is the CRF value in terms of $ml \cdot kg^{-1} \cdot min^{-1}$. For example, a 25-year-old man who walked the mile in 20 min and had a postexercise HR of 140 would have an estimated maximal oxygen uptake of 29.2 $ml \cdot kg^{-1} \cdot min^{-1}$. You can evaluate cardiorespiratory fitness by using that number to compare with the standards presented in Table 9.2. In the example of the 25-year-old man, his maximal oxygen uptake is low, indicating a need for improvement.

Jog/Run Test

One of the most common CRF field tests is the 12-min or 1.5-mi run popularized by Cooper (13). The idea in this test is very much like the walk test mentioned above: Jog or run as fast as possible for 12 min or for 1.5 mi. This test is based on original work by Balke

Steps in Administration of Mile Walk

Step	Activity

Pretest

1. Explain the purpose of the test (i.e., to determine how fast they can walk a mile, which reflects the endurance of their cardiovascular system).
2. Select and mark off (if needed) a level area for the walk.
3. Persons are to walk the mile in the fastest time possible. Only walking is allowed, and the goal is to cover the distance as fast as possible.

Test day

1. Warmup with stretching and slow walking.
2. Several persons walk at the same time.
3. The procedure is explained again.
4. The timer says, "Ready, go" and starts the stopwatch.
5. Each individual has a partner with a watch with a second hand.
6. The partner counts the laps and tells the individual at the end of each lap how many more lap(s) to walk.
7. The timer calls out the minutes and seconds as the persons finish the mile walk.
8. The partner listens for the time when his or her walker finishes the mile and records it (to the nearest second) immediately on a scorecard.
9. The partner takes a 10-s HR immediately after the end of the mile walk.

Table 9.1 Estimated Maximal Oxygen Uptake (ml · kg^{-1} · min^{-1}) for Men and Women, 20-69 Years Old

Heart rate	10	11	12	13	14	15	16	17	18	19	20
					MEN (20-29)						
120	65.0	61.7	58.4	55.2	51.9	48.6	45.4	42.1	38.9	35.6	32.3
130	63.4	60.1	56.9	53.6	50.3	47.1	43.8	40.6	37.3	34.0	30.8
140	61.8	58.6	55.3	52.0	48.8	45.5	42.2	39.0	35.7	32.5	29.2
150	60.3	57.0	53.7	50.5	47.2	43.9	40.7	37.4	34.2	30.9	27.6
160	58.7	55.4	52.2	48.9	45.6	42.4	39.1	35.9	32.6	29.3	26.1
170	57.1	53.9	50.6	47.3	44.1	40.8	37.6	34.3	31.0	27.8	24.5
180	55.6	52.3	49.0	45.8	42.5	39.3	36.0	32.7	29.5	26.2	22.9
190	54.0	50.7	47.5	44.2	41.0	37.7	34.4	31.2	27.9	24.6	21.4
200	52.4	49.2	45.9	42.7	39.4	36.1	32.9	29.6	26.3	23.1	19.8
					WOMEN (20-29)						
120	62.1	58.9	55.6	52.3	49.1	45.8	42.5	39.3	36.0	32.7	29.5
130	60.6	57.3	54.0	50.8	47.5	44.2	41.0	37.7	34.4	31.2	27.9
140	59.0	55.7	52.5	49.2	45.9	42.7	39.4	36.1	32.9	29.6	26.3
150	57.4	54.2	50.9	47.6	44.4	41.1	37.8	34.6	31.3	28.0	24.8
160	55.9	52.6	49.3	46.1	42.8	39.5	36.3	33.0	29.7	26.5	23.2
170	54.3	51.0	47.8	44.5	41.2	38.0	34.7	31.4	28.2	24.9	21.6
180	52.7	49.5	46.2	42.9	39.7	36.4	33.1	29.9	26.6	23.3	20.1
190	51.2	47.9	44.6	41.4	38.1	34.8	31.6	28.3	25.0	21.8	18.5
200	49.6	46.3	43.1	39.8	36.5	33.3	30.0	26.7	23.5	20.2	16.9

Heart rate	Min · mile⁻¹										
	10	11	12	13	14	15	16	17	18	19	20
MEN (30-39)											
120	61.1	57.8	54.6	51.3	48.0	44.8	41.5	38.2	35.0	31.7	28.4
130	59.5	56.3	53.0	49.7	46.5	43.2	39.9	36.7	33.4	30.1	26.9
140	58.0	54.7	51.4	48.2	44.9	41.6	38.4	35.1	31.8	28.6	25.3
150	56.4	53.1	49.9	46.6	43.3	40.1	36.8	33.5	30.3	27.0	23.8
160	54.8	51.6	48.3	45.0	41.8	38.5	35.2	32.0	28.7	25.5	22.2
170	53.3	50.0	46.7	43.5	40.2	36.9	33.7	30.4	27.1	23.9	20.6
180	51.7	48.4	45.2	41.9	38.6	35.4	32.1	28.8	25.6	22.3	19.1
190	50.1	46.9	43.6	40.3	37.1	33.8	30.5	27.3	24.0	20.8	17.5
WOMEN (30-39)											
120	58.2	55.0	51.7	48.4	45.2	41.9	38.7	35.4	32.1	28.9	25.6
130	56.7	53.4	50.1	46.9	43.6	40.4	37.1	33.8	30.6	27.3	24.0
140	55.1	51.8	48.6	45.3	42.1	38.8	35.5	32.3	29.0	25.7	22.5
150	53.5	50.3	47.0	43.8	40.5	37.2	34.0	30.7	27.4	24.2	20.9
160	52.0	48.7	45.4	42.2	38.9	35.7	32.4	29.1	25.9	22.6	19.3
170	50.4	47.1	43.9	40.6	37.4	34.1	30.8	27.6	24.3	21.0	17.8
180	48.8	45.6	42.3	39.1	35.8	32.5	29.3	26.0	22.7	19.5	16.2
190	47.3	44.0	40.8	37.5	34.2	31.0	27.7	24.4	21.2	17.9	14.6
MEN (40-49)											
120	57.2	54.0	50.7	47.4	44.2	40.9	37.6	34.4	31.1	27.8	24.6
130	55.7	52.4	49.1	45.9	42.6	39.3	36.1	32.8	29.5	26.3	23.0
140	54.1	50.8	47.6	44.3	41.0	37.8	34.5	31.2	28.0	24.7	21.4
150	52.5	49.3	46.0	42.7	39.5	36.2	32.9	29.7	26.4	23.1	19.9
160	51.0	47.7	44.4	41.2	37.9	34.6	31.4	28.1	24.8	21.6	18.3
170	49.4	46.1	42.9	39.6	36.3	33.1	29.8	26.5	23.3	20.0	16.7
180	47.8	44.6	41.3	38.0	34.8	31.5	28.2	25.0	21.7	18.4	15.2
WOMEN (40-49)											
120	54.4	51.1	47.8	44.6	41.3	38.0	34.8	31.5	28.2	25.0	21.7
130	52.8	49.5	46.3	43.0	39.7	36.5	33.2	29.9	26.7	23.4	20.1
140	51.2	48.0	44.7	41.4	38.2	34.9	31.6	28.4	25.1	21.8	18.6
150	49.7	46.4	43.1	39.9	36.6	33.3	30.1	26.8	23.5	20.3	17.0
160	48.1	44.8	41.6	38.3	35.0	31.8	28.5	25.2	22.0	18.7	15.5
170	46.5	43.3	40.0	36.7	33.5	30.2	26.9	23.7	20.4	17.2	13.9
180	45.0	41.7	38.4	35.2	31.9	28.6	25.4	22.1	18.9	15.6	12.3
MEN (50-59)											
120	53.3	50.0	46.8	43.5	40.3	37.0	33.7	30.5	27.2	23.9	20.7
130	51.7	48.5	45.2	42.0	38.7	35.4	32.2	28.9	25.6	22.4	19.1
140	50.2	46.9	43.7	40.4	37.1	33.9	30.6	27.3	24.1	20.8	17.5
150	48.6	45.4	42.1	38.8	35.6	32.3	29.0	25.8	22.5	19.2	16.0
160	47.1	43.8	40.5	37.3	34.0	30.7	27.5	24.2	20.9	17.7	14.4
170	45.5	42.2	39.0	35.7	32.4	29.2	25.9	22.6	19.4	16.1	12.8
WOMEN (50-59)											
120	50.5	47.2	43.9	40.7	37.4	34.1	30.9	27.6	24.3	21.1	17.8
130	48.9	45.6	42.4	39.1	35.8	32.6	29.3	26.0	22.8	19.5	16.2
140	47.3	44.1	40.8	37.5	34.3	31.0	27.7	24.5	21.2	17.9	14.7
150	45.8	42.5	39.2	36.0	32.7	29.4	26.2	22.9	19.6	16.4	13.1
160	44.2	40.9	37.7	34.4	31.1	27.9	24.6	21.3	18.1	14.8	11.5
170	42.6	39.4	36.1	32.8	29.6	26.3	23.0	19.8	16.5	13.2	10.0

(Cont.)

Table 9.1   (Continued)

Heart rate	10	11	12	13	14	15	16	17	18	19	20
					Min · mile⁻¹						

Min · mile⁻¹ column spans 10–20.

Heart rate	10	11	12	13	14	15	16	17	18	19	20
MEN (60-69)										
120	49.4	46.2	42.9	39.6	36.4	33.1	29.8	26.6	23.3	20.0	16.8
130	47.9	44.6	41.3	38.1	34.8	31.5	28.3	25.0	21.7	18.5	15.2
140	46.3	43.0	39.8	36.5	33.2	30.0	26.7	23.4	20.2	16.9	13.6
150	44.7	41.5	38.2	34.9	31.7	28.4	25.1	21.9	18.6	15.3	12.1
160	43.2	39.9	36.6	33.4	30.1	26.8	23.6	20.3	17.0	13.8	10.5
WOMEN (60-69)										
120	46.6	43.3	40.0	36.8	33.5	30.2	27.0	23.7	20.5	17.2	13.9
130	45.0	41.7	38.5	35.2	31.9	28.7	25.4	22.2	18.9	15.6	12.4
140	43.4	40.2	36.9	33.6	30.4	27.1	23.8	20.6	17.3	14.1	10.8
150	41.9	38.6	35.3	32.1	28.8	25.5	22.3	19.0	15.8	12.5	9.2
160	40.3	37.0	33.8	30.5	27.2	24.0	20.7	17.5	14.2	10.9	7.7

Note. Calculations assume 170 lb for men and 125 lb for women. For each 15 lb beyond these values, subtract 1 ml. Adapted from Kline et al. (1987).

Table 9.2   Standards for Maximal Oxygen Uptake and Endurance Runs

Age[a]	VO₂max (ml · kg⁻¹ · min⁻¹) Female[b]	Male	1.5-mi run (min:sec) Female	Male	12-min run (mi) Female	Male
GOOD						
15-30	> 40	> 45	< 12	< 10	> 1.5	> 1.7
35-50	> 35	> 40	< 13:30	< 11:30	> 1.4	> 1.5
55-70	> 30	> 35	< 16	< 14	> 1.2	> 1.3
ADEQUATE FOR MOST ACTIVITIES						
15-30	35	40	13:30	11:50	1.4	1.5
35-50	30	35	15	13	1.3	1.4
55-70	25	30	17:30	15:30	1.1	1.3
BORDERLINE						
15-30	30	35	15	13	1.3	1.4
35-50	25	30	16:30	14:30	1.2	1.3
55-70	20	25	19	17	1.0	1.2
NEEDS EXTRA WORK ON CRF						
15-30	< 25	< 30	> 17	> 15	< 1.2	< 1.3
35-50	< 20	< 25	> 18:30	> 16:30	< 1.1	< 1.2
55-70	< 15	< 20	> 21	> 19	< 0.9	< 1.0

Note. From Howley and Franks (1986). These standards are for fitness programs. People wanting to do well in endurance performance need higher levels. For those at the *Good* level, the emphasis is on maintaining this level the rest of their lives. For those in the lower levels, emphasis is on setting and reaching realistic goals.

[a]CRF declines with age.

[b]Women have lower standards because they have a larger amount of essential fat.

(7), who showed that 10- to 20-min running tests could be used to estimate $\dot{V}O_2$max. Balke found the optimal duration to be 15 min. The test is based on the relationship between running velocity and the oxygen uptake required to run at that velocity (Figure 9.1). The greater the running speed, the greater the oxygen uptake required. The reason for the duration of 12 to 15 min is that the running test has to be long enough to diminish the contribution of anaerobic sources of energy (immediate and short-term) to the average velocity. In essence, the average velocity that can be maintained in a 5- or 6-min run overestimates $\dot{V}O_2$max. If the run is too long, the person is not able to run close to 100% of $\dot{V}O_2$max, and the estimate is too low (Figure 9.2).

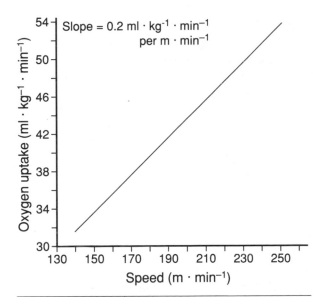

Figure 9.1 Relationship between steady-state oxygen uptake and running speed. Adapted from Bransford and Howley (1977).

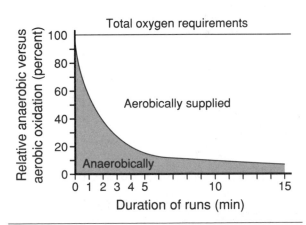

Figure 9.2 The relative role of aerobic and anaerobic energy sources in best-effort runs of various durations. From Balke, B.(1963). Federal Aviation Agency Report, 63:6. Used with permission.

The $\dot{V}O_2$ associated with a specific running speed can be calculated using the following formula (see chapter 8 for details):

$$\dot{V}O_2 = \text{net } O_2 \text{ cost of running} + \text{resting } \dot{V}O_2$$

$$\dot{V}O_2 = 0.2 \text{ ml} \cdot \text{kg}^{-1} \cdot \text{min}^{-1} \text{ per m} \cdot \text{min}^{-1}$$

$$+ 3.5 \text{ ml} \cdot \text{kg}^{-1} \cdot \text{min}^{-1}$$

These estimates are reasonable for adults who jog/run the entire 12 min or 1.5 mi. The formula will underestimate $\dot{V}O_2$max in children because of the higher oxygen cost of running for children (15). In contrast, the formula will overestimate $\dot{V}O_2$max in trained runners, due to their better running economy (14), and in those who walk through the test, because the net oxygen cost of walking is half that of running (see chapter 8).

QUESTION: A 20-year-old female takes the Cooper 12-min-run test following a 15-week walk/jog program and completes 6 laps on a 440-yd (402.3-m) track. What is her $\dot{V}O_2$max?

ANSWER:

$$402.3 \text{ m} \cdot \text{lap}^{-1} \cdot 6 \text{ laps} = 2,414 \text{ m}$$

$$2,414 \text{ m} \div 12 \text{ min} = 201 \text{ m} \cdot \text{min}^{-1}$$

$$\dot{V}O_2 = 0.2 \text{ ml} \cdot \text{kg}^{-1} \cdot \text{min}^{-1} \text{ per m} \cdot \text{min}^{-1}$$

$$+ 3.5 \text{ ml} \cdot \text{kg}^{-1} \cdot \text{min}^{-1}$$

$$\dot{V}O_2 = 0.2 \text{ ml} \cdot \text{kg}^{-1} \cdot \text{min}^{-1} (201 \text{ m} \cdot \text{min}^{-1})$$

$$+ 3.5 \text{ ml} \cdot \text{kg}^{-1} \cdot \text{min}^{-1}$$

$$\dot{V}O_2 = 43.7 \text{ ml} \cdot \text{kg}^{-1} \cdot \text{min}^{-1}$$

The advantage of the 12-min run is that it can be used on a regular basis to evaluate current CRF without expensive equipment. It is easily adapted to cyclists and swimmers, who can evaluate their progress by determining how far they can ride or swim in 12 min. Although no equations exist that can relate cyclists' and swimmers' respective performances to $\dot{V}O_2$max, each participant is able to make a personal judgment about her or his current state of CRF and improvement from training.

As Cooper (13) and others agree, an endurance run should *not* be used at the beginning of an exercise program. A person should progress through the jogging program at low intensities to make some fitness improvements before using an endurance-run field test.

Table 9.2 lists values for CRF as *good, adequate, borderline,* and finally, *needs extra work.* The table takes age and gender into consideration. For example, a 40-year-old woman who runs 1.5 mi in 14 min and

15 s (14:15) would rate between *adequate and good*. This time of 14:15 corresponds to a CRF value of about 35 to 40 ml•kg^{-1}•min^{-1}. We recommend that you should encourage participants to try to achieve and maintain the "*good*" value for age and gender. If persons are not at that level, help them to plan on making small and systematic progress toward that goal using the walking and jogging programs in chapter 14.

Administration of an Endurance-Run Test

The 1-mi run is used in many youth fitness programs. **The following five elements are needed for an endurance run:**

- **A person to start and read the time from a stopwatch**
- **A partner for each runner (perhaps with a sheet to mark off laps)**
- **Running space, marked off**
- **A stopwatch (with a spare ready)**
- **A scoresheet or scorecard**

The Steps in Administration of 1-Mile Run can be used for other endurance runs (e.g., 1.5-mi or 12-min run). The mile run is used as an example.

GRADED EXERCISE TESTS (GXTs)

TYPES OF GRADED EXERCISE TESTS

Many fitness programs use a **graded exercise test (GXT)** to evaluate CRF. These multilevel tests can be administered using a bench, cycle ergometer, or treadmill.

Bench Step

Bench stepping is very economical. It can be used for both submaximal and maximal testing. The disadvantages include the limited number of stages that can be

---

Steps in Administration of 1-Mile Run

Step	Activity

Pretest

1. Explain the purpose of the test (i.e., to determine how fast participants can run a mile, which reflects the endurance of their cardiovascular system).
2. Do **not** administer the test until persons have had several fitness sessions, including some with running.
3. Have persons practice running at a set submaximal pace for one lap, then two, etc., several times prior to test day.
4. Select and mark off (if necessary) a level area for the run.
5. Participants are to run the mile in the fastest time possible. Walking is allowed, but the goal is to cover the distance as fast as possible.

Test day

1. Warm up with stretching, walking, and slow jogging.
2. Several persons run at the same time.
3. The procedure is explained again.
4. The timer says, "Ready, go" and starts the stopwatch.
5. Each individual has a partner (perhaps an older individual, for younger participants).
6. The partner counts the laps and tells the individual at the end of each lap how many more lap(s) to run.
7. The timer calls out the minutes and seconds as the runners finish the mile run.
8. The partner listens for the time when the runner finishes the mile and records it (to the nearest second) immediately on a scorecard.
9. The runners continue to walk one lap after finishing the run.

feasibly included for any one bench height and individual fitness level, and the difficulty of taking certain measurements during the test (e.g., BP). The oxygen cost for stepping at different rates on steps of different heights was presented in chapter 8.

Cycle Ergometer

Cycle ergometers are portable, moderately priced work instruments that allow measurements to be made easily because the upper body is essentially stationary. However, among their disadvantages are that the exercise load is self-paced and that leg-muscle fatigue may be a limiting factor (30). On mechanically braked cycle ergometers such as the Monark models, the work rate can be changed by altering the pedal rate or the resistance on the flywheel. Generally, the pedal rate is maintained constant during a GXT at a rate appropriate to the populations being tested: 50 to 60 rev·min⁻¹ for the low to average fit, 70 to 100 for the highly fit and competitive cyclists (18). The pedal rate is maintained by having the subject attend to a metronome, or by providing some other source of feedback, such as a speedometer. The resistance (load) on the wheel is increased sequentially to systematically overload the cardiovascular system. The starting work rate and the increment from one stage to the next depend on the fitness of the subject and the purpose of the test, as mentioned earlier. $\dot{V}O_2$ can be estimated from a formula that gives reasonable estimates of $\dot{V}O_2$ up to work rates of about 1,200 kpm·min⁻¹ (see chapter 8 for details):

$$\dot{V}O_2 \text{ (ml·min}^{-1}) = [(2 \text{ ml·kpm}^{-1})\cdot(\text{kpm·min}^{-1})]$$
$$+ 300 \text{ ml·min}^{-1}$$

The cycle ergometer differs from the treadmill in that the body weight is supported by the seat and the work rate depends only on pedal rate and the load on the wheel. This means that the relative $\dot{V}O_2$ at any work rate is higher for a small person than for a big person.

QUESTION: What is the relative difficulty of a work rate of 900 kpm·min⁻¹ for two subjects, one 60 kg and the other 90 kg?

ANSWER:

The estimated $\dot{V}O_2$ for 900 kpm·min⁻¹ is 2,100 ml·min⁻¹

2,100 ml·min⁻¹ ÷ 60 kg = 35 ml·kg⁻¹·min⁻¹

2,100 ml·min⁻¹ ÷ 90 kg = 23 ml·kg⁻¹·min⁻¹

In addition, the increments in the work rate, by demanding a fixed increase in the $\dot{V}O_2$ (e.g., an increment of 150 kpm·min⁻¹ is equal to a $\dot{V}O_2$ change of 300 ml·min⁻¹), force the small or unfit subject to make larger cardiovascular adjustments than a large or highly fit subject. As we will see, these factors are considered in the selection of the work rates when a cycle ergometer test is used to evaluate CRF. Table 9.3 summarizes the effects that differences in body weight have on the metabolic responses to weight-supported and weight-carrying work tasks. Thus a larger person does more total work and has the same MET level for tasks in which the body weight is the resistance. In cycling, the same total work is done, but the larger person has a lower MET level.

Treadmill

Treadmill protocols are very reproducible because they set the pace for the subject, whereas the subject may go too slow or too fast on either the bench or the

Table 9.3 Work Differences Based on Body Weight in Work Tasks

Work task	$\dot{V}O_2$ L · min⁻¹	$\dot{V}O_2$ ml · kg⁻¹ · min⁻¹	Total work (kcal)	METs
A **heavier** person will respond with the following differences compared with a **lighter** person when doing the task at the same rate:				
Carry body weight				
Bench	↑	=	↑	=
Walk	↑	=	↑	=
Jog	↑	=	↑	=
Body weight supported				
Cycle	=	↓	=	↓

cycle. Treadmill tests can accommodate the least to the most fit and use the natural activities of walking and running, with the running tests placing the greatest potential load on the cardiovascular system. However, treadmills are expensive, not portable, and make some measurements (BP and blood sampling) difficult (30). The type of treadmill test influences the *measured* $\dot{V}O_2$ max, with the graded running test giving the highest value, a running test at 0% grade the next highest, and the walking test protocols the lowest (6, 22).

For estimates of $\dot{V}O_2$ to be obtained from grade and speed considerations, the grade and speed settings must be correct (21). Further, the subject must carefully follow the directions of not holding onto the treadmill railing during the test, if the estimated $\dot{V}O_2$ values are going to be reasonable (4, 28). For example, it has been observed that HR decreased 17 beats•min^{-1} when a subject who was walking on a treadmill at 3.4 mi•hr^{-1} and a 14% grade held onto the treadmill railing (4). This would result in an overestimation of the $\dot{V}O_2$max, because the HR would be lower at any stage of the test and test duration would be extended. Finally, there is no need to make adjustments to the $\dot{V}O_2$ calculation due to differences in body weight, because treadmill tests require the subject to carry his or her own weight, and the $\dot{V}O_2$ (ml•kg^{-1}•min^{-1}) is therefore proportional to body weight (23).

KEY POINT. CRF responses to different levels of exercise can be determined using a treadmill, cycle ergometer, or bench-stepping protocol.

COMMON VARIABLES MEASURED DURING A GXT

The variables that are commonly measured for resting and submaximal tests include HR, BP, and rating of perceived exertion (RPE). For maximal testing, $\dot{V}O_2$ max, time to exhaustion on a GXT, or time to cover a set distance (or distance run in a set time) is often measured.

Heart Rate

Heart rate (HR) is often used as a fitness indicator at rest and during a standard submaximal work task. Maximal HR is useful for determining the target heart rate (THR) for fitness workouts (see chapter 13), but it is not a good fitness indicator because it changes very little with training. Table 9.4 summarizes the effects

Table 9.4   Effects of Conditioning on HR

Condition	Effects of fitness on HR
Rest	↓
Standard submaximal work (same external work rate)	↓
Maximal work	no change
Set % of maximal	no change

of increasing fitness by training (aerobic exercise or conditioning) on HR in different conditions.

When an ECG is being recorded, the HR can be taken from the ECG strip (see chapter 15). When no ECG is being recorded, HR can be taken by a heart-rate watch, auscultation with a stethoscope, or manual palpation of an artery at the wrist or neck. Heart-rate watches (getting signals similar to ECG from a strap around the chest) have been found to be accurate and are the easiest way to get HR. Fingers (not the thumb) should be used to take HR, preferably at the wrist (radial artery). If a person takes HR at the neck (carotid artery), caution should be used not to apply too much pressure, because it could trigger a reflex that causes the HR to slow down. However, reliable measures are obtained when people are trained in this procedure (26, 29). The HR at rest or during a steady-state exercise should be taken for 30 s for higher reliability. However, when taking HRs after exercise, they should be taken at exactly the same time after work (e.g., 5 s) and taken for 10 or 15 s, because the heart rate changes so rapidly. The 10-s or 15-s rate is multiplied by 6 or 4, respectively, to calculate beats per minute (see Table 9.5).

Blood Pressure

Systolic blood pressure (SBP) and **diastolic blood pressure (DBP)** are often determined at rest, during work, and after work. The proper size of cuff (in which the bladder overlaps two thirds of the arm) and a sensitive stethoscope are required to get accurate values at rest and during work. At rest, the person should have both feet flat on the floor and be in a relaxed position with the arm supported. The cuff should be wrapped securely around the arm, usually with the tube on the inside of the arm. The stethoscope should be below (not under) the cuff—the placement will depend on where the sound can be most easily heard, often toward the inside of the arm. The first and fourth Korotkoff sounds (the first sound heard and the sound when the tone changes or becomes muffled) should be used for SBP and DBP, respectively. During exercise, if SBP fails to

Table 9.5 Heart-Rate Conversion From Beats Per
Minute to Beats in 10, 15, or 30 s

	Number of beats per		
Min	10 s	15 s	30 s
40	7	10	20
45	8	11	23
50	8	13	25
55	9	14	28
60	10	15	30
65	11	16	32
70	12	18	35
75	13	19	38
80	13	20	40
85	14	21	43
90	15	23	45
95	16	24	48
100	17	25	50
105	18	26	53
110	18	28	55
115	19	29	58
120	20	30	60
125	21	31	63
130	22	33	65
135	23	34	68
140	23	35	70
145	24	36	73
150	25	38	75
155	26	39	78
160	27	40	80
165	28	41	83
170	28	43	85
175	29	44	88
180	30	45	90
185	31	46	93
190	32	48	95
195	33	49	98
200	33	50	100
205	34	51	103
210	35	53	105
215	36	54	108
220	37	55	110
225	38	56	113
230	38	58	115

increase, or the DBP increases rapidly with increased work, the work should be stopped.

Rating of Perceived Exertion

Borg introduced the **rating of perceived exertion (RPE)**, based on a scale from 6 to 20 (roughly based on resting to maximal HR, i.e., 60 to 200). Table 9.6 contains this scale as well as Borg's revised 10-point RPE scale (10). Either can be used with a GXT to provide useful information during the test as the person approaches exhaustion and to be a reference point for exercise prescription. The following instructions are recommended to be used when administering the RPE scale (1): "During the graded exercise test we want you to pay close attention to how hard you *feel* the work rate is. This feeling should be your total amount of exertion and fatigue, combining all sensations and feelings of physical stress, effort, and fatigue. Don't concern yourself with any one factor such as leg pain, shortness of breath or exercise intensity, but try to concentrate on your *total, inner* feeling of exertion. Don't underestimate or overestimate, just be as accurate as you can."

Table 9.6 Rating of Perceived Exertion Scales

Original rating scale		New rating scale	
6		0	Nothing at all
7	Very, very light	0.5	Very, very light (just noticeable)
8			
9	Very light	1	Very light
10			
11	Fairly light	2	Light (weak)
12		3	Moderate
13	Somewhat hard	4	Somewhat hard
14			
15	Hard	5	Heavy (strong)
16		6	
17	Very hard	7	Very heavy
18		8	
		9	
19	Very, very hard	10	Very, very heavy (almost max)
20			

Note. From "Psychological Bases of Physical Exertion" by G.A.V. Borg, 1982, *Medicine and Science in Sports and Exercise*, **14**(5). Copyright 1982 by American College of Sports Medicine. Adapted by permission.

Estimation Versus Measurement of Functional Capacity

Functional capacity is defined as the highest work rate (oxygen uptake) reached in a GXT during which time HR, BP, and ECG responses are within the normal range for heavy work. For cardiac patients, the highest work rate does not normally reflect a measure of the maximal capacity of the CR systems, because the GXT might be stopped for ECG changes, angina, claudication pain, and so on. For the apparently healthy person, functional capacity can be called maximal aerobic power or maximal oxygen uptake ($\dot{V}O_2$max). (See chapter 3 for procedures to be used in measurement of oxygen uptake.)

Oxygen uptake increases with each stage of the GXT until the upper limit of CRF is reached. At that point, $\dot{V}O_2$ does not increase further when the test moves to the next stage; the person's $\dot{V}O_2$max has been reached. Given the complexity and cost of these procedures, $\dot{V}O_2$max is usually estimated with equations relating the stage of the GXT to a specific oxygen uptake.

As discussed in chapter 8, a variety of formulas may be used to estimate oxygen uptake on the basis of the stage reached in a GXT. In general, these formulas give reasonable estimates of the $\dot{V}O_2$ achieved in a GXT, if the test has been suited to the individual. However, if the increments in the stages of the GXT are too large relative to the person's CRF, or if the time for each stage is too short, then the person might not be able to reach the steady-state oxygen requirement associated with that stage (16, 20, 24). Failure to achieve the oxygen requirement for a GXT stage results in an overestimation of the $\dot{V}O_2$ at each stage of the test, with the overestimation growing larger with each stage. Inability to reach the oxygen requirement is a common problem with less-fit individuals (e.g., cardiac patients). This inability suggests that more conservative (i.e., smaller increments between stages) GXT protocols should be used to allow the less fit individual to reach the oxygen demand at each stage. A more complete explanation of this problem is found in chapter 3.

Shorter stages and larger increments between stages in a GXT can be used if the purpose of the test is to screen for ECG abnormalities (rather than to estimate $\dot{V}O_2$max). In addition, changes in CRF over time can be determined by periodically using the same GXT on an individual.

KEY POINT. The variables measured during a GXT include heart rate, blood pressure, perceived exertion, and oxygen uptake (often estimated).

EXERCISE TESTING EQUIPMENT AND CALIBRATION

Fitness testing requires the purchase of high-quality equipment that can be calibrated (see chapter 5) and hold that calibration from one test to the next. This section provides an overview of the equipment used in testing centers that conduct submaximal fitness tests. Submaximal tests are used to evaluate a person's HR, BP, and RPE responses either to a single work rate or

to a series of progressive work rates. The test is usually stopped at 70% to 85% of estimated maximal HR. The HR data are then used to estimate $\dot{V}O_2$max by an extrapolation procedure or with specific formulas. **The equipment and supplies used for such tests include**

- **cycle ergometer, step (and metronome), or treadmill;**
- **sphygmomanometer and stethoscope;**
- **clock or stopwatch;**
- **RPE chart; and**
- **recording forms.**

KEY POINT. Equipment to measure and record CRF variables needs to be available and calibrated.

PROCEDURES FOR GRADED EXERCISE TESTING

This section provides information concerning how to administer a GXT and uses examples of different testing protocols. **Before administering any GXT, the tester should**

- **calibrate the equipment,**
- **check supplies and data forms,**
- **select the appropriate test protocol for the participant,**
- **obtain informed consent,**
- **provide instruction in the task, including the cool-down procedure,**
- **have the participant practice the task, if needed,**
- **check to see that pretest instructions were followed, and**
- **follow the test protocol exactly.**

Pretest Instructions

Because resting CRF variables, HR, BP, and RPE responses to submaximal work, and maximal endurance are influenced by a variety of factors, care must be taken to minimize the variation in each from one testing period to the next. These factors include, but are not limited to

- temperature and relative humidity of the room,
- number of hours of sleep,
- emotional state,
- hydration state,
- medication,
- time of day,

- time since last meal, cigarette smoking, caffeine intake, and exercise, and
- psychological environment for the test.

Attention to these factors increases the likelihood that changes in HR, BP, or RPE from one test to the next are caused by changes in physical fitness and physical activity habits. A form such as the Pretest Instructions for a Fitness Test is helpful in assuring that the client will be ready for testing.

Steps During GXT

Typical procedures to follow in doing GXTs are shown in Steps in Administration of GXT.

Termination of GXT

A series of end points should be used to stop a GXT (see Reasons to Terminate a GXT). Some of these guidelines (1) refer specifically to maximal testing, but many can be applied to submaximal testing.

KEY POINT. Careful attention to procedures before and during a test will enhance the safety and accuracy of the test. The tester should know when to stop a test, based on signs, symptoms, or CRF measurements.

Submaximal and Maximal Tests

GXTs have been used to evaluate CRF in fitness programs for healthy populations and in the clinical assess-

ment of ischemic heart disease—a condition in which an inadequate blood flow to the heart muscle can cause changes in the ECG. Exercise is used to place a load on the heart to determine the cardiovascular response and to see if changes occur in the ECG. Some controversy has arisen concerning whether to use submaximal or maximal tests. On the basis of thousands of exercise stress tests conducted over the past 3 decades, it is generally recommended that a maximal exercise test be used to determine the presence of ischemic heart disease. Although submaximal exercise tests are not as effective in identifying disease conditions, they are appropriate for evaluating cardiorespiratory fitness prior to and following exercise programs.

When a fitness center is responsible for both fitness testing and the fitness program, the sequence of testing and activity recommended earlier provides the advantages of each while minimizing the disadvantages. The main objection to maximal tests is the stress they put on a person who has been inactive. Although the risk of a maximal GXT is very small with adequate screening and qualified testing personnel, the discomfort of going to one's maximum without prior conditioning may discourage some people from participating in a fitness program. Objections to the submaximal test include finding fewer abnormal responses to exercise and inaccurately estimating maximal level from submaximal data. In a fitness program for apparently healthy people, the objections against either maximal or submaximal tests given alone are overcome by administering the submaximal test early in the fitness program and waiting until the participant has been involved in a regular exercise program to administer the maximal test. Any of the GXT protocols can be used for submaximal or maximal testing—the only difference is the criterion for stopping the test. Either test is stopped if any of the abnormal responses listed earlier occur. In the

---

Pretest Instructions for a Fitness Test

Name _____ Test date _____ Time _____

Report to _____

Instructions: Please observe the following:
1. Wear running shoes, shorts, and a loose-fitting shirt.
2. No food, drink (except water), tobacco, or medication for 3 hours prior to test.
3. Minimal physical activity on day of test.

Cancellation:
If you cannot keep this appointment, please call _____ or _____

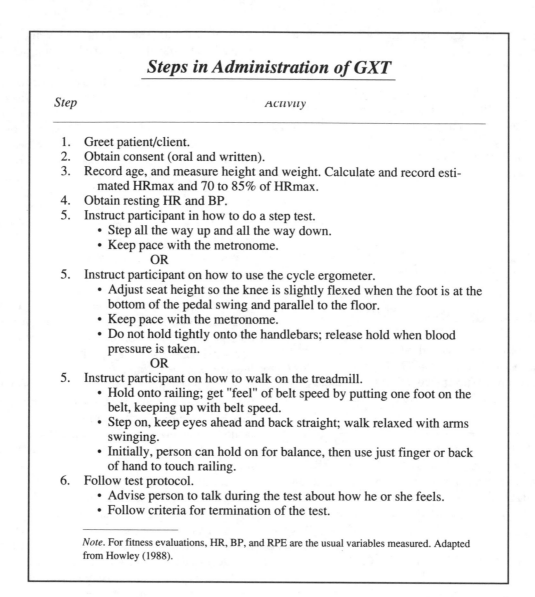

Steps in Administration of GXT

Step	*Activity*

1. Greet patient/client.
2. Obtain consent (oral and written).
3. Record age, and measure height and weight. Calculate and record estimated HRmax and 70 to 85% of HRmax.
4. Obtain resting HR and BP.
5. Instruct participant in how to do a step test.
   - Step all the way up and all the way down.
   - Keep pace with the metronome.
   OR
5. Instruct participant on how to use the cycle ergometer.
   - Adjust seat height so the knee is slightly flexed when the foot is at the bottom of the pedal swing and parallel to the floor.
   - Keep pace with the metronome.
   - Do not hold tightly onto the handlebars; release hold when blood pressure is taken.
   OR
5. Instruct participant on how to walk on the treadmill.
   - Hold onto railing; get "feel" of belt speed by putting one foot on the belt, keeping up with belt speed.
   - Step on, keep eyes ahead and back straight; walk relaxed with arms swinging.
   - Initially, person can hold on for balance, then use just finger or back of hand to touch railing.
6. Follow test protocol.
   - Advise person to talk during the test about how he or she feels.
   - Follow criteria for termination of the test.

Note. For fitness evaluations, HR, BP, and RPE are the usual variables measured. Adapted from Howley (1988).

absence of abnormal responses, the submaximal test is usually terminated when the person reaches a certain HR (often 85% of maximum HR), and the maximal test continues to voluntary exhaustion.

Maximal Exercise Test Protocols

No one GXT protocol is appropriate for all types of people. The time, starting points, and increments between stages should vary with the type of person. Young active, normal sedentary, and people with questionable health status should start at 6, 4, and 2 METs, respectively. The same three groups should increase 2 to 3, 1 to 2, and 0.5 to 1 METs, respectively, for stages of the test. If the test is being used to compare CRF at different times, then 1 or 2 min per stage can be used. However, if trying to predict $\dot{V}O_2max$, the time per stage should be 2 to 3 min. Table 9.7 illustrates how these criteria might be used for a bench, cycle, or treadmill test.

The following testing protocols are examples of tests that could be used for different populations. The first protocol, shown in Table 9.8, could be used with deconditioned subjects by starting at a very low MET level, walking slowly, and increasing 1 MET per stage (25). The Balke Standard (8) protocol (see Table 9.9) could be used for typical inactive adults by progressing at 1 MET per stage and starting at a higher MET level. More active, or younger people could be tested on the Bruce (12) protocol (see Table 9.10), which starts at a moderate MET level and goes up 2 or 3 METs per stage. Unfortunately, some testing centers attempt to use the same testing protocol for all people, with the result that the initial stage is often too high or too low and the work increments for each stage are either too small or too large for the individual being tested.

Reasons to Terminate a GXT

$\dot{V}O_2$max is reached (the normal end point for the healthy individual)
Abnormal signs and symptoms
    Dizziness, mental confusion, staggering, or unsteadiness
    Angina, claudication, or other pain
    Nausea
    Marked dyspnea
    Cyanosis or pallor
    Severe fatigue, facial distress
Subject asks to stop
ECG changes (see chapter 15)
    S–T segment displacement above or below the baseline
    Ventricular arrhythmias
    Ventricular tachycardia
    Ectopic ventricular complexes occurring every second or third beat
    Frequent ventricular complexes
Atrioventricular or ventricular conduction disturbances
    AV block
    Bundle branch block
Abnormal blood-pressure response
    Fall in systolic pressure of 20 mmHg with a stage increase in the GXT, or a systolic pressure of 250 mmHg
    A rise of 20 mmHg in the diastolic pressure, or a diastolic pressure of 120 mmHg
Heart-rate response
    Age-adjusted estimated maximal heart rate can alert the tester that the subject is nearing maximum, but should *not* be used as the end point for maximal test
    A percent of HRmax (e.g., 70% or 85%) can be used to stop submaximal tests
Respiratory response
    Marked dyspnea
Malfunctioning equipment
    Stop the test and reschedule for later time

Note. Adapted from ACSM (1991).

Submaximal Exercise Test Protocols

Any GXT protocol can be used for submaximal or maximal testing. The HFI typically uses a submaximal GXT to estimate a person's $\dot{V}O_2$max or to simply show before-and-after changes in selected variables due to the exercise program. It needs to be emphasized that predicting maximal oxygen uptake from any submaximal test involves substantial error. However, it can provide useful information in a fitness program to estimate a person's functional capacity, and to be used for classification and programming. The only way to determine an individual's functional capacity is to measure it during a maximal test (11). Changes in HR, BP, and RPE as a result of an exercise conditioning program make a submaximal test a good mechanism for showing improvements in CRF.

Treadmill

The initial stage and rate of progression of the GXT should be selected on the basis of the criteria mentioned earlier. In the following example, a Balke Standard protocol (3 mi•hr^{-1}, 2.5% grade increase each 2 min) was used; HR was monitored in the last 30 s of each stage. The test was terminated at 85% of age-adjusted maximal HR. Maximal aerobic power was estimated by extrapolating the HR response to the person's estimated maximal HR. Figure 9.3 presents the results of this test

Table 9.7   Testing Protocol for Different Groups

Stage	METs	Bench Height (cm)	Bench Steps · min⁻¹	Cycle Work rate (kpm · min⁻¹)	RPM	Treadmill Speed (km · hr⁻¹)	Treadmill Grade (%)
				INDIVIDUALS WITH QUESTIONABLE HEALTH			
1	2	0	24	0	50	3.2	0
2	3	16	12	150	50	4.8	0
3	4	16	18	300	50	4.8	2.5
4	5	16	24	450	50	4.8	5.0
5	6	16	30	600	50	4.8	7.5
				"NORMAL" INACTIVE INDIVIDUALS			
1	4	16	18	360	60	4.8	2.5
2	6	16	30	540	60	4.8	7.5
3	7-8	36	18-24	720-900	60	4.8-5.5	10.0
4	9	36	27	900-1080	60	5.5	12.0
5	10-11	36	30-33	1080-1260	60	9.7	0-1.75
				YOUNG ACTIVE INDIVIDUALS			
1	6	16	30	630	70	4.8	7.5
2	9	36	27	1060	70	5.5	12.0
3	12	36	36	1270	70	9.7	3.5
4	15	50	33	1900	70	11.3	7.0
5	17	50	39	2110	70	11.3	11.0

Note. Adapted from Franks (1979).

Table 9.8   Treadmill Protocol for Deconditioned People

Stage	METs	Speed (mi · hr⁻¹)	Grade (%)	Time (min)
1	2.5	2	0	3
2	3.5	2	3.5	3
3	4.5	2	7	3
4	5.4	2	10.5	3
5	6.4	2	14	3
6	7.3	2	17.5	3
7	8.5	3	12.5	3
8	9.5	3	15	3
9	10.5	3	17.5	3

Note. From "Methods of Exercise Testing" by J.P. Naughton and R. Haider. In *Exercise Testing and Exercise Training in Coronary Heart Disease*, by J.P. Naughton, H.R. Hellerstein, and L.C. Mohler (Eds.), 1973, New York: Academic Press.

Table 9.9   Balke Standard Treadmill Protocol for Normal Inactive People

Stage	METs	Speed (mi · hr⁻¹)	Grade (%)	Time (min)
1	4.3	3	2.5	2
2	5.4	3	5	2
3	6.4	3	7.5	2
4	7.4	3	10	2
5	8.5	3	12.5	2
6	9.5	3	15	2
7	10.5	3	17.5	2
8	11.6	3	20	2
9	12.6	3	22.5	2
10	13.6	3	25	2

Note. From "Advanced Exercise Procedures for Evaluation of the Cardiovascular System," *Monograph*, by B. Balke, 1970, Milton, WI: The Burdick Corporation.

with a graph showing the HR response at each work rate. Note that the HR response is rather flat between the 0% and 5% grades. This is not an uncommon finding (see the discussion of the YMCA test); perhaps the subject is too excited, or perhaps the stroke-volume changes are accounting for the changes in cardiac out-

put at these low work rates. The HR response is normally quite linear between 110 beats·min⁻¹ and the subject's 85% of maximal HR cutoff.

To estimate $\dot{V}O_2$max, a line is drawn through the HR points from 7.5% grade to the final work rate. The line is extended (extrapolated) to the person's estimated

Table 9.10   Treadmill Protocol for Young Active People

Stage	METs	Speed (mi · hr⁻¹)	Grade (%)	Time (min)
1	5	1.7	10	3
2	7	2.5	12	3
3	9.5	3.4	14	3
4	13	4.2	16	3
5	16	5.0	18	3

Note. From "Multi-Stage Treadmill Test of Maximal and Submaximal Exercise" by R.A. Bruce. In American Heart Association, *Exercise Testing and Training of Apparently Healthy Individuals: A Handbook for Physicians* (pp. 32-34), 1972, New York: American Heart Association.

maximal HR (183 beats•min⁻¹). A vertical line is dropped from the last point to the baseline to estimate the subject's maximal aerobic power, which is 11.8 METs, or 41.3 ml•kg⁻¹•min⁻¹. Remember that the estimated maximal HR may be inaccurate and that the estimate of maximal oxygen uptake will be influenced by this possible inaccuracy. The subject presented in this figure was later found to have a measured maximal HR of 195 beats•min⁻¹ and was able to finish the 2-min stage equal to 12.8 METs.

KEY POINT. GXT protocols can be used for submaximal tests (early in the testing sequence) or maximal tests (for active persons who have reached minimal fitness levels).

Cyle Ergometer

The steps to be taken for this test are shown in Administration of Submaximal Cycle Ergometer Test.

Our first example of a submaximal cycle-ergometer protocol (Figure 9.4) is taken from *The Y's Way to Physical Fitness* (17). This protocol relies on the observation that there is a linear relationship between HR and work rate ($\dot{V}O_2$) once a HR of approximately 110 beats•min⁻¹ is reached. The test simply requires the person to complete one more stage past the one causing a HR of 110 beats•min⁻¹. The intent of the test is to extrapolate the line describing the HR–work rate relationship out to the person's age-adjusted maximal HR (as was done for the treadmill protocol) to estimate the person's $\dot{V}O_2$max. Each stage of the test lasts 3 min, unless a person's HR has not yet reached a steady state (> 5 beats•min⁻¹ difference between 2nd- and 3rd-min HR). In that case, an extra minute is added to that stage. The pedal rate is maintained at 50 rev•min⁻¹, so that, on a Monark cycle ergometer, a 0.5-kg increase in load is equal to 150 kpm•min⁻¹ (25 W). Seat height is adjusted so that the knee is slightly bent when the pedal is at the bottom of the swing through 1 revolution. The

Name: _____   Age: __37__   Estimated HRmax: __183__   85% HRmax: __155__

Test type: Balke Standard   Ht: _____   Wt: _____   Sex: __Male__
Speed: 3 mph

% grade	Time (min)	Heart rate
0	1	
	2	94
2.5	3	
	4	95
5	5	
	6	100
7.5	7	
	8	118
10	9	
	10	131
12.5	11	
	12	143
15	13	
	14	155

Figure 9.3 Maximal aerobic power estimated by measuring the heart-rate response to a submaximal graded exercise test on a treadmill.

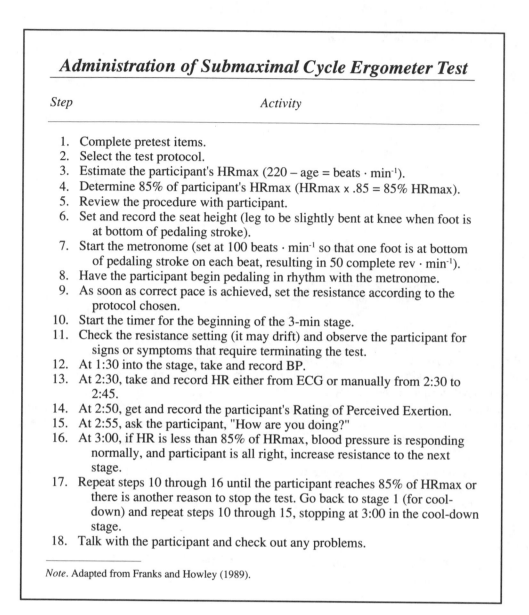

Administration of Submaximal Cycle Ergometer Test

Step   *Activity*

1. Complete pretest items.
2. Select the test protocol.
3. Estimate the participant's HRmax (220 – age = beats · min⁻¹).
4. Determine 85% of participant's HRmax (HRmax x .85 = 85% HRmax).
5. Review the procedure with participant.
6. Set and record the seat height (leg to be slightly bent at knee when foot is at bottom of pedaling stroke).
7. Start the metronome (set at 100 beats · min⁻¹ so that one foot is at bottom of pedaling stroke on each beat, resulting in 50 complete rev · min⁻¹).
8. Have the participant begin pedaling in rhythm with the metronome.
9. As soon as correct pace is achieved, set the resistance according to the protocol chosen.
10. Start the timer for the beginning of the 3-min stage.
11. Check the resistance setting (it may drift) and observe the participant for signs or symptoms that require terminating the test.
12. At 1:30 into the stage, take and record BP.
13. At 2:30, take and record HR either from ECG or manually from 2:30 to 2:45.
14. At 2:50, get and record the participant's Rating of Perceived Exertion.
15. At 2:55, ask the participant, "How are you doing?"
16. At 3:00, if HR is less than 85% of HRmax, blood pressure is responding normally, and participant is all right, increase resistance to the next stage.
17. Repeat steps 10 through 16 until the participant reaches 85% of HRmax or there is another reason to stop the test. Go back to stage 1 (for cool-down) and repeat steps 10 through 15, stopping at 3:00 in the cool-down stage.
18. Talk with the participant and check out any problems.

Note. Adapted from Franks and Howley (1989).

seat height is recorded for future reference. HR is monitored during the later half of the 2nd and 3rd min of each stage.

Proper selection of the initial work rate and the rate of progression of the work rate on the cycle ergometer should take into consideration the person's weight, sex, age, and level of fitness. The ACSM deals with this problem by recommending three cycle-ergometer protocols, depending on body weight and recent pattern of physical activity. Table 9.11 outlines this information. People less than 73 kg (160 lb) would use Protocol A independent of activity status; thus Protocol A would be suitable for most women in our society.

In comparison, the YMCA test starts at 150 kpm•min⁻¹, and subsequent stages are chosen depending on the HR response to the specified work task (see Figure 9.4). A person needs to have only one addi-

tional HR measure past the work rate demanding a HR of 110 beats•min⁻¹.

The HR values for the 2nd and 3rd min of each work rate are recorded, and directions are followed to estimate $\dot{V}O_2$max in liters per minute. These directions and an example are presented in Figure 9.5 for a 50-year-old woman. The stages followed the pattern dictated by the HR response to the initial work rate of 150 kpm•min⁻¹. A line was drawn through the last two HR values and extrapolated to the estimated maximal HR. The $\dot{V}O_2$max was estimated to be 1.77 L•min⁻¹. This value was multiplied by 1,000 to give 1,770 ml•min⁻¹ and divided by the 59-kg body weight to give an estimated $\dot{V}O_2$max of 30 ml•kg⁻¹•min⁻¹.

In contrast to this GXT protocol used to estimate $\dot{V}O_2$max, the Åstrand and Rhyming cycle-ergometer test (5) requires the subject to complete only one 6-

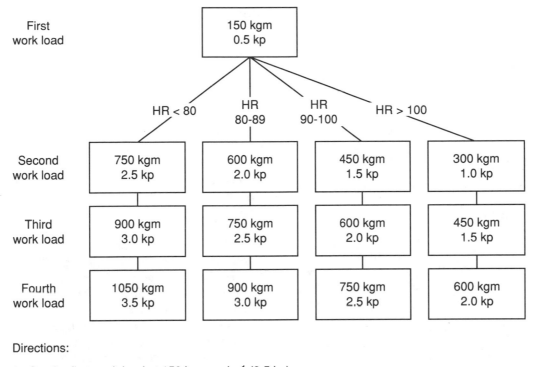

Directions:

1. Set the first work load at 150 kgm · min⁻¹ (0.5 kp).
2. If the HR in the 3rd minute is

   - less than (<) 80, set the second load at 750 kgm (2.5 kp);
   - 80 to 89, set the second load at 600 kgm (2.0 kp);
   - 90 to 100, set the second load at 450 kgm (1.5 kp);
   - greater than (>) 100, set the second load at 300 kgm (1.0 kp).

3. Set the third and fourth (if required) loads according to the loads in the columns below the second loads.

Figure 9.4 Guide for setting power outputs (work loads) for men and women on submaximal cycle ergometer test. *Note.* From Golding, L.A., Myers, C.R., and Sinning, W.E. (Eds.). Reprinted from *Y's Way to Physical Fitness: The Complete Guide to Fitness Testing and Instruction*, 3rd ed., with permission of the YMCA of the USA, 101 N. Wacker Drive, Chicago, IL 60606.

min work rate demanding a HR between 125 and 170 beats·min⁻¹. These investigators observed that for young (18 to 30 years) subjects, the average HR was 128 beats·min⁻¹ for males and 138 beats·min⁻¹ for females at 50% $\dot{V}O_2$max, and at 70% $\dot{V}O_2$max the average HRs were 154 and 164 beats·min⁻¹, respectively. Based on these observations, if you know from a HR response that a person is at 50% $\dot{V}O_2$max at a work rate equal to 1.5 L·min⁻¹, then the estimated $\dot{V}O_2$max would be twice that, or 3.0 L·min⁻¹. Table 9.12 is used to estimate $\dot{V}O_2$max based on the subject's HR response to one 6-min work rate (3).

Using the data collected for the YMCA test displayed earlier, we can see how $\dot{V}O_2$max is estimated in the Åstrand and Rhyming protocol. The 50-year-old woman had a HR of 140 beats·min⁻¹ at a work rate of 450 kpm·min⁻¹. Using Table 9.12, for women, look down the leftmost column to a HR of 140, and look across to the second column (450 kpm·min⁻¹). The estimated

$\dot{V}O_2$max is 2.4 L·min⁻¹. However, because maximal HR decreases with increasing age and the data were collected on young subjects, Åstrand (3) established the following correction factors with which one could multiply the estimated $\dot{V}O_2$max to correct for the lower maximal HR:

Age	Factor
15	1.10
25	1.00
35	0.87
40	0.83
45	0.78
50	0.75
55	0.71
60	0.68
65	0.65

One of the correction factors is multiplied by the estimated $\dot{V}O_2$max to calculate the corrected $\dot{V}O_2$max. For

Table 9.11   Selection Criteria for Cycle Ergometer Protocol

Body weight kg (lb)	Past 3-month activity level Vigorous, > 15 min, 3 days/week?	
	No	Yes
	Test protocol	
< 73 (160)	A	A
74-90 (161-199)	A	B
> 91 (200+)	B	C

Test protocol	Test stages (min)			
	I (1-2)	II (3-4)	III (5-6)	IV (7-8)
A	150[a]	300	450	600
B	150	300	600	900
C	300	600	900	1200

Note. Modified from ACSM (1991).

[a]Work rate is kpm · min⁻¹.

our 50-year-old subject, the correction factor is 0.75, and the corrected $\dot{V}O_2$max is $0.75 \cdot 2.4$ L·min⁻¹ = 1.8 L·min⁻¹. This value compares well with that estimated by the YMCA protocol.

Step Test

A multistage step test can be used to estimate $\dot{V}O_2$max and to show changes in CRF with training or detraining. As always, attention must be given to the initial stage and rate of progression of the stages so that the test is suited to the individual. Table 9.7 presented three examples of step-test protocols. The subject must be instructed to follow the metronome (4 counts per cycle, i.e., up-up-down-down) and step all the way up and all the way down. Each stage should last at least 2 min, with HR monitored in the last 30 s of each 2-min period. HR is more difficult to monitor during a step-test protocol if the palpation technique is used. An alternative is to put a BP cuff on the subject's arm and, when a HR measure is needed, pump the cuff up just above diastolic pressure (around 100 mmHg). With the stethoscope, the pulse rate can be counted for 10 or 15 s. Release the pressure after each measurement. An alternative is to stop the stepping after each stage, taking the HR for a 10-s count 5 s after the stage.

As in most submaximal test protocols, HR is plotted against $\dot{V}O_2$ for each stage, and a line is drawn through the points to the age-adjusted maximal HR. A line is drawn to the baseline to obtain an estimate of $\dot{V}O_2$max. Figure 9.6 shows the results of a step test for a sedentary 55-year-old man prior to a training program. His estimated $\dot{V}O_2$max was about 29 ml·kg⁻¹·min⁻¹, or 8.3 METs.

Form for YMCA Protocol

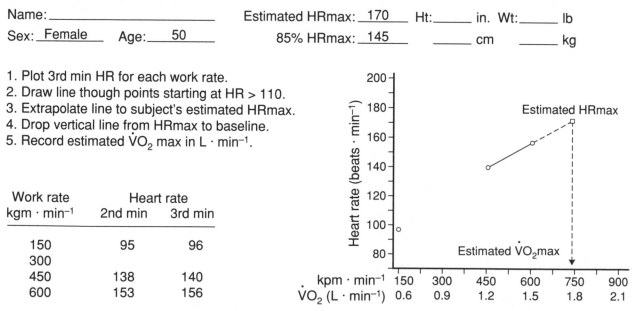

Name: _____   Estimated HRmax: __170__ Ht: _____ in. Wt: _____ lb
Sex: _Female_   Age: __50__   85% HRmax: __145__   _____ cm   _____ kg

1. Plot 3rd min HR for each work rate.
2. Draw line though points starting at HR > 110.
3. Extrapolate line to subject's estimated HRmax.
4. Drop vertical line from HRmax to baseline.
5. Record estimated $\dot{V}O_2$ max in L · min⁻¹.

Work rate kgm · min⁻¹	Heart rate 2nd min	3rd min
150	95	96
300		
450	138	140
600	153	156

Figure 9.5 Maximal aerobic power estimated by measuring the heart-rate response to a submaximal graded exercise test on a cycle ergometer, using the *Y's Way of Fitness* protocol. *Note.* From Golding, L.A., Myers, C.R., and Sinning, W.E. (Eds.). Reprinted from *Y's Way to Physical Fitness: The Complete Guide to Fitness Testing and Instruction*, 3rd ed., with permission of the YMCA of the USA, 101 N. Wacker Drive, Chicago, IL 60606.

Table 9.12   Predicting Maximal Oxygen Uptake From Heart Rate and Work Load During a Bicycle Ergometer Test

	Values for women $\dot{V}O_2$max (L · min⁻¹)						Values for men $\dot{V}O_2$max (L · min⁻¹)				
Heart rate	300 kpm/min	450 kpm/min	600 kpm/min	750 kpm/min	900 kpm/min	Heart rate	300 kpm/min	600 kpm/min	900 kpm/min	1200 kpm/min	1500 kpm/min
120	2.6	3.4	4.1	4.8		120	2.2	3.5	4.8		
121	2.5	3.3	4.0	4.8		121	2.2	3.4	4.7		
122	2.5	3.2	3.9	4.7		122	2.2	3.4	4.6		
123	2.4	3.1	3.9	4.6		123	2.1	3.4	4.6		
124	2.4	3.1	3.8	4.5		124	2.1	3.3	4.5	6.0	
125	2.3	3.0	3.7	4.4		125	2.0	3.2	4.4	5.9	
126	2.3	3.0	3.6	4.3		126	2.0	3.2	4.4	5.8	
127	2.2	2.9	3.5	4.2		127	2.0	3.1	4.3	5.7	
128	2.2	2.8	3.5	4.2	4.8	128	2.0	3.1	4.2	5.6	
129	2.2	2.8	3.4	4.1	4.8	129	1.9	3.0	4.2	5.6	
130	2.1	2.7	3.4	4.0	4.7	130	1.9	3.0	4.1	5.5	
131	2.1	2.7	3.4	4.0	4.6	131	1.9	2.9	4.0	5.4	
132	2.0	2.7	3.3	3.9	4.5	132	1.8	2.9	4.0	5.3	
133	2.0	2.6	3.2	3.8	4.4	133	1.8	2.8	3.9	5.3	
134	2.0	2.6	3.2	3.8	4.4	134	1.8	2.8	3.9	5.2	
135	2.0	2.6	3.1	3.7	4.3	135	1.7	2.8	3.8	5.1	
136	1.9	2.5	3.1	3.6	4.2	136	1.7	2.7	3.8	5.0	
137	1.9	2.5	3.0	3.6	4.2	137	1.7	2.7	3.7	5.0	
138	1.8	2.4	3.0	3.5	4.1	138	1.6	2.7	3.7	4.9	
139	1.8	2.4	2.9	3.5	4.0	139	1.6	2.6	3.6	4.8	
140	1.8	2.4	2.8	3.4	4.0	140	1.6	2.6	3.6	4.8	6.0
141	1.8	2.3	2.8	3.4	3.9	141		2.6	3.5	4.7	5.9
142	1.7	2.3	2.8	3.3	3.9	142		2.5	3.5	4.6	5.8
143	1.7	2.2	2.7	3.3	3.8	143		2.5	3.4	4.6	5.7
144	1.7	2.2	2.7	3.2	3.8	144		2.5	3.4	4.5	5.7
145	1.6	2.2	2.7	3.2	3.7	145		2.4	3.4	4.5	5.6
146	1.6	2.2	2.6	3.2	3.7	146		2.4	3.3	4.4	5.6
147	1.6	2.1	2.6	3.1	3.6	147		2.4	3.3	4.4	5.5
148	1.6	2.1	2.6	3.1	3.6	148		2.4	3.2	4.3	5.4
149		2.1	2.6	3.0	3.5	149		2.3	3.2	4.3	5.4
150		2.0	2.5	3.0	3.5	150		2.3	3.2	4.2	5.3
151		2.0	2.5	3.0	3.4	151		2.3	3.1	4.2	5.2
152		2.0	2.5	2.9	3.4	152		2.3	3.1	4.1	5.2
153		2.0	2.4	2.9	3.3	153		2.2	3.0	4.1	5.1
154		2.0	2.4	2.8	3.3	154		2.2	3.0	4.0	5.1
155		1.9	2.4	2.8	3.2	155		2.2	3.0	4.0	5.0
156		1.9	2.3	2.8	3.2	156		2.2	2.9	4.0	5.0
157		1.9	2.3	2.7	3.2	157		2.1	2.9	3.9	4.9
158		1.8	2.3	2.7	3.1	158		2.1	2.9	3.9	4.9
159		1.8	2.2	2.7	3.1	159		2.1	2.8	3.8	4.8
160		1.8	2.2	2.6	3.0	160		2.1	2.8	3.8	4.8
161		1.8	2.2	2.6	3.0	161		2.0	2.8	3.7	4.7
162		1.8	2.2	2.6	3.0	162		2.0	2.8	3.7	4.6
163		1.7	2.2	2.6	2.9	163		2.0	2.8	3.7	4.6
164		1.7	2.1	2.5	2.9	164		2.0	2.7	3.6	4.5
165		1.7	2.1	2.5	2.9	165		2.0	2.7	3.6	4.5
166		1.7	2.1	2.5	2.8	166		1.9	2.7	3.6	4.5
167		1.6	2.1	2.4	2.8	167		1.9	2.6	3.5	4.4
168		1.6	2.0	2.4	2.8	168		1.9	2.6	3.5	4.4
169		1.6	2.0	2.4	2.8	169		1.9	2.6	3.5	4.3
170		1.6	2.0	2.4	2.7	170		1.8	2.6	3.4	4.3

Note. From *Work Tests With the Bicycle Ergometer* (pp. 24, 25) by Per-Olof Åstrand, 1979, Varberg, Sweden: Monark-Crescent AB. Copyright 1979 by Monark-Crescent AB. Reprinted by permission.

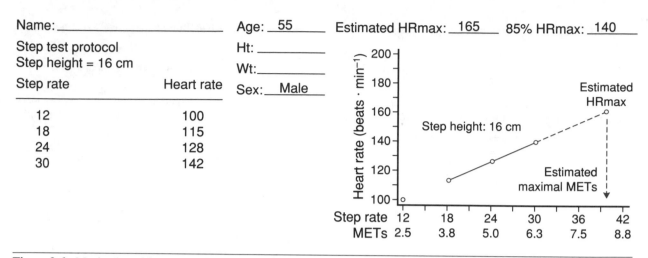

Figure 9.6 Maximal aerobic power estimated by measuring the heart-rate response to a submaximal graded exercise step test.

The StairMaster 4000 shows promise as a stepping ergometer. Work rates (METs) can be selected in a manner similar to setting grade on a treadmill, and the GXT could progress as described earlier, using similar initial settings and rates of progression. However, the true MET value is lower than the setting and can be calculated from the following formula:

True MET values = 0.556 + 0.744 (StairMaster

settings)

If this instrument is used in fitness testing, use 2- to 3-min stages and follow the termination criteria mentioned earlier for the other submaximal GXT protocols.

Posttest Procedures

When the test is over, the tester should conduct a cool-down phase, monitor test variables, and give posttest instructions. The tester should also organize the test data (see Posttest Protocol).

SUMMARY

The evaluation of CRF includes the screening of participants not suitable for CRF testing. Before any testing takes place, the individual signs a consent form that out-

---

Posttest Protocol

Use cool down as programmed per physician and other posttreadmill tests.
Have the subject sit down or lie down depending on posttests (nuclear).
Monitor HR, BP, and ECG immediately and after 1, 2, 4, and 6 min.
Remove cuff and electrodes when double product (HR x systolic BP) is close to
    pretest value.
Provide instructions for showering.
    Ask subject to wait for about 30 min.
    Ask subject to move around in shower, use warm (not hot) water.
    Check for return of person from shower.
Organize test data and discuss test results with person.

Note. Adapted from Howley (1988).

lines the procedures, benefits, and risks. This chapter provides several ways you can evaluate cardiorespiratory fitness levels of fitness participants. CRF evaluation might be in the form of an easily administered field test, such as a 1-mi walking test or the 1.5-m run to estimate maximal aerobic power. It is important to emphasize to the fitness participants that resting and submaximal tests *and a beginning conditioning program* should all precede all-out field tests. You should *not* use a running test to determine cardiorespiratory fitness levels until after the participants have successfully completed a beginning fitness program. Many tests of CRF use a GXT protocol on a treadmill, cycle ergometer, or step. An advantage of a GXT over a field test is the ability to monitor physiological variables (such as BP, HR, and oxygen uptake) at different levels of work. A variety of maximal and submaximal protocols for a treadmill, cycle, or bench step are presented for low-, moderate-, and high-fit individuals. Methods for estimation of maximal oxygen uptake are included. Procedures allowing the HFI to safely obtain accurate data are emphasized.

CASE STUDIES FOR ANALYSIS

9.1 You are contacted by a fitness club to review the test they have used to evaluate cardiorespiratory fitness on middle-aged participants. The club requires the participants to perform the 1.5-mi-run test during their first exercise session. The club director says he uses this test because so much data exists for it—the test has been used for more than 10 years. What is your reaction? (See Appendix A.)

9.2 You do the 1-mi-walk test with a 45-yr-old male client and record the following information: time = 15 min; heart rate = 140 beats$\cdot$min^{-1}; weight = 170 lbs. Calculate his estimated $\dot{V}O_2$max. (See Appendix A.)

REFERENCES

1. American College of Sports Medicine (1991)
2. Åstrand (1960)
3. Åstrand (n.d.)
4. Åstrand (1984)
5. Åstrand and Rhyming (1954)
6. Åstrand and Saltin (1961)
7. Balke (1963)
8. Balke (1970)
9. Blair et al. (1989)
10. Borg (1982)
11. Bouchard, Shephard, Stephens, Sutton, and McPherson (1990b)
12. Bruce (1972)
13. Cooper (1977)
14. Daniels (1985)
15. Daniels, Oldridge, Nagle, and White (1978)
16. Foster et al. (1984)
17. Golding, Myers, and Sinning (1989)
18. Hagberg, Mullin, Giese, and Spitznagel (1981)
19. Hanson (1988)
20. Haskell, Savin, Oldridge, and DeBusk (1982)
21. Howley (1988)
22. McArdle, Katch, and Pechar (1973)
23. Montoye and Ayen (1986)
24. Montoye, Ayen, Nagle, and Howley (1986)
25. Naughton and Haider (1973)
26. Oldridge, Haskell, and Single (1981)
27. Paffenbarger, Hyde, and Wing (1990)
28. Ragg, Murray, Karbonit, and Jump (1980)
29. Sedlock, Knowlton, Fitzgerald, Tahamont, and Schneider (1983)
30. Shephard (1984)
31. Thompson (1988)

SUGGESTED READINGS

American Alliance for Health, Physical Education, Recreation and Dance (1988)
Blair, Painter, Pate, Smith, and Taylor (1988)
Ellestad (1980)
Frohlich et al. (1987)
Kirkendall, Feinlieb, Freis, and Mark (1980)
Kline, Porcari, Hintermeister, Freedson, Ward, McCarron, Ross, and Rippe (1987)
Leblanc, Bouchard, Godbout, and Mondor (1981)
Willerson and Dehmer (1981)

See the Bibliography at the end of the book for a complete source listing.

Chapter 10

Muscular Strength and Endurance, Flexibility, and Low-Back Function

Wendell Liemohn and Gina Sharpe

OBJECTIVES

The reader will be able to:

- Describe the effects and potential risks of using ankle and hand weights
- Describe exercises designed to enhance muscular strength and endurance of the trunk musculature
- Differentiate between isometric, isotonic, and isokinetic strength training, including discussion of fixed- and variable-resistance exercise equipment, steered and unsteered movements (i.e., machine versus free weights), and eccentric contractions
- Describe the types of tests used for assessing muscular strength
- Describe, including advantages and disadvantages of each, the following exercise techniques for enhancing flexibility: dynamic, ballistic, and static stretching, and proprioceptive neuromuscular facilitation
- Describe static stretching and/or proprioceptive neuromuscular facilitation exercises for all major joints
- Explain the importance of flexibility for low-back function
- Describe the types of tests used to assess flexibility
- Describe exercises that may be beneficial in the prevention of low-back pain
- Describe why certain exercises, such as straight and bent-leg sit-ups, are inappropriate
- Differentiate between appropriate and inappropriate flexion, extension, and hyperextension exercises of the spine
- Recognize common errors in body alignment and movement mechanics

TERMS

The reader will be able to define or describe:

Accommodating (variable) resistance
Ballistic stretching
Constant resistance
Dynamic stretching
Hypertrophy
Isokinetic equipment
Isometric
Isotonic
Load
Overload principle
Plyometric exercises

Progressive resistance exercise (PRE)
Proprioceptive neuromuscular facilitation (PNF)
Range of motion (ROM)
Repetitions maximum (RM)
Set
Specificity of training
Static stretching (SS)
Valsalva maneuver
Variable resistance
Viscoelastic

In addition to cardiorespiratory endurance activities, each exercise session should ideally include activities aimed at developing and maintaining desired levels of muscular strength, muscular endurance, and joint flexibility. This chapter defines each of these additional fitness/performance components and discusses their roles in enhancing an individual's ability to perform daily tasks.

Joint flexibility, or particularly maintenance of **range of motion (ROM)**, is an important consideration in exercise programming for all populations, including the elderly. Also of special concern for the elderly is osteoporosis; although this condition is typically considered a concomitant of aging or disuse, exercise programs that develop or maintain strength can play a role in allaying it. This chapter focuses on

- methods for improving muscular strength, endurance, and flexibility,
- factors that may influence muscular development,
- tools that can be used to assess these components, and
- low-back functioning as it relates to these variables.

MUSCULAR STRENGTH AND ENDURANCE

Muscular strength is the maximum amount of force that can be exerted by a muscle. Muscular endurance is the ability of a muscle to exert a force repeatedly over a period of time. Muscular strength and endurance are related; an increase in one of these components usually results in some degree of improvement in the other. A reasonable amount of strength and endurance may help an individual be more efficient in performing daily tasks. Furthermore, the strength and endurance of the trunk musculature can help prevent low-back pain.

Improving Strength and Endurance

The amount of strength desired, beyond that needed to support the weight of the body and perform daily activities, is a personal choice. To become stronger, a muscle or group of muscles must exert a force against a resistance that is greater than what is normally encountered. The term **overload principle** is often used to convey this concept; strength-development programs should focus on the progressive overloading of a muscle. The concept of overload dates back into Greek mythology and the story of Milo of Crotona, who wanted to become the strongest man in Greece. When he was a youth he began lifting a young bull every day; he thereby developed enough strength to lift the bull when it was full grown. A term used today, **progressive resistance exercise (PRE)**, aptly describes Milo's experience and, being generic, applies to most any physical training program; it implies application of the overload principle. For example, in strength training, PRE implies overload; once an individual can easily exert a force against a set resistance, the amount of resistance must be increased to produce further strength gains. Achieving overload is also possible by reducing the total time in which the exercise is performed.

Training programs that emphasize exertion of force against a high resistance for a small number of repetitions enhance gains in strength, muscle size, and, to a lesser extent, endurance. Programs that emphasize a relatively low resistance and a high number of repetitions enhance muscular endurance and, to a smaller degree, strength. These examples exemplify the concept of **specificity of training**; the type of gain relates to the type of regimen followed in the workout. Most individuals who participate in a fitness program can achieve and maintain a desired amount of strength and endurance using the low-resistance, high-repetition approach.

Regular participation in a high-resistance, low-repetition program usually results in **hypertrophy**, or an increase in muscle girth. This increase typically corresponds to an increase in the diameter of the muscle fibers within a muscle. The degree of hypertrophy and the corresponding improvements in strength vary among individuals; however, a linear relationship does exist between strength and a muscle's cross-sectional area. Regular participation in a low-resistance, high-repetition program usually results in an increase in muscle endurance. The latter is related to an increase in muscle

- myoglobin concentration,
- capillary number, and
- mitochondrial size and number.

Some women are concerned that PRE programs may make their muscles larger than they desire. Studies have shown, however, that women tend to increase their strength without great increases in muscle bulk (39). An important factor in this is the relative amounts of testosterone present in males and females. Because endogenous testosterone levels become higher in males than in females after puberty, postpubertal males have a much greater capacity to increase muscle bulk than females. Both sexes appear to reach their strength-gain asymptotes during the late teens and early 20s. Although the trainability difference between sexes is at its maximum at this time, endogenous testosterone levels appear to decrease at a faster rate in males than in females with aging; however, testosterone levels always tend to remain higher in males (17).

Strength- and Endurance-Training Programs

Three basic types of strength-development programs exist; they utilize *isometric, isotonic* (with and without varying resistance), or *isokinetic* protocols. The first type of program to be discussed is **isometric** training; it involves a static muscle contraction wherein the overall length of the muscle does not change during the application of a force against a fixed resistance. An example of an isometric exercise is attempting to move an immovable object. In physics, work is force multiplied by distance (Work = Force × Distance); because the distance the resistance is moved is zero in a static contraction, work per se is not accomplished.

Isometric exercises were very popular in the 1950s and early 1960s; however, because of their inherent limitations and certain contraindications, they are now seldom used. One of the major criticisms of isometric training is that, because it does not require limb movement, strength gains are specific to the angle at which exercise takes place and do not occur equally throughout the entire range of motion (27). These exercises also are potentially dangerous for individuals with cardiovascular symptomatology. A person tends to hold his or her breath during isometric exercises; if this is done with a closed glottis, the increased pressures in the thoracic and abdominal areas can inhibit the return of blood to the heart and cause an increase in blood pressure. This is called the **Valsalva maneuver** (27). Isometric exercises can, however, be a valuable adjunct in the development of the abdominal musculature, as will be discussed in another section of this chapter.

The second type of PRE program is **isotonic** training; in this program, exercises are typically done with free weights (e.g., dumbbells or barbells) or machines in which the resistance is "steered" along a fixed path (e.g., a configuration that includes a lever, a cable or chain, and/or a pulley). Isotonic exercises involve concentric as well as eccentric contractions of muscle. In a concentric contraction, the muscle shortens as the weight is moved against the force of gravity; therefore, positive work is accomplished. In an eccentric contraction, the muscle lengthens as the weight is moved in the direction of the force of gravity; under these circumstances, gravity, rather than muscle contraction, is the force responsible for the movement. The effect of the

lengthening (eccentric) contraction is to slow down the movement. During an arm curl with a dumbbell, a concentric contraction occurs as the weight is lifted; an eccentric contraction occurs as the weight is lowered. More muscle tension can be exerted through eccentric contraction than through either concentric or isometric contraction (18).

Isotonic PREs can include the exertion of a force against a **constant** *or* a **variable resistance**. The previously cited arm-curl exercise with a set weight is an example of an isotonic exercise with a constant resistance; the dumbbell's weight is constant, although the lifter's leverage varies during the exercise and she or he can notice some points in the range of motion that seem to be easier as well as some that seem to be harder. At the easier points, the muscles are not required to contract to their maximum, in part because of the lifter's leverage or mechanical advantage; however, the lifter often elects to accelerate the movement at these points. **Accommodating (variable) resistance** training equipment was designed in an attempt to require the lifter to exert maximum effort throughout the range of movement. This type of equipment theoretically provides greater resistance at the joint angles at which the lifter is stronger, and lower resistance at his or her weaker positions; in other words it accommodates the lifter's leverage or strength. In some equipment (e.g., Nautilus), pulleys, which change the direction of a force, are replaced by cams, which vary the resistance while changing the force's direction. Other equipment (e.g., Universal Gym) achieves accommodating resistance features by altering the lifter's leverage; this is accomplished by varying the length of the moment arm of resistance.

Isokinetic equipment has both accommodating, or variable, resistance and speed-governing features. The performer can choose a speed at which she or he wants to exercise; maximal effort is required when the performer's rate of movement matches the preset speed. Isokinetic equipment typically utilizes a hydraulic form of resistance that is controlled by a speed governor. Because isokinetic equipment controls the rate of muscle contraction, it can potentially train the different muscle-fiber types (e.g., fast-twitch with fast contractions, slow-twitch with slow contractions). This type of equipment is employed in strength-training regimens (e.g., Mini Gym Corporation's Leaper and Charger); isokinetic equipment is also seen extensively in clinical and rehabilitation settings (e.g., Lumex Corporation's Cybex II, Chattecx Corporation's Kin Com).

Despite some inherent limitations of free-weight PRE regimens, free weights are very popular in strength-training programs designed to improve athletic performance. Free weights are often favored because the lifts often

- closely resemble the strength employment seen in athletics,
- require the development of more skill, because the movement is not steered,
- involve complete muscle groups rather than isolated muscles or muscle groups, and
- permit ballistic-type movements that are integral to many sport skills.

However, free-weight PRE programs require much more in the way of coaching and supervision, because incorrect lifting techniques can cause injuries.

All of the aforementioned PREs require minimal to extensive equipment. Items such as books, sandbags, concrete weights, surgical tubing (or commercially available elastic cords) could be substituted for barbells or dumbbells in some applications. A facsimile of accommodating-resistance exercises can be contrived by having partner-type activities wherein each partner provides the accommodating resistance. Strength-development programs can also include activities that use an individual's body weight as the primary resistance—for example, variations of the trunk curl, push-ups, dips, and pull-ups. Fox and Mathews (10) discuss arm sprints and bench blasts (Figure 10.1); these are related to

push-ups and step tests, respectively, and can be most strenuous and challenging.

Plyometric exercises are often used as adjuncts to the more typical PREs in many athletic training programs; their equipment requirements are also negligible. In plyometric exercise, a muscle group is typically put on stretch prior to its contraction (e.g., jumping to the floor from a bench and then immediately jumping for height). However, it is important that the administrator of such programs be cognizant that plyometric exercises often cause muscle soreness when they are used inappropriately.

PRE programs have commonalities regardless of the types of training followed. The terms *load, repetitions maximum*, and *sets* are fundamental to most PRE programs. **Load** is the total number of pounds or kilograms of resistance lifted. **Repetitions maximum (RM)** is the number of consecutive times a specific lift or exercise can be done correctly without interruption or rest. **Set** is the number of times different lifts or exercises in a workout are repeated. An example of a workout regimen is depicted in Figure 10.2.

For optimal strength gains, a training regimen typically follows a 4- to 8-RM protocol; usually three sets are done, and the workout is done every other day (or three times per week). To get maximum strength gains, it is important to follow the overload principle by in-

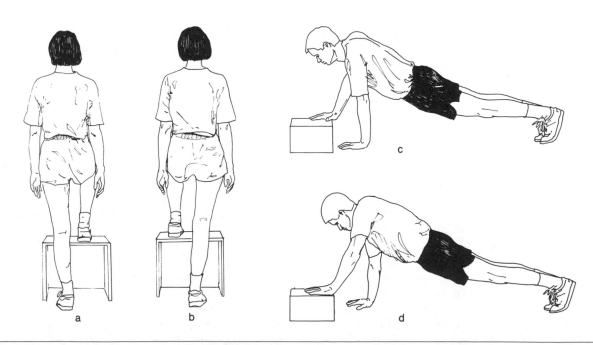

Figure 10.1 Bench blasts and arm sprints. The Whitney Bench Blast can be used for developing leg power. After placing one foot on the bench and the other on the floor (a), the exerciser jumps (blasts) upward; the feet are "switched" in the air so that the opposite is now on the bench and the floor (b). The arm sprints (c-d) can be used for developing arm and shoulder girdle strength; they are similar to bench stepping except the hands are used instead of the feet. Adapted from Fox and Mathews (1974).

creasing the resistance whenever RM exceeds 6 to 8. Overload can also be reached with a lighter load and a greater RM number (e.g., 10 to 25 RM); such a workout places a greater emphasis on muscle-endurance development.

The use of hand and ankle weights in exercises such as walking or aerobic dancing has become popular because

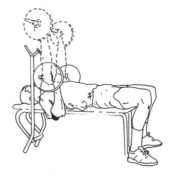

Figure 10.2c Bench press. Hold barbell above chest with hands slightly wider than shoulder width. Lower barbell to chest and push back to starting position. (It is important that the low back maintain contact with the bench.)

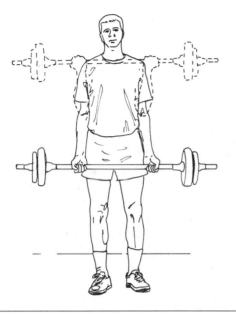

Figure 10.2a Arm curl. With arms extended, hold the barbell with an underhand grip. While keeping the elbows close to the sides, flex the forearms and raise the barbell to the chest; lower to the starting position.

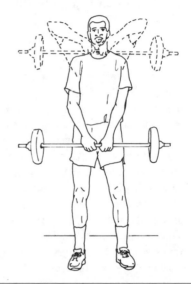

Figure 10.2d Upright rowing. Hold barbell with an overhand grip with hands one to two inches apart. Keep elbows above the bar while raising it to shoulder position; lower to starting position.

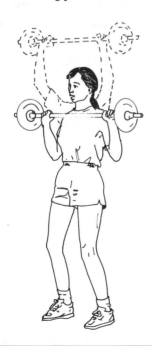

Figure 10.2b Overhead press. Hold the barbell at chest level with an overhand grip. Push the bar straight up to full extension and then lower to the starting position. Do not hyperextend the back.

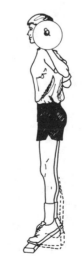

Figure 10.2e Heel lifts. With barbell behind shoulders at the back of the neck, raise upward on toes and then slowly return the heels to the floor.

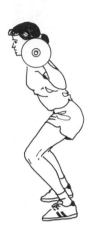

Figure 10.2f Half squats. With barbell behind shoulders at the back of the neck, gradually lower body to the semi-squat position. Keep back straight.

it is believed that the added resistance increases strength and calorie expenditure. However, these possible benefits must be weighed against the increased risk of injury. For example, hand and ankle weights can alter the exerciser's rhythm, balance, and natural movements; the resulting compensatory adjustments can magnify the effective load on the joints and even produce orthopedic problems, including tendon and ligament strains. Furthermore, using ankle weights in locomotion is not recommended, because it increases the already high-impact stresses on the lower extremities. Hand-held weights could theoretically decrease the exerciser's speed and time to exhaustion because of increased energy expenditure.

Assessing Muscular Strength and Endurance

Many tests can be used to assess muscular strength and endurance. A popular test is a one-repetition maximum of a specific activity (e.g., the bench press); this entails utilizing a trial-and-error process to determine the greatest amount of weight an individual can lift. After 1 RM is determined for the specific activity, this value can be divided by the participant's body weight so that interindividual comparisons of strength can be made; Gettman's (11) use of this technique for the seated leg press and the bench press is presented in Tables 10.1 and 10.2, respectively. Isokinetic computerized testing devices are available to provide information about strength throughout the range of movement; although these are very accurate, they are also expensive. At one time dynamometers and cable tensiometers were popular instruments for the measurement of strength; however, except for grip dynamometers, these instruments are seldom used today, because the strength typically measured has little relationship to performance on functional tasks.

FLEXIBILITY

Flexibility is the capacity to move a joint throughout its range of motion (ROM). Although there appears to be a general decline in ROM after adulthood is reached, how much of this diminution is due to aging per se

Table 10.1 Values for Seated Leg Press Strength in 1RM/Body Weight

Rating	\multicolumn{5}{c}{Age (years)}
	20-29	30-39	40-49	50-59	60+
Men
Excellent	> 2.08	> 1.88	> 1.76	> 1.66	> 1.56
Good	2.00-2.07	1.80-1.87	1.70-1.75	1.60-1.65	1.50-1.55
Average	1.83-1.99	1.63-1.79	1.56-1.69	1.46-1.59	1.37-1.49
Fair	1.65-1.82	1.55-1.62	1.50-1.55	1.40-1.45	1.31-1.36
Poor	< 1.64	< 1.54	< 1.49	< 1.39	< 1.30
Women
Excellent	> 1.63	> 1.42	> 1.32	> 1.26	> 1.15
Good	1.54-1.62	1.35-1.41	1.26-1.31	1.13-1.25	1.08-1.14
Average	1.35-1.53	1.20-1.34	1.12-1.25	0.99-1.12	0.92-1.07
Fair	1.26-1.34	1.13-1.19	1.06-1.11	0.86-0.98	0.85-0.91
Poor	< 1.25	< 1.12	< 1.05	< 0.85	< 0.84

Note. Adapted from The Institute for Aerobics Research. 1985 Physical Fitness Norms. (Unpublished Data.) Dallas, TX, 1985, with permission.
Note. The seat should be placed in the middle position for all participants.

Table 10.2 Values for Bench-Press Strength in 1RM/Body Weight

Rating	Age (years)				
	20-29	30-39	40-49	50-59	60+
Men					
Excellent	> 1.26	> 1.08	> 0.97	> 0.86	> 0.78
Good	1.17-1.25	1.01-1.07	0.91-0.96	0.81-0.85	0.74-0.77
Average	0.97-1.16	0.86-1.00	0.78-0.90	0.70-0.80	0.64-0.73
Fair	0.88-0.96	0.79-0.85	0.72-0.77	0.65-0.69	0.60-0.63
Poor	< 0.87	< 0.78	< 0.71	< 0.64	< 0.59
Women					
Excellent	> 0.78	> 0.66	> 0.61	> 0.54	> 0.55
Good	0.72-0.77	0.62-0.65	0.57-0.60	0.53-0.59	0.51-0.54
Average	0.59-0.71	0.53-0.61	0.48-0.56	0.43-0.50	0.41-0.50
Fair	0.53-0.58	0.49-0.52	0.44-0.47	0.40-0.42	0.37-0.40
Poor	< 0.52	< 0.48	< 0.43	< 0.39	< 0.36

Note. Adapted from The Institute for Aerobics Research. 1985 Physical Fitness Norms. (Unpublished Data.) Dallas, TX, 1985, with permission.

or the activity reduction related to aging is unknown. Nonetheless, maintaining a reasonable degree of flexibility is necessary for efficient body movement; being flexible and lithe may also decrease the chances of sustaining muscle injury, muscle soreness, or low-back pain. To move body segments, the muscles opposite (i.e., antagonistic to) those performing the movement (agonist muscles) must lengthen sufficiently. Tight musculature (the tendon and associated connective tissue) limits lengthening of the antagonistic muscles and thus reduces the ROM of body segments. Moreover, soreness or injury may result when tight musculature is subjected to strenuous physical activity.

Because the pelvis is the foundation for the spine, tightness in any muscle that crosses the iliofemoral joint can upset the functional relationship between the lower extremities and the trunk. For example, if any of these "guy wires" is too tight, the abdominal musculature will not be able to control pelvic positioning. The inability of the abdominal musculature to control the position of the pelvis, and hence one's center of gravity, not only will compromise the bioenergetics of gait, but it can also jeopardize spinal integrity, with the end result being low-back dysfunction or pain. Flexibility of joints distal to the hip, as well as of the spine itself, are also keys to the absorption of forces; if they do not provide adequate "give" in activities such as jogging, these forces must be accommodated by the spine. If one is severely limited in any of these joint excursions, not only will the potential to dissipate forces be limited, but compensatory adjustments may result, setting the stage for poorer biomechanics and additional joint damage.

Improving Flexibility

Hartley-O'Brien (16) discusses two approaches to improving flexibility: decreasing the resistance of the target (tight) musculature, and increasing the strength of the antagonistic muscles. Decreasing the resistance of the target musculature can be accomplished by either increasing connective tissue length or attaining a greater degree of relaxation in the target muscle.

Many flexibility regimens employ a prolonged static-stretch technique in an attempt to address both of these factors. **Static stretching (SS)** typically involves slowly lengthening the muscle(s) to a point of slight discomfort; when this point is reached, the position is held for 15 to 30 s, and then repeated 2 or 3 times. Another approach is **dynamic stretching**, which includes active movements that may be bouncy or jerky. If momentum becomes a factor, this type of stretching is referred to as **ballistic stretching**. Should the momentum of the body part become too great in ballistic stretching, the actual movement may exceed joint ROM, and a ligamentous or tendinous sprain may result. Typically when a muscle on one side of a joint rapidly contracts, the muscles opposite the contracting muscle quickly relax to permit lengthening. However, as a protective mechanism against overstretching in some fast, jerky movements, the antagonist muscles may resist lengthening by contracting. This phenomenon, which can actually oppose the desired stretch in some dynamic activities, is called the myotatic, or stretch, reflex.

DeVries (5), who did some of the pioneer research

in the area of flexibility, concludes that both static and dynamic stretching methods are equally effective. However, deVries suggests that the use of static methods might be preferred because (a) there is less chance of stretching beyond the limits of the muscle tissue, (b) the energy requirements are lower, and (c) static stretching may result in less muscle soreness. Although deVries's points should be well taken, for some applications the exercise prescriber must balance the tenets of specificity of training against the likelihood of injury.

As previously explained, if the contractile elements are relaxed, the tendon and its associated connective tissue (i.e., endomysium, perimysium, and epimysium) are usually the major deterrents to good ROM. Tendinous tissue is comparable to ligamentous tissue in that it is **viscoelastic**. The elastic property permits spring-like behavior and allows the musculotendinous unit to return to its original length after a reasonable stretch; the viscous property permits plastic or permanent deformation. For example, a moderate dynamic stretching activity (e.g., a relatively high force of short duration) would permit the elastic tissue of the musculotendinous unit to recover to its resting length, and hence there would be no permanent effect on ROM; however, a more extreme dynamic or ballistic stretching activity could result in either an improvement in ROM because of plastic deformation or a tearing or rupturing of the musculotendinous unit. If permanent increase in ROM is desirable (i.e., plastic deformation), then low-force stretching for a long duration (e.g., a static stretch) is typically used. Although progressively following such a program could result in an improvement of ROM, intuitively, eccentric loading protocols (which by their very nature permit greater force application) could potentially have the greatest effect on tendon length. However, this must be weighed against the greater likelihood of injury with an eccentric stretching regimen.

Hartley-O'Brien's other recommendation for flexibility improvement is to increase the strength of the muscle group antagonistic to the target, or tight, muscle group; a protocol emphasizing this approach should result in an improvement in active ROM. An example of active ROM would be movement resulting from muscle contraction totally controlled by the exerciser, whereas passive ROM would be movement resulting from an outside force (e.g., an exercise partner or gravity). If the difference between active and passive ROM is large, the joint might be vulnerable to injury because the joint musculature is neither controlling nor protecting the joint for this part of the movement. In such a scenario, resistance training to improve active ROM might be appropriate, to enhance joint stability. The latter point should also make it clear that although static stretching might provide an adequate ROM program

for the jogger, it should only be a part of the regimen for the individual who participates in ballistic sports; these individuals also need stretching activities more specific to their sports.

Although athletic trainers often utilize static-stretching (SS) procedures, they often complement these with **proprioceptive neuromuscular facilitation (PNF)** training. In the contract–relax PNF protocol, the limb is moved passively by the trainer to an end point of ROM and held at least 10 s; the exerciser then isometrically contracts the target muscle 6 to 10 s against the resistance provided by the trainer. Although a maximum isometric contraction was recommended in some of the original PNF protocols, a less-than-maximal one is sometimes advised to decrease the chance of injury. Upon relaxation of the target muscle, the trainer slowly moves the limb to the end point of the ROM and holds 15 to 30 s. If in the movement just described the exerciser contracts the agonist after isometrically contracting the antagonist, a greater degree of inhibition may occur in the latter (i.e., the target muscle), while the former increases in strength. This PNF method is called the contract–relax agonist–contract (CRAC) technique; it has been found to improve active ROM to a greater extent than either contract–relax or SS protocols (7, 14).

Although PNF stretching techniques often provide better results than static-stretching protocols (8), the technique is not without its limitations. For example, most PNF protocols require two individuals working together; moreover, injury can result if PNF is done as a partner exercise and the partners are not adequately instructed in the technique (35). Although they did not cite specific research, Hubley-Kozey and Stanish (18) state that athletes are much more apt to injure themselves using this technique and that they may also have to endure significant pain.

For best results, stretching exercises should be performed on a regular basis. Although stretching during the warm-up phase of an exercise bout can be important, the temperature of the muscle and connective tissue should also be considered. For example, if plastic deformation (i.e., lengthening of connective tissue) is the objective, then it is most important that the individual warm up sufficiently before participating in strenuous static or dynamic stretching regimens. However, if plastic deformation is not the goal, and the stretching is done more or less to get the "kinks" out, this factor is less important. If the planned activity is nothing more than a jog or run, a stretching regimen may not be necessary for everyone, and the warm-up may be limited to a slower version of the activity itself.

Stretching exercises at the conclusion of the workout may help decrease muscle soreness, particularly for those who are not regular exercisers. Because connective tissue temperature should be elevated, this would also be a most appropriate time to work on improvement in ROM (i.e., plastic deformation). For limb stretching, we advocate unilateral (one limb at a time) stretching regimens; several are depicted in the flexibility exercises shown in Figure 10.3.

Assessing Flexibility

Because flexibility is joint specific, determining the ROM of a few joints does not necessarily provide an

indicator of flexibility in other joints. Some tests can be used to estimate flexibility of certain body joints. Some of these tests are simple; others are more complex and require specific equipment.

The fingertip-to-floor and the sit-and-reach have sometimes been used to measure lumbar flexibility, but ham-

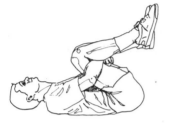

Figure 10.3a Back stretch: flexion. Pull one or both knees toward shoulder(s).

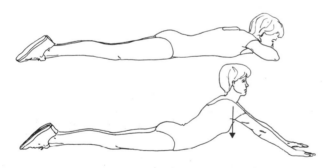

Figure 10.3b Back stretch: extension. 1. Relax back while resting hands on floor. 2. Progress to pressing down in shoulder area with heels of hands while maintaining a relaxed back and keeping pelvis in contact with floor.

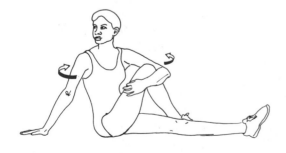

Figure 10.3c Back stretch: rotation. Rotate the trunk while pressing the bent knee across the body and then rotate shoulders (stretch will be felt in hip and back).

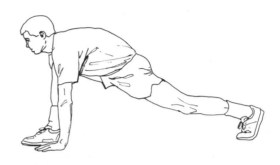

Figure 10.3d Groin stretch. Flex one leg under chest (knee over ankle and foot) and extend opposite one. Lean forward while pushing your hips downward.

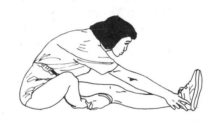

Figure 10.3e Hamstring stretch (#1). By bending from the hip (i.e., keep back straight), this can be particularly effective for stretching the hamstrings. If the hamstrings are tight (e.g., sacral angle less than 80 degrees), the stress would be on the low back instead of the hamstrings; this is *not* desirable.

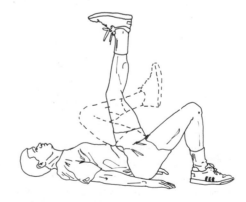

Figure 10.3f Hamstring stretch (#2). Begin from the hook-lying position (on back with both knees bent); bring one knee to chest and then straighten leg vertically. (Note: If the opposite knee is flexed as pictured, the pelvis would be posteriorly rotated approximately 10 degrees, hence 100 degrees of hip flexion is typical; if the opposite leg is extended, while keeping the low back in contact with the floor, only 80 to 90 degrees of hip flexion would be expected.)

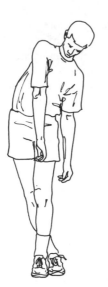

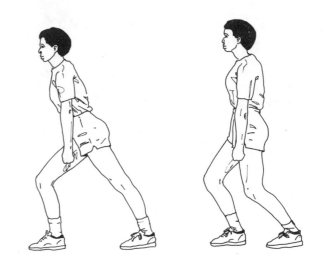

Figure 10.3g Lateral stretch. With right foot firmly planted cross-over in front with the left (left knee slightly bent, keep left foot snug against right) and bend laterally to the left (while keeping shoulders and pelvis in the same plane). This will stretch the iliotibial tract on the right. (Some exercisers may wish to support themselves against a wall as they perform this stretch.)

Figure 10.3i Calf stretch. The left figure depicts stretching the gastrocnemius (a 2-joint muscle); the right figure depicts stretching the soleus.

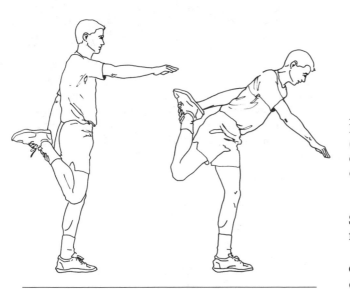

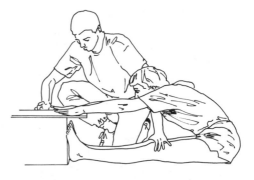

Figure 10.3h Hip-flexor stretch. Grasp contralateral ankle and raise leg while keeping trunk straight. Note incorrect technique of individual on the right; tilting the pelvis precludes stretching the hip flexors. (Some exercisers may wish to support themselves against a wall as they perform this stretch.)

Figure 10.4 Sit-and-reach test of flexibility. Subject's feet (without shoes) are flat against the box; observer holds knees down while subject reaches forward as far as possible with one hand on top of the other.

string extensibility has been found to make the most important contribution to performance on these two items (21, 23). The fingertip-to-floor method is often used in clinical evaluations, sometimes in conjunction with skin-distraction measures (e.g., determining the difference in distance between two non-contiguous vertebrae, T12 and

S1, in upright standing and in forward bending *after* the fingertip-to-floor position is assumed).

The sit-and-reach test warrants further discussion because it is an item seen in many fitness-testing protocols. In one of the more popular versions of this test (Figure 10.4), the person being evaluated sits on the floor with his or her legs extended and feet flat against a box. A meter stick is attached to the top of the box, with the 23-cm mark located above the junction of the feet with the box; the individual being tested is instructed to slowly reach forward as far as possible. Standards for this test are shown in Table 10.3. Although this test can provide a reliable measure of hamstring extensibility, a factor most important to low-back function, the test administrator should also observe the quality of the movement. One quality point to check is the angle of the sacrum with the floor; it should be 80° to 90° (a book or other object with a 90° angle placed

Table 10.3   Standards for Sit-and-Reach Test

Rating	Sit and reach (cm)
Good	> 35
Acceptable	20-30
Needs work	< 20

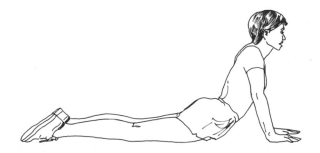

Figure 10.5 Back ROM test (Imrie and Barbuto, 1988). While keeping the pelvis in contact with the floor, the subject elevates the chest with arm action; the score is the distance from the suprasternal notch to the floor. [This test is very similar to one of McKenzie's (1981) therapeutic exercises for patients presenting with LBP.]

Table 10.4   Standards for Back-Extension Test

Rating	Back extension (cm)
Excellent	> 30
Good	20-29
Marginal	10-19
Needs work	< 9

Note. Adapted from Imrie & Barbuto (1988).

next to the sacrum can be the criterion). Conversely, it is also possible that some individuals will exceed 80° on the "book test" but yet be so tight in the lumbosacral area that their score on the sit-and-reach will be poor. And some individuals may be hypermobile in the lumbosacral area and thus able to compensate for tight hamstrings and perform satisfactorily on the sit-and-reach. Although quality factors such as these might be seen only in a minority of individuals tested, they can be vital to the establishment of these individuals' personalized exercise programs.

The fact that a progressive decline in spinal mobility occurs in all planes due to aging or disuse was mentioned previously; it is important to note that this decline is especially seen in spinal extension (6, 36). Unfortunately, spine hyperextension is an issue often ignored or misinterpreted by exercise leaders. (Contributing to this problem are many well-intentioned writers in the exercise area who believe it is more expeditious to label an exercise as being contraindicated rather than attempt to explain its subtleties. However, exercise leaders should be cognizant of the nuances of the specific exercises; this will permit them to do a better job in addressing the specific needs of exercisers.) It is argued that spinal hyperextension is a natural movement and that it is in the best interest of the biomechanics of one's spine to maintain this ability. However, it is also acknowledged that *ballistic*-hyperextension movements of the spine (and particularly ballistic rotation movements) are totally inappropriate. We contend that slow and controlled hyperextension movements are appropriate for inclusion in exercise programs; however, it is important that these movements be carefully taught, because some exercisers do not have a very good kinesthetic awareness of their own biomechanics. In such a scenario it is essential that the exercise leader be able to discriminate between correct and incorrect performance.

A back-extension ROM test from Imrie and Barbuto (20) is presented in Figure 10.5. The individual being tested places the hands under the shoulders as if doing a push-up; however, the pelvis must maintain contact with the floor (possibly with the assistance of the tester) as the individual elevates the chest *with arm* action. It is important to note that this is a passive test of spine extension; the back musculature is *not* to be used. The score is the distance from the suprasternal notch to the

floor; Imrie and Barbuto's scoring protocol is presented in Table 10.4.

In males, in particular, the hamstring muscles tend to restrict ROM at the hip joint more than the hip flexors; however, in some individuals, tightness in the hip flexor musculature precludes adequate ROM. Physical therapists use the Thomas test for determining whether the hip flexors are tight. An example of an administration of this test is presented in Figure 10.6, but the reader is advised to have a very good understanding of the functional anatomy of the hip joint, as well as the nuances of the test, before using the test.

There are several other instruments that fitness leaders might wish to use to appraise ROM. The Leighton Flexometer and the goniometer have been used to assess actual ROM; in the hands of the experienced tester, both devices can provide accurate estimates of joint ROM. In recent years the inclinometer[1] has become a popular instrument (Figure 10.7). Although one manufacturer states that it can replace the goniometer for most any measurement, we find it particularly suited

[1]We have used a model developed by M. I. E. Medical Research, Leeds, U.K.; it is available through: Biokinetics, 9007 Seneca Lane, Bethesda, MD 20817. A comparable model, the Plurimeter-V, is available through Lafayette Instrument, P.O. Box 5729, 3700 Sagamore Parkway North, Lafayette, IN 47903.

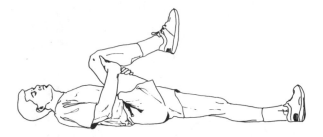

Figure 10.6 Thomas test. While maintaining the left leg in the extended position, the right leg is pulled toward the chest until the pelvis has rotated posteriorly (i.e., lumbar spine snug against floor). If the left leg rises as the right leg is pulled in, this would be indicative of tightness of the hip flexors (e.g., psoas and/or iliacus). (Refer to Kendall and McCreary, 1983, to determine how to use the same test to evaluate for tightness in the rectus femoris.)

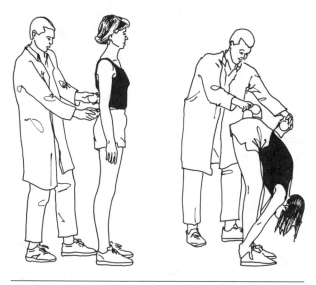

Figure 10.7 Lumbar flexion can be determined by placing inclinometers at the T12-L1 interspace and on the sacrum while the subject is in the neutral standing position. After the inclinometers are set to zero, the individual assumes the "fingertip to floor" position and the readings are taken from both inclinometers. Subtracting the score of the lower inclinometer from that of the upper will give the amount of lumbar flexion; the remainder should be close to agreeing with a goniometric measurement of hamstring flexibility. (Keeley et al., 1986).

for measuring ROM of the axial skeleton, and there is a valid protocol for this measurement (22). A drawback to using instruments such as those just described is that there is little normative data, and much that does exist is based on clinical populations.

LOW-BACK FUNCTION

Low-back pain (LBP) is one of the most common medical complaints among adults in the United States. Prob-

lems related to LBP account for more lost work-hours than any other type of occupational injury and are the most frequent cause of activity limitation in individuals under age 45. Although there are differences of opinion on exact etiology, there are convincing arguments that exercise can be an important factor in decreasing the likelihood of ever having LBP. For the individual succumbing to LBP, exercise can often restore function. Although much has changed since Williams first advocated flexion exercises for LBP approximately 50 years ago, some of his more recent ideas (38) are still used in programs today.

In the earlier discussion on ROM at the hip joint, mention was made of its importance to low-back function. To reiterate, the muscles crossing the hip joint can be viewed as guy wires that support the pelvis; because the sacral component of the pelvis is the foundation for the spine, tightness in musculature crossing the hip joint can severely affect spine biomechanics. For example, if the hamstrings are tight, even strong abdominal muscles may be unable to control the lumbar curve. It is important to understand that the integrity of the spine is dependent upon a functional interrelationship between flexibility and strength. In addition to ROM, aerobic condition and muscular strength are also important fitness factors for the soundness of the spine; each of these components will now be addressed.

Aerobic Condition

Aerobic exercise has established its utility in cardiac rehabilitation; more recently aerobic exercise has been recognized as having potential for decreasing the incidence of LBP (2, 32) and as being important in the rehabilitation of not only the LBP patient but also those with arthritis of the spine (15, 19). Aerobic exercise not only helps control weight but also promotes the nutritional maintenance of those spinal structures implicated in the dysfunction associated with LBP (28).

Trunk Strength and Endurance

Weakened trunk musculature has been known for some time to be an important risk indicator for low-back problems. The muscular system is the only noninvasive mechanism by which an effective and permanent influence can be made on the structure and function of the spine. Although fitness instructors are neither apt to be qualified nor expected to prescribe therapeutic exercises for LBP, an understanding of the functional anatomy of the trunk should enable them to make wise decisions in the selection of general exercises that relate to low-back function. Moreover, the activities they use in their programs have the potential to provide biomechanically sound exercise habits that can, in the long run, decrease the likelihood that those with whom they work will ever succumb to LBP.

One role of the abdominal muscles that is often overlooked is the bracing and stability they provide the trunk. (See chapter 4 for illustrations of the trunk musculature discussed here.) The structure of the abdominal (muscle group is uniquely engineered, with its stratified layers of muscle and aponeurosis forming a strong protective girdle anteriorly and laterally, and even a splinting effect posteriorly. Anteriorly the aponeurosis of the external and internal obliques and the transversus abdominis ensheathes the rectus abdominis; laterally the obliques and the transversus abdominis provide reinforcing layers. Posteriorly the transversus abdominis and a small portion of the internal oblique become contiguous with the thoracolumbar fascia, which in turn ensheathe the bundles of erector spinae and multifidus muscles. This engineering masterpiece has the potential to provide a bracing and corseting effect analogous to a Chinese finger trap. However, when this natural corset is neglected, from an aesthetic viewpoint posture is affected, but from a functional viewpoint the end result might be LBP.

For an understanding of the role of the abdominal muscles in exercise, lumbar movement must be distinguished from movement that occurs at the iliofemoral joint. One key to remember is that lumbar flexion in the sagittal plane is limited to removal of the lordotic curve. What this means, in essence, is that in an activity such as a full sit-up, very shortly after the shoulders are raised from the exercise surface the end ROM of the lumbar spine is reached; thereafter movement occurs at the iliofemoral joint, and the abdominal muscles contract isometrically as the trunk is further elevated by the hip flexors, *regardless* of the position of the knees. Therefore it is unnecessary and usually undesirable to raise the trunk much more than 30° in abdominal strengthening activities. [Further review of the nuances of the bent-leg sit-up appears in (25).]

A partial curl or crunch should be substituted for a full sit-up; such an exercise has been found to make greater utilization of the abdominal muscles in terms of motor-unit recruitment (13), and it also decreases the deleterious involvement of the hip flexors (33). A posterior pelvic tilt should first be emphasized; this is followed by raising the head and shoulders either in the sagittal plane or obliquely. Diagonal curls place greater demands on the oblique musculature; it is particularly desirable to strengthen these muscles, because they are in a position to resist the torsional stresses that are often responsible for LBP symptomatology. Examples of partial curl exercises are presented in Figure 10.8.

Exercises such as these can be done in sets of 10 to 15 repetitions; progressions might include 5-s to 10-s (or longer) isometric holds in some sets as the exerciser

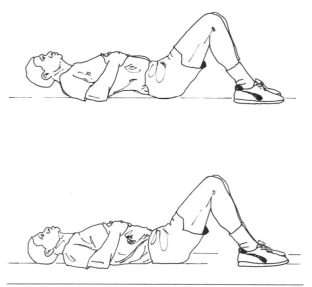

Figure 10.8a Posterior pelvic tilt. The posterior pelvic tilt is either done as an exercise in itself or as the first phase of a trunk curl.

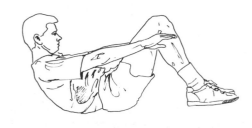

Figure 10.8b Variations of the partial curl (#1). Remember that once the shoulder blades are elevated off of the exercise surface that lumbar flexion has occurred; there is no need to lift the trunk more than 30 degrees unless one wishes to exercise the hip flexors.

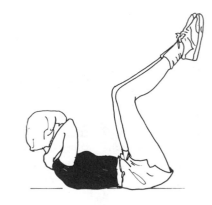

Figure 10.8c Variations of the partial curl (#2).

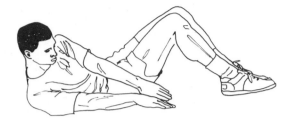

Figure 10.8d Diagonal or oblique curl. Exercise such as the diagonal or oblique curl ensures greater involvement of the internal and external oblique musculature; this is important since these muscles are in the best position to resist the rotational torques that are often responsible for disc problems. In each repetition of this exercise, one shoulder is raised higher than the other.

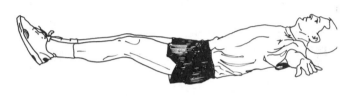

Figure 10.8e Leg lift. The leg lift is not a good exercise and for many individuals it is contraindicated. However, for those individuals who have strong enough abdominal musculature to negate the pull of the psoas by keeping the low back firmly against the exercise surface, this exercise has fewer drawbacks.

becomes stronger. In the last few years an aggressive exercise protocol has been found to be very successful in rehabilitating patients with herniated discs (34); moreover, isometric-type exercises are very prominent in teaching the patient how to brace the trunk with "nature's corset."

Although it is doubtful that anyone who understands the biomechanics of the trunk could endorse utilization of the full sit-up exercise (or test) regardless of knee position, there is less agreement on the positioning of the hands. Obviously the moment arm of resistance is greater if the hands are placed behind the head or neck; however, this is inappropriate *if* it results in hyperflexion in the cervical area. Although neck hyperflexion is perhaps most likely to occur in a timed test when the individual becomes fatigued and body mechanics suffer, if one wishes to maximize the moment arm of resistance this enigma can be resolved simply by having the exerciser place the hands on the forehead or hold the ears. Hyperflexion of the neck is not likely to occur when the oblique curl is performed, if only the hand opposite to the direction of the curling is placed on the neck.

Trunk Strength and Endurance Testing

If it is desirable to incorporate the endurance component with the strength component in testing the abdominal musculature, we endorse use of a recent modification of a protocol developed in Canada (9). In this protocol the individual being tested assumes a hook-lying position with the knees at a 90° angle and the hands palm-down with the fingertips touching strips of masking tape placed perpendicular to the body on each side. Two additional strips of masking tape are placed parallel to the first two at a distance of 8 cm. In the performance of the curl-up, there is an initial "flattening out" of the low-back region followed by a slow "curling-up" of the upper spine, sliding the fingertips along the mat until they touch the second set of tape strips; this is followed by a return to the starting position until the back of the head touches the tester's hands. The movement is always slow, continuous, and well-controlled, with 20 curl-ups per minute (i.e., 3 s per curl-up, with the metronome set at 40 beats·min^{-1}). Subjects perform as many curl-ups as they can without pausing, up to a maximum of 75 (see Figure 10.9). Table 10.5 contains performance standards for women and men of different ages.

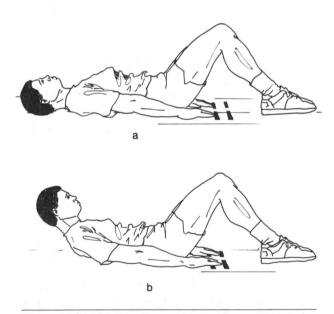

Figure 10.9 The Canadian trunk strength test. The starting position is supine with the knee angle at 90 degrees and the finger tips touching strips of masking tape placed perpendicular to the body (a). After flattening out the low back region the individual curls the upper spine until the finger tips touch the second strips of masking tape (8 cm from the parallel to the first) (b). (See text for further description.)

Table 10.5   Standards for Partial Curl-Up Test

Rating	Number completed					
	Men/Age			Women/Age[a]		
	< 35	35-44	> 45[a]	< 35	35-44	> 45
Excellent	60	50	40	50	40	30
Good	45	40	25	40	25	15
Marginal	30	25	15	25	15	10
Needs work	15	10	5	10	6	4

Note. Adaptation based on research by Faulkner et al. (1988).

[a]The data of Faulkner et al. support use of 8-cm reach rather than 12 cm for subjects > 45 years old and for women.

Even though many exercise programs emphasize development of the abdominal musculature, there is often a more significant decrement in hip and spine extensor strength than in trunk flexor strength (29). For this reason, examples of trunk extension exercises are presented in Figure 10.10; as in any hyperextension movements of the spine, it is important that these exercises be performed smoothly and slowly without any

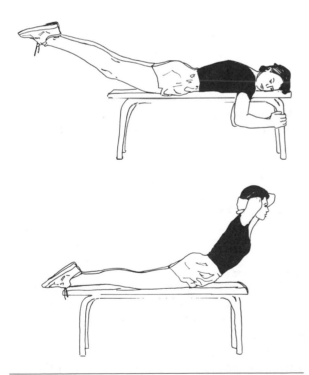

Figure 10.10 ROM extension. Although maintenance of ROM in extension is important, it is imperative that these exercises be done slowly and be very controlled; ballistic movements are contraindicated.

ballistic action. Although extensor muscle strength should not be neglected, the emphasis on abdominal strength development still seems appropriate in view of its potential role in stabilizing the spine in a neutral position.

Biomechanical Considerations of Selected Activities

Stretching

One term permeating much of the preceding discussion is the word *ballistic*; to the ballistic extension and ballistic rotation-extension movements of the spine that were deemed inappropriate, add ballistic flexion. Assume an individual with tight hamstrings were to attempt bouncing (i.e., ballistic) toe touches from either the standing *or* the sitting position; it is probable that the structures of the spine would have to absorb at least part of the forces, and possibly to their detriment, with minimal effect on the length of the hamstrings. Because of this concern, Calliet (3) recommended a unilateral sitting-hamstring stretch under the pretense that it would be less stressful to the spine than the bilateral sit-and-reach for those with tight hamstrings (see Figure 10.11). Although we support the contention that Calliet's stretching activity is potentially less stressful to the spine than the bilateral sit-and-reach, we did not find significant differences in the degree of flexion occurring in the lumbar spine when the two techniques were compared (26).

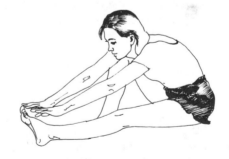

Figure 10.11 Unilateral hamstring stretch. Calliet (1981) contends that this exercise is less stressful on the lower back than the bilateral sit-and-reach since the bending of one knee results in a posterior rotation of the pelvis.

Jogging/Running

Although the aerobic effect of running can have a positive impact on spine function, poor biomechanics in running can exacerbate existing low-back problems as well as bring about new ones as compensatory adaptations are made. For example, poor running technique might include excessive forward lean; this must be counterbalanced by contraction of the back extensors, which may then become overly tired or produce high intersegmental forces on the discs (30). The biomechanics of running are also most important from the perspective of shock absorption and posture. The more forces absorbed by the joints distal to the spine, the fewer that will have to be absorbed by the spine (4).

Posture

Posture is sometimes viewed as being more of aesthetic than of functional importance; however, postural considerations have implications for exercise prescription. Through the use of postural screening instruments (see Figure 10.12), the fitness leader may be able to detect factors that might not otherwise be noticed. Although corrective exercises typically would not be prescribed unless one were extremely knowledgeable in this area, in addition to making referrals for conditions such as scoliosis, there may be other implications. For example, the individual noted to have round shoulders is not going to benefit from a regimen that emphasizes bench presses, for this could further exacerbate his or her condition. There are also biomechanical considerations that relate to functioning of the back. Nachemson (30), on the basis of studies in which intradiscal transducers have been used to measure compressive stresses in the nucleus pulposus of the third lumbar disc, has graphically displayed how a forward lean or a posterior rotation of the pelvis can place stresses on the back.

Lifting

It has long been suspected that the back musculature alone has neither the mass nor the force vectors that would permit lifting heavy objects such as those seen in the performance of the dead lift, and it is a matter of conjecture how the mechanisms of trunk support explain some individuals' ability to lift heavy loads without spine injury. We believe that the mathematical model developed by Gracovetsky and Farfan (12) best explains the phenomenon of lifting heavy weights (e.g., the dead lift). They argue that the passive ligamentous structures of the spine act like "steel cables" as the gluteus maximus and hamstrings provide the force; a review of Gracovetsky and Farfan's research, culminating with their mathematical model, as well as the anatomical basis for its derivation (1), are summarized

elsewhere (24). In part because of the conjecture in the area of lifting, the key guideline given by the National Institute of Occupational, Safety, and Health (37) is that the lifter should attempt to minimize turning movements by keeping the object lifted as close as possible to the body's center of gravity.

Other Aerobic Activity

Nachemson (31) indicates that in addition to jogging, he most commonly recommends backstroke swimming, brisk walking, and stair climbing for LBP. Bicycle riding (stationary or actual) and quality cross-country ski machines would be other good activities; the latter provides an excellent opportunity to develop aerobic conditioning without impact while incorporating tenets of stabilization training (24).

SUMMARY

Muscular strength, muscular endurance, and flexibility exercises should be parts of the total fitness program; each component plays an important role in positive health. Maintaining a reasonable degree of strength and flexibility may

- increase efficiency in performing daily tasks,
- increase resistance to muscle injuries, and
- aid in preventing low-back pain.

Isometric, isotonic, and isokinetic strength-training regimens each have advantages and disadvantages. Several strength-measuring tools are also available. Two basic types of flexibility-development programs are described (i.e., static and dynamic), and a third type is mentioned. Static stretching appears to have advantages in most fitness programs, but training athletes for ballistic sports often requires use of other protocols; flexibility exercises should be performed after the musculotendinous tissue has been warmed sufficiently. Flexibility assessment methods are also discussed. Strength and flexibility have pertinent roles in preventing low-back pain. General exercise principles that may be helpful in preventing or alleviating low-back pain are included in the chapter. In addition, general considerations in developing exercise protocols are mentioned.

In lifting, the individual should keep the load close to the body and avoid lateral flexion and rotation movements. Some individuals may need resistance training for the extensor musculature of the knee and hip to improve their lifting mechanics.

Posture score sheet	Name _____			Scoring dates			
	Good—10	Fair—5	Poor—0				
Head Left Right	Head erect, gravity line passes directly through center	Head twisted or turned to one side slightly	Head twisted or turned to one side markedly				
Shoulders Left Right	Shoulder level (horizontally)	One shoulder slightly higher than other	One shoulder markedly higher than other				
Spine Left Right	Spine straight	Spine slightly curved laterally	Spine markedly curved laterally				
Hips Left Right	Hips level (horizontally)	One hip slightly higher	One hip markedly higher				
Ankles	Feet pointed straight ahead	Feet pointed out	Feet pointed out markedly, ankles sag in (pronation)				
Neck	Neck erect, chin in, head directly above shoulders	Neck slightly forward, chin slightly out	Neck markedly forward, chin markedly out				
Upper back	Upper back normally rounded	Upper back slightly more rounded	Upper back markedly rounded				
Trunk	Trunk erect	Trunk inclined to rear slightly	Trunk inclined to rear markedly				
Abdomen	Abdomen flat	Abdomen protruding	Abdomen protruding and sagging				
Lower back	Lower back normally curved	Lower back slightly hollow	Lower back markedly hollow				
			Total scores				

Figure 10.12 New York Posture Rating Chart. *Note.* From *The New York Physical Fitness Test: A Manual for Teachers of P.E.*, New York State Education Dept. (Division of HPER) 1958. Reprinted by permission.

REFERENCES

1. Bogduk and Macintosh (1984)
2. Cady, Bischoff, O'Connell (1979)
3. Calliet (1981)
4. Cappozzo (1983)
5. deVries (1980)
6. Einkauf, Gohdes, Jensen, and Jewell (1987)
7. Etnyre and Abraham (1986)
8. Etnyre and Lee (1987)
9. Faulkner, Sprigings, McQuarrie, and Bell (1988)
10. Fox and Mathews (1974)
11. Gettman (1988)
12. Gracovetsky and Farfan (1986)
13. Halpern and Bleck (1979)
14. Hardy (1985)
15. Harkcom, Lampman, Banwell, and Castor (1985)
16. Hartley-O'Brien (1980)
17. Hettinger (1961)
18. Hubley-Kosay and Stanish (1984)
19. Ike, Lampman, and Castor (1989)
20. Imrie and Barbuto (1988)
21. Jackson and Baker (1986)
22. Keeley, Mayer, Cox, Gatchel, Smith, and Mooney (1986)
23. Kippers and Parker (1987)
24. Liemohn (1990)
25. Liemohn, Snodgrass, and Sharpe (1988)
26. Liemohn, Sharpe, and Wasserman (1990)
27. Mathews and Fox (1976)
28. Mayer (1990)
29. Mayer, Smith, Keeley, and Mooney (1985)
30. Nachemson (1975)
31. Nachemson (1990)
32. Nutter (1988)
33. Robertson and Magnusdottir (1987)
34. Saal and Saal (1989)
35. Surburg (1983)
36. Tanii and Masuda (1985)
37. U.S. Department of Health and Human Services (1981)
38. Williams (1974)
39. Wilmore (1982)

SUGGESTED READINGS

Kendall and McCreary (1983)
McKenzie (1981)
Sharpe, Liemohn, Wasserman, Hungerford, and Lewis (1990)
White and Panjabi (1978)

See the Bibliography at the end of the book for a complete source listing.

Chapter 11

Personality, Stress, and Health

OBJECTIVES

The reader will be able to:

- Describe how the HFI deals with different personalities in an exercise setting
- Describe how physical activity may affect stress
- Describe the positive and negative aspects of stress
- Describe how aging may affect response to stressors
- Describe recommendations for healthy stress levels
- Describe ways to increase relaxation

TERMS

The reader will be able to define or describe:

Aggression

Anxiety

Assertiveness

Catharsis

Depression

Euphoria

Fear

Goal orientation

Hostility

Motivations

Personality

Play orientation

Rationalizations

Rejection

Stress

Stressor

Types A and B

This book emphasizes physical fitness, but mental, physical, psychological, social, and spiritual aspects of life are all intertwined. This chapter deals with one of those areas that bridges the psychological and physiological aspects of fitness.

After a recent review of exercise, fitness, and mental health, Brown (4) reported that 25% of our population may be functioning at less than optimal levels as a result of stress and stress-related emotions such as anxiety and depression. Robinson (6) reported that in the U.S., two-thirds of visits to primary-care physicians are stress-related; 112 million people take medication for stress, and industry loses more than $150 billion annually on stress-related problems. Exercise and fitness play a role in promoting positive mental health and preventing negative mental health.

RELAXATION/AROUSAL BALANCE

The healthy life involves the ability to relax and disregard irrelevant stimuli during quiet times. The fit person can also work and play with vigor and enthusiasm. Relaxation (parasympathetic nervous system dominance) and vitality (sympathetic nervous system dominance) are both enhanced by physical conditioning. One of the keys to a healthy life is a balance between arousal and relaxation. People who are always relaxed and easygoing do not accomplish very much. On the other hand, people who at all moments have the go-get-'em attitude toward all aspects of life exhibit "coronary-prone" behavior. This chapter describes the relationships among personality, physical activity, stress, and health. Dealing extensively with all psychological aspects of fitness is beyond the scope of this chapter. Those with pathological traits or behaviors (i.e., mental illness) should be referred to appropriate health or psychological professionals. We are dealing with mental health in terms of different levels of "normal" personality and stress, with an emphasis on their implications for fitness programs.

KEY POINT.　Stress is a major psychophysiological fitness concern. Achieving a balance between arousal and relaxation is one aspect of the healthy life.

PERSONALITY-RELATED VARIABLES AND PHYSICAL ACTIVITY PROGRAMMING

Providing definitive comments about the psychophysiological effects of a specific external stimulus is impossible, because individuals perceive and react to the same situation differently. The same movie may evoke anger, laughter, or no emotion from three different people. Playing in front of a crowd might cause best and worst performances in different people.

Part of the different perception of and reaction to the same situation is related to **personality**. Although completely characterizing someone's personality or predicting exactly how that personality will interact with physical activity or other stimuli is not possible, some generalizations aid the HFI in dealing with individuals in fitness programs.

Type A and Type B Behavior

There is general agreement that one's personality and ability to cope with stress are related to CHD. However, the exact characteristics that cause the higher risk are difficult to enumerate or measure. One attempt to do this separates people's behaviors into Type A and Type B. **Type A** behavior (i.e., the go-getter, hard-driving, time-conscious, hostile, impatient person) is coronary-prone behavior. A Type A person has a greater stress response to psychological stressors. Therefore this person should learn to relax, should be cautious about overdoing exercise, and should be engaged in more relatively noncompetitive activities. The Type A person often has to learn to deal with anger and hostility. The **Type B** person (easygoing, nonaggressive, "laid-back"), on the other hand, may need more

stimulation and motivation to begin and continue in the exercise program.

Anger

Some evidence suggests a relationship between anger and CHD. People who keep their anger "bottled up" inside rather than expressing it (e.g., talking to a close friend about it) have increased risk of CHD. Three recommendations can be made to help people with anger:

1. Try to develop positive attitudes toward self, others, and the world in general, so that anger is less frequent.
2. Express emotions, such as anger, rather than denying the emotions or keeping them inside.
3. Develop the kinds of relationships with others in which emotions can be shared.

By being open about her or his own feelings (e.g., "that . . . really made me angry yesterday") and by being sensitive about the fitness participants' moods (e.g., "you seem upset today"), the HFI can help people acknowledge their emotions.

Aggression, Assertiveness, Hostility, and Denial

Aggression, assertiveness, hostility, and denial may all, for different reasons, cause a person to do too much. **Aggressive** or **hostile** individuals may try to do too much exercise because they get so involved in the activity that they don't pay attention to signs of discomfort or danger. Some people try to deny that they have pain and thus tend to do too much. One of the distinctions between **assertiveness** and aggression or hostility is that the assertive person is sensitive to others, whereas the aggressive or hostile person tends to be less concerned with others' feelings. The HFI needs to protect other members of the group from aggressive or hostile behavior.

Anxiety, Depression, and Fear

Postcardiac patients have high levels of **anxiety, fear**, and **depression**. Others with low fitness levels may also be bothered by one or more of these conditions. People who are unduly worried or afraid need support. They must be able to ease into activity and to see that positive results can occur with minimum risks; gradually they can be introduced to higher levels of exercise. The feeling of lack of control is often a part of anxiety, fear, or depression, and a person who is becoming physically active and adopting other healthy behaviors may have increased perception of control over her or his own life.

KEY POINT.   Various personality traits, such as Type A, anger, and hostility, increase the risk of health problems. Other emotional problems, such as anxiety and depression, may result from health problems and low fitness levels. Individuals with these characteristics need special attention in exercise situations.

Rationalization

One of the difficult skills in dealing with people is to be able to differentiate between real reasons for behavior and **rationalizations** that are given that sound better than the real reasons. It will not be possible to help a person deal with exercise or other health behaviors until the real reasons for the current behaviors are known. The HFI hears many excuses for why someone can't develop healthy activities or discontinue unhealthy behaviors. One technique to help the person deal with the underlying reasons for his or her inactivity is to keep asking questions aimed at uncovering the real reasons. Chapter 12 provides assistance for helping people modify behavior.

Rejection

Rejection is relevant in two ways for the HFI. Some people in the fitness program have rejected exercise in the past or feel that active people have rejected them (e.g., they have usually been the last ones chosen to play games). The HFI must be sensitive to this feeling and help the person feel included and welcome. On the other hand, the HFI should realize that she or he will not be 100% successful in helping people become active. Some potential fitness participants will reject fitness programs; it is important for the HFI not to take that rejection personally.

Catharsis

Some people use exercise for **catharsis**—that is, as a cleansing agent for the mind and emotions. Fitness activities are used to erase the cluttered state and allow the person to start fresh following the exercise. After a minimum level of fitness is reached, the fitness program should accommodate activities that allow individuals to

"let go." Chapter 14 describes a variety of activities that might be utilized in this type of atmosphere.

Euphoria

Numerous reports show that some people experience a special emotional state (e.g., "runner's high") while exercising. This state of **euphoria** resembles a deep religious experience or some of the emotional states achieved by drugs. It cannot be planned, nor can it serve as the basis for motivation, because not all people will experience it. However, people can develop a positive addiction to exercise as they achieve the common state of *feeling good* as a result of appropriate exercise. One of the HFI's main purposes is to help people progress to the fitness levels where they become "addicted" to exercise in the sense that they look forward to their regular workouts. On the other hand, as with all healthy behaviors, it is possible to go to the extreme, so that instead of a healthy addiction to exercise as one part of life, some may become obsessed and overemphasize its importance, spending time exercising that should be spent on other parts of their lives. The HFI assists at both extremes, helping inactive people become active and discouraging exercise fanatics from spending excessive amounts of time in physical fitness activities.

KEY POINT.   A number of psychological traits may promote or interfere with exercise. An understanding of rationalization, rejection, catharsis, and euphoria will assist in helping individuals with their exercise program.

Motivation

The HFI is concerned with the **motivations** for exercise, at two levels. The first level is, How can we get people to begin a fitness program? What kind of contact can be made with people in our communities to encourage them to begin fitness programs? The public has been educated about healthy behaviors (e.g., most people agree that they should exercise on a regular basis). However, convenient programs that provide personal contact and concern by exercise professionals are needed to complement information about the healthy life. The second level of motivation deals with the things that can be done to get people to continue exercise as a part of their lifestyles. Individual attention, realistic goals that are periodically tested, options for group participation, involvement of spouse or important others, contracts, and programs that minimize injury all seem to help adherence to fitness programs. Chapter 12 deals with characteristics of people who tend to drop out of fitness programs and suggests ways to enhance regular exercise behavior. Whether the HFI is motivating a participant to begin or to continue activity, fitness has to achieve priority status (like eating and sleeping) in a person's life. Efforts at increasing motivation must have that end in sight at all times. Thus, external (extrinsic) rewards must be viewed as a temporary means to change behavior, but the behavior can only be maintained over the long haul with internal (intrinsic) motivation.

Empathy

It is difficult for the HFI to understand the feelings of many people who join fitness programs. The HFI must try to understand and appreciate how it feels to have a low self-esteem about one's body, to be unable to perform well on many physical tasks, and to be slow at learning new physical skills. For example, the HFI should pay attention to his or her own emotional feelings when in uncomfortable situations. Many potential fitness participants have similar feelings when involved in fitness tests and exercise. An HFI's sensitivity to all emotional feelings of participants is part of the individual attention and concern that is important for motivation.

Play and Goal Orientation

One of the key elements in achieving a balance between arousal and relaxation and in defusing the Type A or Type B personality is to help people appreciate a balance of work and play. The Type A individual has difficulty taking time just to play and enjoy an activity (that is not directly related to productivity); the Type B person has a problem in getting down to a task and getting it done. People who try to pattern fitness programs after military or athletic models often have the **goal orientation** without the play. Others who are not discriminating about the selection of activities, as long as everyone is happy, have a **play orientation** and may achieve the playfulness without fitness gains. The good fitness program achieves this balance by including activities designed to improve all fitness components (goal orientation) and a playful atmosphere where participating is fun for its own sake (play orientation).

Traits and States

A distinction between the usual (trait) personality characteristics and the specific situational (state) personality characteristics is helpful in dealing with people. For example, a person who is normally very quiet and introverted (has that trait) may become an extrovert (be in that state) during competitive games. Or a person who is normally very relaxed (trait) may get anxious (state) during an exercise class.

Generally, personality traits do not change very much or very quickly. An HFI should use an understanding of traits to work with individuals on a long-term basis. Emotional states vary with situations and are more susceptible to change. For example, people who are afraid of or anxious about exercise need to be introduced to activity in a way that helps them become relaxed and unafraid when exercising.

KEY POINT.   Motivation to begin and continue exercise can be enhanced by a sensitivity to personality traits and states, along with a fitness program that includes a balance of play and work approaches to exercise.

HFI AND PERSONALITY OF PARTICIPANTS

Understanding the different personalities and interests of individual fitness participants will assist the HFI in providing fitness alternatives in an atmosphere that will motivate participants to adopt and continue healthy lifestyles. Two ways motivation is enhanced are by

- being more sensitive to individuals, and
- providing fitness activities that will be appealing to people with diverse interests.

The HFI learns to respond to specific behaviors. For example, participants with Type A, angry, aggressive, or hostile behavior need to be directed to more relaxing, noncompetitive activities. Participants with Type B behavior need to be motivated, and participants with fearful behavior need encouragement to ease into activities that can be easily learned, taking small steps in trying new activities.

The way the HFI communicates with fitness participants can assist in providing a good atmosphere for the program. Taylor and Miller (9) list four types of communication skills needed:

1. Noncommittal acknowledgment
2. Door openers
3. Content paraphrase
4. Confrontation

In the first form of communication, the HFI indicates acceptance of the participant by comments like, "I see," or nodding her or his head. In the second, the HFI asks the participant to continue expressing a thought. The third form of communication suggests that the HFI may want to repeat what the participant has said in different words to demonstrate that she or he has been listening and to check for accuracy. These first three types of communication are especially helpful for participants who are uncomfortable or withdrawn in the exercise setting. These skills would be helpful in talking with persons who are not participating on a regular basis. The HFI can use the suggestions in chapter 12 to help this person become a regular exerciser. The fourth type of communication skill is needed for inappropriate behavior. Participants who are disrupting the class or threatening the safety of themselves or other participants should be dealt with directly and firmly. Persons who are not ready for exercise either physically or mentally should be excused from class and told that they are welcome to return when they are ready and able to participate. Those who disrupt the program by finding fault with everything, being a "clown," doing too much above the recommended intensity, or trying to take over the class often need special individual attention. It is important to spend some additional time with these individuals to help them identify their goals for the program and what is and is not appropriate behavior.

To provide for persons with varying personalities, fitness programs should include options for individual or group, controlled or uninhibited, competitive or cooperative activities, with an "it's OK to choose any of the options" atmosphere.

KEY POINT. An understanding of personality and communication skills and a comprehensive fitness program will allow the HFI to enhance the exercise experience for diverse individuals.

STRESS CONTINUUMS

Personality is related to stress, in that a person's perception of a stimulus or situation largely determines how stressful the situation is for that person. No uniform agreement exists on definitions of stress terms. For our purposes, a **stressor** is defined as any stimulus or condition that causes physiological arousal beyond what is necessary to accomplish the activity. This excessive arousal is called **stress**.

Stress has three major components. A complete description of a stressful event includes the amount by which the stress response exceeds the functional demand, how pleasant it is to the individual, and whether it causes development or deterioration. The following sections expand on each of these bases for understanding stress.

Functional-to-Severe Stress Continuum

The physiological response at any one time lies on a continuum from what is essential to provide the energy for that task to an extreme physiological response beyond what is needed. Physiological responses (8) include increased

- heart rate,
- blood pressure,
- catecholamine levels,
- ventricular arrhythmia,
- levels of free fatty acids and serum cholesterol, and
- platelet adhesion

Table 11.1 illustrates how typical resting and submaximal HRs include not only the HR needed to provide energy for the body, but also the increased HR (stress) due to chronic stressors (e.g., excess fat) and acute stressors (e.g., certain emotional states).

Table 11.1   Stress Components of Heart Rate (beats · min^{-1})

	Activity		
Component of heart rate	Sitting	Climbing stairs	Running
HR needed to do task	30	50	100
Additional HR due to chronic stress			
Poor aerobic fitness	+15	+20	+40
Excess fat	+ 5	+15	+20
Additional HR due to acute stress			
Not relaxed	+10	+ 5	0
Emotional state	+15	+10	0
Total HR	75	100	160

Note. This HR model shows the contribution of the heart rate necessary to do various tasks plus the additional HR response caused by chronic and acute stressors. The actual HR values will vary with the individual depending on body size, fitness level, and type and severity of stressors.

Enjoyable-to-Unpleasant Stressors Continuum

Another aspect of stress is how the stressor is perceived by the individual. A person might have similar stress responses to an exciting concert and to taking the Health Fitness Instructor Certification examination but perceive the concert as more enjoyable.

Development-to-Deterioration Continuum

The third aspect of stress is what happens to the person as a result of the stressful experience. This is, of course, the main criterion for determining whether the stressful event was positive or negative. The positive stressor results in a healthier, stronger person. The negative stressor leads to a weaker individual. The end result of stress is somewhat independent of the other two aspects of stress. For example, a very stressful event (i.e., causing a large stress response beyond what is essential physically) could result in a person's being inspired to achieve great things, or it might destroy a person's initiative. On the other hand, conditions that cause small stress responses might lead to steady development or gradually wear down a person's desire to excel. In addition, a person might grow and develop from stressors that are both pleasant (e.g., positive reinforcement) and unpleasant (e.g., deadline to have a project done). Either pleasant or unpleasant stressors might tempt a person to escape from dealing with important areas of life. Thus the HFI should be cautious in identifying a specific stressor as being healthy or unhealthy based on the degree of physiological and psychological stress response or how much the individual liked the situation. A better criterion is to determine whether the experience led the person toward higher levels of mental, social, or physical health.

KEY POINT.   Excessive response (stress) to a situation (stressor) is described in terms of level of arousal, degree of unpleasantness, and most importantly, whether it results in a positive or negative shift in health status.

PHYSICAL ACTIVITY AND STRESS

One of the advantages of separating functional stimuli from stressors is that they interact with physical activity differently. Separating the effects of immediate and long-term physical activity on stress responses is also helpful.

Response to Acute Exercise and Other Functional Stimuli

The physiological response to acute physical activity and other functional stimuli is additive. Numerous stimuli such as exercise, heat, altitude, and pollution cause a functional increased physiological response (see chapter 3). If more than one of these is present, the physio-

logical response is greater than if only one stimulus were present. Thus, when people exercise in hot, humid, or polluted conditions, or at high altitude, they must do less exercise for the same physiological response (e.g., target heart rate). The one exception is exercising in the cold, because the heat by-product of exercise helps deal with the cold.

Response to Acute Exercise and Psychological Stressors

The physiological response to acute exercise and psychological stressors varies with the intensity of exercise, but generally it is not additive. Nonfunctional stimuli appear to affect the physiological response at rest and during light exercise but have little effect on the response to moderate or hard exercise. Nonfunctional stimuli also affect a person's decision about when to stop during a maximal task. Thus, if a person is very angry or happy, the HR and BP at rest and during light exercise may be elevated, and the person may decide to continue exercising longer or quit early. If the person is sad or relaxed, the HR and BP during light work may be depressed, and the decision to stop exercising may come earlier or later than usual. Thus emotional state, such as anxiety about taking the test, during a graded exercise test may affect some of the physiological and psychological measurements taken early in the test, as well as the length of time until voluntary exhaustion.

KEY POINT.   Exercise and physical stimuli, such as heat or altitude, interact to produce increased cardiorespiratory response at all levels of exercise intensity. Psychological stressors affect physiological and psychological responses at rest and during light work, as well as time to exhaustion, but have little influence on physiological response to moderate work.

Physical Activity for Stress Reduction

Many writers have justified exercise programs partly on the basis of stress reduction. Although the claims have often exceeded the evidence, there is some basis for a relationship between stress reduction and acute (immediate) and chronic (long-range) exercise.

Acute Activity

Acute exercise results in a positive mood change and has been shown to reduce state anxiety and muscle tension (4). Five factors are related to single bouts of exercise helping reduce stress.

Distraction. As with many other activities, exercise can serve as a temporary distraction from stressors. Stepping away from a problem and then coming back to it at a later time is often helpful. This technique is healthy as long as exercise does not become an escape from the problem. The ultimate reduction of stress must come from coping with the stressor. However, one part of the coping strategy can be the distraction of physical activity.

Control of the Situation. One of the primary concepts in a person's ability to cope with stressors is the perception of personal control. In some cases, exercise enhances this feeling of control. For example, increased practice and skill acquisition causes less stress in playing a game in the presence of others. One of the benefits of a postcardiac program is that it reduces the fear that any exertion will cause another heart attack (thus exercise increases feelings of control).

Feeling Good. The subjective reports of "feeling good" after exercise last as long as 6 hours postexercise and are related to reduction in depression, anxiety, and tension (7).

Interaction With Others. Another way acute exercise may influence stress is by providing a time to have more or less interaction with others. Stress reduction can result when the exercise session provides a time to be alone, for people who experience daily stress from constant contact with other people (e.g., the working parent who must spend almost every waking moment in the presence of others, such as children, spouse, employees, employer, and colleagues, all demanding time and attention). That person can use a walk/jog program as a time to be alone with his or her own thoughts. At the other extreme is the person who has little contact with other people during the typical day and has loneliness as a potential stressor. Doing activities and having time to talk with other people in an exercise program can aid that person. The HFI needs to be aware of the needs of individuals in terms of the amount of social interaction during the exercise sessions.

Physiological Changes. There are changes that take place as a result of exercise that may effect stress. For example, endorphins (i.e., endogenous, morphine-like chemicals) are increased as a result of exercise. One of the effects of this change is to lessen our perception of pain. The increased arousal (sympathetic nervous system) may cause some individuals to feel good. Following exercise, there is often an increased relaxation (parasympathetic nervous system), resulting in reduced muscle tension.

KEY POINT. Single bouts of activity may reduce stress through distraction, increased perception of con-

trol, positive mood shift, interaction with others, and physiological changes in the body.

Chronic Activity

The long-term effects of a regular exercise program also provide bases for stress reduction. Reduced arousal prior to, during, and after exposure to stressors, quicker recovery from stressors, and improved emotional reactions to some stressors are related to habitual exercise (2).

Repeated Acute Activity. Regular acute bouts of exercise provide substantial time when persons are less affected by stressors, thus providing an additional benefit for conditioning. This includes an improved glucose tolerance (chapter 13), positive mood changes, and reduction in tension.

Reduction of Chronic Stressors. Increased CRF and decreased body fat cause the person to be less stressed throughout the day. Further, these changes reduce the risk of CHD, hypertension, glucose intolerance, and the risk of sudden death.

Exercise Becoming Less of a Stressor. With increased fitness levels, physical activity itself becomes less of a stressor. For example, numerous studies have shown that a fit person can do the same amount of external work with lower HR, BP, catecholamines, and so forth. Thus the functional response to the work (the energy necessary to accomplish the task) remains the same, but the stress response is reduced.

Cross-Adaptation. Some people believe, with some support, that increased adaptation to physical activity provides a basis for better adaptation to other stressors. Others believe, with some support, that increased adaptation is specific to different stimuli and stressors. This question needs additional research before definitive claims can be made.

KEY POINT. Chronic exercise (conditioning) may reduce stress through a series of acute activities, reduction of chronic stressors, lessening the stress of exercise, and perhaps some cross-adaptation.

RELATIONSHIP BETWEEN STRESS AND HEALTH

Stress is important for both positive and negative aspects of health. No discussion of the highest quality of life possible or of serious health problems would be complete without including the relevance of stress.

Positive Stress

People often think of stress as primarily a negative influence on their lives, but it has many positive features. Having a great variety of stimuli and stressors provides the interesting experiences essential to a full life. People develop, learn, grow, and strive for their optimal potential through encountering stress. Even peak experiences, those special emotional moments of "the good life" that are remembered forever, are usually stressful. Without stress, life would be bland indeed.

KEY POINT.   Stress is a factor in positive health. Stressors are involved in having varied experiences, special moments in life, and accomplishment of goals.

Negative Stress

Stress is considered a risk factor for many major health problems (e.g., CHD, hypertension, cancer, ulcers, low-back pain, and headaches). Although inability to cope with stress probably is not sufficient to cause any of these problems if no predispositions exist, stress seems to manifest itself wherever the "weak link" is found. So for some people, stress results in a myocardial infarction (MI); for others, it results in hypertension, ulcers, low-back pain, or headaches.

An inability to cope with one stressor can be transferable to other stressors. Many people, because of stressors in other areas of their lives, find themselves getting upset (stressed) over something else that normally would not bother them. Two aspects of the inability to cope are perception of and reaction to a potential stressor. Although the positive transfer of adaptation to one stressor to other stressors is an open question, there is little doubt about negative transfer: An inability to cope in one area leads to coping problems in other areas of life.

The health problems caused by lack of exercise can also be sources of stress, and negative physiological and psychological changes (stressors) have also been related to excessive exercise [e.g., exercising more than 5 days per week, longer than 30 min per workout, or higher than THR (4)]—including increased injury risk, soreness, obsession, impatience, strain on relationships, neglect of work, and withdrawal symptoms when one cannot exercise (4, 7).

KEY POINT.   Inability to cope with stress is related to major health problems as a secondary risk factor and can cause problems in other areas of one's life. Both too little and too much exercise can be related to stress.

Aging

It is difficult to separate the effects of aging, itself, from things that typically happen as a person gets older. Certain experiences are more likely to have happened (more often) as a person becomes older. Positive aspects of aging include increased opportunities to deal with a variety of stressors. From this, many people develop a varied repertoire of coping behaviors.

On the negative side, the longer a person lives, the more likely it is that she or he will develop a serious health problem (although not living longer does not appear to be an attractive alternative). Some of the special life events that appear to cause stress (e.g., death of a loved one) obviously become more frequent with age.

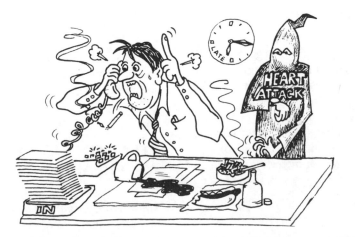

Figure 11.1   Negative aspects of stress.

There is often dramatic change in store for parents when all of the children leave home and for people when they retire. Lifestyle patterns developed over decades undergo major modifications, sometimes with additional financial difficulties. Evidence shows that people are more likely to have a number of health problems following a series of stressful life events.

Older people often become less active, causing more deterioration in fitness and performance than would occur simply because of increased age. Careful warm-up, safety precautions, cool-down, and gradual progression in activity become even more important in older populations because of the higher risk of health problems and injury and decreased fitness and performance skills. The good news is that an active lifestyle can slow down the physical deterioration of aging. It's never too late to start, and previously sedentary elderly individuals show remarkable fitness improvements as a result of initiating fitness programs.

RECOMMENDATIONS FOR HEALTHY STRESS LEVELS

People can do many things to maximize the positive aspects of stress while minimizing stress's negative side. In a fitness program, the HFI can help participants learn to fill their lives with healthy stress.

Seek Exposure to a Variety of Stimuli and Stressors

Simply being exposed to a wide range of experiences helps a person become better educated and less stressed by new situations. A good fitness program provides a variety of experiences, including cooperative, problem-solving, competitive, individual, partner, and team activities. This variety enriches the participant by improving fitness and improving the ability to cope with different physical and social experiences.

Develop a Range of Coping Abilities

People should observe the different strategies that seem to enhance coping with a potentially stressful situation. Facing the problem, looking at alternatives, talking about the problem with close friends, seeking professional or technical advice when needed, stepping back or away from it for a brief time, and so on, are all behaviors that people use to cope with stress. Which ones are better suited for particular situations? Do some behaviors help but feel uncomfortable to the individual? The HFI might encourage people to practice coping behaviors in "easy" settings. In terms of fitness, the variety of activities in a good program require different coping strategies. In addition, the HFI should be sensitive to participants who need help just coping with physical activity itself. After easing these people into exercise, the HFI can use a variety of fitness activities found in chapter 14 to develop coping abilities.

Maintain Social Support

Coping with stressors is often aided by positive connections between an individual and her or his social surroundings: family, close friends and relatives, and groups to which one belongs, such as churches, clubs, unions, and other social groups. The support for one's health is related to a special kind of relationship in these types of social settings (3).

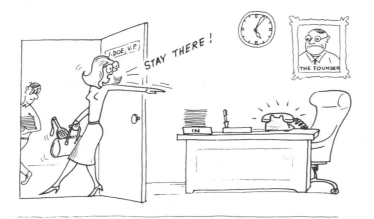

Figure 11.2 Coping with stressors.

Develop Optimal Fitness

Developing physical, mental, and social fitness characteristics causes potential stressors to be less threatening. For the person who can do hard physical work, physical stressors are not dreaded. For people who are accustomed to the mental processes that lead to problem solving, having a difficult problem is less stressful. Social fitness can be enhanced by doing such things as establishing meaningful relationships with other people, therein developing a support group that helps one respond positively to stressful situations.

KEY POINT.   Coping with stress can be aided by exposure to many stimuli, developing a social network, and increased levels of fitness.

Gain Control of as Much of Life as Possible

Perception of control repeatedly looms as a major element in coping with stress. Therefore, whatever a person can do to help gain control of her or his life diminishes the stress of potentially stressful conditions.

Adopt Healthy Behaviors

One of the by-products of exercising, eating nutritious foods, and refraining from use of harmful drugs is the feeling that one is taking responsibility for one's own life. Not only do the healthy behaviors reduce stress, but the fact that one has "taken charge" also reduces stress levels. Chapter 12 recommends ways to increase healthy behaviors.

Gain Competence in Important Areas

People should give attention to the things, tasks, and relationships that are important to them, so that they increase their skills in those areas and gain enhanced self-confidence that they can be successful in things they find important. In the fitness program, the HFI helps people improve skills in the activities they are interested in.

Be Assertive in Resisting Unreasonable Demands

People must learn to recognize unreasonable demands, whether imposed by themselves or by someone else, and to work with others (e.g., boss, spouse) to try to accomplish common goals in a reasonable way within an appropriate time frame; this is essential to good health. The HFI must be careful not to place unrealistic

goals or demands for future activities and fitness gains on the participant. The HFI can also help individuals set goals that will not be sources of stress.

Learn to Relax

Techniques can be learned to help people relax. Benson (1) and others have demonstrated the benefits of the "relaxation response," including increased parasympathetic dominance resulting in decreased HR, BP, and muscle tension. The HFI should include relaxation techniques as part of the program, perhaps including a short relaxation period following the cool-down.

Methods.   Many different methods have been used to increase relaxation (7), including

- biofeedback-assisted relaxation,
- autogenic training,
- breathing strategies,
- quieting-reflex training,
- cognitive restructuring,
- sensory awareness, and
- progressive relaxation.

Biofeedback includes focusing on something (e.g., heart rate, muscle tension) and learning to decrease it through relaxation. Autogenic training involves learning to relax by concentrating on heaviness, warmth, heart, respiration, solar plexus, and forehead. Participants are asked to think and say to themselves phrases such as *my left leg is feeling heavy* or *my right arm is feeling warm*. Attention to respiration can help one relax. The participant is asked to use primarily the abdomen (rather than chest) in breathing and to relax during exhalation. Quieting-reflex training involves a combination of other methods, such as self-talk (toward an alert mind and a calm body), relaxed breathing, conscious relaxation during exhalation, and imagining a wave of warmth and heaviness. Cognitive restructuring helps the participant become more positive about her- or himself through self-talk. Sensory awareness can be used with other relaxation techniques, by helping the person realize that the sensation of pressure from contact with objects has diminished during the relaxation.

Progressive Relaxation.   One technique (progressive relaxation) introduced by Jacobsen (5) is aimed at having people recognize the feelings produced by tension. The HFI should have participants get into comfortable positions with their eyes closed. We recommend that the technique be done with the participants lying on mats, but they can be sitting. The procedure is to have people tense a specific area of the body, hold for about 20 s, then relax; then tense a larger segment, hold, relax, and so forth. The HFI talks in a calm voice, asking the people to feel the tension during the hold period and to feel the tension leave the area during the relax period. The following sequence can be used:

Right toes	Left arm below the elbow
Left toes	Right arm below the shoulder
Right foot	
Left foot	Left arm below the shoulder
Right leg below the knee	
Left leg below the knee	Both arms below the shoulders
Right leg below the hip	
Left leg below the hip	Chest
Both legs below the hips	Neck
Abdomen and buttocks	Jaw
Right fingers	Forehead
Left fingers	Entire head
Right arm below the elbow	Entire body

Extend this last relaxation period; have people feel the tension leaving their bodies, feel their breathing, then be silent for several minutes.

KEY POINT.   The concept of gaining control of one's life is important in learning to cope with stress. Gaining control includes exhibiting healthy behaviors, getting rid of unhealthy habits, increasing competence in important areas, becoming assertive related to unreasonable demands, and learning how to relax.

SUMMARY

One aspect of a healthy lifestyle is a balance between arousal and relaxation. Personality characteristics can influence a person's response to a situation. The HFI can aid individuals by expressing emotions and being sensitive to the moods of participants. The HFI must be concerned with motivating people to begin the exercise program and continue in it.

A stressor is a situation that causes physiological arousal beyond what is necessary to accomplish an activity. The response of the individual to the stressor, and whether or not the stressor caused development or deterioration, help evaluate a stressful event. The physiological response to physical activity and environmental stimuli (e.g., altitude) are additive. Psychological stressors may influence a person's physiological responses at rest and during light work and time to voluntary exhaustion. Acute exercise may reduce stress by being a distraction and increasing a sense of control. Conditioning causes a reduction in chronic stressors.

Stress can provide variety and excitement in a person's life, or it can be a secondary risk factor for CHD.

Ways to emphasize the positive aspects of stress and minimize the negative aspects include exposing oneself to a variety of stimuli, developing a range of coping abilities, increasing fitness, gaining control of more of one's life, becoming competent in important areas, being assertive in resisting unreasonable demands, and learning to relax.

CASE STUDIES FOR ANALYSIS

11.1 Jim Jones, a former long-distance runner, is trying to get everyone in the Jonestown exercise program to run in 10K races on Saturday morning. Jim entered the exercise class as a team in a race coming up, without asking anyone, and is now trying to get 100% of the members to run. You get the feeling that some of the participants would enjoy running but would be embarrassed by their times, and that others prefer to spend their weekend doing other things. What would you do? (See Appendix A.)

11.2 Jennifer Jones, a single parent with three young children, has an executive position dealing with personnel in the local government. She joined the fitness center several months ago and seemed to enjoy the walking and jogging programs. After she had advanced in her jogging to 3 mi per day, 4 days per week, you suggested that she might enjoy participating in the coed games group 2 days per week. She tried it a couple of weeks and then quit coming to the center. You called her and asked her to come to see you. What do you think might be the problem? How would you proceed with the conversation with her? (See Appendix A.)

REFERENCES

1. Benson (1975)
2. Bouchard, Shephard, Stephens, Sutton, and McPherson (1990b)
3. Breslow (1990)
4. Brown (1990)
5. Jacobsen (1938)
6. Robinson (1990)
7. Sime (1990)
8. Sime and McKinney (1988)
9. Taylor and Miller (1988)

See the Bibliography at the end of the book for a complete source listing.

Part IV

Activity Recommendations

Chapter 12

Behavior Modification

Mark Hector

OBJECTIVES

The reader will be able to:

- List the steps in the General Model for modifying behavior
- Identify three strategies for increasing adherence to exercise
- Identify three models that have been proposed to explain smoking behavior
- Describe a danger of the rapid-smoking strategy
- Describe the debate over appropriate goals for the alcoholic
- List the eight components of successful weight-loss programs
- List the three stages of the stress inoculation model

TERMS

The reader will be able to define or describe:

Behavioral contract	Private speech
Negative-change goals	Role model
Nicotine addiction	Social support
Opponent process	Stress inoculation

Everyone has times when she or he wants to change some behavior. Having participants indicate their current level of satisfaction and things that bother them (see checklists for Degree of Satisfaction with Different Levels of Fitness and Things That Bother Me) will provide a start for deciding what areas of life they should consider changing. In working with participants, you can have them use the forms from *Fitness Facts*, or you can copy the forms from this book for their use.

Although you can assist persons in making healthy changes, they have to decide what changes to make. Honest answers to the Plans for Change Behavior form will assist you and the participant in establishing the goals for a fitness program.

This chapter focuses on five behaviors that are directly related to positive health: reductions in smoking, alcoholic drinking, weight, and stress, and an increase in exercise. The chapter starts with general points that the HFI should consider in trying to help individuals modify any behavior. The subsequent sections deal with some of the reasons for and ways to help people deal

with inactivity, smoking, alcoholism, obesity, and stress. Specific procedures for resolving these problems are recommended.

GENERAL PLAN FOR MODIFYING BEHAVIOR

Some general steps can be recommended for helping individuals adopt healthy behaviors. This General Model for Changing Behavior includes several components; it is not intended that the HFI should use all of these components with all of the individuals who seek help. A single set of procedures would not work for all people and the varieties of problems that they face. The HFI needs to be familiar with different strategies and combinations of strategies. Effectively helping an individual requires the helper to be knowledgeable, creative, and flexible. The steps found in the General Model provide a plan from which steps can be eliminated, added, or modi-

211

Degree of Satisfaction
With Different Aspects of Fitness

Circle the best number for each area, using this scale:
  4 = Very satisfied
  3 = Satisfied
  2 = Dissatisfied
  1 = Very dissatisfied

Amount of energy	4	3	2	1
Cardiovascular endurance	4	3	2	1
Blood pressure	4	3	2	1
Amount of fat	4	3	2	1
Strength	4	3	2	1
Ability to cope with tension and stress	4	3	2	1
Ability to relax	4	3	2	1
Ability to sleep	4	3	2	1
Posture	4	3	2	1
Amount of low-back problems	4	3	2	1
Physical appearance	4	3	2	1
Overall physical fitness	4	3	2	1
Level of regular medication	4	3	2	1

Things That Bother Me

List the things that bother you about yourself:

  Specific physical problem:

  Appearance of particular part of body:

  Ability to play specific sport:

  Risk of a health problem:

  Other:

fied depending on the individual case. The general plan also provides a preview of the procedures discussed in terms of modifying specific behaviors in later portions of this chapter.

The HFI needs to do whatever can reasonably be done to help an individual adopt healthy behaviors by being a facilitator, consultant, advocate, and encourager. However, it must be realized that the change of behavior is basically the responsibility of the person whose behavior is being changed.

Initially, the HFI helps the individual analyze the problem, including when the behavior started, what the

---

Plans to Change Behavior

Circle your plans to change each area:

Behavior	Plan to change		
Exercise	Now	Soon	No plans
Weight	Now	Soon	No plans
Use of drugs and medications	Now	Soon	No plans
Pattern of sleeping	Now	Soon	No plans
Use of tobacco	Now	Soon	No plans
Handling of tension and stress	Now	Soon	No plans
Diet	Now	Soon	No plans
Use of seat belts	Now	Soon	No plans
Other, list:	Now	Soon	No plans

General Model for Changing Behavior

Desire change.
Analyze history of problem.
Record current behavior.
Analyze current status.
Set long-term goal.
Set short-term goals.
Sign contract with friend(s).
List many possible strategies that could be used.
Select one or two strategies to be used.
Learn new coping skills.
Contact helper regularly.
Outline potential maintenance problems after goal is reached.
Learn new coping skills.
Contact helper periodically.

---

conditions were, why it continues, and when it last happened and under what conditions (22, 23). The individual and the HFI need to reach a mutual understanding of the problem. This analysis is often aided with the collection of some baseline data concerning the extent of the behavior over a period of several days. After the initial analysis, the participant should be able to clearly describe the current status of the problem.

The past and present having been analyzed, the future is addressed by a discussion of goals. Goal statements are about future conditions, and they often include time constraints (22, 23). The participant suggests the desired goal, and the HFI assists in making the goal realistic and clear. When a large amount of behavior change is desired, subgoals are advisable. Success with a single day may encourage the participant to persist for 2 days, 3 days, a week, and so forth. To increase the chances

of achieving the goal, a reward can be made contingent on its successful accomplishment. The reward is obtained only if the goal is reached. Another procedure that has helped individuals achieve goals is the signing of a **behavioral contract**. The written agreement, specifying conditions to be met and the rewards or consequences if it is not met, is more successful if made between the individual desiring to change and a close friend. In some cases, contracts are made with groups of individuals, forming a support group that can provide encouragement and increase the level of commitment of the participants.

Once a problem has been analyzed and a goal has been agreed upon, the next step is to determine a plan for reaching the goal (22, 23). The first step in developing a plan is for the HFI and participant to list as many different plans as possible without taking time to

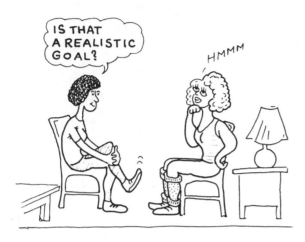

Figure 12.1 Setting realistic goals.

evaluate each one as it is mentioned (brainstorming). From this list, the participant can pick the one or two strategies that seem to have the best chance of success.

Depending on the strategy selected, the participant might need to learn new coping behaviors, such as new social skills, increasing professional competence, learning how to relax, or learning how to be assertive. The coping behaviors focused upon depend on the goals and strategies selected.

Individuals who have had difficulty changing their behaviors in the past often have such feelings as fear and helplessness when they try to change again. Throughout the process, the HFI can be an effective facilitator. Becoming a respected and effective helper largely depends on the HFI being accepting, friendly, aware of the feelings of the participants, and a good **role model**.

After an individual has reached a goal of change, a very difficult stage begins: namely, How can long-term results be maintained? Participants need practice in recognizing the environmental conditions under which old behaviors are likely to occur. Being able to recognize the onset of these potentially dangerous conditions increases the likelihood that steps will be taken to avoid them. Long-term contacts between the HFI and the participant also help to maintain change over time.

EXERCISE ADHERENCE

Exercise is good for people. The health objectives for the United States for the year 2000 include a threefold increase in the adult population (from 20% to 60%) in appropriate aerobic exercise. The HFI is in a position to help that goal become a reality. Exercise seems to be good both physiologically (see chapter 3) and psychologically (see chapter 11). Chapter 13 deals with specific factors (e.g., intensity) needed for improvement in health-related fitness. Chapter 14 presents a variety of activities that can be used for fitness.

The current emphasis on and interest in exercise assists fitness programs in attracting participants, even though new ways must be found to motivate many sedentary people to become active. A major problem for the HFI is to keep up the involvement (adherence) of those who do start, because up to 50% quit within 6 months in many programs. People who are more likely to drop out tend to smoke and have low self-motivation, lack of social reinforcement, and the belief that additional exercise is not needed. Reasons often given for quitting exercise are inconvenience and lack of time. Several strategies have been suggested to increase adherence to exercise (1, 2, 6, 8, 14).

Availability of the Program

Change is facilitated by accessible programs. The times and locations of the programs need to be convenient for the targeted population.

Social Support

The fitness program should include **social support** by including family and significant others (i.e., people who are important to the individual such as a spouse or partner, work colleagues, or friends) so that others can encourage and support participation in the fitness program (16).

Emphasis on Enjoyable Activities and Health Benefits

Learning new behaviors must be pleasurable, if old behaviors are to be discarded. Physical fitness programs need to recognize that fitness changes need to happen in an enjoyable atmosphere. The performance models (e.g., military or athletic) aimed only at producing results regardless of the enjoyment of the participant will not work in a lifelong fitness program. Education for a new behavior should direct attention to potential gains more than to losses. A contract (see Sample Contract to Begin Exercise) between the individual and a program leader that focuses on these gains is an effective route to behavior change in this area (24).

Program Characteristics

Qualified and enthusiastic personnel, regular assessment of important fitness components, relevant personal and general communication, and participant

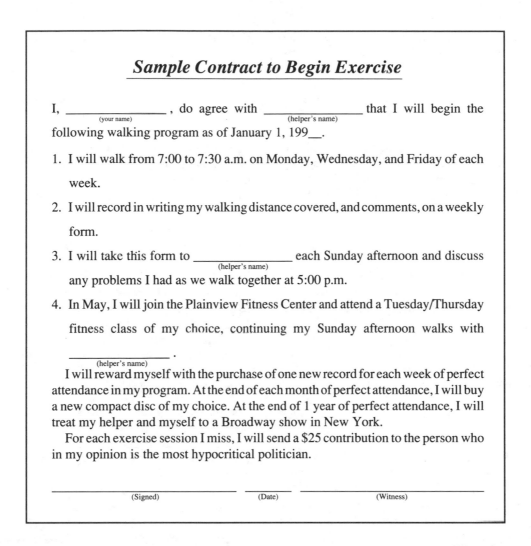

Sample Contract to Begin Exercise

I, _____ , do agree with _____ that I will begin the
_(your name) _(helper's name)
following walking program as of January 1, 199__.

1. I will walk from 7:00 to 7:30 a.m. on Monday, Wednesday, and Friday of each week.

2. I will record in writing my walking distance covered, and comments, on a weekly form.

3. I will take this form to _____ each Sunday afternoon and discuss
_(helper's name)
any problems I had as we walk together at 5:00 p.m.

4. In May, I will join the Plainview Fitness Center and attend a Tuesday/Thursday fitness class of my choice, continuing my Sunday afternoon walks with

_____ .
_(helper's name)

I will reward myself with the purchase of one new record for each week of perfect attendance in my program. At the end of each month of perfect attendance, I will buy a new compact disc of my choice. At the end of 1 year of perfect attendance, I will treat my helper and myself to a Broadway show in New York.

For each exercise session I miss, I will send a $25 contribution to the person who in my opinion is the most hypocritical politician.

_____   _____   _____
(Signed)   (Date)   (Witness)

choice of a variety of group and individual exercises, games, and sports are all qualities of a good fitness program. Physical exercise and socializing make a profitable combination, as evidenced by the success of many dance and physical fitness groups. Many enjoy the social interaction with others, and a support group develops to help continue the exercise.

Role Models

People learn from each other and from others they admire (3). The importance of an HFI who displays healthy behaviors cannot be overemphasized.

SMOKING CESSATION

There is little disagreement outside cigarette-producing circles that smoking is bad for health. Ample data show that smoking is the largest avoidable cause of death in the United States. Through warning labels on packages and in advertisements, virtually everyone has been

made aware of the dangers. Millions have quit smoking. However, the overall number of smokers has remained almost constant since the late 1960s because of the increases in the number of new smokers, especially young females.

Why People Smoke

Three models that have been proposed to explain smoking behavior are

- social learning,
- nicotine addiction, and
- opponent process.

The social learning theory indicates that smokers often acquire the habit with social reinforcement, usually with peer pressure (3). This positive reinforcement of smoking and the decreased aversion to the smoke itself produce a habit difficult to break.

The second model, **nicotine addiction**, holds that the smoker acquires an addiction to smoking similar to addictions to other drugs.

The "rewards" of smoking include the nicotine

reaching the brain a few seconds after inhaling, giving the smoker a series of "highs." Withdrawal symptoms and a smoker's craving for nicotine, make the habit resistant to change (15).

The **opponent process** model proposes that two opposing processes (one pleasurable and one aversive) interact to continue the smoking habit. For example, the social reinforcement and the nicotine highs cause a pleasant emotion, whereas attempts to quit smoking cause unpleasant withdrawal symptoms that can be eliminated by having a smoke. Thus the positive effects of smoking and negative effects of not smoking combine to encourage a continuation of the habit (15).

A Plan for Smoking Cessation

The three stages of the following plan for stopping smoking are

1. preparation,
2. cessation, and
3. maintenance.

Stage 1—Preparation

Smokers need to gain confidence that they can successfully quit smoking. Confident, organized, sensitive, nonsmoking leaders can foster smokers' self-confidence through clear presentation of goals, procedures, and rationale for the program. During this stage, participants self-monitor their current frequency of smoking. This self-observation often temporarily helps reduce the smoking behavior.

Stage 2—Cessation

An abrupt end to the smoking behavior has been found to be more effective than gradually cutting down (7). An effective method is to have a contract (see Sample Contract to Stop Smoking) to quit on a specific date. The behavioral contract involves a specific agreement between the smoker and some other person. The goal is specified in precise behavioral terms. For example, no cigarette will be smoked by Robert Jones between the dates of January 1, 199x and January 1, 199y. The behavior, or lack of behavior, should be specifically described and linked to a time constraint. The contract also specifies what contingency comes into effect if the contract is broken. For example, if Robert Jones is a liberal democrat, his contract might specify that for each cigarette smoked during 199x, he will send a $100 political contribution to Senator Jesse Helms of North Carolina (a political figure he particularly dislikes). The contract is individually tailored to the capabilities and needs of the individual who is to abide by the contract.

How long does Robert Jones feel that he has to refrain from smoking for him to believe that he has quit? To whom should the donation be sent to make the penalty especially aversive? What is the maximum amount of money he can send and still be able to abide by the conditions of the contract? Robert Jones will most likely feel committed and motivated if he is involved in the development of the contract. He knows best what contingencies will help him abide by the conditions of the contract. Frequent contact between the abstaining smoker and the leader of the program during the early part of the contract is needed for encouragement and discussion of unanticipated problems.

Another smoking-cessation strategy that has a good record of success is rapid smoking. This strategy is based on the principle of satiation, whereby an individual is encouraged to smoke as rapidly and continuously as possible until he or she becomes sick and has to quit. Because of the possibility of nicotine poisoning, along with physiological abnormalities, this method should include careful screening and supervision (5, 10).

Stage 3—Maintenance

Contact with the leader and the development of new behavioral skills are essential ingredients of maintaining the behavioral change. Communication with the leader should include learning the advantages of a smokeless life (e.g., a lower risk of major health problems, less stress in daily activities). The nonsmoker should be helped to learn new skills for dealing with old stimuli that were associated with cigarette smoking. If drinking coffee at the end of a meal was an old cue to light up, then avoid coffee. If cigarette smoke in the lobby of a basketball arena provided a cue for lighting up, then either remain seated in the arena or chew gum in the lobby as new behaviors. Once again, it needs to be emphasized that the determination of what new behaviors are needed and what will be effective involves both the participant and the leader. It is unlikely that leaders who rigidly prescribe what *must* be done will be as effective as those who mutually work out the strategies with the new nonsmoker.

ALCOHOLIC DRINKING HABITS

Alcoholism is one of our nation's leading public health problems. There are an estimated 5 to 15 million alcoholics in the United States (17). The problems of family disruption, lost time at work, bodily injury, and death that are directly and indirectly caused by excessive drinking are not disputed even by the producers of these beverages. The drinking problem exacts a heavy toll on

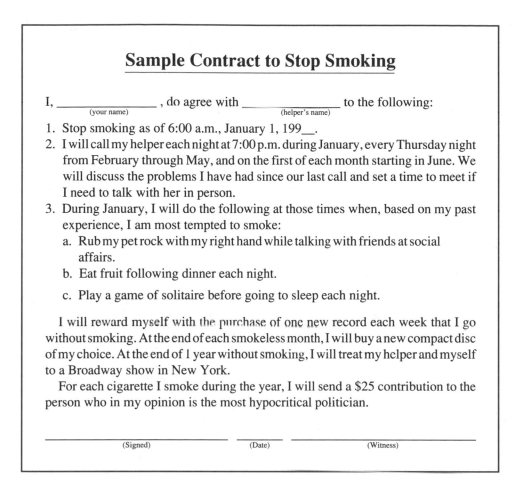

Sample Contract to Stop Smoking

I, _____ , do agree with _____ to the following:
(your name)   (helper's name)

1. Stop smoking as of 6:00 a.m., January 1, 199__.
2. I will call my helper each night at 7:00 p.m. during January, every Thursday night from February through May, and on the first of each month starting in June. We will discuss the problems I have had since our last call and set a time to meet if I need to talk with her in person.
3. During January, I will do the following at those times when, based on my past experience, I am most tempted to smoke:
   a. Rub my pet rock with my right hand while talking with friends at social affairs.
   b. Eat fruit following dinner each night.
   c. Play a game of solitaire before going to sleep each night.

   I will reward myself with the purchase of one new record each week that I go without smoking. At the end of each smokeless month, I will buy a new compact disc of my choice. At the end of 1 year without smoking, I will treat my helper and myself to a Broadway show in New York.

   For each cigarette I smoke during the year, I will send a $25 contribution to the person who in my opinion is the most hypocritical politician.

_____   _____   _____
(Signed)   (Date)   (Witness)

the health and financial well-being of the people of our nation.

Although there is no debate on the reality of the alcoholism problem, there is heated debate on the appropriate goals for treatment of the problem. Should the alcoholic person strive for controlled moderate drinking or complete abstinence? Those who feel that abstinence is the correct goal tend to conceptualize the problem as a disease (12). Alcoholics Anonymous (AA) is a successful treatment group with an approach based on the disease concept. One fundamental precept of AA is that once a person has the disease of alcoholism, he or she will always have it—there is no cure. To combat the disease, total abstinence is required. Individuals are helped to achieve this goal by the support of other alcoholics in person-to-person contacts and regular group meetings.

Others contend that alcoholism is not a disease and that no crucial difference distinguishes the social drinker from the problem drinker other than the amount of alcohol consumed (18). It has been proposed that four factors determine the probability of excessive drinking: (a) the degree to which the individual feels controlled, (b) the availability of an adequate coping response, (c) expectations about the results of the drink-

ing, and (d) the availability of alcohol and situational constraints. For example, at a New Year's Eve party, the individual may feel strong pressure to drink (Factor a), may lack an adequate coping response (e.g., "I'd like a ginger ale on the rocks") (Factor b), may have pleasant memories of previous New Year's Eve parties that included excessive drinking (Factor c), and finds plenty of alcohol available for party-goers to consume (Factor d).

Social Skills Training

Social skills training to reduce excessive drinking normally includes instruction in assertive responding, refusing alcohol, preventing a relapse, and obtaining reinforcement other than drinking (21). In assertiveness training an individual learns how to communicate feelings in a productive and caring manner (4). This type of training is helpful to some problem drinkers because the excessive drinking behavior is related to an inability to communicate feelings to friends and other associates. Helping individuals learn how to refuse alcoholic drinks is important. Some alcoholics simply lack the cognitive awareness of verbalized sentences or words that can be used to refuse a drink. Role playing is a technique widely used to learn and practice ways of refusing a drink.

Relapse prevention is probably the most important component of the social skills training plan. Many techniques can enable a person to abstain or drink less for a given period of time. However, maintaining these improvements over a long period of time is difficult (15). One of the key elements in maintaining the desired behavior is to be able to anticipate problem situations. Prior planning of ways to avoid problems can lead to discovering that there are behaviors other than excessive drinking that can provide positive reinforcement from peers and important others. For example, improving one's conversation or storytelling skills can substitute for excessive drinking habits in some situations. Once again, role playing can be used to avoid relapses. The leader works with the person to discuss feelings and coping behaviors in potential problem situations.

Choice Between Abstinence and Controlled Drinking

The choice of an appropriate goal for problem drinkers must involve the individual working with the leader. In general, people who have long-standing chronic problems with alcohol abuse and who have developed serious life problems associated with their drinking may be more suited to the complete abstinence approach. But younger people who are open to learning new social skills may respond well to the controlled drinking approach.

WEIGHT REDUCTION

Obesity seems to be more difficult to overcome than smoking or problem drinking. Less than 5% of obese individuals successfully maintain a lower weight for a year, whereas, 20% to 25% report success at quitting smoking or alcohol abuse. One problem seems to be an emphasis on **negative-change goals** rather than developing healthy substitute behaviors (13). For example, instead of concentrating on eating less cheese, why not encourage a plan to promote eating fruit at snack time. Another problem is the disregard for either energy intake or energy expenditure. Both decreased caloric intake and increased exercise (caloric expenditure) are normally essential for maintaining desired weight; either one by itself is doomed to failure for most people. Another problem is directing attack at the behavior rather than at the reasons for the behavior. Thus if a particular cue results in poor eating behavior, the person should either avoid the cue or learn to react to it differently. Ready access to food and drink, and the

mass media message that there is a direct relationship between happiness and what is consumed, contribute to the problem for people trying to change their eating behaviors.

Chapter 7 deals with methods for determining percent fat and estimating ideal weight. The participant should be counseled to work toward the goal gradually in ways that can be accepted physiologically and psychologically.

No one weight-loss program can be recommended for all people. However, the following seven components appear to be common ingredients for successful programs. Much of the success depends on the leader working with the participant to decide what steps are likely to work for that person, then working with the person to make it happen.

1. Before any specific steps are implemented, the participant keeps a daily diary. The 2-week diary should describe quantity of food eaten and the eating environment (see chapter 6 for a form that can be used).
2. The participant, in consultation with the leader, determines the ultimate weight goal, then sets weekly weight-loss goals (from 0.5 to 2 lb). Extremely obese people should be referred for medical supervision.
3. A dietary plan that specifies food types and portions and calorie amounts needs to be agreed upon. Several sound diets are available (see chapter 6).
4. Certain situations or cues often are strongly related to eating patterns (e.g., watching a movie or TV). The participant needs to agree to eat only at certain places (e.g., at the dining room table) at certain times (e.g., breakfast, lunch, supper, and one snack time).
5. Some people are helped by providing small rewards for progress toward their goals (such as a new cassette tape for each 3-lb loss), and a larger reward (e.g., an evening out at a Broadway show) when the final goal is reached. The rewards should be consistent with healthy behaviors, something desired by the person, and things for which there are no acceptable alternatives.
6. The first section of this chapter dealt with ways to begin and continue regular exercise. Although not everyone who begins an exercise program needs to begin a diet-reduction program, most people who need to lose fat need to begin diet and exercise programs simultaneously (9).
7. The awareness and support of a spouse, partner, or other important person greatly assists the participant in adhering to the program. Involvement of friends or family members early in the program enhances its possibility of success.

STRESS REDUCTION

Attempts to understand human stress (see chapter 11) and to develop plans to alleviate it are relatively recent. Three approaches have been used. Some emphasize the stress response itself, using Selye's (20) stages of alarm, resistance, and exhaustion. A second approach focuses on the stimulus (stressor), dealing primarily with changes in the environment; life crises such as the death of a loved one, the loss of a job, serious injury, or even holidays or vacations can be stress-producing events. The third approach deals with the interaction of the person and the environment. Studies showing stress reactions of people with various personality traits (e.g., Type A) to psychological stressors (e.g., a work deadline) are examples of the interaction approach.

Three stages in the **stress-inoculation** model are cognitive preparation, skill acquisition, and application training (11). In cognitive preparation, the stressed individual is prepared mentally for the coming stressful situation. The leader provides a manual that deals with a particular stressor. The participant keeps a diary of the frequency and conditions surrounding the stressor.

In the skill acquisition stage, the main emphasis is on learning basic cognitive and behavioral coping skills. One of the skills is **private speech**, where individuals learn sentences to say to themselves before, during, and following the stressor (e.g., before taking a major test one might say, "It's going to be hard, but I have prepared for it"; during the event, "If I stay calm I will be less likely to block on a question" and/or "I'm getting tense—relax and take it easy"; and following, "I did as well as I could because I stayed calm").

A second component of the skill acquisition stage is relaxation training (19). Chapter 11 includes an example of tensing and relaxing specific muscle groups. With practice, a relaxed state can be achieved rapidly in a potentially stressful situation.

In the application training, or final stage of the stress-inoculation training program, the stressed individual is guided through a series of practice situations that help him or her learn to apply the previously taught skills. The sequence of situations progresses from relatively mild to more severe, so that the participant can experience success and gain confidence in using the skills.

SUMMARY

One of the primary responsibilities of the HFI is to help participants modify lifestyle behaviors. The focus of attention is on increasing exercise, but it should be clear that other unhealthy behaviors need to be decreased. These behaviors include smoking, alcohol consumption, overeating and sedentarism that lead to obesity,

and inadequate coping with stress. Each of these behaviors is discussed in terms of what causes them to occur and methods that can be used to change them. Some commonalities exist among the behavior-change techniques; the following is a set of guidelines to follow in helping people change behavior. Analyze the history of the problem and record the current status of the behavior; set a long-term goal and several short-term goals, and sign a contract with a friend; list as many strategies as possible, selecting one or two that will be effective; learn new coping skills and have regular meetings with the HFI; once the goal is reached, outline a maintenance schedule, including periodic contacts with the HFI.

CASE STUDIES FOR ANALYSIS

12.1 Sara True had lived in the Atlanta area for 10 years. As a real estate appraiser, she spent a lot of time in office work and making short trips to real estate sites. She had always desired to keep up a regular exercise schedule, but to her the thought of exercise was always associated with the word *drudgery*. As a result of this association, she had joined five health/fitness centers. Upon joining each new center, Sara hoped that exercise would become enjoyable. Overall, she exercised very irregularly and very little. At the sixth health/fitness center Sara joined, things were different. She became a regular and happy participant in the center's dance exercise and swimming programs. What was different from all the other centers? Sara felt that the HFI was the most important factor, but she was not exactly sure why.

Describe how the HFI might have related to Sara to help her develop her new pleasure in exercising. (See Appendix A for one strategy that worked.)

12.2 Carl Brown was looking forward to his second marriage. His prospective bride, Terry Wood, put a condition on the marriage that was causing Carl some genuine concern, however. She was not going to live with a person who smelled of cigarette smoke. Her parents and first husband had smoked, and she was fed up with all that goes with the habit. Carl never smoked around Terry, but that was not good enough for her. If they were going to live in the same house, he had to give it up for good. Carl never enjoyed smoking, but he had never had a strong enough reason to quit. He was afraid that he could never break the habit.

Carl's sister was in a fitness program. She asked the HFI for ideas of how Carl could deal with this problem. What would you have suggested? (See Appendix A.)

REFERENCES

1. Allen and Iwata (1980)
2. Andrew et al. (1981)
3. Bandura (1969)
4. Cormier and Cormier (1979)
5. Danaher (1977)
6. Dishman, Ickes, and Morgan (1980)
7. Flaxman (1978)
8. Gettman, Pollock, and Ward (1983)
9. Gormally and Rardin (1981)
10. Horan, Linberg, and Hacket (1977)
11. Hussina and Lawrence (1978)
12. Jellinek (1960)
13. Kincey (1983)
14. Martin (1982)
15. Miller (1980)
16. Murphy et al. (1982)
17. National Institute on Alcohol Abuse and Alcoholism (1978)
18. Pattison, Sobell, and Sobell (1977)
19. Rimm and Masters (1974)
20. Selye (1956)
21. Sobell and Sobell (1978)
22. Watson and Tharp (1977)
23. Williams and Long (1983)
24. Wysocki, Hall, Iwata, and Riordan (1979)

See the Bibliography at the end of the book for a complete source listing.

Chapter 13

Exercise Prescription for Cardiorespiratory Fitness

OBJECTIVES

The reader will be able to:

- Identify the physiological principles related to warm-up and cool-down
- Develop an exercise prescription for correct exercise intensity, frequency, and duration to achieve and maintain cardiorespiratory fitness goals
- State the error in estimating maximal heart rate from formulas based on age
- Express exercise intensity in terms of energy production, heart rate, and rating of perceived exertion
- Incorporate warm-up, aerobic stimulus, muscular strength and endurance, flexibility, and cool-down phases into a complete exercise session
- Modify the exercise prescription for the following conditions or groups: orthopedic limitation, obese, hypertensive, asthmatic, pregnant, cardiac, diabetic, chronic obstructive pulmonary disease, seizure disorder, and elderly
- Explain the concepts of overload, specificity, and reversibility, related to training programs
- Describe the effects of high temperature and humidity, altitude, and pollution on the exercise prescription

TERMS

The reader will be able to define or describe:

Asthma

Carbon monoxide (CO)

Chronic obstructive pulmonary disease (COPD)

Coronary artery bypass graft surgery (CABGS)

Dry-bulb temperature

Duration

Exercise-induced asthma (EIA)

Frequency

Globe temperature

Glucagon

Heart-rate reserve (HRR)

Hyperglycemia

Hypertension

Hyperthermia

Hypertrophic obesity

Hypoglycemia

Hypothermia

Insulin

Intensity

Mast cells

Myocardial infarction (MI)

Obesity

Orthopedic

Osteoporosis

Overload

Ozone

Percentage of the maximal heart rate (%HRmax)

Percentages of the maximal $\dot{V}O_2$ (%$\dot{V}O_2$max)

Percutaneous transluminal coronary angioplasty

Rating of perceived exertion (RPE)

Reversibility

Specificity

Sulfur dioxide (SO_2)

Target heart rate (THR)

Threshold

Total work
Training intensity
Type I diabetes

Type II diabetes
Wet-bulb globe temperature (WBGT)
Windchill index

Physical inactivity is regarded as a risk factor not only for coronary heart disease (CHD) but for hypertension, glucose intolerance (adult-onset diabetes), elevated serum lipids (cholesterol and triglycerides), low-HDL cholesterol, and hyper-reactivity to stress (7). Because each of these problems is, in itself, a risk factor for CHD, physical activity, both directly and indirectly, decreases the risk of CHD. In fact, one of the main nonpharmacological interventions used to treat hypertension, adult-onset diabetes, hyperlipidemia, and stress is to systematically increase the person's physical activity (7).

Given the prevalence of inactivity in the general population, there is a general consensus that the greatest gains in public health would occur by having sedentary people become moderately active—expending approximately 200 to 300 kcal every other day, equivalent to walking 4 to 5 mi or jogging 2 to 3 mi (38, 73). However, individuals who expend more than 2,000 kcal per week, or who possess a high $\dot{V}O_2$max, show the lowest death rate from all causes (11, 67). Consequently, there are benefits to be gained not only when a sedentary person becomes active, but also as a person engages in more vigorous exercise that increases functional capacity ($\dot{V}O_2$max). The purpose of this chapter is to lead you through the steps involved in developing an exercise prescription for various groups of participants, including those with known problems or special characteristics. But first a brief review of the major principles of training.

BASIS FOR PHYSIOLOGICAL CHANGES: EXERCISE PRINCIPLES

The degree to which a tissue such as bone, skeletal muscle, or cardiac muscle functions depends on the activity to which it is exposed. This statement summarizes the two major principles underlying training programs: *overload* and *specificity*.

Overload

The principle of **overload** describes a dynamic characteristic of living creatures: *use increases functional ca-*

pacity. If a tissue or organ system is caused to work against a load to which it is not accustomed, instead of wearing out and becoming weaker, it becomes stronger. The slang is "use it or lose it." The corollary of the overload principle is the principle of **reversibility**, which indicates that physiological gains are lost when the load against which it is working is reduced. The variables that contribute to an overload in an exercise program include the intensity, duration, and frequency of the exercise. As we will see, it is the combination of these elements that results in a sufficient amount of *total work*, or energy expenditure, to cause an increase in the functional capacity of the cardiorespiratory (CR) systems.

Specificity

The principle of **specificity** states that the training effects derived from an exercise program are specific to the exercise done and the muscles involved. For example, a person who runs as a primary form of exercise shows little change in the arm muscles, just as the person who exercises at a low intensity that recruits only Type I muscle fibers will have little or no training effect in the fast-twitch fibers in the same muscle groups—if the fibers are not used, they cannot adapt, and consequently they will not become "trained." Finally, the type of adaptation that occurs as a result of training is specific to the type of training taking place (e.g., running vs. heavy resistive strength training). Running causes an increase in the number of capillaries and mitochondria in the muscle fibers involved in the exercise, and makes them more resistant to fatigue. Strength training causes a hypertrophy of the muscles involved, due to an increase in the amount of contractile proteins, actin and myosin, in the muscle (42, 82).

KEY POINT. Tissues adapt to the load to which they are exposed; to increase the functional capacity of a tissue, it must be *overloaded*. The type of adaptation is *specific* to the muscle fibers involved and types of exercise. Endurance exercise increases mitochondria and capillary number, and strength training increases the contractile protein and size of the muscle.

GENERAL GUIDELINES FOR CARDIORESPIRATORY FITNESS PROGRAMS

To apply these two principles to cardiorespiratory fitness (CRF), activities that overload the heart and respiratory systems need to be used in exercise programs. Activities that use the large muscle groups contracting in a rhythmic manner and on a continuous basis are the types that specifically overload the CR systems. Activities involving a small muscle mass, and weight-training exercises, are less appropriate because they tend to generate very high cardiovascular loads relative to energy expenditure (see chapter 3). Activities that improve CRF are high in caloric cost and therefore help to achieve a relative leanness goal. How do you get someone started?

Screen Participants

If the person has not already done so, have him or her fill out one of the health status forms. Chapter 2 provides guidelines for who should and should not seek medical clearance before exercising.

Encourage Regular Participation

Exercise must become a valuable part of a person's lifestyle. It is not something that can be done sporadically, nor will doing it for a few months or years build up a fitness reserve. Dramatic gains accomplished through fitness activities are lost quickly with inactivity (see chapter 3, "Detraining"). Only people who continue activity as a way of life receive its long-term benefits (remember the principle of reversibility).

Provide Different Types of Activities

A fitness program starts with easily quantified activities, such as walking or cycling, so that the proper exercise intensity can be achieved. After a minimum level of fitness is achieved, a variety of activities are included in the program. Chapter 14 outlines three phases of activities: (a) Work up to walking briskly for 4 mi per workout; (b) gradually begin jogging, and work up to jogging continuously for 3 mi; and (c) introduce a variety of activities.

Program for Progression

Given the importance of helping sedentary persons become active, the emphasis in any health-related fitness

program that includes such individuals should be to *start slowly* and, when in doubt, do too little rather than too much. Participants should begin at work levels that can be easily completed and should be encouraged to *gradually* increase the amount of work they can do during a workout. For example, a sedentary participant who is interested in jogging as a goal should begin a training program by walking a distance that she or he can complete without feeling fatigued or sore. With time, the participant will be able to walk a greater distance at a faster pace without discomfort. After this person can walk 4 mi briskly without stopping, she or he can gradually work up to jogging 3 mi continuously per workout. For the participant who is ready to begin jogging, you might introduce the interval-type workout with walking-jogging-walking-jogging. As individuals adapt to the interval workouts, they will be able to gradually increase the amount of jogging while decreasing the distance walked (see the walking and jogging programs in chapter 14).

Adhere to Format for a Fitness Workout

The main body of the fitness workout consists of dynamic large-muscle-group activities at an intensity high enough and a duration long enough to accomplish enough total work to specifically overload the CR systems. Stretching and light endurance activities are included before the workout (warm-up) and after the workout (cool-down) for safety and to improve low-back function.

There are physiological, psychological, and safety reasons for including warm-up and cool-down (28). In general the warm-up and taper-down consist of

- activities similar to the activities done in the main body of the workout, but done at a lower intensity (e.g., walking, jogging, or cycling below THR);
- stretching exercises for the muscles involved in the activity, as well as those in the midtrunk area; and
- muscular endurance exercises, especially for the muscles in the abdominal region.

These activities help the participants ease into and out of a workout and provide activities for a healthy low back. If a workout is going to be shorter than usual, the reduction in time should take place in the main body of the workout, retaining the warm-up and cool-down.

Conduct Periodic Tests

Routine testing to determine a participant's progress can be motivational and may help alter programs that are not achieving desired results. The HFI can help by setting realistic goals for the next testing session when discussing test results. A rule of thumb would be a 10% improvement in 3 months in the test scores that need to change. Once the person has reached a desirable level, the goal is to maintain that level.

FORMULATION OF THE EXERCISE PRESCRIPTION

The CRF training effect is dependent on the degree to which the systems are overloaded—that is, upon intensity, duration, and frequency of training. Improvements in CRF have been shown to occur with fitness programs conducted at intensities of 50% to 85% $\dot{V}O_2$max, frequencies of 2 to 5 times per week, and durations of 15 to 60 min (2). The blend of intensity and duration should result in an energy expenditure (**total work**) of 200 to 300 kcal per session. This latter variable, total work, seems to be crucial in developing and maintaining a CRF training effect (2). Why recommend that someone do four workouts per week, if two would suffice?

Frequency

Figure 13.1 shows that gains in CRF increase with the **frequency** of exercise, but begin to level off at 4 days

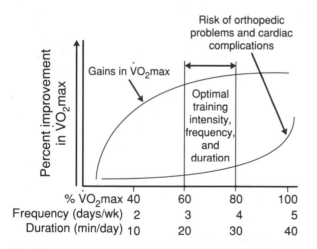

Figure 13.1 Effects of increasing the frequency, duration, and intensity of exercise on the increase in $\dot{V}O_2$max in a training program. This figure demonstrates the increasing risk of orthopedic problems due to exercise sessions that are too long, or conducted too many times per week. The probability of cardiac complications increases with exercise intensity beyond that recommended for improvements in cardiorespiratory fitness. From Powers and Howley (1990). Drawing based on M.M. Dehn and C.B.Mullins (1977), and H.K. Hellerstein and B.A. Franklin (1984).

per week (2). People who start a fitness program should plan to exercise three or four times per week. The long-recommended work-a-day-then-rest-a-day routine has been validated on the basis of improvements in CRF, low incidence of injuries, and achievement of weight-loss goals (2). Although exercising for fewer than 3 days per week can cause some CRF improvements, the participant would have to exercise at a higher **intensity**, and weight-loss goals may be difficult to achieve (71). Exercising for more than 4 days per week for previously sedentary people seems to be too much and results in more dropouts and injuries and less psychological adjustment to the exercise (21, 71).

KEY POINT. The optimum frequency of training, based on improvements in CRF and a low risk of injuries, is three to four times per week at a moderate intensity.

Duration

How many minutes of exercise should a person do per session? Figure 13.1 also shows that improvements in $\dot{V}O_2$max increase with the **duration** of the exercise session. However, the optimum duration of an exercise session depends on the intensity. The total work accomplished in a session is the most important variable determining CRF gains, once the minimal intensity threshold is achieved (3). If the goal is to accomplish 300 kcal of total work in an exercise session in which the individual is working at 10 kcal·min^{-1} (2 L O_2 per min), the session would have to be 30 min long. If the person is working at half that intensity, 5 kcal·min^{-1}, the duration would have to be twice as long. Thirty minutes of exercise can be taken as one 30-min session, two 15-min sessions, or three 10-min sessions. Figure 13.1 also shows that when the duration of moderately strenuous exercise (75% $\dot{V}O_2$max) exceeds 30 min, the risk of orthopedic injury increases (71).

KEY POINT. The duration of an exercise session should balance the exercise intensity to result in an energy expenditure of 200 to 300 kcal.

Intensity

The **training intensity** question is, "How hard does a person have to work to provide sufficient overload for the cardiovascular and respiratory systems to increase their functional capacities?" As mentioned in the introduction, gains in CRF have been shown to occur in exercise programs in which the intensity is at 50% to 85% $\dot{V}O_2$max (2). However, it is generally believed that the intensity threshold for a training effect is at the low end of this continuum for those who are sedentary, and at the high end of the scale for those who are fit (3). For most people who are cleared to participate in moderate exercise, 60% to 80% $\dot{V}O_2$max seems to be the optimum range of exercise intensities. Figure 13.1 shows that exercise at the high end of the scale has been associated with more cardiac complications (21, 41). Exercise intensity must be balanced against the duration so that the person can exercise long enough to expend 200 to 300 kcal per session, consistent with achieving CRF and body-composition goals. If the exercise intensity is too high, the person may not be able to exercise long enough to achieve the total work goal.

KEY POINTS.

- CRF is improved with exercise intensities of 50% to 85% $\dot{V}O_2$max.
- The intensity threshold for a training effect is lower for those who are sedentary
- The optimal intensity for the average individual is approximately 60% to 80% $\dot{V}O_2$max.

Metabolic load

How is exercise intensity set? The most direct way to determine the appropriate exercise intensity is to use a percentage of the measured maximal oxygen consumption. Remember, the optimum range of exercise intensities associated with improvements in CRF is 60% to 80% $\dot{V}O_2$max. The advantage of using this method for determining exercise intensity is that the method is based on the criterion test for CRF—maximal oxygen consumption. The major disadvantages are the expense and difficulty of measuring oxygen consumption for each individual and trying to suit specific fitness activities to meet the specific metabolic demand for each person.

QUESTION: A 75-kg man completes a maximal GXT, and his $\dot{V}O_2$max is 3.0 L•min^{-1}. This is equal to 15 kcal•min^{-1} (5 kcal•L^{-1} • 3 L•min^{-1}), 40 ml•kg^{-1}•min^{-1}, and 11.4 METs. At what exercise intensities should he work to be at 60% to 80% $\dot{V}O_2$max?

ANSWER:

1. 60% of 3.0 L•min^{-1} = 1.8 L•min^{-1}; 80% of 3.0 L•min^{-1} = 2.4 L•min^{-1}.
   60% of 15 kcal•min^{-1} = 9 kcal•min^{-1}; 80% of 15 kcal•min^{-1} = 12 kcal•min^{-1}.

2. 60% of 40 ml•kg^{-1}•min^{-1} = 24 ml•kg^{-1}•min^{-1}. 80% of 40 ml•kg^{-1}•min^{-1} = 32 ml•kg^{-1}•min^{-1}.
3. 60% of 11.4 METs = 6.8 METs; 80% of 11.4 METs = 9.1 METs.

He should use activities that require

1.8 to 2.4 L•min^{-1}
9 to 12 kcal•min^{-1}
24 to 32 ml•kg^{-1}•min^{-1}
6.8 to 11.4 METs

When these values are known, appropriate activities can be selected from tables listing the caloric cost of activities (see chapter 8 for these tables). However, this is a very cumbersome method to use to prescribe exercise. Prescribing on the basis of the caloric cost of the activity does not take into consideration the effect that environmental (heat, humidity, altitude, cold, pollution), dietary (adequate hydration), fatigue, and other variables have on a person's response to some absolute exercise intensity. The participant's ability to complete a workout will depend on her or his perception of the effort associated with the activity, rather than the activity itself. Fortunately, by using specific heart-rate values that are approximately equal to 60% to 80% $\dot{V}O_2$max, there is a way to prescribe exercise that takes many of these factors into consideration. These HR values are called the **target heart rate (THR)** range. How is the THR range determined?

THR—Direct Method

As was described in chapter 3, HR is linearly related to the metabolic load. In the direct method for determining THR, HR is monitored at each stage of a *maximal GXT*. HR is then plotted on a graph against the $\dot{V}O_2$ (or MET) equivalents of each stage of the test. The HFI determines the THR range by taking appropriate **percentages of the maximal $\dot{V}O_2$ (%$\dot{V}O_2$max)** at which the person should train and finds what the HR responses were at those points. Figure 13.2 shows this method being used for a subject with a functional capacity of 10.5 METs. Work rates of 60% to 80% of max METs demanded HR responses of 132 to 156 beats•min^{-1}, respectively. The HR values become the intensity guide for the subject and represent the THR range (3).

THR—Indirect Methods

In contrast to the direct method, which requires the participant to complete a maximal GXT, two indirect methods have been developed to estimate an appropriate THR.

Heart-Rate-Reserve Method. The **heart-rate reserve (HRR)** is the difference between resting and maximal

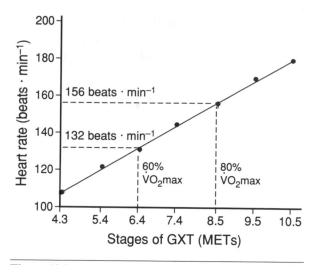

Figure 13.2 Direct method of determining the target heart rate zone when maximal aerobic power (functional capacity) is measured during a graded exercise test. Adapted from the American College of Sports Medicine (1980). *Guidelines for Graded Exercise Testing and Exercise Prescription.*

heart rate. For a maximal heart rate of 200 beats•min^{-1} and a resting HR of 60 beats•min^{-1}, the HRR is 140 beats•min^{-1}. Further, as shown in Figure 13.3, the percentage of the HRR is approximately equal to the percentage of $\dot{V}O_2$max. For example, 60% of the HRR is equal to about 60% $\dot{V}O_2$max (72). **The HRR method of determining the THR range, made popular by Karvonen, requires a few simple calculations (53):**

> 1. **Subtract resting HR from maximal HR to obtain HR reserve.**
> 2. **Take 60% and 80% of the HR reserve.**
> 3. **Add each value to resting HR to obtain the THR range.**

QUESTION: A 40-year-old male participant has a maximal HR of 175 beats•min^{-1} and a resting HR of 75 beats•min^{-1}. What is his THR range, calculated by the Karvonen (HRR) method?

ANSWER:

1. HRR = 175 beats•min^{-1} − 75 beats•min^{-1} = 100 beats•min^{-1}
2. 60% of 100 = 60 beats•min^{-1} + 75 beats•min^{-1} = 135 beats•min^{-1} for 60% $\dot{V}O_2$max
   80% of 100 = 80 beats•min^{-1} + 75 beats•min^{-1} = 155 beats•min^{-1} for 80% $\dot{V}O_2$max

The advantage of this procedure for determining exercise intensity is that the recommended THR is always between the person's resting and maximal HRs. Although the resting HR is variable and can be influ-

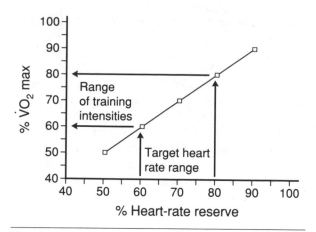

Figure 13.3 Relationship of percent heart-rate reserve and percent of maximal aerobic power ($\dot{V}O_2$max). Based on Pollock and Wilmore (1990).

enced by factors such as caffeine, lack of sleep, dehydration, emotional state, and training, this does not introduce a serious error into the calculation of the THR (37). Consider the following example.

QUESTION: The 40-year-old subject mentioned above becomes trained, and his resting HR decreases to 65 beats•min^{-1}. Because maximal HR (175 beats •min^{-1}) is not affected by training, what happens to his THR range?

ANSWER:

1. The HRR now equals 175 beats•min^{-1} − 65 beats •min^{-1} = 110 beats•min^{-1}
2. 60% of 110 beats•min^{-1} = 66 beats•min^{-1} + 65 beats•min^{-1} = 131 beats•min^{-1}
   80% of 110 beats•min^{-1} = 88 beats•min^{-1} + 65 beats•min^{-1} = 153 beats•min^{-1}.

Consequently, the change in resting HR had only a minimal effect on the THR range.

Percentage of Maximal HR Method. Another method of determining THR is to take a fixed **percentage of the maximal HR (% HRmax)**. The advantage of this method is its simplicity and the fact that it has been validated across many populations (41, 58). Figure 13.4 shows the relationship between %HRmax and %$\dot{V}O_2$max. It is clear that they are linearly related, and the %HRmax can be used to estimate the metabolic load in training programs. The usual guideline used to estimate a reasonable exercise intensity is 70% to 85% HRmax. These HR values are equal to approximately 55% and 75% $\dot{V}O_2$max, respectively, and represent a slightly more conservative intensity prescription than that generated by the HRR method (60% to 80% $\dot{V}O_2$max). The following example shows how to use the %HRmax method of calculating the THR range.

QUESTION: How can I calculate a target-heart-rate range if I don't know what the resting heart rate is?

ANSWER:

1. Consider the 40-year-old subject mentioned above who had a maximal HR of 175 beats·min^{-1}.
2. Take 70% and 85% of that value:
   70% of 175 beats·min^{-1} = 122 beats·min^{-1}
   85% of 175 beats·min^{-1} = 149 beats·min^{-1}.

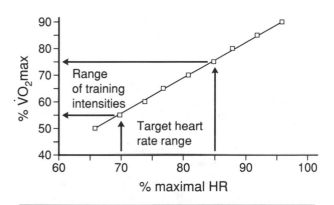

Figure 13.4 Relationship of percent of maximal heart rate and percent of maximal aerobic power ($\dot{V}O_2$max). Data from Londeree and Ames (1976).

If 55% and 75% of the HRR were used in the Karvonen calculation (to simulate the values for the %HRmax method) for this subject who had a maximal HR of 175 beats·min^{-1} and resting HR of 65 beats·min^{-1}, the THR range would be 125 to 147 beats·min^{-1}, very close to that calculated by the %HRmax method.

Remember, these two indirect methods for estimating exercise intensity provide *guidelines* to use in an exercise program, and small differences between methods are not important. They must be viewed as guidelines, because, as for any prediction equation, there is an error involved in the estimate provided by the equation. For example, two standard deviations of the estimate of %$\dot{V}O_2$max determined from HR is ±11.4% $\dot{V}O_2$max (58). Therefore, for 95% of the subjects, when we use HR to predict a work intensity that is 60% $\dot{V}O_2$max, the true intensity is somewhere between 48.6% and 71.4% $\dot{V}O_2$max! This is why we need to use other indicators of exercise intensity (see later in this chapter).

Relationship of Percentages of $\dot{V}O_2$max, HRR, and HRmax

One area of potential confusion about the calculation of exercise intensity by the two indirect methods is that the percentage value used in the HRR method is about 10% to 15% lower than the values used in the %HRmax

procedure for the same work level. Table 13.1 presents values for both of these methods versus work rates expressed as a percentage of maximal oxygen consumption.

Table 13.1   Relationship of %HRmax, %HRR, and %$\dot{V}O_2$max

%$\dot{V}O_2$max	%HRR[a,b]	%HRmax[c]
50	50	66
55	55	70
60	60	74
65	65	77
70	70	81
75	75	85
80	80	88
85	85	92
90	90	96

[a]HRR is the difference between HRmax and resting HR.
[b]From Londeree and Ames (1976).
[c]From Pollock & Wilmore (1990).

Threshold

As was mentioned above, the intensity of exercise that provides an adequate stimulus for cardiorespiratory improvement varies with activity level and age. For most of the population, the intensity **threshold** is in the following ranges:

- 60% to 80% of $\dot{V}O_2$max
- 60% to 80% of HRR
- 70% to 85% of HRmax

The threshold is toward the lower part of the range for older sedentary populations, and toward the upper part of the range for younger healthy populations. There is a need to go below this range (i.e., <60% $\dot{V}O_2$max) for diseased and extremely deconditioned people, and above it (i.e., >80% $\dot{V}O_2$max) for very active people. The middle of the range (70% $\dot{V}O_2$max, 70% HRR, or 80% HRmax) is an *average training intensity* and is appropriate for the typical apparently healthy person who wishes to be involved in a regular fitness program. Participating in activities at this intensity places a reasonable load on the cardiorespiratory system to constitute an overload, resulting in an adaptation over time.

KEY POINT.   The *average* training intensity for apparently healthy persons is

- 70% $\dot{V}O_2$max

- 70% HRR
- 80% HRmax

Earlier editions of the ACSM *Guidelines* presented a sliding-scale method to estimate the average training intensity (3). This method is quite consistent with the previous discussion. An exercise intensity equal to 60% of max METs is taken as the baseline in this calculation. The HFI adds to this a value equal to the subject's maximal METs (e.g., for a person with a functional capacity of 5 METs, the calculation is 60% + 5% = 65%). The 65% value is then multiplied by either the subject's maximal METs or the HRR to obtain the average conditioning intensity. In the previous example, the person would exercise at an average intensity of 3.3 METs (65% of 5 METs). Given that the vast majority of apparently healthy individuals have functional capacities between 8 and 12 METs, the sliding-scale method would yield a value similar to 70% max METs (i.e., 60% + 8 METs = 68% max METs, and 60% + 12 METs = 72% max METs).

Maximal Heart Rate

The indirect methods for determining exercise intensity utilize maximal HR. It is recommended that the maximal HR be measured directly (by GXT) when possible. If it cannot be measured, then any estimation must consider the effect of age on maximal HR. Maximal HR can be estimated by the formula

$$HRmax = 220 - age$$

That estimate is a potential source of error for both the HR reserve and the %HRmax methods. For example, given that one standard deviation of this estimate of maximal heart rate is about 11 beats$\cdot$min^{-1}, a 45-year-old person's true HRmax may be anywhere between 142 and 208 rather than the estimated 175. However, 68% ($\pm$ 1 SD) of the population would be between 164 and 186 beats$\cdot$min^{-1}. If the maximal HR is known (e.g., from a GXT), it should be used to determine THR, rather than using the estimate with its potential error (59). This is another reason for using caution when relying solely on the THR range as an indicator of exercise intensity. There is error both in the estimate of maximal heart rate and in the equations in which various percentages of HRmax are used to predict %$\dot{V}O_2$max (see the earlier discussion).

Use of Target Heart Rate

This concept of an intensity threshold provides the basis for the importance of regular fitness workouts. Low-intensity activity around the house, yard, and office are to be encouraged, but specific workouts above the intensity threshold are necessary to achieve optimum CRF results. At the other extreme, a person who pushes himself or herself near maximum does not have a fitness advantage, because the same results can be obtained at a moderate intensity that is above the threshold.

The THR can be used as an intensity guide for large-muscle-group, continuous, whole-body types of activities such as walking, running, swimming, rowing, cycling, skiing, and dancing. However, the same training results may not occur from activities using small-muscle-groups or resistive exercises, because these exercises elevate the HR much higher for the same metabolic load.

People who are less active and have more risk factors should use the lower part of the THR range. More active people with fewer risk factors should use the upper part of the THR range. The THR can be divided by 6 to provide the desired 10-s THR. If the person's HRmax is unknown, the estimated THR for 10 s, by age and activity level, can be found in Table 13.2. People can learn to exercise at their THRs by walking or jogging for several minutes and then stopping and *immediately* taking a 10-s HR. If the person's HR is not within the target range, then an adjustment is made in intensity (by going slower or faster to try to get within the THR range) for a few minutes and again taking a 10-s count. **Using the THR to set exercise intensity has many advantages:**

- **It has a built-in individualized progression** (i.e., as a person increases fitness, harder work has to be done to achieve the HR).
- **It takes into account environmental conditions**

Table 13.2 Estimated 10-s THR, for People Whose HRmax is Unknown

Population	Intensity %$\dot{V}O_2$max	\multicolumn{7}{c}{Age (years)}						
		20	30	40	50	60	70	80
Inactive	50	22	21	20	18	17	16	15
with several	55	23	22	21	19	18	17	16
risk factors	60	24	23	22	20	19	18	17
Normal activity	65	25	24	23	21	20	19	18
with few	70	26	25	24	22	21	20	18
risk factors	75	28	26	25	24	22	21	19
	80	29	28	26	25	23	22	20
Very active	85	30	29	27	26	24	23	21
with low	90	31	30	28	27	25	24	22
risk								

(e.g., a person decreases the intensity while working in very hot temperatures).

- **It is easily determined, learned, and monitored.**

These recommendations are appropriate for most people, but individuals differ in terms of threshold, maximal level, and other factors that influence exercise intensity. The HFI must use *subjective judgment*, based on observation of the person exercising, to determine whether the intensity should be higher or lower. If the work is so easy that the person experiences little or no increase in ventilation and is able to do the work without effort, then the intensity should be increased. At the other extreme, if a person shows signs of maximal work and is still unable to reach THR, then a lower intensity should be chosen. In this case the top part of the THR range might be above the person's true HRmax, because the 220−age formula provides only an *estimate* of the value. The HFI should not rely on the THR as the only method of judging whether or not the participant is exercising at the correct intensity. Attention should be paid to other signs and symptoms of overexertion, and Borg's *rating of perceived exertion* might be useful in this regard.

Rating of Perceived Exertion

The Borg **rating of perceived exertion (RPE)** scale that is used to indicate the subjective sensation of effort experienced by the subject during a graded exercise test (see chapter 9) can be used in prescribing exercise for the apparently healthy individual (12). Exercise perceived as "somewhat hard," a rating of 12 to 14 on the original RPE scale (4 on the new RPE scale) approximates 60% to 80% of $\dot{V}O_2$max (66, 72). In this way, if the maximal heart rate is not known, and the THR range is perceived as too low or too high, an RPE rating can provide an estimate of the overall effort experienced by the individual, and the exercise intensity can be adjusted accordingly. Further, as a participant becomes accustomed to the physical sensations experienced when exercising at the THR range, there will be less need for frequent pulse-rate measurements.

KEY POINT.   Exercise at 12 to 14 on the original RPE scale to approximate 60% to 80% $\dot{V}O_2$max.

EXERCISE RECOMMENDATIONS FOR THE UNTESTED MASSES

Certain general recommendations can be made for any person wanting to begin a fitness program. Although the HFI might wish to have each individual go through a complete testing protocol before beginning exercise, that simply is not realistic. In addition, people without known health problems who follow the general guidelines mentioned above can begin to exercise at low risk. In fact, continuing not to exercise places a person at a higher risk for CHD than if he or she begins a modest exercise program. The left side of Figure 13.5 provides a good summary of the recommendations for achieving fitness goals.

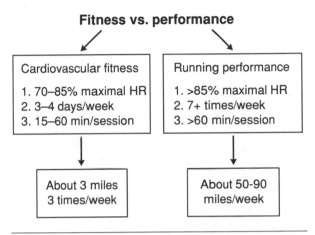

Figure 13.5   Contrast of demands of training for fitness versus performance.

EXERCISE PROGRAMMING FOR THE FIT POPULATION

Exercise recommendations written for people who possess reasonably high levels of fitness tend to be associated with less risk, and the participant requires less supervision. In fact, people in this group may focus on performance, in contrast to health maintenance, as the primary goal. A wide variety of programs, activities, races, and competitions are available to address the needs of this group.

The THR range will be calculated as described above, but these people will function at the top part of the range (≥85% of $\dot{V}O_2$max, or ≥90% of HRmax). As was mentioned earlier, a less fit person can be started at the low end of the range and experience a training effect. The more fit individual needs to work at the top end of the range to maintain a high level of fitness.

Training for competition demands more than the training intensity needed for CRF. Individuals who do interval-type training programs have peak HRs close to maximum during the intervals. The recovery period between the intervals should include some work at a lower intensity (near 40% to 50% of functional capacity) to help metabolize the lactate produced during the interval (22) and to reduce the chance of cardiovascular complications that can occur when a person comes to a complete rest at the end of a strenuous exercise bout (72).

For people who participate in sports that are intermittent in nature but that still require high levels of aerobic fitness for success, a running/jogging program is a good way to maintain general conditioning when not playing the activity. However, given the specificity of training, there is no substitute for the real activity when conditioning for a sport.

As Figure 13.5 shows, people interested in performance who work at the top end of the THR range, exercise 5 to 7 times per week, and for longer than 30 min each exercise session are doing much more than the person interested in fitness, and it should be no surprise that they tend to experience more injuries. When this is coupled with the inherent risks associated with competitive activities, a need exists to build in alternative activities that can be done when participation in the primary activity is not possible. This reduces the chance of becoming detrained when injuries do occur.

EXERCISE PRESCRIPTIONS USING COMPLETE GXT RESULTS

In the previous section, the exercise recommendation was made on the basis of little or no specific information about the person involved. In many adult fitness programs, potential participants have had a general medical exam or a GXT with appropriate monitoring of the HR, BP, and possibly ECG responses. Unfortu-

nately, this information is sometimes not used in designing the exercise program; instead, the measured maximal HR is used in the THR formulas, and the rest of the data are ignored. **This section outlines the steps that should be followed when making the exercise recommendation based on information about the person's functional capacity and the cardiovascular responses to graded exercise.** The HFI is not directly involved in the clinical evaluation of a GXT, but an understanding of the steps and the procedures used to make clinical judgments clearly enhances communication between the HFI and the Program Director, Exercise Specialist, and medical doctor. The following sections on Steps in GXT Analysis and Designing an Exercise Program were written with this intent. A series of case studies follows, representing submaximal and maximal GXT responses of individuals ranging from the apparently healthy to those people with identified disease.

PROGRAM SELECTION

Exercise program options include exercising alone, in small groups, in fitness clubs, and in clinically oriented settings. The HFI must consider a variety of factors before recommending participation in a supervised or unsupervised program.

Supervised Program

The risk factors, the response to the GXT, the health and activity history, and personal preference influence

---

Steps in GXT Analysis for Exercise Prescription

1. Analyze the person's history and list the known risk factors for CHD; also, identify those factors that might have a direct bearing on the exercise program, such as orthopedic problems, previous physical activity, current interests, and so forth.
2. Determine if the functional capacity is a true maximum or if it is sign- or symptom-limited. Express the functional capacity in METs, and record the highest HR and RPE achieved without significant signs or symptoms.
3. If it was monitored, itemize the person's ECG changes as indicated by the physician.
4. Examine the HR and BP responses to see if they are normal.
5. List the symptoms reported at each stage
6. List the reasons why the test was stopped (e.g., ECG changes, falling systolic pressure, dizziness).

Steps in Designing an Exercise Program on the Basis of a GXT

1. Based on the overall response to the GXT, make a decision to either refer for additional medical care or initiate an exercise program.
2. Identify the THR range and approximate MET intensities of selected activities needed to be within that THR range.
3. Specify the frequency and duration of activity needed to meet the goals of increased cardiorespiratory fitness and weight loss.
4. Recommend that the person participate in either a supervised or unsupervised program, be monitored or unmonitored, do group or individual activities, and so forth.
5. Select a variety of activities at the appropriate MET level that allow the person to achieve THR. Consider environmental factors, medication, and any physical limitations of the participant when making this recommendation.

---

the type of program in which an individual should participate. Generally, the higher the risk, the more important it is that the person participate in a supervised program. People at high risk for CHD and those who have diseases such as diabetes, hypertension, asthma, CHD, and so on should be encouraged to participate under supervision, at least at the beginning of an exercise program. The personnel in the supervised program are trained to provide the necessary instruction in the appropriate activities, to help monitor the participant's response to the activity, and to administer appropriate first aid or emergency care. Supervised programs run the continuum from those conducted within a hospital for patients with CHD and other diseases, to programs conducted in fitness clubs for people at low risk for CHD. In general, as a person moves along the continuum from "in-patient" to "out-patient," less formal monitoring is required. In addition, the background and training of the personnel tend to vary. The exercise programs aimed at maintaining the fitness level of the CHD patients who went through a hospital-based program have medical personnel and emergency equipment appropriate for the population being served. Supervised fitness programs for the apparently healthy have an HFI who can focus more on the appropriate exercise, diet, and other lifestyle behaviors needed to increase positive health.

The supervised program offers a socially supportive environment for individuals to become and stay active. This is important, given the difficulty of changing lifestyle behaviors. The group program allows for more variety in the types of activities to be used (games) and reduces the chance of boredom. To be effective in the long run, the program should try to wean the partici-

pants from the group in a way that encourages them to maintain their activity patterns when they are no longer in the program.

Unsupervised Program

In spite of the risks just described, the vast majority of people at risk from or possessing CHD participate in unsupervised exercise programs. Reasons for this include the limited number of supervised programs, the level of interest of the participant and physician in such programs, and the financial resources required to bring them about.

Participation in an unsupervised exercise program requires clear communication of correct information from the HFI or physician about how to begin and maintain the exercise program. The emphasis in beginning an unsupervised exercise program is on low intensity, at or below 60% functional capacity (70% HRmax), because the threshold for a training effect is lower in deconditioned people. The goal is to increase the duration of the activity, with exercise frequency approaching every day. This reduces the chance of muscular, skeletal, or cardiovascular problems caused by the exercise intensity, and increases muscle function with the expenditure of a relatively large number of calories. Quite importantly, the regularity of the exercise program encourages a habit. The outcome of such programs results in the individual being able to conduct her or his daily affairs with more comfort and sets the stage for people who would like to exercise at higher levels.

In an unsupervised exercise program, the person

needs to be provided with explicit information about the intensity (THR), duration, and frequency of exercise so that no doubt remains about what should be done. For example, the exercise recommendation might read, "Walk 1 mi in 30 min each day for 2 weeks. Monitor and record your heart rate." The person has to receive information about how to take the pulse rate and be encouraged to follow through on the recording.

UPDATING THE EXERCISE PROGRAM

During participation in an endurance-training program, an individual's capacity for work increases. The best sign of this is that the "regular" exercise is no longer sufficient to reach THR. This is clear evidence that the person is adapting to the exercise. Taking the HR during a regular activity session provides a sound basis for upgrading the intensity or duration of the exercise session.

The exercise program, including the THR, should be periodically updated. The need to update is greater, the lower the initial level of fitness and the higher the number of risk factors. An individual who has a low functional capacity because of heart disease, orthopedic limitations, or chronic inactivity, which might include prolonged bed rest, has difficulty reaching a true maximum on a first treadmill test, and she or he experiences the greatest improvements in the shortest period of time in a fitness program. This individual benefits from frequent retesting because the test allows progress (or the lack of) to be monitored, and it may give new information that influences the exercise prescription. If the person has had a change in medication that influences the HR response to exercise, a special need exists for a reevaluation of the exercise program.

For people who reach a true maximum in the first test, actual THR will change little during a fitness program, because the maximal heart rate is affected very little by regular endurance exercise. However, they still benefit from an evaluation of the overall exercise program on a regular basis, given that their activity interests may change or they may develop orthopedic problems that did not exist before. The reevaluation allows the HFI to probe for information that may enable her or him to refer the person for treatment at a time when treatment will do the most good. Lastly, such contact increases the chance that the person will stay involved in an activity program—which is the most important factor in maintaining aerobic fitness.

At the end of this chapter, we include a variety of case studies on individuals varying in age, fitness, disease, and orthopedic limitations. The case studies have been selected to give you an idea of the variety of responses to a GXT and how the exercise recommendations would be made.

SPECIAL CONSIDERATIONS IN MAKING EXERCISE RECOMMENDATIONS

The HFI must be knowledgeable about a wide variety of common conditions of circumstances that can affect an exercise prescription, or a participant's response to exercise might be compromised. This section examines the issues that must be addressed in planning exercise programs for those with orthopedic limitations and certain diseases, the elderly, and the pregnant. Several of these summaries have been adapted from Powers and Howley's *Exercise Physiology* (74).

Orthopedic Limitations

Orthopedic limitations (e.g., ankle, knee, or hip pain when walking or jogging) must be considered on a case-by-case basis when designing an exercise program. The exercise recommendation still indicates the THR range, but the participant should be advised to stay at the low end of the THR range while the problem exists. The emphasis should be on light work interspersed with rest periods. The type of activity recommended is somewhat dependent on the interests and abilities of the participant; however, weight-supported activities (e.g., cycle ergometer, rowing) and aquatic activities tend to reduce the chance of aggravating the problem. Chapter 16 outlines procedures to follow in caring for chronic injuries. The participant should be informed of proper procedures for warm-up, cool-down, and immediate care of the affected part following an activity session.

Diabetes

Diabetes is a disease characterized by a chronically elevated blood glucose concentration. It is the third largest cause of death by disease in the United States, with more than 12 million having the disease. Diabetes causes blindness, kidney disease, heart disease, stroke, and peripheral vascular disease that can lead to the amputation of a leg or foot (4). Table 13.3 indicates that diabetics are classified into two groups on the basis of whether the diabetes is caused by a lack of **insulin (Type I diabetes)** or by a resistance to insulin (**Type II diabetes**). Type I, insulin-dependent diabetes, occurs primarily in young persons, with the rapid development of signs or symptoms, including (4)

- frequent urination,
- unusual thirst,
- extreme hunger,
- rapid weight loss,
- weakness and fatigue,
- irritability,
- nausea, and
- vomiting.

To counter the pancreas's lack of natural insulin, Type I diabetics are dependent on injected insulin to maintain the blood glucose concentration within normal limits.

Table 13.3   Summary of the Differences Between Type I and Type II Diabetes

Characteristics	Type I insulin dependent	Type II non–insulin dependent
Another name	Juvenile-onset	Adult-onset
Proportion of all diabetics	~10%	~90%
Age at onset	< 20	> 40
Development of disease	Rapid	Slow
Family history	Uncommon	Common
Insulin required	Always	Common, but not always
Pancreatic insulin	None, or very little	Normal or higher
Ketoacidosis	Common	Rare
Body fatness	Normal/lean	Generally obese

Note. From Berg (1986) and Cantu (1982).

About 90% of all diabetics have Type II, non–insulin dependent diabetes, which occurs later in life than Type I diabetes and is linked to obesity (8). The Type II diabetic displays a resistance to insulin, which is usually available in adequate amounts. However, some may require injectable insulin or an oral medication that stimulates the pancreas to produce additional insulin. The primary treatment of Type II diabetics includes diet and exercise to reduce body weight and help control blood glucose. Before describing the role that exercise plays in the treatment of diabetes, let's review the means by which the blood glucose concentration is regulated at rest and during exercise.

Control of Blood Glucose: Rest and Exercise

Blood glucose is the primary fuel for the brain, and the concentration of blood glucose is maintained within close limits to assure a constant supply. If the concentration of blood glucose is falling, the pancreas releases the hormone **glucagon** to stimulate the liver to release glucose and bring the blood level back to normal. If the blood glucose concentration is too high (e.g., following a meal), the pancreas releases insulin, which, when bound to receptors at various tissues, allows glucose to be taken up at a faster rate to be used as a fuel or stored for later use. The blood glucose concentration then returns to normal.

KEY POINTS.

- Insulin facilitates the removal of glucose from the blood to lower the blood glucose concentration.
- Glucagon mobilizes glucose from the liver to elevate the blood glucose concentration.

During exercise, additional glucose must be released from the liver to replace that taken up by muscle, which has been using it as a fuel for energy production. To facilitate this, the plasma insulin level decreases during exercise and the glucagon level increases. These changes favor the mobilization of glucose from the liver. What must be noted is that *during and following* exercise, the muscles have an increased *sensitivity* to the avilable insulin; that is, for any insulin level, blood glucose is taken into the muscle faster during and following exercise. This could be due to changes in the way receptors bind insulin or in the events that occur after insulin is bound to the receptor (96). This increased sensitivity is what makes exercise useful in the treatment of diabetes, in that it reduces the need for insulin and helps to lower the blood glucose concentration. However, there is more to the story.

Exercise and Insulin

Knowing that exercise increases the rate at which glucose leaves the blood, one can see that it can be a useful part of the treatment to maintain blood glucose control, because less insulin is required. However, this depends on whether or not the diabetic's blood glucose is "under control." Having it under control means that *prior to exercise* the diabetic has eaten the proper quantity of carbohydrates and injected the proper amount of insulin to keep the blood glucose concentration close to normal values. The Type I diabetic who is in control maintains normal values *during exercise* because the liver production of glucose is balanced by the increased uptake by the muscles. On the other hand, too little or too much insulin injected before exercise can cause problems. The diabetic with an inadequate level of insulin experiences only a small increase in glucose utilization by muscle but has the "normal" increase in glucose release from liver; this causes a **hyperglycemia**, an elevation of the plasma glucose. When an insulin-dependent diabetic starts exercise with too much insulin, blood glucose is used by muscle faster than it is released from the liver; this causes a very dangerous condition called **hypoglycemia**, a low blood-glucose concentration (80). This information is important in understanding the use of exercise as part of a program to help diabetics control the blood glucose concentration. Type I diabetics are primarily the ones confronted with the problem of a variable insulin level, because they must inject the insulin; Type II diabetics tend to have normal or slightly elevated insulin levels. Because of this we will discuss each type separately.

KEY POINTS.

- Exercise + adequate insulin = control
- Exercise + inadequate insulin = hyperglycemia
- Exercise + too much insulin = hypoglycemia

Type I Diabetes

For many years the treatment for Type I diabetics was based on the triad of insulin, diet, and exercise (9). However, consider the difficulty a sedentary Type I diabetic has at the start of an exercise program. Dietary carbohydrate and injected insulin would not only have to achieve a balance between each other, they would have to be balanced against an exercise session whose intensity and duration would demand a variable amount of the body's carbohydrate store. Given this problem, and the success that modern intensified insulin therapies have in maintaining blood glucose control, some feel that exercise should no longer be regarded as a necessary part of the treatment to achieve control *at rest* (9, 80). On the other hand, these same authorities recognize the fact that many Type I diabetics believe that participating in exercise and sports is a normal part of life, and that they must deal with the complications brought on by exercise. What steps should the Type I diabetic follow in starting an exercise program?

The Type I diabetic should have a careful medical exam before starting an exercise program, because strenuous exercise can aggravate any retina, kidney, or peripheral nerve problems that are already present. The exam might include a graded diagnostic exercise test, if the person is over 30 years of age or has had diabetes for 10 years or more. In addition, peripheral nerve damage may block signals coming from the foot, so that serious damage may occur before it is perceived. The diabetic should wear supportive shoes during exercise, and the exercise should not aggravate existing problems

(29). The primary concern for the Type I diabetic who is starting an exercise program is that blood glucose should already be adequately controlled. The emphasis is on educating the diabetic about the potential for blood glucose problems during *and* after exercise, and the need for self-management or self-monitoring of blood glucose.

KEY POINTS.

- Type I diabetics should have a thorough medical exam, possibly including a stress test, before starting the exercise program.
- Educate the diabetic about control and self-monitoring of blood glucose.

Studies have shown that, for diabetics in control, a reduction in insulin of 30% to 50% before exercise, or the ingestion of 15 g of glucose before exercise and 15 to 30 g following exercise, prevents hypoglycemia for a 45-min exercise session at 55% $\dot{V}O_2$max. For more prolonged exercise, a greater reduction in insulin or a greater intake of carbohydrate is needed to prevent hypoglycemia (96).

Another recommendation aimed at reducing the chance of hypoglycemia during exercise is to vary the site of injection away from the muscles involved in the exercise. If insulin is injected into one of the active limbs prior to exercise, the higher muscle blood-flow during exercise might increase the movement of insulin from the site of injection into the blood and increase the chance of hypoglycemia (96). Recently, however, others have suggested that to maintain control during exercise, attention should be focused on reducing the amount of insulin injected and increasing the quantity of carbohydrates ingested, rather than on varying the site of injection (9).

It is difficult to provide a standard set of guidelines to follow, because of the variation in the severity of the disease within the diabetic population (96), but the following suggestions provide an approach to prevent hypoglycemia during exercise (29):

- For a leisurely walk, there is no need to increase carbohydrate intake if blood glucose is >100 mg• dl^{-1} (5.6 mM).
- For moderate activity with blood glucose of 100 to 180 mg•dl^{-1} (5.6 to 10 mM), 10 to 15 g of carbohydrate is taken before exercise. If blood glucose is >180 (10mM) and <300 mg•dl^{-1} (16.6 mM), no additional carbohydrate is needed. If >300 mg•dl^{-1}, exercise is not recommended until blood glucose is brought under control.
- For strenuous exercise of 1 to 2 hr with blood

glucose in the normal range, consumption of 25 to 50 g of carbohydrate is recommended before exercise.

- For prolonged exercise, including day-long hikes, insulin intake is decreased, even though carbohydrate intake is increased. The decrease can be from 20% to 75% of the normal dose (8).
- Additional carbohydrate should be consumed *during recovery* from exercise. Interestingly, hypoglycemia might occur following exercise if this is not done, because dietary carbohydrate is also being used to replace the depleted muscle glycogen store.

In addition, the Type I diabetic should increase fluid intake, carry a readily available form of carbohydrate and adequate identification, and follow the "buddy system" by exercising with someone who can help in an emergency.

KEY POINT. To maintain control during exercise, the Type I diabetic

- decreases the dose of insulin injected, and/or
- increases the consumption of carbohydrate.

Type II Diabetes

Type II diabetes occurs later in life (>40 years), and patients generally have a variety of CHD risk factors in addition to glucose intolerance: hypertension, hyperlipidemia, and obesity (9, 96). As a result, these individuals need a thorough physical exam before starting an exercise program. However, in contrast to the Type I diabetic's potential trouble with trying to maintain control at the start of an exercise program, exercise is a primary recommendation for the Type II diabetic to help deal with the obesity that is usually present, as well as to help control blood glucose. The combination of exercise and diet may decrease or eliminate the need for insulin or the oral medication taken to stimulate insulin secretion (20). With Type II diabetics representing about 90% of the whole population of diabetics, it is not surprising to find such individuals in adult fitness programs. It is important that clear communication exists between the participant and the exercise leader, to reduce the chance of a "surprise" hypoglycemic response. Even though Type II diabetics do not experience the same fluctuations in blood glucose during exercise as do Type I diabetics, Type II diabetics taking insulin or oral medication may have to reduce the dosage to maintain their glucose concentration, as does the Type I diabetic (80). As with the recommendations for the Type I diabetic, clear identification and a readily

available source of carbohydrate should be carried along during an exercise session. In addition, it is reasonable to recommend that the buddy system be followed.

For any overweight, deconditioned individual, it is better to do too little than to do too much at the start of an exercise program. In addition, for the Type II diabetic it may be more important to do daily activity to maintain the increased insulin sensitivity effect, which is short-lived (96). By starting with light activity and gradually increasing the duration, diabetics can exercise each day. Daily activity provides an opportunity to learn how to control blood glucose while minimizing the chance of a hypoglycemic response. In addition, a habit of exercise may develop that is crucial if one is to realize long-term improvement in glucose tolerance.

There are specific dietary guidelines for the diabetic, not only for dealing with the problem of maintaining blood glucose, but also for reducing the risk of heart disease, which is much greater for the diabetic. **The American Diabetes Association (5) recommends that**

- **caloric intake should be adjusted to achieve and maintain ideal weight,**
- **carbohydrates should approach 55% to 60% of caloric intake,**
- **fiber should be increased and refined carbohydrates decreased,**
- **one should consume only 0.8 g protein per kilogram of body weight,**
- **fat should be limited to 30% of caloric intake, with saturated fats being ≤10%,**
- **sodium intake should be limited to 1 g per 1,000 calories, not to exceed 3 g per day, and**
- **alcohol should be used only in moderation.**

These recommendations should sound familiar. They are the same recommendations presented in chapter 6 for all of us to reduce the chance of developing CHD. They are doubly important for the diabetic, who has a much higher risk of heart disease. The combination of the recommended diet and regular exercise not only improves the diabetic's chance of maintaining control over blood glucose, it lowers body fat and weight, increases HDL cholesterol and $\dot{V}O_2$max, and improves self concept (8, 96). These changes will reduce the overall risk associated with CHD (80).

Asthma

Asthma is a respiratory problem characterized by labored breathing (dyspnea) and a shortness of breath accompanied by a wheezing sound. It is due to a spasmodic contraction of the smooth muscle around the bronchi, a swelling of the mucosal cells lining the bronchi, and an excessive secretion of mucous. Asthma attacks can be initiated by allergic reactions, exercise, aspirin, dust, pollutants, and emotions (64). Before presenting the guidelines to follow in providing recommendations for exercise, we need to outline the causes of and ways to prevent an asthma attack.

Causes

A variety of factors, such as dust, chemicals, antibodies, and exercise, cause asthma attacks by increasing the calcium level in the **mast cells** lining the bronchial tubes, resulting in a release of chemical mediators such as histamine. These chemical mediators cause

- bronchoconstriction, leading to a narrowing of the airway, and
- an inflammation (swelling) of the bronchial tubes.

Most people do not experience an asthma attack on exposure to the above factors; a "sensitivity" or hyperirritability of the respiraotry tract is a necessary prerequisite to initiate the asthma attack (64).

Prevention and Relief of Asthma

A variety of drugs and procedures are used to either prevent the asthma attack or provide relief when one occurs. For those with allergies, simple avoidance of the allergen prevents the attack. If exposure is unavoidable, immunotherapy helps the person become less sensitive to the allergen. Drugs are now available to alter the activity of the mast cells, which is where the asthma attack begins, as well as relax the bronchiolar smooth muscle that decreases the airway diameter. These include

- *cromolyn sodium*, which reduces chemical mediator release from the mast cells;
- *beta-receptor agonists* (ß₂-agonists), epinephrine-like drugs that cause a relaxation of bronchiolar smooth muscle as well as a decrease in chemical mediator release by stimulating ß-adrenergic receptors; and
- *theophylline*, a caffeine-like compound that relaxes bronchiolar smooth muscle.

The net result of using these drugs is that both the inflammation response and the constriction of the bronchiolar smooth muscle are blocked. With that background, let's discuss exercise-induced asthma.

Exercise-Induced Asthma

A form of asthma of particular interest to the HFI is **exercise-induced asthma (EIA)**. The attack is initiated by exercise and can occur 5 to 15 min (early phase) or 4 to 6 hr (late phase) following exercise. Approximately 80% of asthmatics experience EIA, versus only 3% to 4% of the nonallergic population (95). Interestingly, 67 members (11%) of the 1984 Olympic team had EIA, and 41 of them (61%) won Olympic medals (56, 95), showing that EIA can be controlled.

The following have been identified as causes of EIA: cold air, hypocapnia (low PCO_2), respiratory alkalosis, and specific intensities and durations of exercise. Scientists are now studying the role that *cooling and drying* of the respiratory tract have on the initiation of EIA. When large volumes of dry air are breathed during the exercise session, moisture is evaporated from the surface of the airways, which becomes cooled (24, 87). When dry air removes water from the surface of the mast cells, an increase in osmolarity occurs, and this triggers the influx of calcium that leads to the increased release of chemical mediators and the narrowing of the airways (24, 55, 56, 87). This proposed mechanism has received support from observations showing that EIA can be prevented by breathing warm, humidified air.

The chance that an exercise-induced bronchospasm will occur is related to the

- type of exercise done,
- time since the previous bout of exercise,
- interval since medication was taken, and
- temperature and humidity of the inspired air.

It has been observed that running causes more attacks than cycling or walking, which cause more than swimming (87). Exercise prescriptions should be guided by observations that (24, 56, 87)

- attacks are associated with strenuous, long-duration exercise, and
- exercising within 60 min of a previous EIA attack reduces subsequent bronchospasms.

What do these observations suggest to the HFI who is prescribing exercise for someone with EIA?

The asthmatic should follow a medication plan to *prevent* the occurrence of an EIA attack. This is done by the physician working with the individual to fine-tune the medications to prevent the problem without interfering with the person's response to exercise. The HFI should structure the exercise session to include a conventional warm-up and mild to moderate activity organized into 5-min segments. Swimming is better than other types of exercise, because the air above the water tends to be warmer and contain more moisture. A scarf or face mask can be used to help trap moisture when exercising outdoors in cold weather. The participant should carry an inhaler with a ß₂-agonist and use it at the first sign of wheezing (32, 55, 69). As for the diabetic, the buddy system is a good plan to follow in case a major attack occurs.

KEY POINTS.   Persons with asthma who engage in exercise should

- pretreat with medication,
- warm up and use 5-min intermittent bouts of light to moderate activity,
- carry a ß$_2$-agonist, and
- follow the buddy system.

Obesity

Obesity is linked to a variety of CHD risk factors such as glucose intolerance (Type II diabetes), hypertension, and hyperlipidemia, as well as to CHD itself (51, 77, 81). Chapter 7 provided an introduction to obesity and the role that diet and exercise programs play in the achievement of weight-loss goals. Does research, though, support the idea that exercise is an effective part of an obesity treatment?

Studies on the effect of exercise in the treatment of obesity show inconsistent results (13), due to a variety of factors, including

- length of study—short-duration studies do not allow for sufficient caloric expenditure through added exercise to distinguish itself from a diet-only group;
- sample size—larger samples are needed to account for differences in the ways different types of obese individuals respond to exercise;
- type of obesity—those with **hypertrophic** (large fat-cell size) **obesity** respond better to exercise than those with hyperplastic (high fat-cell number) obesity;
- caloric expenditure—the exercise intensity and duration must result in the expenditure of enough calories for an exercise effect to show, compared to a diet-alone treatment; and
- dropout rate—conclusions drawn from a small number remaining at the end of a study can provide misleading results.

As a result of these confounding variables, it is difficult to make clear statements about the importance of exercise and diet, compared to diet alone, in achieving *weight loss* (13, 30). However, all authorities emphasize the importance of exercise in the treatment of obesity (13, 14, 30). Why the apparent conflict in these conclusions?

The following reasons have been offered for using a combination of diet and exercise, rather than diet alone, in treating obesity; some reasons have stronger support than others (9, 13, 14, 30, 34, 96). **Diet + exercise**

- **maintains lean body mass and resting metabolic rate,**
- **improves glucose tolerance,**
- **decreases blood pressure,**
- **improves lipid profile (e.g., elevates HDL cholesterol),**
- **improves self-esteem, and**
- **maintains weight loss in the long run.**

Whether exercise accomplishes a faster rate of weight loss than diet alone is not the important issue. The obese person's overall risk of CHD is lower, and the probability of keeping the weight off is greater, when exercise is part of the treatment. How, then, does one prescribe exercise for the obese?

As for any other risk factor, the level of risk is directly related to the magnitude of the problem, and recommendations for exercise vary accordingly. Those who are borderline obese (19% to 24% fat for males and 26% to 31% for females) differ in the probability of risk factors from those with moderate obesity (25% to 30% fat for males, and 32% to 37% fat for females) and massive obesity (>30% fat for males and >37% fat for females). It would be appropriate for obese individuals to have medical exams to determine whether they have glucose intolerance, hypertension, hyperlipidemia, or other risk factors, because medication might be required to deal with the problems.

The emphasis in the exercise prescription is on low-intensity activities that can be done anywhere, at any time, alone or with others, and with a low risk of musculoskeletal injury; this will maximize the chance of adhering to the exercise program (13, 17). Walking fits these requirements, and a typical walking program is presented in chapter 14. The HFI should be careful to set initial goals (e.g., to walk 400 m) that clearly can be achieved. These goals will obviously be set on a case-by-case basis and should be adjusted over time to maintain progress and interest. The pace should be self-selected, and it will vary from very slow (less than 1 mi•hr^{-1}) to moderate (3+ mi•hr^{-1}) speeds, depending on the degree of obesity (17). The net caloric cost of the walk can be estimated from tables found in chapter 8.

Some obese individuals will have a difficult time starting an exercise program, and working on a one-on-one basis or in a small-group setting may be helpful. The HFI should educate the obese participants about the possibility that they will experience heat-related disorders when they are walking outdoors in the heat and humidity (see later). Further, special attention should be paid to those on medication for hypertension and Type II diabetes, to avoid hypotensive and hypoglycemic responses, respectively.

Other activities that would reduce the chance of musculoskeletal problems include those in which body weight is supported (e.g., swimming, cycling, and rowing). With regard to swimming, time in the water should not be the variable used to estimate energy expenditure. The HFI should set distance goals, whether for swimming laps or for walking across the width of the shallow end of the pool. Water aerobic programs, which would include a wide variety of activities in addition to moving through the water, would be suitable, depending on interest. The newer stationary cycles and rowing machines that offer a caloric-expenditure summary for each exercise session might prove useful in setting goals and possibly in motivating the participant to achieve those goals. Remember, the emphasis is on low-intensity activities that can be done with success and lead to a lifelong habit. The guideline we presented earlier fits here: the person should be able to walk 4 mi at a brisk pace before becoming involved in more strenuous activities.

Hypertension

The risk of coronary heart disease increases with increases in either diastolic or systolic blood pressure (50). **Hypertension** is an enormous problem, with 30 million people classified as hypertensive if a cutoff of 160/95 is used, and 60 million if 140/90 is used (52). Typically hypertension is treated with drugs, but this form of treatment has its own risks, both medically and personally. Studies indicate that death rates are higher for hypertensives with ECG abnormalities who were treated with diuretic medications than for those treated with other medications. Further, simply classifying a person as a "patient" due to the presence of hypertension increases symptoms of other diseases and can actually alter a person's lifestyle (52). Consequently, although there is little disagreement that those with blood pressures of >160/>105 should be treated with medication, many believe that for those with mild hypertension, 140-160/90-104, nonpharmacological interventions should be considered (34, 50, 52, 99).

The presence of mild hypertension must be verified by several independent measurements taken days apart (99). If mild hypertension is identified, the person needs a complete physical exam to determine whether other risk factors are present that would increase the overall risk of CHD. Although a decision might be made to medicate someone with multiple risk factors (smoking, high cholesterol, obesity, etc.), Kannel (50) pointed out that getting a hypertensive patient to quit

smoking confers more immediate benefit against CHD risk than any known medication. It should be no surprise that dietary, weight-control, and exercise recommendations would be included in any nonpharmacological treatment package (6, 7, 34, 99).

Dietary change includes a reduction in sodium intake that has been shown to independently reduce systolic and diastolic blood pressures by approximately 5 and 3 mmHg, respectively (6, 34, 52). Obesity is linked to hypertension, and a review of various studies indicated that a loss of 9.8 kg resulted in a decrease in systolic and diastolic pressures of 15 and 10 mmHg, respectively (34, 52). Finally, participation in an endurance-exercise program has been shown to cause decreases in systolic and diastolic pressures of 10 mmHg (34, 52).

Hagberg's (34) review of the use of exercise in the treatment of hypertension indicates that low-intensity exercise, at 40% to 60% of $\dot{V}O_2max$, may be the best choice. Further, for those with higher blood pressures who are taking medication, such an exercise program can also be used along with other lifestyle changes in diet, smoking, and body weight to lower blood pressure. In these cases, blood pressure should be checked frequently to allow medications to be reduced as needed. Further, the gradual establishment of appropriate diet and exercise habits would improve the chance that a person will maintain normal blood pressure once it has been normalized. If a person is being treated with beta-adrenergic blocking drugs, the ordinary calculation of the THR using the 220−age formula to estimate the maximal HR should not be used, because beta-blocking drugs lower the maximal HR (see chapter 15). Using an RPE rating of 10 to 12 on the original scale (2 on the new scale) to establish light exercise (40% to 60% of $\dot{V}O_2max$) is a reasonable alternative (2).

KEY POINTS.

- Nonpharmacological treatment of mild hypertension (140–160/90–104) includes changes in diet (including sodium intake), smoking, body fatness, and exercise.
- Light exercise (at 40% to 60% of $\dot{V}O_2max$; 10 to 12 on the original RPE scale) is recommended.
- The patient's blood pressure should be evaluated regularly to alter medication, if necessary.

Seizure Susceptibility

Individuals with controlled seizure disorders (e.g., epilepsy) are able and encouraged to lead normally active lives. In many cases, the individual is aware of the unique circumstances that might trigger a seizure and can avoid the situation. The HFI should be aware of any member of an exercise group that has a seizure disorder. Recommendations include participation in a variety of activities with little or no restriction. Suggestions for safety include exercising with another person who can physically support and aid the individual in case of a seizure in potentially dangerous situations, such as jogging on a road or swimming.

Chronic Obstructive Pulmonary Disease

Chronic obstructive pulmonary diseases (COPDs) cause a reduction in airflow that can dramatically affect one's ability to perform daily activities. These diseases include chronic bronchitis, emphysema, and bronchial asthma, alone or in combination. Each disease causes an obstruction to airflow, but the underlying reason is different for each (10, 49, 86):

- Bronchial asthma—bronchial smooth-muscle contraction and increased airway reactivity
- Chronic bronchitis—persistent production of sputum due to a thickened bronchial wall with excess secretions
- Emphysema—loss of elastic recoil of alveoli and bronchioles and enlargement of those pulmonary structures

COPD is considerably different from the controlled asthmatic condition mentioned above. Asthma is reversible; chronic bronchitis and emphysema are not. The patient with developing COPD perceives an inability to do normal activities without experiencing dyspnea, but tragically, by the time this occurs the disease is already well advanced (10).

Testing and Evaluation

A patient with COPD receives a thorough medical examination as well as a variety of tests to help classify the degree of disability associated with the disease. One of the most important pulmonary function tests is the FEV_1, a measure of the maximum volume of air that can be moved in one second. Unfortunately, due to the progressive nature of this disease, by the time the person is aware of symptoms, the FEV_1 is already less than 60% of predicted (49). Exercise tests are also used in the assessment of those with COPD. The tests may be the standard graded exercise test (GXT) or a simple 6- or 12-min walk on a flat surface. During the GXT, cardiovascular, pulmonary, metabolic, and power-output measurements are obtained and used to evaluate the severity of disability on a 4-point scale. Table 13.4 presents the standards for each of the four grades of disability (49).

Treatment

COPD is characterized by a gradual decrease in the ability to exhale, and because of the narrowed airways, a "wheezing" sound is made. The person with COPD experiences a decreased capacity for work, which may influence employment, but he or she may also experience an increase in psychological problems, such as anxiety regarding the simple act of breathing and depression related to a loss of sense of self-worth (10, 49, 65).

Given the complex problems associated with this disease, it should be no surprise that treatment of COPD includes more than simple medication and O_2 inhalation therapy. A typical COPD rehabilitation program has

Table 13.4 Guide to Grading Disability (Based on 40-Year-Old Man)

Grade	Cause of dyspnea	FEV_1 (%pred)	Max $\dot{V}O_2$ ($ml \cdot min^{-1} \cdot kg^{-1}$)	Exercise Max V_E ($L \cdot min^{-1}$)	Blood gases
1	Fast walking and stair climbing	> 60	> 25	Not limiting	Normal PCO_2, S_aO_2
2	Walking at normal pace	< 60	< 25	> 50	Normal P_aCO_2; S_aO_2 above 90% at rest and with exercise
3	Slow walking	< 40	< 15	< 50	Normal P_aCO_2; S_aO_2 below 90% with exercise
4	Walking limited to less than 1 block	< 40	< 7	< 30	Elevated P_aCO_2; S_aO_2 below 90% at rest and with exercise

Note. From "Chronic Obstructive Respiratory Disorders" by N.L. Jones, L.B. Berman, P.D. Bartkiewicz, and N.B. Oldridge. In *Exercise Testing and Exercise Prescription for Special Cases* (p. 181) by J.S. Skinner (Ed.), 1987, Philadelphia: Lea & Febiger. Copyright 1987 by Lea & Febiger. Reprinted by permission.

the patient's self-care as its goal, and to achieve that goal, physicians, nurses, respiratory therapists, psychologists, exercise specialists, and clergy are recruited to deal with the various manifestations of the disease process (65, 92). The COPD patient receives education about the different ways to deal with the disease, including breathing exercise, ways to approach the activities of daily living at home, and how to handle work-related problems. The latter can be so affected that new on-the-job responsibilities may have to be assigned, or if the person cannot meet the requirements, retirement may be the only outcome. To help deal with these problems, counseling by psychologists and clergy may be needed for patient and family. The extent of these problems is directly related to the severity of the disease. Those with minimal disease may require the help of only a few of these professionals, while others with severe disease may require the assistance of all. It is therefore important to understand that the rehabilitation program is very individualized (65).

The exercise component of the rehabilitation program varies with the level of disability. Those with Grade 1 disability (see Table 13.4) can follow the normal exercise prescription process. However, additional guidelines are needed for those with Grade 2 or Grade 3 disability. Those with Grade 2 disability are limited to exercises that demand only 60% to 80% of ventilatory capacity and a breathing frequency of 30 breaths·min^{-1}. A THR may be prescribed relative to those goals. The person should do several short-duration exercise bouts each day, and with time, gradually increase the duration of each exercise bout as tolerance improves (49).

Those with Grade 3 disability follow the intermittent-exercise recommendation of the Grade 2 guidelines, but the exercise intensity is very low, and oxygen supplementation may be needed. Breathing exercises are also included. Unfortunately, those with Grade 4 disability are probably in respiratory or cardiovascular failure, and the emphasis is on counseling the person on how to conserve energy to accomplish daily tasks, which may require supplemental oxygen (49).

The goals of the exercise component of the COPD rehabilitation program are very pragmatic: ability to do home or work activities, ability to climb two flights of stairs, and so on (10, 65). Generally, COPD patients achieve an increase in exercise tolerance without dyspnea and an increase in the sense of well-being, but without a reversal of the disease process (65, 86). The changes in the psychological variables are very important in the long run, given that the person's willingness to continue the exercise program is a major factor that will dictate the rate of decline during the course of the disease.

Cardiovascular Disease

Exercise training is now an ordinary part of the treatment of individuals with CHD. The details of how to structure such programs, from the first steps taken after being confined to a bed to the time of returning to work and beyond, are spelled out clearly in books such as *Exercise in Health and Disease* (72) and *Rehabilitation of the Coronary Patient* (97). This section is meant as a brief introduction to various aspects of such programs.

Populations

Cardiac rehabilitation programs include patients who have experienced angina pectoris, myocardial infarctions (MI), coronary artery bypass graft surgery (CABGS), and angioplasty (26). *Angina pectoris* refers to the chest pain that is due to ischemia of the ventricle resulting from an occlusion of one or more of the coronary arteries. The pain appears when the oxygen requirement (work) of the heart (estimated by the double product = systolic BP • HR) exceeds a value that coronary blood flow cannot meet. Nitroglycerin can prevent an angina attack or relieve the pain by relaxing the smooth muscle in veins to reduce venous return and, thus, the work of the heart. Angina patients may also receive a beta- (ß-) adrenergic blocking drug like propranolol (Inderal®) to reduce the HR and/or BP responses to work; the angina symptoms would then occur at a later stage into work (see chapter 15 for medications). Exercise training supports this drug effect, in that as the person becomes trained, the HR response and double product are reduced at any work rate. More strenuous tasks can then be done without experiencing chest pain.

Myocardial Infarction.   **Myocardial infarction (MI)** patients have actual heart damage (loss of ventricular muscle) due to the occlusion of one or more of the coronary arteries. The degree to which left-ventricular function is affected depends on the mass of the ventricle permanently damaged. MI patients usually take medications (ß-blockers) to reduce the work of the heart and control the irritability of the heart tissue so that dangerous *arrhythmias* (irregular heart beats) do not occur. Generally, these patients experience a training effect similar to those who did not have an MI (26).

Coronary Artery Bypass Graft Surgery.   **Coronary artery bypass graft surgery (CABGS)** patients have had surgery to bypass one or more blocked coronary arteries. In this procedure a saphenous vein or mammary artery is sewn into existing coronary arteries above and below the blockage. Those with chronic angina pectoris prior to CABGS find a relief of symptoms, with 50% to 70% having no more pain. Generally, with an increased blood flow to the ventricle there is an improvement in left-ventricular function and the capacity for work (98). These patients benefit from systematic exercise training, because most are deconditioned prior to surgery as a result of activity restrictions related to chest pain. The cardiac rehabilitation program also helps the patient differentiate angina pain from chest-wall pain related to the surgery. The overall result is a smoother and less traumatic transition back to full function.

Percutaneous Transluminal Coronary Angioplasty.

Some CHD patients undergo a special procedure, **percutaneous transluminal coronary angioplasty**, to open occluded arteries. In this procedure the chest is not opened; instead, a balloon-tipped catheter (a long slender tube) is inserted into the coronary artery, where the balloon is inflated to push the plaque back toward the arterial wall. These patients tend not to have as severe disease as those who undergo CABGS (94).

Testing

Testing of patients with CHD is much more involved than for the apparently healthy person described in chapter 9. There are classes of CHD patients for whom exercise or exercise testing is inappropriate and dangerous (3). For those who can be tested, a 12-lead electrocardiogram (ECG) is monitored at discrete intervals during the GXT while a variety of leads are displayed continuously on an oscilloscope. Blood pressure, RPE, and various signs or symptoms are also noted. The criteria for terminating the GXT focus on various pathological signs (e.g., S–T segment depression) and symptoms (e.g., angina pectoris) rather than on achieving some percentage of age-adjusted maximal HR. On the basis of the response to the GXT, the person may be referred for additional testing: use of radioactive molecules to evaluate perfusion ([201]thallium) and the capacity of the ventricle to eject blood ([99]technetium), or direct *angiography*, in which a radiopaque dye is injected into the coronary arteries to determine the blockage directly (72).

Exercise Program

The basic cardiac rehabilitation exercise program resembles the one mentioned earlier for the apparently healthy, in that it includes warm-up with stretching, endurance exercise at a THR, muscle-strengthening activities, and a cool-down period. However, due to the fact that CHD patients are generally very deconditioned, only light exercise is required to achieve their THR. In addition, because these patients are on a wide variety of medications, some of which will decrease maximal HR, the THR zone is determined from their GXT results; the 220–age formula is not used. The patients usually begin with intermittent low-intensity exercise (1 min on, 1 min off) and with time increase the duration of the work period. Given that CABGS and post-MI patients have had direct damage to their hearts, the exercise should facilitate, and not interfere with, the healing process. As you might guess, given the nature of the patients and the risks involved, cardiac rehabilitation programs take place in hospitals and clinics where there is direct medical supervision and the capacity to deal with emergencies, should they occur. After a patient completes an 8- to 12-week Phase II program, the person may continue in a Phase III program away from the hospital, with less supervision but the same capacity to respond to emergencies (72). What are the benefits of such programs to the patient with CHD?

Effects

There is no question that CHD patients have improved cardiovascular function as a result of exercise programs. This is shown in higher $\dot{V}O_2$max values, higher work rates achieved without ischemia, as shown by angina pectoris or S–T segment changes, and an increased capacity for prolonged submaximal work (72, 97). The improved lipid profile (lower total cholesterol and higher HDL cholesterol) is a function of more than the exercise alone, given that weight loss and the saturated-fat content of the diet can modify these variables (6, 68). It must be mentioned that a cardiac rehabilitation program should not be viewed simply as an exercise program. It is a multi-intervention effort involving exercise, medication, diet, and counseling.

The Elderly

Maximal aerobic power decreases in the average population after the age of 20 at the rate of about 1% per year (17). However, this decrease is due to both inactivity and weight gain, as well as to an "aging effect." Recent studies show that this decline can be reversed by a physical activity program, and middle-aged men who maintain their activity and body weight show little change in $\dot{V}O_2$max over a 22-year period (54). Unfortunately, most people experience the steady decline in $\dot{V}O_2$max with age, so that by the time they are ready to retire, their ability to engage in normal physical activities has been compromised. This reduced capacity for work can lead to a vicious cycle, resulting in lower and lower levels of cardiorespiratory fitness that may not allow them to perform activities of daily living. This, of course, affects the elderly's quality of life and independence, and they may end up having to rely on others. Regular physical activity is useful in dealing not only with this downward spiral of cardiorespiratory fitness but with osteoporosis and the related sudden hip fractures that can lead to more inactivity and death (89).

Osteoporosis is a loss of bone mass that is responsible for 1.2 million fractures annually. *Type I osteoporosis* is related to fractures of the vertebra and distal radius in 50- to 65-year-olds, and is 8 times more common in women than men. *Type II osteoporosis*, experienced by those aged 70 and above, results in hip, pelvic, and distal humerus fractures and is twice as common in women (48). Osteoporosis is more common in women over 50, due to the lack of estrogen after menopause. If estrogen treatment is instituted early in menopause, it may prevent bone loss. However, if the treatment is initiated years after menopause, it cannot replace the lost bone; it will only maintain existing bone (57). To prevent the problem, attention is focused on adequate dietary calcium (40) and exercise (89). Dietary calcium is important in preventing and treating osteoporosis. However, because most women take in less than the RDA (see chapter 6), they must focus more attention on taking in an adequate amount of calcium, especially if the requirements for the premenopausal and immediate postmenopausal women are actually greater than the RDA (40).

Bone structure is maintained by the downward force due to gravity (upright posture) and the lateral forces generated by muscle contraction. Unfortunately, although research has shown that exercise programs can slow or reverse bone loss, the optimal training program to prevent osteoporosis has yet to be defined (90). Weight-bearing activities (such as walking and jogging) are better than bicycling and swimming for maintaining spine and hip mineral, but for the low fit or those with previous fractures, these latter activities are recommended (89). Two to 3 hr of exercise a week may reduce or reverse the bone mineral loss that occurs with age (89).

With respect to making exercise recommendations for fitness, Smith (88) indicates the need to distinguish among the aged populations:

- Athletic old—>55 years of age; $\dot{V}O_2max = 9$ to 10 METs
- Young old—55 to 75 years of age; $\dot{V}O_2max = 6$ to 7 METs
- Old old—>75 years of age; $\dot{V}O_2max = 2$ to 3 METs

The $\dot{V}O_2max$ values of the "athletic old" allow for a variety of activities that would be similar to those suitable for the ordinary younger and more sedentary population. The "young old" subject's $\dot{V}O_2max$ of 6

to 7 METs is similar to that of a cardiac patient, and the structure and routine of this subject's exercise program would not be too different from that of the cardiac patient. However, prescribing activities for the "old old" group, whose members have extremely low functional capacities, demands creativity in terms of both exercise testing and prescription (88).

Smith and Gilligan's chair-step test (89) provides an interesting substitute for traditional treadmill and cycle ergometer testing of the elderly. In this test the person remains seated on a chair and alternates leg lifts to raise the heel of the foot 6, 12, or 18 in., pausing momentarily on a step. The recommended cadence results in work increments of only 0.5 METs. Although exercise prescription follows the procedures described earlier, the HFI must implement unique, low-intensity, *controlled* exercises focusing on the low end of the MET scale and using support (91). The "old old" individual can do these exercises while lying or seated, or holding onto a chair while standing. The exercises include foot, leg, and arm movements that will increase flexibility and muscular endurance and expend calories. Given the rapid increase in the number of individuals in this age group, the HFI will be required to develop competence with such exercise programs.

Pregnancy

Pregnancy places special demands on a woman, given the developing fetus's needs for calories, protein, minerals, vitamins, and of course, the physiologically stable environment needed to process these nutrients. The fitness program must be evaluated against these diverse needs. The pregnant woman should begin with a thorough medical examination by her physician to rule out pregnancy-related complications such as glucose intolerance and hypertension, and to obtain specific information about diet, alcohol and drug use, and the signs and symptoms to watch for during the course of the pregnancy.

In general, moderate exercise does not appear to interfere with oxygen delivery to the fetus, and the HR response of the fetus shows no signs of "distress." For women in excellent condition before pregnancy, exercise does not appear to have any negative or positive effects in terms of fetal outcome (60, 61). The guidelines for exercise during pregnancy have been developing over the past decade, but not without some disagreement. On the one hand, some physicians believe that women should not start a new exercise program after becoming pregnant, whereas others feel that people should not all be held to the same standard (e.g., "Don't allow the HR to exceed 140 beats•min^{-1} during exercise") (19, 31). This latter view is countered with the need for conservative guidelines most likely to protect mother and fetus (31). See the American College of Obstetricians and Gynecologists Guidelines. The recommendation is for moderate exercise (HR ≤140 beats·min^{-1}) of short duration (15 min) that would not require a Valsalva maneuver. Given that high body temperatures have been linked to tetrogenic damage to the fetus, the guidelines emphasize short-duration exercise, adequate hydration, and not exercising in hot, humid weather, to keep the body temperature below 38 °C. However, the relations between heat stress and tetrogenic damage have not been systematically studied (60,

American College of Obstetricians and Gynecologists Guidelines for Exercise During Pregnancy and Postpartum

1. Regular exercise (at least three times per week) is preferable to intermittent activity. Competitive activities should be discouraged.
2. Vigorous exercise should not be performed in hot, humid weather or during a period of febrile illness.
3. Ballistic movements (jerky, bouncy motions) should be avoided. Exercise should be done on a wooden floor or a tightly carpeted surface to reduce shock and provide a sure footing.
4. Deep flexion or extension of joints should be avoided because of connective tissue laxity. Activities that require jumping, jarring motions, or rapid changes in direction should be avoided because of joint instability.
5. Vigorous exercise should be preceded by a 5-min period of muscle warm-up. This can be accomplished by slow walking or stationary cycling with low resistance.
6. Vigorous exercise should be followed by a period of gradually declining activity that includes gentle stationary stretching. Because connective-tissue laxity increases the risk of joint injury, stretches should not be taken to the point of maximum resistance.
7. Heart rate should be measured at times of peak activity. THRs and limits established in consultation with the physician should not be exceeded.
8. Care should be taken to gradually rise from the floor to avoid orthostatic hypotension. Some form of activity involving the legs should be continued for a brief period.
9. Liquids should be taken liberally before and after exercise to prevent dehydration. If necessary, activity should be interrupted to replenish fluids.
10. Women who have led sednetary lifestyles should begin with physical activity of very low intensity and advance activity levels very gradually.
11. Activity should be stopped and the physician consulted if any unusual symptoms appear.

Pregnancy only

1. Maternal HR should not exceed 140 beats · min^{-1}.
2. Strenuous activities should not exceed 15 min in duration.
3. No exercise should be performed in the supine position after the 4th month of gestation is completed.
4. Exercises that employ the Valsalva maneuver should be avoided.
5. Calorie intake should be adequate to meet the extra energy needs not only of pregnancy, but also of the exercise performed.
6. Maternal core temperature should not exceed 38 °C.

Note. The American College of Obstetricians and Gynecologists. *Exercise During Pregnancy and the Postnatal Period* ACOG home exercise programs. Washington, DC © 1985. Reprinted by permission.

61). Finally, the guidelines suggest that the pregnant woman should not exercise in the supine position after the 4th month of gestation. These guidelines are viewed as a good starting place for a conversation between the woman and her physician. However, those who were physically active before pregnancy can exercise safely at higher intensities and longer durations (19, 31).

ENVIRONMENTAL CONCERNS

Target heart rate is used as an indicator of the proper exercise intensity in health-related fitness programs. However, there are environmental factors such as heat, humidity, pollution, and altitude that can cause HR and the perception of effort to increase during an exercise session. This could shorten the exercise session and reduce the chance of expending sufficient calories and experiencing a training effect. Fortunately, by decreasing the exercise intensity we can "control" these environmental problems to provide a safe and effective exercise prescription. The purpose of this section is to discuss the effects different environmental factors have on the exercise prescription, and what we can do about them.

Environmental Heat and Humidity

Chapter 3 described the increases in body temperature (**hyperthermia**) that occurs with exercise, the heat-loss mechanisms called into play, and the benefits of becoming acclimatized to the heat. Our core temperature (37 °C, or 98.6 °F) is within a few degrees of a value that could lead to death by heat injury. However, as described in chapter 16, heat injury includes a series of stages from heat cramps to heat stroke, that need to be recognized and attended to, to prevent a progression from the least to the most serious. Although treatment of these problems is important, prevention is a better approach.

Figure 13.6 shows the major factors related to heat injury. Each of the following factors influences susceptibility to heat injury and can alter the HR and metabolic responses to exercise.

- Fitness—Fit people have a lower risk of heat injury (33), can tolerate more work in the heat (23), and acclimatize faster (17).
- Acclimatization—Seven to 10 days of exercise in the heat increases our capacity to sweat, initiates sweating at a lower body temperature, and reduces salt loss. Body temperature and HR responses are lower during exercise, and the chance of salt depletion is reduced (17).
- Hydration—Inadequate hydration reduces sweat

rate and increases the chance of heat injury (17, 83, 84). Generally, during exercise the focus should be on replacing water, not salt or carbohydrate stores.
- Environmental temperature—Exercising in temperatures greater than skin temperatures results in a *heat gain* by convection and radiation. Evaporation of sweat must compensate, if body temperature is to remain at a safe value.
- Clothing—As much skin surface as possible should be exposed, to encourage evaporation. Materials should be chosen that will "wick" sweat to the surface for evaporation; materials impermeable to water will increase the risk of heat injury and should be avoided.
- Humidity (water vapor pressure)—Evaporation of sweat is dependent on the water vapor pressure gradient between skin and environment. In warm and hot environments, the relative humidity is a good index of the water vapor pressure, with a lower relative humidity facilitating the evaporation of sweat.
- Metabolic rate—During times of high heat and humidity, decreasing the exercise intensity decreases the heat load, as well as the strain on the physiological systems that must deal with it.
- Wind—Wind places more air molecules into contact with the skin and can influence heat loss in two ways. If there is a temperature gradient for heat loss between the skin and the air, wind will increase the rate of heat loss by convection. In a similar manner, wind increases the rate of evaporation, assuming the air can accept moisture.

Recommendations for Fitness

The members of a fitness program need to be educated about all of the above factors. The HFI might suggest

- information on heat-illness symptoms: cramps, lightheadedness, and so on, and how to deal with them (see chapter 16);
- exercising in the cooler parts of the day to avoid heat gain from the sun or from building or road surfaces heated by the sun;
- gradually increasing exposure to high heat and humidity to safely acclimatize over a period of 7 to 10 days;
- drinking water before, during, and after exercise, and weighing in each day to monitor hydration;
- wearing only shorts and a tank top to expose as much skin as possible, but being careful to use a sunblock to reduce the chance of skin cancer; and
- taking HR measurements several times during the activity and reducing exercise intensity to stay in the THR zone.

The last recommendation, regarding THR, is most important. HR is a sensitive indicator of dehydration, en-

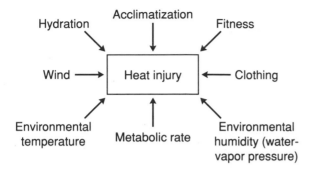

Figure 13.6 Factors affecting heat injury. *Note.* From *Exercise Physiology* (p. 508) by S.K. Powers and E.T. Howley, 1990, Dubuque, IA: Wm. C. Brown Publishers. Copyright 1990 by Wm. C. Brown Publishers. Reprinted by permission.

vironmental heat load, and acclimatization. Variation in any of these factors will modify the HR response to any fixed submaximal exercise. It is therefore important for fitness participants to monitor HR on a regular basis and slow down to stay within the THR zone. The RPE can also be used in this regard, in that it provides an index of the overall physiological strain being experienced by the participant.

Implications for Performance

Any athlete performing in an environment that is not conducive to heat loss is at an increased risk of heat injury. This has been a major problem for football, but the increased number of people running 10K races, marathons, and triathlons has shifted our focus of attention (35, 47). In response to this problem, and on the basis of sound research, in 1985 the American College of Sports Medicine developed a position stand, "The Prevention of Thermal Injuries During Distance Running" (1). The elements in the position stand are consistent with what was presented earlier.

Environmental Heat Stress

The preceding discussion mentioned high temperature and relative humidity as factors increasing the risk of heat injuries. To quantify the overall heat stress associated with any environment, a **wet-bulb globe temperature (WBGT)** guide has been developed (1). This overall heat-stress index is composed of the following measurements:

- **Dry-bulb temperature (Tdb)**—ordinary measure of air temperature taken in the shade
- **Black-globe temperature (Tg)**—measure of the radiant heat load measured in direct sunlight
- **Wet-bulb temperature (Twb)**—measurement of air temperature with a thermometer whose mercury bulb is covered with a wet cotton wick [making it sensitive to the relative humidity (water-

vapor pressure) and providing an index of the ability to evaporate sweat]

The formula used to calculate the WBGT temperature shows the importance of the wet-bulb temperature, being 70% (0.7) of the WBGT index, in determining heat stress (1). This is related to the role the wet-bulb temperature plays in estimating the ability to evaporate sweat, the most important heat-loss mechanism in most situations. The formula is

$$WBGT = 0.7\ Twb + 0.2\ Tg + 0.1\ Tdb$$

The risk of heat stress is given by the following color-coded flags on race courses:

Red flag = High risk
WBGT = 23 to 28 °C (73-82 °F)

Amber flag = Moderate risk
WBGT = 18 to 23 °C (65-73 °F)

Green flag = Low risk (of heat injury)
WBGT < 18 °C (<65 °F)

White flag = Low risk (of hyperthermia, but possibility of hypothermia)
WBGT < 10 °C (<50 °F)

Table 13.5 provides another estimate of heat stress, using just temperature and relative humidity. Because

Table 13.5 Interaction of Temperature and Relative Humidity in Causing Heat Stress

% relative humidity	Temperature								
	60	65	70	75	80	85	90	95	100
0									
10	59	62	64	67	69	72	74	77	79
20	59	62	65	68	70	73	76	79	82
30	59	62	65	68	72	75	78	81	84
40	59	63	66	69	73	76	79	83	86
50	59	63	67	70	74	76	81	85	88
60	60	63	67	71	75	79	83	87	91
70	60	64	68	72	76	81	85	88	93
80	60	64	69	73	78	82	86	91	95
90	60	65	69	74	79	84	88	93	98
100	60	65	70	75	80	85	90	95	100

Caution / Extreme caution

Note. Use as a conservative guide, because the radiant heat load is not considered. From *On the Ball* by B.A. Franklin, N.B. Oldridge, K.G. Stoedefalke, and W.E. Leochel, 1990, Carmel, IN: Benchmark Press. Reprinted with permission from Brown and Benchmark.

this table does not include radiant heat load (**globe temperature**), it should be used conservatively in estimating heat load.

Exercise and Cold Exposure

Exercising in the cold can create problems, if certain precautions are not taken. As mentioned in the White Flag category of heat stress, a WBGT of 10 °C (50 °F) or less is associated with hypothermia. **Hypothermia** is a decrease in body temperature that occurs when heat loss exceeds heat production. In cold air, there is a larger gradient for convective heat loss from the skin; cold air also is ''dry'' (has a low water vapor pressure) and facilitates the evaporation of moisture from the skin to further cool the body. The combined effects can be deadly, as shown in Pugh's report of three deaths during a walking competition over a 45-mi distance (75).

Figure 13.7 shows the factors related to hypothermia. These include *environmental factors*, such as temperature, water vapor pressure, wind, and whether air or water are involved; *insulating factors*, such as clothing and subcutaneous fat; and the capacity for sustained *energy production*. We will now comment on each of these, relative to hypothermia.

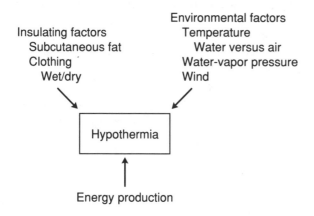

Figure 13.7 Factors affecting hypothermia. *Note.* From *Exercise Physiology* (p. 511) by S.K. Powers and E.T. Howley, 1990, Dubuque, IA: Wm. C. Brown Publishers. Copyright 1990 by Wm. C. Brown Publishers. Reprinted by permission..

Environmental Factors

Conduction, convection, and radiation are dependent on a temperature gradient between the skin and the environment; the larger the gradient, the greater the rate of heat loss. What is surprising is that the environmental temperature does not have to be below freezing to cause hypothermia. There are other environmental factors that interact with temperature to create the dangerous

condition by facilitating heat loss—namely, wind and water.

Windchill Index. The rate of heat loss at any given temperature is directly influenced by wind speed. Wind increases the number of cold air molecules coming into contact with the skin, increasing the rate of heat loss. The **windchill index** indicates what the ''effective'' temperature is for any combination of temperature and wind speed (see Table 13.6) and allows you to properly gauge the conditions for a variety of wind velocities and temperatures. Keep in mind that if you are running, riding, or cross-country skiing into the wind, you must add your speed to the wind speed to evaluate the full impact of the windchill. For example, cycling at 20 mi•hr^{-1} into calm air at 0 °F has a windchill value of −35 °F! However, wind is not the only factor that can increase the rate of heat loss at any given temperature.

Water. You can lose heat 25 times faster in water compared to air of the same temperature. Unlike air, water offers little or no insulation at the skin–water interface, so heat is rapidly lost from the body. Movement in cold water would increase heat loss from the arms and legs, so the recommendation is to stay as still as possible in *long-term* immersions (44).

Insulating Factors

The rate at which heat is lost from the body is inversely related to the insulation between the body and the environment. The insulating quality is related to the thickness of subcutaneous fat, the ability of clothing to trap air, and whether or not the clothing is wet or dry.

Body Fat. Subcutaneous fat thickness is an excellent indicator of total body insulation per unit surface area through which heat is lost (39). For example, a fat man was able to swim for 7 hr in 16 °C water with no change in body temperature; but a thin man had to leave the water in 30 min with a core temperature of 34.5 °C (76). For this reason, long-distance swimmers tend to be fatter than short-course swimmers, and the higher body fatness provides more buoyancy, requiring less energy to swim at any set speed (43).

Clothing. Clothing can extend our natural subcutaneous fat insulation, allowing us to endure very cold environments. The insulation quality of clothing is given in ''clo'' units, where 1 clo unit is the insulation needed at rest (1 MET) to maintain core temperature when the environment is 21 °C (70 °F), the RH = 50%, and the air movement is 6 m•min^{-1} (0.2 mi•hr^{-1}) (15). As the air temperature falls, clothing with a higher clo value must be worn to maintain core temperature, because the gradient between skin and environment is increasing. Figure 13.8 shows the insulation needed at different energy expenditures across a broad range of environ-

Table 13.6   Windchill Index

Wind speed (mi · hr⁻¹)	Actual thermometer reading (°F)											
	50	40	30	20	10	0	–10	–20	–30	–40	–50	–60
	Equivalent temperature (°F)											
Calm	50	40	30	20	10	0	–10	–20	– 30	– 40	– 50	– 60
5	48	37	27	16	6	– 5	–15	–26	– 36	– 47	– 57	– 68
10	40	28	16	4	– 9	–21	–33	–46	– 58	– 70	– 83	– 95
15	36	22	9	– 5	–18	–36	–45	–58	– 72	– 85	– 99	–112
20	32	18	4	–10	–25	–39	–53	–67	– 82	– 96	–110	–124
25	30	16	0	–15	–29	–44	–59	–74	– 88	–104	–118	–133
30	28	13	– 2	–18	–33	–48	–63	–79	– 94	–109	–125	–140
35	27	11	– 4	–20	–35	–49	–67	–82	– 98	–113	–129	–145
40	26	10	– 6	–21	–37	–53	–69	–85	–100	–116	–132	–148

(Wind speeds greater than 40 mi · hr⁻¹ have little additional effect)	Little danger (for properly clothed person)	Increasing danger	Great danger
		Danger from freezing of exposed flesh	

Note. From *Physiology of Fitness* (3rd ed.) (p. 226) by B.J. Sharkey, 1990, Champaign, IL: Human Kinetics. Copyright 1990 by Brian J. Sharkey. Reprinted by permission.

mental temperatures, from −60 to +80 °F (15). It is clear that as energy production increases, insulation must decrease to maintain core temperature. When clothing is worn in layers, insulation can be removed as needed to maintain core temperature. By following these steps, sweating, which can rob the clothing of its insulating value, will be minimized. If the clothing becomes wet, the insulating quality decreases, because the water can now conduct heat away from the body about 25 times better than air (44). A primary goal, then, is to avoid wetness due to either sweat or weather. This problem is exacerbated by the cold environment's very dry air, which would cause a greater evaporation of moisture. When this problem of cold, dry air and wet clothing is coupled with windy conditions, the risk is even greater. The wind not only provides for greater convective heat loss, as described in the windchill, but it also accelerates evaporation (36).

KEY POINT.   When exercising in cold weather

- wear clothing in layers,
- remove layers to minimize sweating, and
- stay dry.

Energy Production

Energy production can modify the amount of insulation needed to maintain core temperature and prevent hypothermia (see Figure 13.8). When thin (<16.8% fat) male subjects were immersed in cold water, the drop in body temperature that occurred at rest was prevented when they did exercise at an energy expenditure of about 8.5 kcal·min⁻¹ (62, 63).

Table 13.7 shows the progression of signs and symptoms that occur as body temperature decreases in hypo-

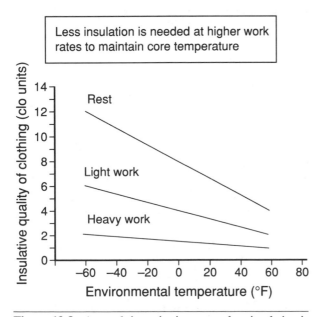

Figure 13.8 As work intensity increases, less insulation is needed to maintain core temperature. Data from Burton and Edholm (1955).

Table 13.7   Clinical Symptoms of Hypothermia

Core temperature (°C)	Symptoms and signs
37	Feeling of cold; skin cooling; decreased social interaction
36	Goose pimples
35	Shivering; muscle tension; fatigue
34.5	Deep cold
	Numbness
	Loss of coordination
	Stumbling
	Dysarthria
	Muscle rigidity
32	Disorientation
	Decreased visual acuity
31-30	Semicoma—coma
28	Ventricular fibrillation and cardiovascular death

Note. From "Environmental Considerations for Exercise" by L.E. Hart and J.R. Sutton, 1987, *Cardiology Clinics*, **5**, p. 246. Copyright 1987 by W.B. Saunders. Reprinted by permission.

thermia (93). It is important to deal with these problems "on site" rather than wait until the person can be taken to an emergency room. Following Sharkey (85), one should

- get person out of the cold, wind, and rain;
- remove all wet clothing;
- provide warm drinks, dry clothing, and a warm, dry sleeping bag for a mildly impaired person;
- keep the person awake, if semiconscious, undress the person, and put him or her into a sleeping bag with another person; and
- find a heat source, such as a campfire.

Effect of Air Pollution

Air pollution includes a variety of gases and particulates that are products of the combustion of fossil fuels. The smog that results when these pollutants are in high concentration can have detrimental effects on health and performance. The gases can affect performance by decreasing the capacity to transport oxygen, increasing airway resistance, and altering the perception of effort required when the eyes burn and the chest hurts.

Physiological responses to these pollutants are related to the amount, or "dose," received. The major factors determining the dose are the

- concentration of the pollutant,
- duration of the exposure to the pollutant, and
- volume of air inhaled.

The volume of air inhaled is clearly large during exercise, and this is one reason why physical activity is curtailed during times of peak pollution levels (25). The following discussion will focus on the major air pollutants: ozone, sulfur dioxide, and carbon monoxide.

Ozone

The **ozone** in the air we breathe is generated by the reaction between ultraviolet (UV) light and emissions from internal combustion engines. There is evidence that a single 2-hr exposure to a high ozone concentration, 0.75 ppm (parts per million), decreases $\dot{V}O_2max$, and recent studies show that a 6- to 12-hr exposure to a concentration of only 0.12 ppm (the U.S. air-quality standard) produces a decrease in lung function and an increase in respiratory symptoms. Interestingly, subjects can become adapted to ozone exposure, showing diminished responses to subsequent exposures during the "ozone season." However, concern about long-term lung health suggests that it would be prudent to avoid heavy exercise during the time of day when ozone and other pollutants are elevated (25).

Sulfur Dioxide

Sulfur dioxide (SO_2) is produced by smelters, refineries, and electrical utilities that use fossil fuel for energy generation. SO_2 does not affect lung function in normal subjects, but it causes bronchoconstriction in asthmatics—a response influenced by the temperature and humidity of the inspired air, as mentioned in the earlier section dealing with the asthmatic. Nose breathing is encouraged, to "scrub" the SO_2, and drugs like cromolym sodium and ß$_2$-agonists can partially block the asthmatic's response to SO_2 (25).

Carbon Monoxide

Carbon monoxide (CO) is derived from the burning of fossil fuel, coal, oil, gasoline, and wood, as well as from cigarette smoke. Carbon monoxide can bind to hemoglobin (HbCO) and decrease the capacity for oxygen transport. The carbon monoxide concentration in blood is generally less than 1% in nonsmokers, but may be as high as 10% in smokers (79). As mentioned in chapter 3, beyond a HbCO concentration of 4.3% there is a 1% reduction in $\dot{V}O_2max$ for each 1% increase in the HbCO concentration. In contrast, when one exercises at about 40% $\dot{V}O_2max$, the HbCO concentration can be as high as 15% before endurance is affected. The cardiovascular system simply has a greater capacity to respond with a larger cardiac output when the O_2 concentration of the blood is reduced during submaximal work (45, 78, 79). This, of course, requires a higher HR for the same work task, and a participant needs to reduce the intensity of exercise during exposure to CO to stay in the THR range. Because it takes about 2 to 4 hr to remove half the CO from the blood once the exposure has been removed, CO can have a lasting effect on performance (25). Unfortunately, it is difficult to predict what the actual CO concentration will be in any given environment. Because we must consider the previous exposure to the pollutant, as well as the length of time and rate of ventilation associated with the current exposure, the following guidelines are provided for exercising in an area with air pollution (79).

- Reduce exposure to the pollutant prior to exercise, because the physiological effects are time and dose dependent.
- Stay away from areas where one might receive a "bolus" dose of CO: smoking areas, high traffic areas, urban environments.
- Do not schedule activities during the times when pollutants are at their highest levels: 7 to 10 a.m. and 4 to 7 p.m., due to traffic.

Effect of Altitude

An increase in altitude decreases the partial pressure of oxygen and reduces the amount of oxygen bound to hemoglobin. As a result, the volume of oxygen carried in each liter of blood decreases. As mentioned in chapter 3, maximal aerobic power steadily decreases with increasing altitude, so that by 2,300 m (7,500 ft) the value is only 88% of that measured at sea level. This means that an activity that demanded 88% of $\dot{V}O_2$max at sea level now requires 100% of the "new" $\dot{V}O_2$max.

More than maximal aerobic power is affected by altitude exposure. Any submaximal work rate is going to demand a higher HR at altitude compared to sea level

(shown in Figure 13.9). The reason is quite simple. Because each liter of blood has less oxygen, more blood is required to deliver the same quanity of oxygen to the tissues. Consequently, the HR response is elevated at any given submaximal work rate. To stay within the THR range, a person must cut back on the intensity of the exercise when at altitude. Just like exercise in high heat and humidity, the THR allows the modification of the intensity of the activity relative to any additional environmental demand (46).

KEY POINT.   When exercising at altitude or during exposure to carbon monoxide, decrease work intensity to stay within the THR zone.

SUMMARY

Two major principles of training related to the improvement of cardiovascular function are overload and specificity. The apparently healthy but sedentary participant should start out slowly, with a goal to become a regular exerciser. Each exercise session should start with a warm-up and finish with a cool-down. Exercise sessions should be scheduled three to four times per week, and each workout should be long enough to expend about 200 to 300 kcal. The intensity of the exercise session should be about 60% to 80% of functional capacity. The exercise intensity is usually set by identifying HR values equivalent to these work loads. The THR can be obtained directly by seeing what HRs were equivalent to 60% and 80% of the functional capacity measured on a GXT. Two indirect means of estimating the THR are the heart–rate–reserve (HRR) method and the simple percentage-of-maximal HR (%HRmax) method. In the HRR method, the HFI takes 60% to 80% of the HR reserve (HRR = maximal HR − resting HR) and adds the result to resting HR. In the %HRmax method, the HFI takes 70% to 85% of maximal HR. Maximal HR is determined from a GXT, or it can be estimated to be equal to 220 − age. However, there is considerable variability (SD = ±11 beats·min⁻¹) in the estimated, compared with the measured, value. The average person experiences a cardiovascular training effect at an average training intensity of 70% of $\dot{V}O_2$max (70% HRR or 80% HRmax). Extremely deconditioned individuals experience some training effect at relatively low intensities (<60% of $\dot{V}O_2$max). Very fit people, on the other hand, must train at the upper end (80% to 90% of $\dot{V}O_2$max) to improve CRF. Exercise recommendations are provided for the following conditions and groups: orthopedic limitation, obese, hypertensive, asthmatic, pregnant, cardiac, diabetic, chronic

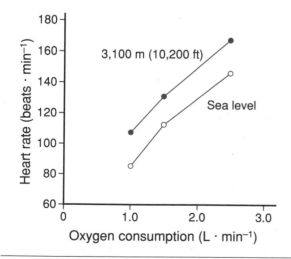

Figure 13.9   The effect of altitude on the heart-rate response to submaximal exercise. Based on data of R. Grover et al. (1967).

obstructive pulmonary disease, seizure disorder, and elderly. In general, these populations require more thorough physical examinations and physician direction, and should engage in low-intensity activities. Heat, humidity, altitude, and pollution can all cause a higher-than-expected HR response to submaximal work. Under these circumstances, the HFI should recommend a decrease in the intensity of exercise to keep the person within the THR zone. The participant should be educated about needed precautions for exercising in extremely hot, humid, or cold conditions, to prevent heat illness and hypothermia, respectively.

REFERENCES

1. American College of Sports Medicine (1985)
2. American College of Sports Medicine (1990)
3. American College of Sports Medicine (1991)
4. American Diabetes Association (1985)
5. American Diabetes Association (1987)
6. American Heart Association Committee Report (1982)
7. Bassett and Zweifler (1990)
8. Berg (1986)
9. Berger and Kemmer (1990)
10. Berman and Sutton (1986)
11. Blair et al. (1989)
12. Borg (1982)
13. Bray (1990)
14. Brownell (1988)
15. Burton and Edholm (1955)
16. Buskirk (1987)
17. Buskirk and Bass (1974)
18. Buskirk and Hodgson (1987)
19. Caldwell and Jopke (1985)
20. Cantu (1982)
21. Dehn and Mullins (1977)
22. Dodd, Powers, Callender, and Brooks (1984)
23. Drinkwater, Denton, Kupprat, Talag, and Horvath (1976)
24. Eggleston (1986)
25. Folinsbee (1990)
26. Franklin, Hellerstein, Gordon, and Timmis (1986)
27. Franklin, Oldridge, Stoedefalke, and Loechel (1990)
28. Franks (1983)
29. Franz (1987)
30. Garfinkel and Coscina (1990)
31. Gauthier (1986)
32. Gerhard and Schachter (1980)
33. Gisolfi and Cohen (1979)
34. Hagberg (1990)
35. Hanson and Zimmerman (1979)
36. Hardy and Bard (1974)
37. Haskell (1978)
38. Haskell, Montoye, and Orenstein (1985)
39. Hayward and Keatinge (1981)
40. Heaney (1987)
41. Hellerstein and Franklin (1984)
42. Holloszy and Coyle (1984)
43. Holmer (1979)
44. Horvath (1981)
45. Horvath, Raven, Dahms, and Gray (1975)
46. Howley (1980)
47. Hughson et al. (1980)
48. Johnson and Slemenda (1987)
49. Jones, Berman, Bartkiewig, and Oldridge (1987)
50. Kannel (1990)
51. Kannel and Gordon (1979)
52. Kaplan (1986)
53. Karvonen, Kentala, and Mustala (1957)
54. Kasch, Boyer, Van Camp, Verity, and Wallace (1990)
55. Katz (1986)
56. Katz (1987)
57. Lindsay (1987)
58. Londeree and Ames (1976)
59. Londeree and Moeschberger (1982)
60. Lotgering, Gilbert, and Longo (1985)
61. Lotgering, Gilbert, and Longo (1984)
62. McArdle, Magel, Gergley, Spina, and Toner (1984)
63. McArdle, Magel, Spina, Gergley, and Toner (1984)
64. Middleton (1980)
65. Miracle (1986)
66. Noble, Borg, Cafarelli, Robertson, and Pandolf (1982)
67. Paffenbarger, Hyde, and Wing (1986)
68. Physician and Sportsmedicine (1987)
69. Pierson, Covert, Koenig, Namekta, and Shin Kim (1986)
70. Pollock et al. (1972)
71. Pollock et al. (1977)
72. Pollock and Wilmore (1990)
73. Powell and Paffenbarger (1985)
74. Powers and Howley (1990)
75. Pugh (1964)
76. Pugh and Edholm (1955)
77. Rabkin, Mathewson, and Hsu (1977)
78. Raven (1980)
79. Raven et al. (1974)
80. Richter and Galbo (1986)
81. Rimm and White (1979)
82. Saltin and Gollnick (1983)
83. Sawka, Francesconi, Young, and Pandolf (1984)
84. Sawka, Young, Francesconi, Muza, and Pandolf (1985)

85. Sharkey (1984)
86. Shephard (1976)
87. Sly (1986)
88. Smith (1984)
89. Smith and Gilligan (1987)
90. Smith, Smith, and Gilligan (1990)
91. Smith and Stoedefalke (1978)
92. Stockdale-Woolley, Haggerty, and McMahon (1986)
93. Sutton (1990)
94. Tommaso, Lesch, and Sonnenblick (1984)
95. Voy (1986)
96. Vranic and Wasserman (1990)
97. Wenger and Hellerstein (1984)
98. Wenger and Hurst (1984)
99. World Health Organization (1986)

SUGGESTED READINGS

Åstrand and Rodahl (1986)
Grover et al. (1967)
Lamb (1984)
Nutrition and your health: Dietary guidelines for Americans (1980)
Vranic and Berger (1979)

See the Bibliography at the end of the book for a complete source list.

CASE STUDIES

13.1 Paul is a white male, 46 years of age, 88 kg, and 178 cm tall, and he has 28% body fat. Blood chemistry values indicate that total cholesterol = 270 ml·dl^{-1} and HDL cholesterol = 38 mg·dl^{-1}. His mother died of a heart attack at the age of 63, and his father had a heart attack at the age of 78. He is sedentary and has engaged in no endurance-training program since college. The following are the results of maximal GXT conducted by his physician.

Test: Balke, 3 mi·hr^{-1}; 2.5% per 2 min

Grade (%)	METs	SBP	DBP	HR	ECG	Symptoms
	Rest	126	88	70	—	—
2.5	4.3	142	86	142	—	—
5	5.4	148	88	150	—	—
7.5	6.4	162	86	160	—	—
10	7.4	174	84	168	—	—
12.5	8.5	186	84	176	—	—
15	9.5	194	84	190	—	Calf tight
17.5	10.5	198	84	198	—	Fatigue

If a person has a normal response to a GXT, HR and systolic blood pressure increase with each stage of the test, whereas the diastolic pressure remains the same or decreases slightly. In addition, the ECG response shows no significant S–T segment depression or elevation, and no significant arrhythmias occur. In these cases it can be assumed that the last load achieved on the test represents the true functional capacity (max METs). The above GXT is representative of such a test.

Paul has normal resting BP and a negative family history for CHD. Risk factors include a relatively high percent body fat (indicating obesity), sedentary lifestyle, and a poor blood lipid profile. Based on these findings, a THR range of 139 to 168 beats·min^{-1} was calculated (70 to 85% HRmax). This HR range corresponds to work rates equal to 4 to 7.5 METs. Initially, he will work at the low end of this THR range, with the emphasis on the duration of activity. As he becomes more active he will work at the upper end of the THR range, depending, of course, on his interests. He was referred for nutritional counseling to improve his blood lipid profile.

Paul has an estimated HRmax of 174 beats•min^{-1}; his measured HR was 24 beats•min^{-1} higher. Given the inherent biological variation in the estimated HRmax, use the measured values when they are available.

13.2 In some instances a physician may confirm the existence of an old "functional" ECG abnormality on a resting ECG tracing and feel the need for a more complete picture of how the individual's ECG would respond with the heart under stress. John's case is such an example. John is a 44-year-old white male who has been active in sports most of his life but has not recently engaged in any regular endurance-training program. His blood chemistry values indicate the following: glucose = 100 mg•dl^{-1}, cholesterol = 220 mg•dl^{-1}, HDL cholesterol = 53 mg•dl^{-1}, and triglycerides = 87 mg•dl^{-1}. His resting ECG shows that he has Left Bundle Branch Block (LBBB), and his physician thinks John should have a maximal GXT before increasing his activity level.

Test: Balke, 3 mi•hr^{-1}; 2% per minute

Grade (%)	METs	SBP	DBP	HR	ECG	Symptoms
	Rest	128	90	76	LBBB	—
0	3.3	146	90	95	LBBB	—
2.5	4.3	152	90	100	LBBB	—
5	5.4	154	90	107	LBBB	—
7.5	6.4	154	90	113	LBBB	—
10	7.4	164	90	125	LBBB	—
12.5	8.5	172	90	144	LBBB	—
15	9.5	184	90	156	LBBB	—
17.5	10.5	190	90	164	LBBB	Fatigue

The results show that John has normal HR and BP responses to the GXT. Further, the test was judged to be a true maximal test. His blood chemistry values are considered normal with the exception of a slightly elevated total cholesterol value. A THR range was calculated to be 114 to 140 beats•min^{-1} (70 to 85% HRmax), representing activities in the range of 6 to 8 METs. The beginning of his exercise program will emphasize an exercise intensity at the low end of his THR range, progressing toward the upper end to facilitate his participation in a variety of sports.

13.3 Mary is a 38-year-old white female, 170 cm tall, and 61.4 kg, and she has 30% body fat. Blood chemistry values indicate a total cholesterol of 188 mg•dl^{-1} and a HDL cholesterol of 59 mg•dl^{-1}. Her resting blood pressure is 124/80. Family history indicates that her father suffered a nonfatal heart attack at the age of 67. She has smoked 1 pack-a-day of cigarettes for the past 13 years. The following is the result of her submaximal cycle ergometer test.

Test: Y Way of Fitness

Work rate (kgm•min^{-1})	HR (Min 2)	HR (Min 3)
150	118	120
300	134	136
450	152	156

Note. Pedal rate = 50 rpm, predicted HRmax = 182 beats•min^{-1}, seat height = 6, and 85% HRmax = 155 beats•min^{-1}.

Mary's maximal aerobic power was estimated to be 1.65 L•min⁻¹ by extrapolating the HR/ work rate relationship to the predicted maximal heart rate (see chapter 9). This is equivalent to a $\dot{V}O_2$max of 27 ml•kg⁻¹•min⁻¹, or 7.7 METs.

Her blood chemistry values and BP are normal. Her family history is negative for CHD. Her HR response to the test is normal and indicates poor cardiorespiratory fitness. The low maximal aerobic power is related to the sedentary lifestyle, the cigarette smoking (carbon monoxide), and the 30% body fatness. She was encouraged to participate in a smoking-cessation program and was given the names of two local professional groups.

The recommended exercise program emphasized the low end of the THR zone (70% HRmax: 127 beats•min⁻¹) with long duration. She preferred a walking program to begin with, because of the freedom it gave her schedule. She was given the walking program in chapter 14 and was asked to record her HR response to each of the exercise sessions.

A body-fatness goal of 22% resulted in a target body weight of 121 lb (55 kg). She did not feel the need for dietary counseling at this time, but she agreed to record her food intake for 10 days to determine the patterns of eating behavior that would be beneficial to change (see chapter 6). She made an appointment for a meeting with the HFI in 2 weeks to discuss the progress with her program.

13.4 Chris is a white female, 49 years of age, 164 cm tall, and 93 kg, and she has 40% body fat. Her serum total cholesterol is 190 mg•dl⁻¹, serum triglycerides are 100 mg•dl⁻¹, blood glucose is 92 mg•dl⁻¹, and resting blood pressure is 130/84. She had been active in swimming and tennis in college but has led a relatively sedentary lifestyle since that time. Her goal is to lose weight and become active again. The following are the results of a submaximal GXT taken to 85% of predicted maximal heart rate:

Test: Balke, 3 mi•hr⁻¹; 2.5% per 2 min

Grade (%)	METs	SBP (mmHg)	DBP (mmHg)	HR	RPE
2.5	4.3	134	90	122	11
5	5.4	140	90	132	13
7.5	6.4	162	80	143	14

Note. Predicted HRmax = 171 beats•min⁻¹, and 85% HRmax = 145 beats•min⁻¹.

Chris has normal HR, BP, and RPE responses to the GXT. The HR/MET relationship was extrapolated to predicted HRmax, and her functional capacity is estimated to be 9.3 METs.

Her blood chemistry values and resting BP are normal. The major problem is the 40% body fat. Given this fatness, a $\dot{V}O_2$max of 9.3 METs is surprisingly high. A gradual reduction in body fatness would increase her functional capacity and increase the variety of physical activities in which she could participate.

A weight-reduction plan was designed to result in a weight loss of about 1 to 2 lb per week. In spite of her reasonably high functional capacity, activities were selected to keep her at the low end of the THR zone (70% HRmax: 120 beats•min⁻¹) and to put only a small load on the weight-bearing joints. She was given a walking program to do at home (see chapter 14) and a swimming program to do at the fitness club. The emphasis was on a level of work that would not cause fatigue.

She was given a dietary recall form (see chapter 6) to record her daily food intake for 1 week. She was instructed to not make changes in her diet during that week, but to simply record the information. At the end of the week she discussed the results with the HFI to see what major "junk food" items could be eliminated from her diet. In addition, she was given the name of three weight-control programs in the community to contact for additional advice.

13.5 Walt is a 38-year-old male, 71 in. tall (180 cm), and 212 lb (96.2 kg), and he has 24% body fat. Two years ago he shifted jobs, and now he works for a well-known brokerage house. He is also finishing up the last year of a 6-year evening law school program. He got married 1.5 years ago, and his wife is 5 months pregnant. He played most American sports in high school and was involved in long-distance bicycle rides (> 50 mi) as recently as 2 years ago. His weight has fluctuated from 185 to the present value over the past few years. He desires to get back to a regular program of activity. The following are the results of a submaximal GXT:

Test: Y Way of Fitness

Work rate (kgm•min^{-1})	Minute 3 heart rate (beats•min^{-1})
300	116
600	127
750	Skipped
900	141

Note. Pedal rate = 50 rpm, predicted HRmax = 182 beats•min^{-1}, seat height = 8, and 85% HRmax = 155.

The heart rate/work rate line was extrapolated to the predicted maximal heart rate, and functional capacity was estimated to be 4.0 L/min, which is 41.6 ml•kg^{-1}•min^{-1}, or 11.9 METs.

In the interview with this person it became clear that the last 2 years were full of stressful life events that were not yet under control. It was recommended that he talk with the stress management counselor at his place of employment. Further, his schedule of travel to work and the evening law school program left little time in the day to add one more thing. He agreed to exercise on his own with a walk/jog program until the law school program ended. At that time he would join a structured exercise program aimed at increasing his ability to participate in vigorous activities and sports at a health club. His calculated THR range is 127-155 beats/min (70-85% HRmax). He was given the walk/jog program and asked to record his heart rate and comments following each run (see chapter 14).

The following four cases represent a sample of the types of people who are tested prior to entry into an in-hospital cardiac rehabilitation program. The severity of their diseases varies, and the recommendations that follow each GXT are consistent with the subjects' responses to the GXTs.

Sometimes the subjects demonstrate inappropriate signs (ECG change or an inappropriate blood-pressure response) or experience symptoms (angina or claudication pain) during the course of a GXT. It is very important to consider these when writing the exercise prescriptions. The end point used in such a test may be quite different from the last measurements made on a test. Case Study 13.6 demonstrates this point. Note that these tests were done with a physician present.

13.6 Susan is a 50-year-old woman that recently experienced chest pain while climbing stairs. The following GXT was used to determine the extent of limitation before admission into an in-hospital cardiac rehabilitation program.

Test: Balke, 3 mph (80 m/min); 2.5% per 2 min

Grade (%)	METs	SBP	DBP	HR	ECG	Symptoms
	Rest	140	86	83	—	—
0	3.3	150	84	96	—	—
2.5	4.3	156	84	108	—	—
5	5.4	166	92	120	—	—
7.5	6.4	160	96	130	—	Chest pain
10	7.4	154	96	135	—	Chest pain/dizziness

Calculating a THR range for Susan using the 220-minus-age formula gives the values of 119 to 145 beats·min⁻¹ (70% and 85% HRmax). This presents some problems, because Susan did not achieve a HR of 145! The second choice might be to use her measured HRmax, and a THR range of 95 to 115 would be calculated. On the surface this might appear to be appropriate, but the 5% grade is the last stage in which she did not experience chest pain and where the BP response might still be considered normal. After that, the systolic pressure fell and the diastolic pressure increased. By checking the BP responses and her symptoms, the true "functional" limit was achieved at the 5% grade. The THR calculated would be based on the HR measured at the 5.4 METs stage. A THR range of 96 to 108 beats·min⁻¹ (60% to 80% of functional capacity) includes work rates in which Susan was sign- and symptom-free. The emphasis would be on light work of long duration. The THR could be adjusted upward on subsequent retesting if the response merited a change.

If the %HRmax method were used to calculate a THR (70% to 85% HRmax) in this test, the bottom part of the THR zone would equal resting HR. In GXT where the HR response is blunted, the direct THR method (60 to 80% of functional capacity) is the method of choice.

13.7 Nelson is a 56-year old black male who had unstable angina for several weeks. He had paroxysmal atrial fibrillation, which was converted to a normal sinus rhythm by Digitalis. His physician recommended an 8-week in-hospital rehabilitation program. His GXT follows:

Test: 2 mph; 3.5% per 2 min

Grade (%)	METs	SBP	DBP	HR	ECG
Rest	—	112	74	77	—
0	2.5	100	78	110	1 mm S–T seg depression
3.5	3.5	114	80	112	3 mm S–T seg depression

Based on the results of this treadmill test, Nelson was referred for coronary angiography and subsequently had 3-vessel bypass surgery.

13.8 Jake is a 59-year-old white male who is 75 kg and 178 cm tall. He had been a 1.5-pack-a-day cigarette smoker for 38 years prior to experiencing chest pain and then a myocardial infarction. After being discharged from the hospital, he experienced angina from mild exertion. Coronary angiography was carried out, and triple-bypass surgery followed. An in-hospital cardiac rehabilitation program was recommended; the GXT that follows represents his status as he entered the program. He was not taking any medication at the time of the GXT.

Test: 2 mph; 3.5% per 2 min

Grade (%)	METs	SBP	DBP	HR	ECG	Symptoms
Rest	—	120	68	83		—
0	2.5	154	80	119	*[a]	—
3.5	3.5	170	86	122	*	—
7	4.5	184	84	132	*	—
10.5	5.5	196	95	135	*	Mild fatigue

[a]* = no changes from the resting ECG.

The symptom of fatigue and the elevation of the diastolic pressure in the last stage suggest that 5.5 METs is Jake's functional capacity. Work rates equal to 60% and 80% of this value are approximately the 3.5% and 7% grades, corresponding to a THR range of 122 to 132 beats·min^{-1}. Calculation of the THR by the usual procedure (70% to 85% HRmax) yields a THR range of 95 to 115 beats·min^{-1}. The reason for the discrepancy in the THR range between the methods is a somewhat nonlinear HR response in addition to a contracted HR response, which is a change of only 16 beats·min^{-1} across a 3-MET work-rate change. The change is typically 25 to 30 beats·min^{-1}. The upper limit of the THR, calculated by taking 80% of the highest work rate, yielded a HR of 132 beats·min^{-1}, or 98% of the highest HR measured. Clearly one must examine the reasonableness of the THR independent of the method of calculation.

13.9 Andy is a 56-year-old white male who is 80 kg and 180 cm tall. His mother died at age 72 of a heart attack, and his father died at age 92 of congestive heart failure. All other family members are healthy. Prior to his myocardial infarction, he was a 2-pack-a-day cigarette smoker; he has had none since the MI. The following stress test was administered prior to an in-hospital exercise program. He was taking Lanoxin, Isordil, and nitroglycerine at the time of the test.

Test: 2 mi·hr^{-1}; 3.5% per 2 min

Grade (%)	METs	SBP	DBP	HR	ECG
Rest	—	116	84	51	PVC[a]
0	2.5	140	84	83	—
3.5	3.5	152	96	96	—
7	4.5	162	88	109	PVC
10.5	5.5	172	100	116	1 mm S–T seg depression
14	6.5	168	110	126	2 mm S–T seg depression

[a]PVC = preventricular contraction

Andy's HR response was normal, but the BP and ECG responses were not. These abnormal changes must be used in choosing the real end point for the test. The HR, BP, and ECG could be considered normal at 7% grade. A THR range of 83 to 96 beats·min^{-1} (60% to 80% of functional capacity) was calculated for this subject. This THR range is achieved at MET values of 2.5 to 3.5. A supervised, in-hospital program was recommended to allow close monitoring of progress. Beginning exercises included walking on a treadmill at 2 mi·hr^{-1}, 0% grade; pedaling a cycle ergometer 150 kg·min^{-1}; and stepping at a rate of 12 steps·min^{-1} on a 6-in. step. The work was done intermittently at first (1 min work, 1 min rest) until he could sustain 3 to 5 min of work comfortably and within the THR range.

Chapter 14

Exercise Leadership and Exercise Programs

OBJECTIVES

The reader will be able to:

- Distinguish between low-intensity exercise programs recommended for everyone, systematically structured exercise programs for those interested in improving functional capacity, and programs aimed at achieving performance goals
- Describe the characteristics of a good exercise leader
- Describe the factors related to a high and low probability of participation
- Describe safety and clothing considerations relative to walking and running programs
- Describe the balance between duration and intensity in a typical walking program, and indicate activities used in walking programs to improve enjoyment and adherence
- Outline appropriate walk-jog-walk intervals used at the beginning of a jogging program
- Describe the activities done in a swimming pool, other than lap swimming, that can be an effective part of an aerobic exercise program
- Provide recommendations regarding low- and high-impact dance-exercise programs relative to the beginner, and indicate the typical kinds of exercises included in such programs
- Indicate how exercise intensity is monitored in an exercise session
- Describe a circuit-training program using aerobic and strength-training equipment

Terms

The reader will be able to define or describe:

Circuit training	Health Fitness Director
Exercise Leader	Health Fitness Instructor (HFI)
Exercise Specialist	Leadership
Exercise Test Technologist	Program Director

The purpose of a fitness program must be kept uppermost in the HFI's mind. The HFI is trying to help people include appropriate physical activity as a vital part of their lifestyles. This assumes that the participants understand what is appropriate, have sufficient skills to achieve satisfaction from the activities, and have the intrinsic motivation to continue to be active for the rest of their lives. Thus HFIs try to help people increase their physical fitness levels in ways that are psychologically, mentally, and socially relevant and appealing.

EFFECTIVE LEADERSHIP

To obtain and maintain cardiorespiratory fitness, a person must participate regularly in some form of dynamic, aerobic, physical activity. The problem is that over 50% of those who begin a fitness program drop out, and at present only 10% of Americans are involved in regular vigorous physical activity (2). Why are so few people involved? Why is the dropout rate so high?

Figure 14.1a summarizes the factors related to a high probability of participation, and Figure 14.1b, the factors associated with a low probability of participation. What must be clear to the HFI *and* the exercise leaders is that there are a wide variety of factors affecting people's involvement in personal or supervised exercise programs. In general, better educated, self-motivated individuals who enjoy physical activity and believe in the health outcomes associated with physical activity are more likely to exercise on a regular basis (see Figure 14.1a). In contrast, individuals with a high risk of CHD and who hold blue-collar jobs are less likely to be involved (see Figure 14.1b). It would appear that the ones with the greatest need to exercise are the least likely to become involved. However, more than personal characteristics are involved in the decision.

Support from one's spouse or partner, family, physician, and peers seems to drive involvement, but this must be viewed against the variable of perceived convenience of facilities. Those with poor time-management and goal-setting skills are less likely to be successful (Figures 14.1a and 14.1b). What does this say about the HFI's role in providing exercise leadership? It is clear that exercise leadership involves much more than exercise!

Henry Kissinger is cited as saying that a leader is one who can take people from where they are to where they have not been (11). This is very true for the exercise

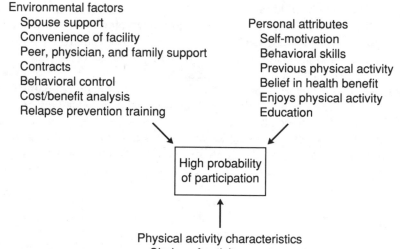

Figure 14.1a summarizes content (Environmental factors, Personal attributes, Physical activity characteristics → High probability of participation)

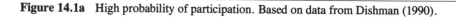

Figure 14.1a   High probability of participation. Based on data from Dishman (1990).

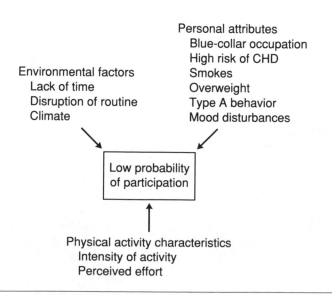

Figure 14.1b   Low probability of participation. Based on data from Dishman (1990).

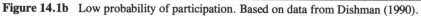

leader, who must counter the negative influences bearing on the portion of the population most in need of physical activity. We normally think that a HFI

- **screens** individuals relative to health status,
- **evaluates** various fitness components,
- **prescribes** activities at the appropriate intensity, duration, and frequency consistent with test results and personal goals,
- **leads** individuals or groups in appropriate activities,
- **monitors** participants' responses within an exercise session,
- **modifies** activities depending on environmental and other factors,
- **records** progress and problems,
- **responds** to emergencies, and
- **refers** problems to appropriate health professionals.

Leadership means more than simply taking a class through its paces. There is a need to make the participant feel welcome, generate motivation within the person or group, and be a friend. To do all these things, the exercise leader must develop interpersonal skills. A summary of these leadership abilities follows.

Certification

Over the past 15 years a variety of organizations have developed certification and education programs to promote exercise programming in preventive and rehabilitative settings. One of the earliest to do so was the American College of Sports Medicine (ACSM). Qualification in these certification areas requires the applicant to have a specific knowledge base and demonstrate specific behaviors. The current certification programs (1) include

- **Exercise Leader**—qualified to lead exercise "on the floor";
- **Health Fitness Instructor (HFI)**—qualified in exercise testing, prescription, and leadership in preventive programs;
- **Health Fitness Director**—qualified as a HFI and responsible for administration in preventive programs;
- **Exercise Test Technologist**—qualified in exercise testing in preventive and rehabilitative programs;
- **Preventive/Rehabilitative Exercise Specialist**—qualified in exercise testing, prescription, and leadership for all populations; and
- **Preventive/Rehabilitative Program Director**—qualified as an Exercise Specialist and responsible for administration, community education programs, research and development, and so forth, in preventive and rehabilitative programs.

These certifications are considered the "standard" by many in the fitness and cardiac-rehabilitation areas. However, there are a variety of other certification programs, some especially related to unique aspects of exercise leadership. We will mention these as specific areas of exercise are discussed.

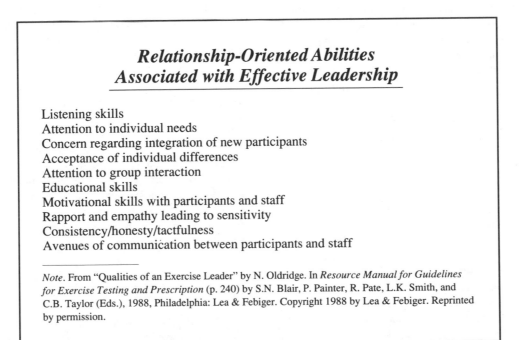

Relationship-Oriented Abilities Associated with Effective Leadership

Listening skills
Attention to individual needs
Concern regarding integration of new participants
Acceptance of individual differences
Attention to group interaction
Educational skills
Motivational skills with participants and staff
Rapport and empathy leading to sensitivity
Consistency/honesty/tactfulness
Avenues of communication between participants and staff

Note. From "Qualities of an Exercise Leader" by N. Oldridge. In *Resource Manual for Guidelines for Exercise Testing and Prescription* (p. 240) by S.N. Blair, P. Painter, R. Pate, L.K. Smith, and C.B. Taylor (Eds.), 1988, Philadelphia: Lea & Febiger. Copyright 1988 by Lea & Febiger. Reprinted by permission.

Role Model

The authors of this book clearly support the notion that the HFI should be a role model. The idea of an overfat, out-of-shape exercise leader is one whose time has passed. A leader must plan appropriate activities, evaluate the progress of the participants, provide incentives, and so forth, but the leadership associated with many exercise programs is in the form of quiet subtle value statements that do not require words. The HFI's presence and behaviors, consistent with a healthy lifestyle, add much meaning and value to her or his words and programs.

Program Planning

All activity programs must have daily, weekly, and monthly plans to provide appropriate activities, meet the needs of the participants, and reduce the chance of boredom. This planning allows the HFI to judge the usefulness of the activity and encourage systematic modification from one month to the next. If the HFI is working with individuals who exercise on their own, then the reasonableness of detailed activities becomes obvious. The value of the feedback received from these individuals depends on the information they were originally given at the start of their program. The following comments can be applied to both group and individual exercise programs.

Variety

A program needs to have variety built in as a cornerstone. Some elements are a part of each exercise session: warm-up and stretching, a stimulus phase, and cool-down. The variety comes in the form of different exercises used in each part of a session, short educational messages presented to the class while they are stretching or cooling down, or the use of games to add spice to routine exercises. The most important thing is to plan the activity sessions far enough in advance to minimize repetition and maximize variety.

Control

The exercise leader must have control over the exercise session. This is especially true in the use of games, where the intensity is not as easily controlled as in jogging. Control implies an ability to modify the session as needed to meet the THR and total work goals of each individual. Some people will have to slow down, and others may need encouragement to increase intensity. The element of control (at a distance) for people who exercise on their own can be provided by using written guidelines about what to do and when to move from

one stage to the next. In addition, specific information should be provided about symptoms that indicate inappropriate responses to exercise.

Monitoring and Record Keeping

Keeping track of a participant's response to the exercise session will give clues about that individual's adaptation to that particular session and about overall, day-to-day changes. This information is important for updating exercise prescriptions and answering specific questions the participant may raise. Each exercise class should have regular pauses to check HR and determine whether individuals are close to their THRs. Rather than keeping track of a large number of 10-s THRs, ask each participant to indicate the number of beats over or under the 10-s goal. This increases the participant's awareness of the THR and indicates how the intensity of the exercise should be adjusted to stay on target.

Each person's HR response is probably the best and most objective indicator of his or her adjustment to an exercise session, but do not stop with that. Elicit information about how the participant feels in general; ask about any new pains, aches, or strange sensations. Record keeping should include a daily attendance check, a weekly weighing, a regular BP check (if appropriate), and a column asking for comments (e.g., THR, rating of perceived exertion, symptoms). An example of such a form is the Daily Activity Form. This information allows the HFI to make better recommendations about the participants' exercise programs and refer them to appropriate professionals if needed.

The point we have emphasized throughout this section on exercise leadership is the need for the leader to help the participant. The HFI who is interested in ways to increase leadership qualities should find the Behavioral Strategies list helpful.

PROGRESSION OF ACTIVITIES

Sedentary people who want to begin a fitness program should follow a logical sequence of fitness activities. Low-intensity activity should be encouraged for everyone, and a systematic program of activities should be provided to help participants achieve an increase in functional capacity. The following paragraphs summarize our recommendations on how this can be accomplished.

Phase 1—Regular Walking

The first phase, for sedentary individuals, is to get them in the habit of including exercise as a part of their weekly patterns. The major fitness goal is to be able to

Daily Activity Form

Name: _____

Target weight: _____   Target-heart-rate zone: _____

Week	Day	Weight	Resting BP	Resting HR	Exercise HR	RPE	Signs	Symptoms	Comments
1	Mon								
	Wed								
	Fri								
2	Mon								
	Wed								
	Fri								
3	Mon								
	Wed								
	Fri								
4	Mon								
	Wed								
	Fri								

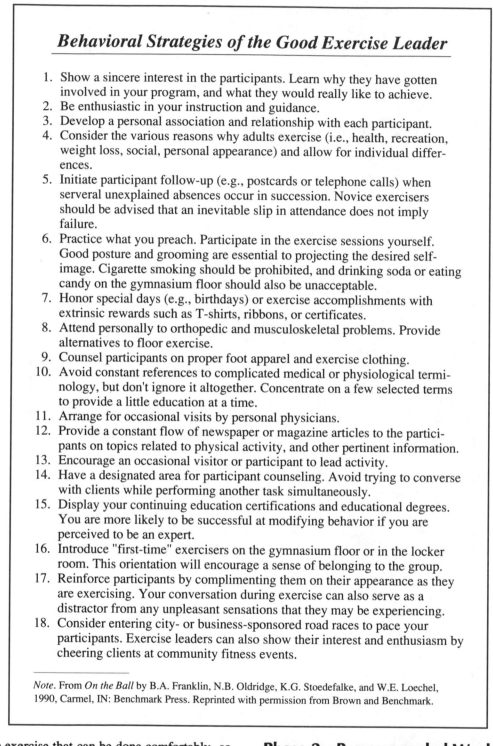

Behavioral Strategies of the Good Exercise Leader

1. Show a sincere interest in the participants. Learn why they have gotten involved in your program, and what they would really like to achieve.
2. Be enthusiastic in your instruction and guidance.
3. Develop a personal association and relationship with each participant.
4. Consider the various reasons why adults exercise (i.e., health, recreation, weight loss, social, personal appearance) and allow for individual differences.
5. Initiate participant follow-up (e.g., postcards or telephone calls) when serveral unexplained absences occur in succession. Novice exercisers should be advised that an inevitable slip in attendance does not imply failure.
6. Practice what you preach. Participate in the exercise sessions yourself. Good posture and grooming are essential to projecting the desired self-image. Cigarette smoking should be prohibited, and drinking soda or eating candy on the gymnasium floor should also be unacceptable.
7. Honor special days (e.g., birthdays) or exercise accomplishments with extrinsic rewards such as T-shirts, ribbons, or certificates.
8. Attend personally to orthopedic and musculoskeletal problems. Provide alternatives to floor exercise.
9. Counsel participants on proper foot apparel and exercise clothing.
10. Avoid constant references to complicated medical or physiological terminology, but don't ignore it altogether. Concentrate on a few selected terms to provide a little education at a time.
11. Arrange for occasional visits by personal physicians.
12. Provide a constant flow of newspaper or magazine articles to the participants on topics related to physical activity, and other pertinent information.
13. Encourage an occasional visitor or participant to lead activity.
14. Have a designated area for participant counseling. Avoid trying to converse with clients while performing another task simultaneously.
15. Display your continuing education certifications and educational degrees. You are more likely to be successful at modifying behavior if you are perceived to be an expert.
16. Introduce "first-time" exercisers on the gymnasium floor or in the locker room. This orientation will encourage a sense of belonging to the group.
17. Reinforce participants by complimenting them on their appearance as they are exercising. Your conversation during exercise can also serve as a distractor from any unpleasant sensations that they may be experiencing.
18. Consider entering city- or business-sponsored road races to pace your participants. Exercise leaders can also show their interest and enthusiasm by cheering clients at community fitness events.

Note. From *On the Ball* by B.A. Franklin, N.B. Oldridge, K.G. Stoedefalke, and W.E. Loechel, 1990, Carmel, IN: Benchmark Press. Reprinted with permission from Brown and Benchmark.

increase the exercise that can be done comfortably, so no emphasis on intensity is necessary at this point. The person starts with the distance that can be walked easily without pain or fatigue, then gradually increases the distance and pace until about 4 mi can be walked briskly every other day. Those with an orthopedic limitation can substitute a weight-supported activity such as cycling, rowing, or swimming.

Phase 2—Recommended Work Levels for a Fitness Base

Once Phase 1 is accomplished, the person is taught about recommended levels of work for fitness changes (see chapter 13). A work-relief interval-training program is introduced—jogging is the work, and walking is the relief. So the person walks, jogs a few steps, then walks, and so forth. Gradually, jogging covers more distance than walking, until the person can jog continuously for 2 to 3 mi at target heart rate (THR). This can also be done for those interested in cycling and swimming (see later). For those interested in aerobic dance, the transition should be from the walking program to a low-intensity, low-impact class.

Phase 3—Variety of Fitness Activities

The first two phases are generally recommended for everyone (with alternative activities for people who cannot or choose not to jog—such as cycling, dancing, or running in water). Phase 3, on the other hand, is quite individualized, based on the person's interests. The purpose is to promote the continued activity habit. Some people prefer to continue to stretch, walk, and jog, some prefer to exercise alone, and others (the majority) enjoy working out with others. Some people like cooperative and relatively low-level competitive activities, and others like the thrill of competition. Some enjoy a variety of different movement forms; others enjoy repeating the same activity. The HFI must provide an atmosphere where people feel free to try new things without embarrassment and allow individuals to choose from among a variety of options for their fitness activities.

WALK/JOG/RUN PROGRAMS

During walking, at least one foot is in contact with the ground at all times. In jogging and running, more muscular force is exerted to propel the body completely off the ground, causing a nonsupport phase. The distinction between jogging and running is not as clearly defined. Some people view the speed as being the difference, but no commonly accepted speed criterion for running exists, although 6 mi $\cdot$ hr^{-1} is often mentioned. Others distinguish between the two by the intent of the participant—a jogger is simply interested in exercise, whereas a runner trains to achieve performance goals in road races.

General Considerations

There are a variety of factors common to both walking and jogging that need to be discussed before we begin a presentation of how to institute walking and jogging programs.

Footwear

Any comfortable pair of good, well-supported shoes can be worn for a beginning walking program. The serious walker and all joggers should invest in appropriate shoes having well-padded heels that are higher than the soles, and a fitted heel cup. The shoes should be flexible enough to bend easily. The same kind of socks that will be worn while exercising should be worn during the fitting to ensure a comfortable and proper fit. Only the serious competitive runner needs racing shoes, which are a lighter weight and offer less cushioning.

Clothing

The weather conditions and vigorousness of the activity determine the amount and type of clothing to be worn. Warm weather dictates light, preferably cotton, loose-fitting clothing. Nothing should be worn that prevents perspiration from reaching the outside air. A brimmed hat should cover the head on hot, sunny days. For the jogger, long pants are probably not needed until the temperature (windchill factor considered) drops below 40 °F.

During cold weather, the jogger should dress in layers for the flexibility of removing or adding clothing when necessary. Wool and the new polypropylene fabrics are good choices for extreme cold, but most joggers have a tendency to overdress. A hat, preferably a wool stocking cap, that can be pulled down over the forehead and ears also should be worn. Gloves or mittens are also a necessity. Cotton socks worn as mittens are useful not only to keep hands warm but also to act as "wipers" for the sniffling nose that often accompanies cold-weather jogging.

Surface

The surface for walkers is not as crucial as it is for joggers, although some walkers need a soft surface, such as grass or a running track with a shock-absorbent surface. Many people prefer exercising off of the track, but regular jogging on hard surfaces such as concrete or blacktop can lead to stress problems in the ankle, knee, and hip joints and in the lower back. Joggers need to observe special precautions when running on the road: jog facing traffic, assume cars at crossroads do not see joggers, and beware of cracks and curbs. Running cross-country usually means running on a softer surface, but joggers must be aware of the uneven terrain and the increased potential for ankle injuries.

KEY POINT. Educate your participants that for safety when walking or jogging, they should

- move toward the oncoming traffic,
- yield the right of way (cars are bigger and can hurt them),
- not listen to music while exercising on a busy street, and listen for the traffic, and
- use well-lighted streets, or running tracks on school grounds.

Walking

The advantages of walking include its convenience, practicality, and naturalness. Walking is an excellent activity, especially for people who are overfat, and poorly conditioned and whose joints cannot handle the stresses of jogging.

As with all exercise programs, the participants begin with warm-up activities and perhaps some static stretching before the actual walk. The walk should begin at a slow speed and gradually increase to a pace that feels comfortable to the participant. The arms should swing freely, and the trunk should be kept erect with a slight backward pelvic tilt. The feet should be pointing forward at all times. Many walkers have taken to malls, which provide air-conditioned comfort and a smooth surface and are usually within a short, convenient drive.

Walking programs can progress by increasing the distance and/or the speed. Participants should gradually increase their distances until they can easily walk 4 mi at a brisk pace. Thinking about jogging or achieving the THR in an aerobic dance class is not necessary until the 4-mi walking goal can be reached. The following Walking Program is graduated and leads to an activity level needed for those who wish to start a jogging program.

The question is, can you make walking interesting for a class of 30 to 40 participants? An exercise leader must emphasize variety to keep interest high in such situations. Some ways you might do this are to

- have participants follow the leader over hill and dale, up and down steps or slopes, with the walking speed changing from time to time;
- have the group do "line-walking" on a track, in which the person at the end of the line must walk faster to catch up to the front of the line, which, as a whole, moves at a steady pace—giving each person an interval-type workout;
- add a ball to the front of the line-walking line, and have participants pass it to the side or overhead until it reaches the end of the line, at which time the last person dribbles to the front and restarts the process;

- vary the activity used to reach the front of the line-walking line, with people skipping, jogging, and so on;
- vary the length of the line-walking line so that "teams" can be formed, and control the overall pace by balancing the teams and checking the THR;
- plan a game of "it" in a gym or field where all participants must walk, and exert control by defining the boundaries; and
- establish a distance goal for a 15-week walking class—such as "we will walk to Nashville (180 mi)"—and use a large map to monitor each participant's progress from week to week, using stick pins, and award T-shirts or hold a country-western party when everyone finishes.

Jogging

No single factor determines when an individual can begin jogging. A person who can walk about 4 mi briskly but is unable to reach the THR range by walking should consider a jogging program to make additional improvements in CRF. A slow to moderate walker whose HR is within the THR zone should increase the distance and/or speed of walking rather than begin jogging. Also, the ability of the individual's joints to withstand the additional stresses of jogging should be considered. Remember, walking may be the first and only activity for a large number of people, and it is more important that they stay active than move up the scale to more intense activities.

The techniques of jogging are basically the same as walking. In jogging, there is a greater flexion of the knee of the recovery leg, and the arms are bent more at the elbows. The arm swing is exaggerated slightly but should still be in the forward/backward direction. The heel makes the first contact with the ground; then the foot immediately rolls forward to the ball of the foot and then to the toes. As speed increases, the landing foot may contact the ground closer to a flat-footed position. Breathing is done through both the nose and mouth. Common faults of the beginning jogger include breathing with the mouth closed, insufficiently bending the knee during the recovery phase, and swinging the arms across the body.

Many people begin jogging at too high a speed, which results in an inability to continue for a sufficient length of time to accomplish the desired amount of total work; often this causes a dislike of the activity. This problem can be prevented by jogging at a speed slow enough to allow conversation, and using work-relief intervals, which for beginners is slow jogging for a few

Walking Program

Rules

1. Start at a level that is comfortable to you
2. Be aware of new aches or pains.
3. Don't progress to the next level if you are not comfortable.
4. Monitor your heart rate and record it.
5. It would be healthful to walk at least every other day.

Stage	Duration	Heart rate	Comments
1	15 min		
2	20 min		
3	25 min		
4	30 min		
5	30 min		
6	30 min		
7	35 min		
8	40 min		
9	45 min		
10	45 min		
11	45 min		
12	50 min		
13	55 min		
14	60 min		
15	60 min		
16	60 min		
17	60 min		
18	60 min		
19	60 min		
20	60 min		

Note. From *Fitness Leader's Handbook* by B.D. Franks and E.T. Howley, 1989, Champaign, IL: Human Kinetics. This form may be copied by the fitness leader for distribution to participants.

seconds, then walking, then slow jogging, and so forth. Participants should be reassured that they will be walking less and/or jogging more as they become more fit. An example of such a progression is shown in the Jogging Program.

After a person has progressed to the point where 2 or 3 mi can be jogged continuously within the THR zone, several approaches to a jogging program are available. A person can just go out and jog 3 or 4 times a week, with the only plan being to exercise at an

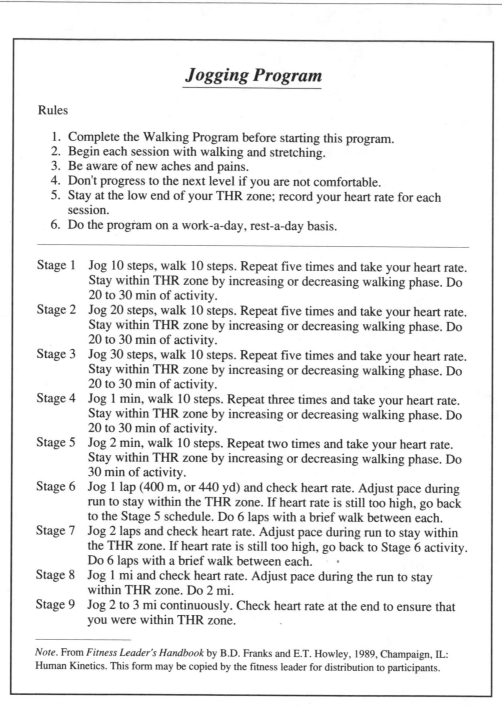

Jogging Program

Rules

1. Complete the Walking Program before starting this program.
2. Begin each session with walking and stretching.
3. Be aware of new aches and pains.
4. Don't progress to the next level if you are not comfortable.
5. Stay at the low end of your THR zone; record your heart rate for each session.
6. Do the program on a work-a-day, rest-a-day basis.

Stage 1   Jog 10 steps, walk 10 steps. Repeat five times and take your heart rate. Stay within THR zone by increasing or decreasing walking phase. Do 20 to 30 min of activity.

Stage 2   Jog 20 steps, walk 10 steps. Repeat five times and take your heart rate. Stay within THR zone by increasing or decreasing walking phase. Do 20 to 30 min of activity.

Stage 3   Jog 30 steps, walk 10 steps. Repeat five times and take your heart rate. Stay within THR zone by increasing or decreasing walking phase. Do 20 to 30 min of activity.

Stage 4   Jog 1 min, walk 10 steps. Repeat three times and take your heart rate. Stay within THR zone by increasing or decreasing walking phase. Do 20 to 30 min of activity.

Stage 5   Jog 2 min, walk 10 steps. Repeat two times and take your heart rate. Stay within THR zone by increasing or decreasing walking phase. Do 30 min of activity.

Stage 6   Jog 1 lap (400 m, or 440 yd) and check heart rate. Adjust pace during run to stay within the THR zone. If heart rate is still too high, go back to the Stage 5 schedule. Do 6 laps with a brief walk between each.

Stage 7   Jog 2 laps and check heart rate. Adjust pace during run to stay within the THR zone. If heart rate is still too high, go back to Stage 6 activity. Do 6 laps with a brief walk between each.

Stage 8   Jog 1 mi and check heart rate. Adjust pace during the run to stay within THR zone. Do 2 mi.

Stage 9   Jog 2 to 3 mi continuously. Check heart rate at the end to ensure that you were within THR zone.

Note. From *Fitness Leader's Handbook* by B.D. Franks and E.T. Howley, 1989, Champaign, IL: Human Kinetics. This form may be copied by the fitness leader for distribution to participants.

intensity that will elevate the HR to the training zone for a predetermined minimum length of time (or distance), with the option to go longer (or farther) on days when so desired. Other people do better with a specific program to follow that gives progressive speed and distance goals, even if they do not have plans for competition.

As for the walking class mentioned earlier, the HFI should include variety in a jogging program, and the same types of modifications cited earlier for the walking program would be appropriate. In addition, in some communities where there are established exercise or fitness trails, one can combine walking/jogging with specific exercises for all parts of the body. "Fun runs" are often held in many communities; the goal is to finish the distance, and a small prize is usually awarded.

Joggers who are not fast enough to compete successfully in road races may enjoy other types of competition, such as prediction runs, in which speed does not determine the winner. The purpose of a prediction run is to see which jogger comes closest to her or his predicted time of finishing, which is declared before the race. A "handicapped" run does require joggers to know and declare their previous fastest times for the distance. A percentage (80% to 100%) of the time difference between the fastest runner's declared time and each other runner's time is subtracted from each runner's actual finish time. For example, suppose runner A's fastest previous time is 18 min for 3 mi; runner B's, 19 min; and runner C's, 20 min. Forty-eight seconds (0.8 × 60-s difference between A and B) is subtracted from B's finish time, and 96 s (0.8 × 120-s difference) is subtracted from runner C's. Suppose runner A completes the race in 17:50, runner B in 18:30, and C in 20:10. The adjusted finish times would be runner A = 17:50 (actual time); runner B = 17:42 (18:30 − 48); and C = 18:34 (20:10 − 96). Runner B is the winner. Another method of handicapping a race is to stagger the start according to each jogger's previous best time, with the slowest runner starting first, the fastest last. The first one over the finish line is the winner. Teams can be formed in which each four-member team, for example, could have one runner from each of four groups classified by running speed.

Competitive Running

In almost all communities there are road races sponsored by track clubs and service organizations as a means of raising funds, many for worthy purposes. Each entrant pays a registration fee, and most of the races have gender and age divisions, with prizes awarded to the top finishers, both overall and in each division. Usually every finisher receives an award, such as a certificate or T-shirt. The race distances range between 1 mi (often considered a "fun run") and 100 mi, but the most common are the 5K (3.1 mi) and 10K (6.2 mi). Remember that fitness participants should not be pressured to enter road races by those who enjoy them.

KEY POINT.   The HFI should consider entering races with interested participants to help them select a starting spot and establish a pace, and to provide encouragement. This may help them make a good transition from a jogging group to an individualized jogging program.

It must be remembered that those who train for performance goals will be working at the top part of the THR range, 6 to 7 days per week, and for more than 30 to 40 min per exercise session. Such programs are bound to result in more injuries, and the HFI should encourage those with such goals to have an alternative activity that can be done when they are recovering from injuries.

CYCLING

Riding a bicycle or stationary exercise cycle is another good fitness activity. Some people who have problems walking, jogging, or playing sports may be able to cycle without difficulty. The Cycling Program follows the guidelines (chapter 13) for making CRF improvements. Although bicycles and terrains vary widely, checking THR allows the cyclist to adjust the speed so that she or he is working at the appropriate intensity. Generally, a person covers three to four times the distance cycling compared to jogging. (e.g., a person works up to 3 mi jogging or 9 to 12 mi cycling per workout). The seat should be comfortable, and its height should be adjusted so that the knee is slightly bent at the bottom of the pedaling stroke.

GAMES

One of the characteristics of children that is often lost in adulthood is a sense of playfulness. A child does not feel a need to justify spending time playing a game just for the fun of it. One of the attributes that seems to be present in coronary-prone behavior is the inability to appreciate play for its own sake. Perhaps one of the things a good fitness program can do for people is provide them with activities that increase both fitness and playfulness.

For games to be an effective part of a fitness program, certain elements must be present:

- **Enjoyment.** This requires a balance of cooperation and competition, continued participation by everyone, and the chance for everyone to be a winner.
- **Inclusion.** A key ingredient for a fitness game is that everyone is included. This may mean modifying the rules.
- **Vigor.** The main body of the workout should include games in which all people are continuously active in the THR range.
- **Cooperation.** Having small groups solve problems together to accomplish fitness tasks can be enjoyable and healthy.
- **Competition.** Competition is not to be avoided, but little emphasis should be put on winning, and the game should not be used to exclude people from participating.
- **Skill.** Some fitness games may require certain minimum levels of skill that can be taught as part of the fitness program.

Cycling Program

Rules

1. Seat is comfortable for you.
2. Use either a regular bicycle or a stationary exercise cycle.
3. If you are starting at Stage 1, simply get used to riding 1 or 2 mi. Don't be concerned about time or reaching the lower end of your THR zone.

Stage	Distance (mi)	THR (% HRmax)	Time (min)	Frequency (days/week)
1	1-2	—	—	3
2	1-2	60	8-12	3
3	3-5	60	15-25	3
4	6-8	70	25-35	3
5	6-9	70	25-35	4
6	10-15	70	40-60	4
7	10-15	80	35-50	4-5

Note. From *Fitness Leader's Handbook* by B.D. Franks and E.T. Howley, 1989, Champaign, IL: Human Kinetics. This form may be copied by the fitness leader for distribution to participants.

Special Considerations

The warm-up and cool-down activities can be done for people at any fitness level. However, the more vigorous games usually involve high-intensity bursts, stopping, starting, and quickly changing directions. They are not recommended for the early stages of a fitness program. Some additional stretching and easy movements in different directions should be included as part of the warm-up. Obviously the space, number of people, equipment, and so forth have to be considered in the selection of activities. The leader must emphasize safety and should change the rules immediately when something is not working. A variety of games should be offered, so that people with different skill levels can participate. When large groups are involved in activities, the activities should be changed frequently to maintain interest. Finally, in addition to warm-up and cool-down activities, higher and lower intensity activities should be alternated to prevent undue fatigue. People should be encouraged to go at their own paces. THR should be checked periodically to ensure that people are within their ranges.

Fitness Games

The classes of Fitness Games and Activities are summarized in Box 14.6 (5). In general, the level of control varies from that associated with circle and line activities to those with few rules, such as keep-away. Games can involve diverse muscle groups, using the body weight as a resistance, and simultaneously encourage the continued development of balance and coordination, which are not necessarily outcomes of walking, jogging, or exercising with fixed equipment. *On the Ball* (3), a book written specifically to encourage games in a fitness setting, should be a part of every exercise leader's library. In addition, *The New Games Book* (10) provides a playful, fun, and inclusive approach to games for various numbers of people.

AQUATIC ACTIVITIES

Aquatic activities can be a major part of a person's exercise program or can be the needed relief from other forms of exercise, especially when a person is injured. The intensity of the activity can be graded to suit the needs of the least and the most fit, from the recent postmyocardial infarction patient to the endurance athletes. HR can be checked at regular intervals to see whether THR has been reached, and a caloric expenditure goal can be achieved, given the high energy requirement associated with aquatic activities. Individuals with orthopedic problems who cannot run, dance, or play games, can exercise in water. The water supports the

Fitness Games and Activities

1. Skills and games with balls of various sizes.
   The size and type of ball can lead to innovative use—for instance, the cage ball can be used as a substitute for a basketball. Examples of other balls include tennis balls, volleyballs, playground balls, basketballs, medicine balls, handballs, softballs, mush balls, and nerf balls.
2. Activities with apparatus. Examples include hoola hoops, frisbees, paddle rackets, skip ropes, skittles, "quoits," surgical tubing, culverts, and play bouys.
3. Chasing games. Examples include tag, chain tag, fox and geese, and dodge ball.
4. Relays with and without apparatus. Examples such as running, hopping, rolling, crawling, and dribbling with hands and feet.
5. Stunts and contests. Including dual activities such as balancing stunts, forward rolls, backward rolls, strength moves, push-ups, sit-ups, and limited combatives such as rooster fights and partner sparring.
6. Lead-up games for major sport games. Examples are soccer, tennis, basketball, volleyball, handball, and football, often with rules adjusted to fit the level of skill and capacity of the participants.
7. Children's games. Activities such as skittle ball, four square, and bounce ball.

Note. From "Organization of an Exercise Testing Session" by Michael Geise. In *Resource Manual for Guidelines for Exercise Testing and Prescription* (p. 246) by S.N. Blair, P. Painter, R. Pate, L.K. Smith, and C.B. Taylor (Eds.), 1988, Philadelphia: Lea & Febiger. Copyright 1988 by Lea & Febiger. Adapted by permission.

person's body weight, and problems associated with weight-bearing joints are minimized.

Target Heart Rate

One consistent finding is that the maximal HR response to a swimming test is about 14 beats • min^{-1} lower than that found in a maximal treadmill test. This suggests that for swimming, THR should be shifted downward (2 beats less for a 10-s count) to achieve the 60% to 80% $\dot{V}O_2$max goal associated with an endurance training effect (8).

Progression

Swimming activities can be graded not only by varying the speed of the swim, but also by varying the activity. A postmyocardial infarction patient with an extremely low functional capacity benefits from simply walking through the water. People with recent bypass surgery benefit from moving the arms as they walk across the pool. The following are examples of the types of activities that can be used in aquatic exercise programs. The reader is referred to the book *Hydroaerobics* by Krasevec and Grimes (7) and to the Aquatic Exercise Association (P.O. Box 497, Port Washington, WI 53074) for information on certification programs for this speciality.

Side-of-Pool Activities

A wide variety of activities can be done while holding on to the side of the pool. These range from simple movements of the legs to the side, front, or back while holding on to the side of the pool with one hand, to practicing a variety of kicks that can ultimately be used while swimming. Range-of-motion-type movements are a good way to warm up before undertaking the more vigorous activities of walking or jogging across the pool.

Walking and Jogging Across the Pool

A person with a low functional capacity can begin an aquatic program by simply walking across the shallow end of the pool. The water offers resistance to the movement while supporting the body weight, resulting in a reduced downward load on the ankles, knees, and hips. The arms can be involved in the activity to simulate a swimming motion; this increases the range of motion of the arms and shoulder girdle. The speed and form of the walk can be changed as the person becomes accustomed to the activity. The person can walk with long strides with the head just above the water or do a side step across the pool. Lastly, the person can practice jogging across the pool with the water at chest height. Remember to check to see whether THR has been achieved.

Floatation Devices

People with limited skill can use floatation devices (e.g., a life jacket or kick board). The extra resistance offered by the jacket compensates for the extra buoyancy it provides. The participant can stop periodically to determine whether THR has been reached.

Lap Swimming

The participant must be skilled, to use swimming as a substitute activity for running or cycling. An unskilled swimmer operates at a very high energy cost, even when moving slowly, and may become too fatigued to last for the whole workout. But this doesn't mean that swimming should be eliminated as an option in personal fitness programs. A person can learn to swim over a period of several months, gradually adjusting during that time to the exercise, and become able to use swimming as the primary activity, even if elementary strokes are used. Increasing the number of activities a person can do increases the chance that the person will remain active when something interferes with a primary activity.

Lap swimming should be approached the same way as lap running: warming up with stretching activities, starting slowly, taking frequent breaks to check the pulse rate, and gradually increasing the distance. Remember, the caloric cost of swimming compared to the cost of running is about a 1:4 ratio. If jogging a total distance of 1 mi is a reasonable goal in someone's physical activity program, then swimming 400 m is equivalent in terms of energy expenditure. The Swimming Program describes a series of stages that could be included in an endurance swimming program, beginning with walking across the pool. All steps assume that a warm-up has preceded the activity and that a cool-down follows.

The HFI should not view the stages in the Swimming Program as discrete steps that must be followed in a particular order. Two stages can be combined, or games can be introduced, to make the walk-and-jog and width swims more enjoyable. The major point to keep in mind is to gradually increase the intensity and duration of the aquatic activities.

EXERCISE TO MUSIC (AEROBICS, AEROBIC DANCE)

Moving to the rhythm of music is an enjoyable way to participate in exercise. One can join a group at a fitness club or do individual workouts at home with videotapes.

Advantages

Exercise to music has provided an enjoyable fitness activity for many participants—especially women, who have been the majority of those choosing this type of activity, though an increasing number of men are coming to prefer this kind of fitness activity.

Motivation

Music provides motivation to continue exercising. The variety of tempos and rhythms of the different songs keeps the workout exciting and challenges participants to keep up with the beat. Music makes routine exercises fun.

Achievement of Target Heart Rate

Aerobic dance programs can develop all the fitness components. The recommended frequency, intensity, and total work (see chapter 13) can be achieved in exercise-to-music programs and cause gains in $\dot{V}O_2max$ (12). THR can easily be monitored following a music segment, but beginners need to be cautioned about doing too much too soon. A recent review indicated that THR can be achieved with either low- or high-impact routines. Although the energy cost of high-intensity, high-impact aerobic dance was higher than that of low-impact programs for the same routines and music, the activities were not very different when multidirectional movements were included in the low-impact routines (12).

Low Skill Requirements

Movement to music can be adapted to any skill level, because no competition is involved. The only rule is to keep moving at a pace needed to achieve THR. The routines can also be adapted for all ages. Gradual progression within each session, as well as from one workout to the next, is needed to enhance enjoyment.

Swimming Program

Rules

1. Start at a level that is comfortable for you.
2. Don't progress to the next stage if you are not comfortable with current one.
3. Monitor and record your heart rate.

Stage 1   In chest-deep water, walk across the width of the pool four times and see if you are close to THR. Gradually increase the duration of the walk until you can do two 10-min walks at THR.

Stage 2   In chest-deep water, walk across and jog back. Repeat twice and see if you are close to THR. Gradually increase the duration of the jogging until you can complete four 5-min jogs at THR.

Stage 3   In chest-deep water, walk across and swim back (any stroke). Use kickboard or flotation device if needed. Repeat this cycle twice and see if you are at THR. Keep up this pattern of walk-swim to do about 20 to 30 min of activity.

Stage 4   In chest-deep water, jog across and swim back (any stroke); repeat and check THR. Gradually decrease the duration of the jog and increase the duration of the swim until four widths can be completed within the THR zone. Accomplish 20 to 30 min of activity per session.

Stage 5   Slowly swim 25 yd, rest 30 s, slowly swim another 25 yd, and check THR. On the basis of the heart rate response, change the speed of the swim and/or the length of the rest period to stay within the THR zone. Gradually increase the number of lengths you can swim (three, then four, etc.) before checking THR.

Stage 6   Increase the duration of continuous swimming until you can accomplish 20 to 30 min without a rest.

Note. From *Fitness Leader's Handbook* by B.D. Franks and E.T. Howley, 1989, Champaign, IL: Human Kinetics. This form may be copied by the fitness leader for distribution to participants.

The HFI needs to be familiar with the types of aerobic dance programs offered in his or her community, because some (e.g., Jazzercize®) may require more knowledge and skill of "dance" movements than other forms. One needs also to be aware of the programs that would be appropriate for different age, skill, and interest groups.

Disadvantages

Injury is always a potential risk in fitness programs, and aerobic dance is no different. A recent review found that about 44% of students and 76% of instructors reported injuries resulting from aerobic dance, with the injury rate being 1 injury per 100 hr of activity for students, and 0.22 to 1.16 injuries per 100 hr for the instructors. However, the severity of the injuries were such that only once in 1,092 to 4,275 hr of participation did an individual have to seek medical attention (4). **It is our recommendation that people should participate in aerobic dance programs only after they can walk about 4 mi without discomfort.** Further, they should move from low-intensity, low-impact sessions to more strenuous sessions using THR as a guide.

Other ways to minimize the risk of injury in aerobic dance are to

- **warm up and cool down with walking and static stretching,**
- **include calf stretching throughout the session,**
- **avoid hyperextension of the back,**
- **bend at least one knee in front hip-flexion exercises,**
- **concentrate on correct standing posture (i.e., pelvis forward, buttocks tight, head and chin up, with shoulders back)**
- **avoid deep knee bends,**

- **keep the knees aligned directly over the feet,**
- **wear shoes with good cushioning and support, and**
- **come all the way down on the heels when jumping.**

Music Selection

Selection of music for different phases of the exercise session sets the tone for the appropriate intensity of warm-up, aerobic phase, and cool-down (6, 9). The music can vary, depending on choice, from top-40 hits to instrumental Muzak. The warm-up starts slowly, with the music tempo about 100 beats $\cdot$ min^{-1}. The cardiorespiratory endurance phase includes increasingly intense aerobic exercises at a faster pace (about 140 beats $\cdot$ min^{-1}). The muscular-fitness phase is at a slower tempo. In the final cool-down, the music tempo and volume decrease to invoke a relaxing conclusion.

An easy way to keep variety of movement within the program is by using one particular music selection for a specific area of the body. Exercises for a specific area of the body can be kept in mind when choosing an appropriate song. For example, the first selection might be used for upper body flexibility, and the second song might be used for lower-body flexibility exercises. As the program progresses in duration or difficulty, two or more music selections can be used for one area of the body. Music selections should be periodically changed for more variety.

Components

There are no set routines; the program can be individualized by the instructor. Suggested components of an exercise session include

- a full-body warm-up (including static and dynamic flexibility exercises),
- exercises for muscular endurance and strength for the arms, legs, thighs, and abdominal region,
- exercises for cardiorespiratory endurance, using a variety of muscle groups; and
- cool-down.

In some programs, the cardiorespiratory segment precedes the muscular-fitness segment. In that case, a short cool-down precedes muscular-fitness exercises.

An easy progression for beginners would include 25 to 30 min of mostly flexibility activities, with light muscular- and cardiorespiratory-endurance activities. A more advanced program would last 45 to 60 min, with longer duration for all of the fitness components (see Exercise to Music outlines).

Warm-Up

For a gradual progression, the program should begin with static stretches for the whole body before dynamic flexibility exercises are performed. Examples of static stretches include neck, arm across the chest, arm to side, crossed-leg hamstring, and achilles/calf (see chapter 10 for additional low-back stretches). Dynamic flexibility includes exercises such as arm circles, side bends, and half-knee bends. The warm-up should continue for 5 to 10 min.

Muscular Endurance

Once the warm-up (or cardiorespiratory and cool-down) activities are completed, the muscular-endurance exercises can be performed for 10 to 20 min. These include variations of side-lying leg lifts, curl-ups, and push-ups.

Cardiorespiratory Endurance

In this segment, movement is done while on the feet, using large muscles (legs) and movements with the arms. Hops, strides, skips, kicks, and jogging variations are used in addition to moving hands and arms to get the HR within the THR zone. Variety in this segment can be accomplished by using stationary exercises on the spot or in a circle, crossing the floor in a line together, or introducing variations with two participants moving down the area between parallel lines or with jogging variations around the room. Other exercises include jumping jacks, step-hops, cross-over steps, toe-heel kicks, and so forth. The duration of this section is 15 to 30 min, with THR taken after every couple of songs. The intensity of this segment can be increased by using more vigorous arm movements or higher hops. Intensity can be decreased by using fewer body parts, slowing the pace, and walking rather than jogging through the movement.

Cool-Down

A cool-down should follow the cardiorespiratory segment. It should start with a lower intensity activity, such as walking, to get the HR back below the THR. Dynamic flexibility exercises should be included, ending with static stretching. If the muscular-fitness phase follows the cardiorespiratory phase, the final cool-down may consist of mainly static stretches.

Aerobic Dance Organizations

There are many aerobic dance organizations that provide opportunities to be certified, as well as educational and professional support materials. They include

Exercise-to-Music Outline for Beginners

Duration (min)	Song (no.)	Exercises
2-3	1	Sitting/standing static flexibility (lower body)
2-3	2	Sitting/standing static flexibility (upper body)
2-3	3	Standing dynamic flexibility
5-6	4	Side-lying flexibility and muscular endurance
	5	Hands and knees flexibility
12	6	Aerobic—stationary
	7	Aerobic—moving
	8	Aerobic—stationary and moving
2-3	9	Cool-down—dynamic
2-3	10	Cool-down—static

Exercise-to-Music Outline for Advanced Participants

Duration (min)	Song (no.)	Exercises
2-3	1	Sitting/standing static flexibility (lower body)
2-3	2	Sitting/standing static flexibility (upper body)
4-5	3	Standing dynamic flexibility
3-4	4	Side-lying muscular endurance
3-4	5	Hands and knees muscular endurance
3-4	6	Sit-ups and push-ups
20-30	7	Aerobic—stationary
	8	Aerobic—crossing
	9	Aerobic—jogging
	10	Peel off
	11	Stationary walk
2-3	12	Cool-down—dynamic
2-3	13	Cool-down—static

- **IDEA**, 2431 Morena Blvd., San Diego, CA 92110
- **AFFA**, 15250 Ventura Blvd., Sherman Oaks, CA 91403-3201
- **Aerobex**, Fort Sanders Medical Center, 1805 Laurel Ave., Knoxville, TN 37916
- **Jazzercize**, 2808 Roosevelt Blvd., Carlsbad, CA 92008

EXERCISE EQUIPMENT

The tradition of walk, jog, run, and dance programs offered by an exercise leader have been supplanted in many fitness clubs by exercise equipment. The equipment includes treadmills, cycle ergometers, ski machines, rowers, climbing ergometers, and stepping devices. The variety of equipment can help a participant stay with an exercise program, as well as provide feedback about the number of calories used. Those with orthopedic limitations can choose weight-supported activities, and those who wish to train for specific performance goals can do so in air-conditioned comfort—although air conditioning may be a problem for participants who plan to engage in races scheduled for hot days, and the issue of acclimatization needs to be addressed for reasons of performance and safety (see chapters 13 and 16).

If a participant plans to buy exercise equipment for

home use, the HFI can help with the decision by encouraging experimentation with all types of equipment and, within each type (e.g., cycle ergometers), as many brands as possible. The cost of the equipment may appear high in the short term, but it may be a wise investment in the long run in terms of health care costs, *provided it is used*.

Generally, fitness clubs provide a variety of strength-training equipment that can be used as part of an overall workout, or as a separate strength-training workout on another day. Recommendations for gains in muscular strength and endurance were presented in chapter 10. The emphasis at the start of a program must be on endurance, low resistance, and high repetitions. As strength and interest increase, for some participants the emphasis may shift to high-resistance, low-repetition workouts.

CIRCUIT TRAINING

Circuit training can be an effective way to conduct an exercise program. The point is to maximize the variety of exercise, distribute the work over a larger muscle mass than could be accomplished with a single form of exercise, and include exercises for all aspects of a fitness session. Circuits can include the following:

- Moving from one piece of exercise equipment to another with a brief rest period between each. A person might exercise for 5 to 10 min (or 50 to 100 kcal) on a cycle ergometer, then on a treadmill, then on a rower, then on a stepper, and so on.
- A typical workout for muscular strength and endurance, in which 2 or 3 sets are done on a specific machine, before moving to the next.
- A circuit set up around the perimeter of a large room with signs posted in discrete locations describing specific exercises that the participant would do during one trip around the circuit. The circuit could include warm-up activities, flexibility activities, strengthening exercises using body weight as a resistance, and, of course, aerobic activities. Beginning, intermediate, and advanced goals specifying the number of repetitions (or duration) can be posted at each station. Build in a station to check the THR following the aerobic exercise stations.

Good examples of walk/jog/run circuits have been in place for the past decade. We are all aware of jogging trails that have signposts along the way indicating specific exercises to do at each stop. They can be found in many cities, and they provide a break in the regular routine of steady jogging or running, while focusing attention on flexibility and strengthening exercises.

SUMMARY

Exercise leaders should be role models for the participants, plan classes to reduce boredom, maintain a high level of control to ensure safety, and monitor and keep records of the participants' responses to each session. The programs themselves should begin with regular walking, progress to rhythmical activities needed to achieve THR, and finally, include games and sport activities to provide enjoyment and variety. Walking programs should be structured to provide clear guidelines to the participant about knowing how much to do, being aware of signs of overexertion, and recording the HR achieved. The jogging program follows the walking program, beginning with short jog/walk intervals and slowly, over weeks, building up to continuous jogging. The HFI should learn to use games as a part of a regular exercise session. They provide variety and are a good distraction from the exercise. Games at appropriate intensities must include, not exclude, participants; so care must be taken in the selection of games. Exercise sessions can be conducted in a pool, even if swimming will not be used as a primary activity. Participants can progress from poolside activities to walking and jogging across the pool, to lap swimming. A series of steps in such a program is provided. Exercise to music has become a popular fitness activity. The music seems to provide motivation to keep up with the activity, and exercise can be adapted to any skill level. Participants must be alert for lower leg problems and must keep track of THR. Music selection should be consistent with the warm-up/stimulus/cool-down phases of the session. Programs for different levels are presented. Circuit-training programs can be designed indoors or outdoors to deal with the components of fitness, add variety to the workout, and distribute the workout over a larger muscle mass.

CASE STUDIES FOR ANALYSIS

14.1. You are making a presentation to a group of adults who have their own neighborhood walking program. What topics should you address to emphasize safety and comfort? (See Appendix A.)

14.2. A participant who has been involved in your walking program for the past 10 weeks asks your advice regarding an aerobic dance class. What would you recommend? (See Appendix A.)

REFERENCES

1. American College of Sports Medicine (1991)
2. Dishman (1990)
3. Franklin, Oldridge, Stoedefalke, and Loechel (1990)
4. Garrick, Requa (1988)
5. Giese (1988)
6. Kisselle and Mazzeo (1983)
7. Krasevec and Grimes (1984)
8. Londeree and Moeschberger (1982)
9. Mazzeo (1984)
10. New Games Foundation (1976)
11. Peters and Waterman (1982)
12. Williford, Scharff-Olson, and Blessing (1989)

SUGGESTED READINGS

Oldridge (1988)

See the Bibliography at the end of the book for a complete source listing.

Chapter 15

ECG and Medications

Daniel Martin

OBJECTIVES

The reader will be able to:

- Describe the basic anatomy of the heart
- Describe the basic electrophysiology of the heart
- Identify the basic electrocardiograph complexes
- Calculate heart rate from electrocardiograph rhythm strips
- Identify the various types of atrioventricular conduction defects and their probable impact on a subject's exercise response
- Identify the normal and abnormal cardiac rhythms and their significance, and predict the probable impact of the abnormal rhythms on exercise performance
- Identify S–T segment depression, and discuss the significance of this abnormality
- Contrast the characteristics of anginal pain and musculoskeletal pain
- List the common categories of prescription medications used to treat cardiovascular and related diseases, some of the members of each category, and the probable impact of these medications on exercise performance

TERMS

The reader will be able to define or describe:

Aneurysm	Myocardial ischemia
Angina pectoris	Myocardium
Anti-arrhythmics	Nicotine gum
Anticoagulants	Premature atrial contraction
Antiglycemic agents	Premature junctional contraction
Antihypertensives	Premature ventricular contraction (PVC)
Atrial fibrillation	P–R interval
Atrial flutter	P–R segment
Atrioventricular (AV) node	Pulmonary valve
Beta-adrenergic blocking medications	Purkinje fibers
(β-blockers)	P wave
Bronchodilators	QRS complex
Bundle branch	Q–T interval
Bundle of His	Q wave
Calcium antagonists	R–R interval
Coronary arteries	R wave
Digitalis	Second-degree AV block
First-degree AV block	Sinus arrhythmia
J point	Sinus bradycardia
Mobitz Type I AV block	Sinus rhythm
Mobitz Type II AV block	Sinus tachycardia
Myocardial infarction (MI)	S–T segment

S–T segment depression
S–T segment elevation
S wave
Third-degree AV block

Tricuspid valve
T wave
Ventricular fibrillation
Ventricular tachycardia

This chapter is not intended to be a complete guide to ECG interpretation and cardiovascular medications; several excellent texts on these topics are listed in the reference section. The purposes of this chapter are to provide the HFI with background information on the basics of ECG analysis and cardiovascular medications as they relate to exercise testing and prescription.

STRUCTURE OF THE HEART

The heart is a muscular organ composed of four chambers. Blood flow through the heart is directed by pressure differences and valves between the chambers. Venous blood from the body enters the right atrium via the inferior and superior vena cava (Figure 15.1). From the right atrium, blood passes through the **tricuspid**

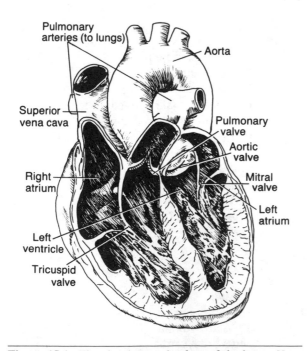

Figure 15.1 The chambers and valves of the heart. *Note.* From *Living Anatomy* (2nd ed.) (p. 199) by J.E. Donnelly, 1990, Champaign, IL: Human Kinetics. Copyright 1990 by Joseph E. Donnelly. Reprinted by permission.

valve into the right ventricle. The right ventricle pumps blood through the **pulmonary valve** into the pulmonary arteries to the lungs. In the lungs, blood gives up carbon dioxide and picks up oxygen. The oxygen-rich blood is returned to the heart via the pulmonary veins emptying into the left atrium. From the left atrium, blood passes through the mitral valve into the left ventricle. The left ventricle pumps oxygenated blood past the aortic valve and into the aorta, coronary arteries, and to the rest of the body. The left ventricle, which generates more pressure than the right ventricle, is thicker and requires a greater blood supply.

Coronary Arteries

The heart muscle, the **myocardium**, does not receive a significant amount of oxygen directly from blood in the atria or ventricles. Oxygenated blood is supplied to the myocardium via the coronary arteries, which branch off from the aorta at the coronary sinus. The two coronary artery systems are the right and left **coronary arteries**. The left main coronary artery follows a course between the left atria and pulmonary artery and branches into the left anterior descending and left circumflex arteries. The left anterior descending artery follows a path along the anterior surface of the heart and lies over the interventricular septum, which separates the right and left ventricles (Figure 15.2). The left circumflex artery follows the groove between the left atrium and left ventricle on the anterior and lateral surfaces of the heart. The right coronary artery follows the groove that separates the atria and ventricles around the posterior surface of the heart, and forms the posterior descending artery or posterior interventricular artery. Numerous smaller arteries branch off from each of the major arteries and form smaller and smaller arteries, finally forming the capillaries in the muscle cells where gas exchange occurs. A major obstruction in any of these coronary arteries results in a reduced blood flow to the myocardium (*myocardial ischemia*) and decreases the ability of the heart to pump blood. If the coronary arteries become blocked and the heart muscle does not receive oxygen, then a portion of the heart muscle might die, which is known as a *myocardial infarction*, or heart attack.

Coronary Veins

Venous drainage of the right ventricle is supplied via the anterior cardiac veins, which normally have two or three major branches and eventually empty into the right atrium. The venous drainage of the left ventricle is primarily provided by the anterior interventricular vein, which roughly follows the same path as the left anterior descending artery, and eventually forms the coronary sinus and empties into the right atrium (Figure 15.2).

OXYGEN USE BY THE HEART

The myocardium is very well-adapted to use oxygen to generate adenosine triphosphate (ATP). Approximately 40% of the volume of a heart muscle cell is composed of mitochondria, the cellular organelle responsible for producing ATP with oxygen. The oxygen consumption of the heart in a resting person is about 8 to 10 ml·min^{-1} per 100 g of myocardium, and the resting oxygen consumption for the body is about 0.35 ml·min^{-1} per 100 g of body mass (1). Myocardial oxygen consumption can increase six- to sevenfold during heavy exercise; in young people the total body oxygen consumption can

easily increase 12 to 15 times. The myocardium has a limited capacity to produce energy via anaerobic pathways; it depends on the delivery of oxygen to the mitochondria to produce ATP. At rest, the whole body extracts only about 25% of the oxygen present in each 100 ml of arterial blood, and the body can meet its need for oxygen by simply extracting more from the blood. In contrast, the heart extracts about 75% of the oxygen available in arterial blood. Consequently, the heart muscle's oxygen needs must be met by increasing the delivery of blood via the coronary arteries. An adequate oxygen supply to the heart is needed not only to allow the heart to pump blood, but to help maintain normal electrical activity, which is covered in the next section.

ELECTROPHYSIOLOGY OF THE HEART

At rest, the insides of myocardial cells are negatively charged and the exteriors of the cells are positively charged. When the cells are depolarized (stimulated), the insides of the cells become positively charged and the exteriors of the cells become negatively charged. If a recording electrode is placed so the wave of stimulation spreads toward the electrode, the ECG records a

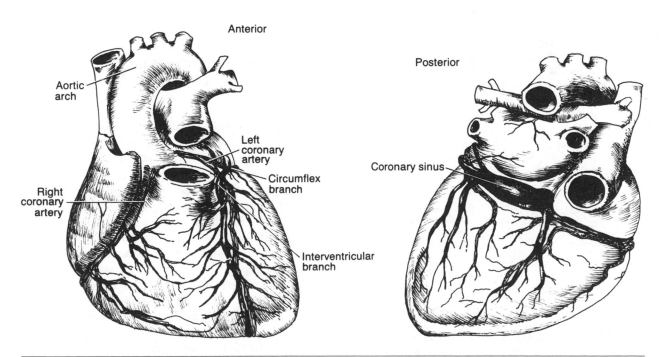

Figure 15.2 Coronary blood vessels. *Note.* From *Living Anatomy* (2nd ed.) (p. 202) by J.E. Donnelly, 1990, Champaign, IL: Human Kinetics. Copyright 1990 by Joseph E. Donnelly. Reprinted by permission.

positive deflection. If the wave of depolarization spreads away from the recording electrode, a negative deflection occurs. When the myocardial muscle cell is completely at rest, or completely stimulated, the electrocardiogram records a flat line, known as the isoelectric line. Following depolarization, the myocardial cell undergoes repolarization to return its electrical state to what it was at rest. The steps leading from rest to complete stimulation to repolarization are shown in Figures 15.3 to 15.7.

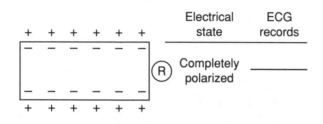

Figure 15.3 Completely polarized. The myocardial cell is at rest and is completely polarized. The electrocardiogram records the isoelectric line.

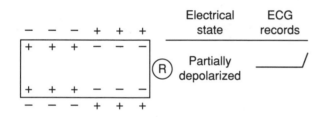

Figure 15.4 Partially depolarized. The heart muscle cell has been stimulated on the left end, and the wave of depolarization (depolarization equals negative charges extracellularly) spreads from the left to the recording electrode on the right. The depolarization moves from the interior of the myocardium to the surface of the heart muscle, and the ECG records a positive deflection. The amplitude of the deflection is proportional to the mass of the myocardium undergoing depolarization.

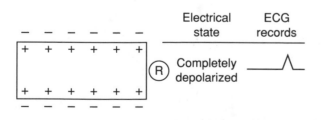

Figure 15.5 Completely depolarized. Depolarization is now complete. The ECG has recorded a positive deflection corresponding to depolarization and is now recording no electrical activity, or the isoelectric potential.

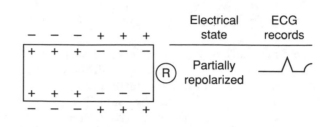

Figure 15.6 Partially repolarized. Repolarization has started from the right and moves to the left. The recording electrode senses a wave of positivity moving away from it, and a positive deflection results. Repolarization is thought to occur in the opposite direction (surface to interior) from depolarization in the human heart and is the reason the ECG complexes for depolarization and repolarization are both normally positive. If repolarization had started on the left and moved to the right, the ECG deflection would have been negative.

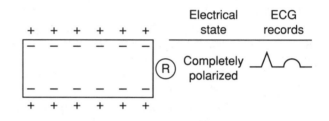

Figure 15.7 Completely polarized. The myocardial cell is now completely repolarized, or in the resting state, and the ECG records the isoelectric line. The myocardial cell is now ready to be depolarized again.

THE CONDUCTION SYSTEM OF THE HEART

The **sinoatrial node** is the normal pacemaker of the heart and is located in the right atrium near the vena cava (see Figure 15.8). Depolarization spreads from the sinoatrial node across the atria and results in the P wave. There are also three intra-atrial conduction tracts within the atria that conduct the wave of depolarization to the **atrioventricular (AV) node**. Impulses travel from the sinoatrial node through the atrial muscle and intra-atrial tracts and enter the atrioventricular node, where the speed of conduction is slowed to allow the atrial contraction to empty blood into the ventricles before the start of ventricular contraction. The **bundle of His** is the conduction pathway that connects the atrioventricular node with bundle branches in the ventricles. The right **bundle branch** splits off the bundle of His and forms ever-smaller branches that serve the right ventricle. The left bundle splits into two major branches

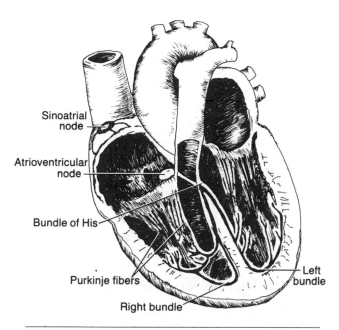

Figure 15.8   The electrical conduction system of the heart. These are the normal pathways used to ensure the rhythmical contraction and relaxation of the chambers of the heart.

that serve the thicker left ventricle. **Purkinje fibers** are the terminal branches of the bundle branches and form the link between the specialized conductive tissue and the muscle fibers.

ELECTROCARDIOGRAM

This section on the analysis of the ECG may appear to be beyond what an HFI should know about the topic. In fact, the physician is the person to make judgments about whether or not an ECG response is normal. However, the HFI must be aware of the basic information related to ECG interpretation to facilitate communication with the physician, program director, and exercise specialist.

A systematic approach to ECG evaluation allows the examiner to determine the heart rate, rhythm, and conduction pathways and to search for signs of ischemia or infarction. Physicians normally evaluate a 12-lead ECG, but for our purposes a single ECG lead is adequate (Figure 15.9). The most commonly used single ECG lead for exercise testing is the CM5, which looks very similar to lead V5 on a 12-lead ECG.

Time and Voltage

ECG paper is marked in a standard manner to allow measurement of time intervals and voltages (Figure

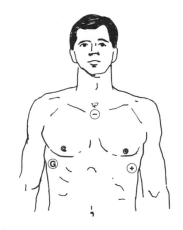

Figure 15.9   Lead placement for CM5: (−) negative electrode, (+) positive electrode, (G) ground. Adapted from Ellestad (1980).

15.10). Time is measured on the horizontal axis, and the paper normally moves at 25 mm (millimeters) per second. Most ECG machines can be set to run at 50 or 25 mm per s, so one must know the paper speed when measuring the duration of ECG complexes. ECG paper is marked with a repeating grid. Major grid lines are 5 mm apart, and at a paper speed of 25 mm per s, 5 mm corresponds to 0.20 s. Minor lines are 1 mm apart, and at a paper speed of 25 mm per second, 1 mm equals 0.04 s. Voltage is measured on the vertical axis, and the calibration of the machine must be known to evaluate the ECG. The standard calibration factor is normally 0.1 mV (millivolt) per millimeter of deflection.

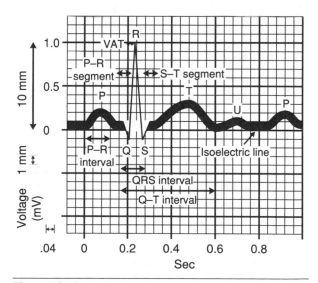

Figure 15.10   ECG complex with time and voltage scales. *Note.* From *Principles of Clinical Electrocardiography* (11th ed.) by M.J. Goldman, 1982, Cambridge, MD: Lange Medical. Copyright 1982 by Lange Medical Publications, Los Altos, CA. Reprinted by permission.

Most ECG machines can be adjusted to reduce this factor by 50% or double it. As with paper speed, the voltage calibration should be known before evaluating an ECG. All ECG measurements in this book refer to a paper speed of 25 mm per second and a voltage calibration of 0.1 mV per mm.

Basic Electrocardiographic Complexes

The **P wave** is the graphical representation of atrial depolarization. The normal P wave is less than 0.12 s in duration and has an amplitude of 0.25 mV or less. The Ta wave is the result of atrial repolarization. It is not normally seen, because it occurs during ventricular depolarization, and the larger electrical forces generated by the ventricles "hide" the Ta wave. The **Q wave** is the first downward deflection after the P wave; the Q wave signals the start of ventricular depolarization. The **R wave** is a positive deflection after the Q wave and is the result of ventricular depolarization. If more than one R wave occurs in a single complex, then the second occurrence is called R' (R prime). The **S wave** is a negative deflection preceded by Q or R waves and is also the result of ventricular depolarization.

The **T wave** follows the QRS complex and represents ventricular repolarization.

Electrocardiograph Intervals

The **R–R interval** is the time between successive R waves. An approximate HR can be determined by dividing 1,500 (60 s•25 mm•sec^{-1}) by the number of millimeters between adjacent R waves, provided the heart is in normal rhythm.

The **P–P interval** represents the time between two successive atrial depolarizations.

The **P–R interval** is measured from the start of the P wave to the beginning of the QRS complex. The interval is called P–R even if the first deflection following the P wave is a Q wave. The P–R interval represents the time from the start of atrial depolarization, through delay through the AV node, and to the start of ventricular depolarization. The upper limit for the P–R interval is 0.20 s, or 5 small blocks.

The **QRS complex** represents the time for depolarization of the ventricles. A normal QRS complex lasts less than 0.10 s, or 2.5 small blocks on the ECG paper.

The **Q–T interval** is measured from the start of QRS complex to the end of the T wave and corresponds to the duration of ventricular systole.

Segments and Junctions

The **P–R segment** is measured from the end of the P wave to the beginning of the QRS complex. This segment forms the isoelectric line, or baseline, from which S–T segment deviations are measured.

The RS–T segment, or **J point**, is the point at which the S wave ends and the S–T segment begins.

The **S–T segment** is formed by the isoelectric line between the QRS complex and the T wave. This segment is closely examined during an exercise test for depression, which may indicate the development of myocardial ischemia. **S–T segment depression** is usually measured 60 or 80 ms after the J point.

Atrioventricular Conduction Disturbances

There are three categories of atrioventricular (AV) conduction defects: first-, second-, and third-degree blocks. Atrioventricular conduction defects are present when electrical impulses are slowed or completely blocked while passing through the atrioventricular node.

First-Degree Atrioventricular Block

When the P–R interval exceeds 0.20 s and all P waves result in ventricular depolarization, a **first-degree AV block** exists (Figure 15.11). Causes of a first-degree AV block can include medications, such as digitalis and quinidine; infections; or vagal stimulation.

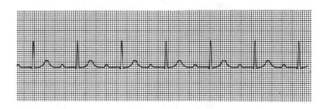

Figure 15.11   First-degree atrioventricular block.

Second-Degree Atrioventricular Block

The main distinguishing factor of the **second-degree AV block** is that some, but not all, P waves result in ventricular depolarization. There are two types of second-degree AV blocks: Mobitz Type I, or Wenchebach, and Mobitz Type II. **Mobitz Type I**, or Wenchebach, **AV block** (Figure 15.12) is a form of second-degree atrioventricular block characterized by

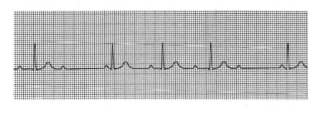

Figure 15.12 Mobitz Type I atrioventricular block.

a progressively lengthening P–R interval until an atrial depolarization fails to initiate a ventricular depolarization. This type of conduction disturbance is most commonly seen after a myocardial infarction. The site of the block is within the AV node and is probably the result of reversible ischemia.

Mobitz Type II AV block (Figure 15.13) is the more serious of the second-degree atrioventricular blocks and is characterized by atrial depolarization, occasionally not resulting in ventricular depolarization, but with constant P–R intervals. The site of the block is beyond the bundle of His and is usually the result of irreversible ischemia of the interventricular conduction system.

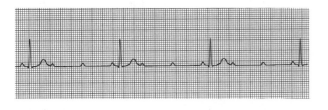

Figure 15.13 Mobitz Type II atrioventricular block.

Third-Degree Atrioventricular Block

Third-degree AV block is present when the ventricles contract independently of the atria (Figure 15.14). The P–R interval varies and follows no regular pattern. The ventricular pacemaker may be either the atrioventricular node, the bundle of His, the Purkinje fibers, or the ventricular muscle, and almost always results in a slow ventricular rate of less than 50 beats·min^{-1}.

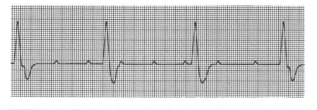

Figure 15.14 Third-degree atrioventricular block.

Rhythms and Arrhythmias

The HFI needs a general understanding of the various rhythms and arrhythmias, to communicate effectively with the health care team members. The following section contains examples of normal rhythms, the more common arrhythmias, and explanations of their significance.

Sinus Rhythm

Sinus rhythm is the normal rhythm of the heart (Figure 15.15). The rate is 60 to 100, and the pacemaker is the sinoatrial node.

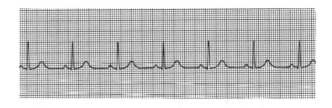

Figure 15.15 Normal sinus rhythm.

Sinus Arrhythmia

Sinus arrhythmia is a normal variant and is defined as a sinus rhythm in which the R–R interval varies by more than 10%, beat to beat. Sinus arrhythmia is often seen in highly trained subjects and occasionally in patients taking beta-adrenergic-receptor-blocking medications (ß-blockers), such as Inderal. The rhythm may be associated with respiration, because HR increases with inspiration and decreases with expiration.

Sinus Bradycardia

The pacemaker is the sinoatrial node, and the rate in **sinus bradycardia** is 60 or less (Figure 15.16). This is a normal rhythm and is often seen in trained subjects and patients taking ß-blockers.

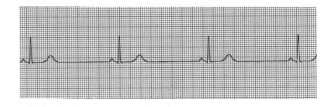

Figure 15.16 Sinus bradycardia.

Sinus Tachycardia

Sinus tachycardia (Figure 15.17), heart rates of 100 or more, may be seen at rest in deconditioned people or in apprehensive individuals prior to exercise testing.

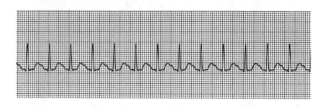

Figure 15.17   Sinus tachycardia.

Premature Atrial Contraction

In **premature atrial contraction**, the rhythm is irregular and the R–R interval is short between a normal sinus beat and the premature beat (Figure 15.18). The origin of the premature beat is somewhere other than the sinoatrial node and is known as an *ectopic focus*. Premature atrial contractions may be caused by stimulants such as coffee or tea and may be seen prior to exercise testing in apprehensive subjects.

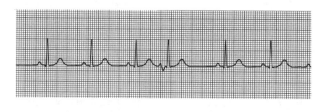

Figure 15.18   Premature atrial contraction.

Atrial Flutter

During **atrial flutter**, the atrial rate may be 200 to 350, with a ventricular response of 60 to 160 beats·min⁻¹. The atrial rhythm is usually irregular, whereas the ventricular rhythm is either regular or irregular. The pacemaker site during atrial flutter is not the sinoatrial node, and as a result normal P waves are not present. F waves, resembling a sawtooth pattern, may be seen (Figure 15.19). The causes of atrial flutter include increased sympathetic drive, hypoxia, and congestive heart failure.

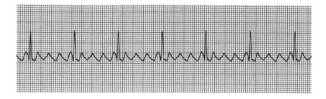

Figure 15.19   Atrial flutter.

Atrial Fibrillation

During **atrial fibrillation**, the atrial rate is 400 to 700, and the ventricular rate is usually 60 to 160 beats·min⁻¹ and is irregular. Multiple pacemaker sites are present in the atria, and P waves cannot be discerned (Figure 15.20). The significance of atrial fibrillation in an exercise-testing and training setting lies in its effect on ventricular function. During atrial fibrillation, the atria and ventricles do not work together in a coordinated fashion, and the ability of the left ventricle to maintain an adequate cardiac output may be impaired. The causes of atrial fibrillation are essentially the same as for atrial flutter.

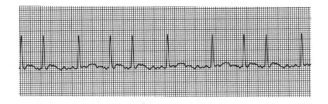

Figure 15.20   Atrial fibrillation.

Premature Junctional Contraction

A **premature junctional contraction** results when an ectopic pacemaker in the atrioventricular junctional area depolarizes the ventricles. Inverted P waves are frequently seen with premature junctional contractions as the atrial depolarization proceeds in an abnormal direction (Figure 15.21). If the AV nodal tissue is still in the refractory phase after a premature junctional contraction, then normally conducted waves of depolarization initiated from the sinoatrial node are not conducted into the ventricles, and a compensatory pause develops. Premature junctional contractions usually result in a QRS complex of normal duration, or they may slightly prolong the QRS complex. The causes of premature junctional contractions include catecholamine-type medications, increased parasympathetic tone, or damage to the AV node. Premature junctional contractions are of little consequence unless they occur very frequently (more than 4 to 6 premature junctional contractions per minute) or compromise ventricular function.

Arrhythmias originating above the ventricles (*supraventricular*) may cause concern among exercise leaders

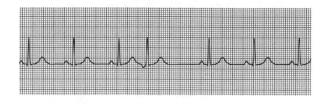

Figure 15.21   Premature junctional contraction.

and patients, but Ellestad (4) has found that the long-term survival of CAD patients with exercise-induced supraventricular arrhythmias does not seem to be compromised. The significance of the supraventricular arrhythmias lies in the uncoupling of coordination between the atria and ventricles and the resulting effect on the ability of the ventricles to maintain an adequate cardiac output. Recurrent atrial fibrillation may have little effect on the exercise response of an individual with good left-ventricular function, but may cause significant symptoms in a person with poor ventricular function.

Premature Ventricular Contractions

Premature ventricular contractions (PVCs) are the result of an abnormal impulse (ectopic focus), arising in the His-Purkinje system, that initiates a ventricular contraction. Premature ventricular contractions last more than 0.12 s, and the T wave is usually oriented in the opposite direction from the QRS complex (Figure 15.22). Premature ventricular contractions often result in the ventricles being in the refractory phase of depolarization when the normal sinus depolarization wave reaches the ventricles, and a compensatory pause develops. Premature ventricular contractions are among the most common arrhythmias seen with exercise testing and training in coronary artery disease patients. If PVCs have the same shape, they originate from the same site (ectopic focus) and are called *unifocal*. Multiple-shape PVCs that originate from multiple sites in the ventricles are called multifocal and are much more serious than unifocal PVCs. The rhythm of normal contractions alternating with PVCs is called *bigeminy*; if every third contraction is a PVC, the rhythm is called *trigeminy*. Three or more consecutive premature ventricular contractions are known as **ventricular tachycardia**. If a single premature ventricular contraction falls on the descending portion of the T wave, the "vulnerable time," then the ventricles may be thrown into fibrillation. Premature ventricular contractions have an adverse effect on the survival of CAD patients; generally, the more complex the premature ventricular contractions, the more serious the problem. Ellestad (4) and co-workers have shown that the combination of S–T segment depression and premature ventricular con-

tractions increase the incidence of future cardiac events.

KEY POINT.   If PVCs occur during pulse counting, a person may report that the heart "skipped a beat" and may undercount his or her HR. They should be instructed not to increase the exercise intensity in an attempt to keep the HR in the target zone as a result of skipped beats. They should immediately reduce the exercise intensity and report the appearance or increase in the number of skipped beats to the exercise leader and physician.

Ventricular Tachycardia

Ventricular tachycardia is present whenever three or more consecutive PVCs occur (Figure 15.23). This is an extremely dangerous arrhythmia that may lead to ventricular fibrillation. The ventricular rate is usually 100 to 220 beats $\cdot$ min^{-1}, and the heart may be unable to maintain adequate cardiac output during ventricular tachycardia. Ventricular tachycardia may be caused by the same factors that initiate PVCs; it requires immediate medical attention.

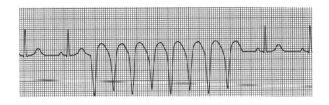

Figure 15.23   Ventricular tachycardia.

Ventricular Fibrillation

Ventricular fibrillation is a life-threatening rhythm and requires immediate cardiopulmonary resuscitation (CPR) until a defibrillator can be used to restore a coordinated ventricular contraction; otherwise, death will result. A fibrillating heart contracts in an unorganized, quivering manner (Figure 15.24) and is unable to maintain significant cardiac output. P waves and QRS complexes are not discernible; instead, the electrical pattern is a fibrillatory wave.

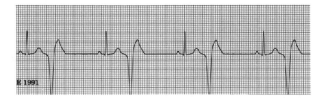

Figure 15.22   Premature ventricular contraction.

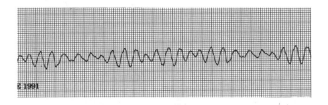

Figure 15.24   Ventricular fibrillation.

Myocardial Ischemia

Myocardial ischemia is a lack of oxygen in the myocardium caused by inadequate blood flow. Obstruction of the coronary arteries is the most common cause of myocardial ischemia. A coronary artery is significantly obstructed if more than 50% of the opening is blocked (6). A 50% reduction in diameter is equal to a loss of 75% of the arterial lumen. An obstructed coronary artery may be able to supply an adequate blood supply at rest, but may be unable to provide enough blood and oxygen during periods of increased demand, such as exercise. Ischemia often, but not always, results in angina pectoris.

Angina pectoris is pain or discomfort caused by temporary, reversible ischemia of the myocardium that does not result in death or infarction of the heart muscle. The pain is often located in the center of the chest, but may occur in the neck, jaw, or shoulders or radiate into the arm(s) and hand(s). Angina pectoris tends to be reproducible, often appearing at roughly the same level of exertion. During exercise, an individual experiencing anginal discomfort may deny pain, but upon further questioning will admit to the sensation of burning, tightness, pressure, or heaviness in the chest or arms. Anginal pain is frequently confused with musculoskeletal pain. Anginal pain generally is not altered by movements of the trunk or arms, while musculoskeletal pain may be increased or decreased by trunk or arm movement. Discomfort is probably not angina if the pain is changed in quality or intensity by pressing on the affected area.

Myocardial ischemia may cause S-T segment depression on the ECG during an exercise test. S-T segment depression usually occurs at a relatively constant double product. The double product equals the HR times systolic BP and is a good estimate of the amount of work the heart is doing. Three types of S-T segment depression are recognized: upsloping, horizontal, and downsloping (Figure 15.25). Ellestad (4) and co-workers have shown

that individuals with upsloping and horizontal S-T segment depressions have roughly similar life expectancies, and that downsloping S-T segment depression has a more adverse impact on survival.

S-T segment elevation may also occur during exercise testing. S-T segment elevation during an exercise test usually indicates the development of an **aneurysm**, or an area of noncontracting myocardium and/or scar tissue.

Myocardial Infarction

If the myocardium is deprived of oxygen for a sufficient length of time, a portion of the myocardium dies; this is known as a **myocardial infarction (MI)**. Pain is the hallmark symptom of a myocardial infarction. It is often very similar to anginal pain, only more severe, and may be described as a heavy feeling, squeezing in the chest, or a burning sensation. Other symptoms that may accompany a myocardial infarction are nausea, sweating, and shortness of breath.

Information from the Framingham project indicates that up to 25% of MIs may be silent infarctions, meaning that the infarction does not cause sufficient symptoms for the victim to seek medical attention (7). These silent infarctions may be recognized during routine ECG examinations.

CARDIOVASCULAR MEDICATIONS

A wide variety of medications are used to treat people with heart disease. Some medications control BP, others control the heart rate or rhythm, and still others affect the force of contraction of the ventricles. Other drugs likely to be encountered by the HFI include medications for diabetics to control the blood glucose concentration, and bronchodilators for individuals with

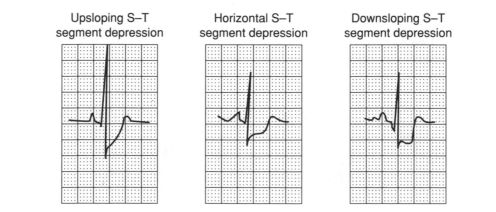

Figure 15.25   S-T segment depression.

asthma. The HFI will not be prescribing medications, or dealing on a day-to-day basis with patients taking these medications, but he or she will eventually encounter participants taking some of these medications. The purpose of this section is to summarize the major classes of drugs, describe how they affect the exercise HR response, and indicate possible side effects.

Beta-Adrenergic Blockers

Beta-adrenergic blocking medications (ß-blockers) are commonly prescribed for patients with coronary artery disease and apparently healthy subjects with hypertension and, occasionally, for migraine headaches. All of these medications compete with epinephrine and norepinephrine for the limited number of ß-adrenergic receptors; thus ß-blockers blunt the effect of these hormones. ß-blockers are generally used to reduce the heart rate and vigor of myocardial contraction, which reduces the oxygen need of the heart. Because of the effect these medications have on submaximal and maximal HR, these beta-blockers have a profound impact on the exercise prescription. Subjects should be tested on ß-blockers if they will be training on these medications. All ß-blockers lower HR at rest and particularly during exercise, as seen in Figure 15.26.

Two types of ß-adrenergic receptors are recognized, β_1 and β_2. β_1 receptors are found mainly in the heart, and β_2 receptors are primarily located in the smooth muscle in the lungs. Some ß-blockers selectively block the β_1 receptors in the heart. The β_1-selective blockers include Sectral, Tenormin, Brevibloc, and Lopressor. Other ß-blockers are less selective and exert action on both β_1 and β_2 receptors. The less specific ß-blockers include Inderal, Trandate, Corgard, Visken, and

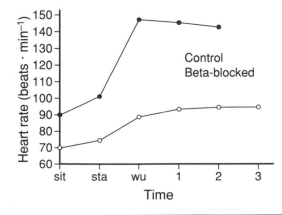

Figure 15.26 The heart rate before and after beta blockade (2 days of 40 mg of Inderal per day) in a very apprehensive patient during treadmill testing (sit = sitting, sta = standing, wu = warmup @ 1.0 mph, 0% grade. Minutes 1 and 2 are 2.0 mph, 0% grade. Minute 3 was at 2.0 mph and 3.5% grade).

Blockadren. An undesirable side-effect of the nonselective beta-blockers is contraction of the smooth muscle surrounding the airways in the lungs, which reduces the airway lumen and increases the work of breathing. This can result in labored breathing, shortness of breath, and other asthma-like symptoms.

Indications for the use of ß-blockers include hypertension, angina pectoris, and supraventricular arrhythmias. In addition, some ß-blockers are sometimes used to treat migraine headaches. As a general rule, nonspecific ß-blocking medications are not recommended for use in patients with asthma, bronchitis, or similar lung problems. ß-blocking medications may also blunt some of the symptoms of hypoglycemia in insulin-dependent diabetics.

The use of Inderal and presumably other ß-blockers does not invalidate the THR method of prescribing exercise intensity. Hossack, Bruce, and Clark (5) have shown that the regression equations relating %HRmax to %$\dot{V}O_2$max are similar in ß-adrenergic blocked and nonblocked CAD patients. There has been little work in the area, but it is assumed that the THR method of exercise prescription is valid with the other ß-blocking medications.

Because ß-blocking medications lower maximal HR, the use of these medications *invalidates* estimating THR based on taking 70% to 85% of age-adjusted, predicted HRmax (predicted HRmax = 220 − age). For example, a 40-year-old individual has a predicted HRmax of about 180, with an estimated 70% to 85% THR of 126 to 153 beats•min^{-1}. If this individual were given a ß-blocking medication, HRmax could easily be reduced to 150 beats•min^{-1}. If the estimated THR of 126 to 153 beats•min^{-1} were used for training, this individual would be training at maximal heart rate. Measurement of HRmax is required, to calculate an appropriate THR for anyone taking ß-blocking medications, and testing should be repeated following any change in ß-blocking medication dosage.

There has been some question as to whether the use of ß-blocking medicines reduces or blocks the effectiveness of endurance training. Sable et al. (9) have reported that chronic use of Inderal diminishes the effects of endurance training in healthy, young subjects. Pratt and co-workers (8), using patients with coronary artery disease, have found that chronic use of ß-blockers does not prevent the typical endurance-training effects.

Nitrates

This class of drugs exists in several forms, including patches applied to the skin, long-acting tablets, and sublingual tablets, and is used to prevent or stop attacks of angina pectoris. The physiological mechanism of action is the relaxation of vascular smooth muscle, which reduces venous return and the quantity of blood the heart has to pump. Arterial smooth muscle is also relaxed, although to a lesser degree than venous smooth muscle, which reduces the resistance against which the heart has to pump. Both of these actions help reduce the work and oxygen requirements of the heart. Many patients use nitroglycerine (NTG) on a 24-hr basis with ointment or patches. Longer acting tablet forms of NTG (Cardilate, Sorbitrate, and Isordil) may be taken prior to activities that are likely to provoke anginal attacks; sublingual tablets (Nitrostat) are used to treat acute anginal episodes. Headaches, dizziness, and hypotension are the main side-effects of NTG use. Beta-adrenergic blocking medications may potentiate the hypotensive actions of NTG.

Calcium Antagonists

This class of drugs currently has three members: Isoptin, Procardia, and Cardizem. These drugs interfere with the slow calcium currents during depolarization in cardiac and vascular smooth muscle. Isoptin is used primarily to treat atrial and ventricular arrhythmias; Procardia and Cardizem are used in the treatment of exertional angina and variant angina pectoris, or angina pectoris attacks that occur at rest.

The effects of **calcium-antagonist** medications on exercise prescription and training has received little attention. Chang and Hossack (2) have shown that the regression equations relating %HRmax and %$\dot{V}O_2$max are the same in patients taking Cardizem and non-medicated patients. Isoptin and Procardia are assumed to not alter the relationship between %HRmax and %$\dot{V}O_2$max. Calcium antagonists are not thought to adversely affect endurance training in healthy subjects or CAD patients. Duffey and co-workers (3) have shown that Procardia does not diminish training responses in healthy, young subjects.

Anti-Arrhythmic Medications

Some of the more commonly used **anti-arrhythmics** are Pronestyl, Norpace, Cardioquin, Quinaglute, Tambacor, Sectral, Cordarone, Tonocard, and the digitalis preparations. The ß-blocking medications are also used to treat some types of arrhythmias. With the exception of the ß-blockers, these medications will have little influence on the HR response to exercise, but the reduction in arrhythmias may improve work capacity.

Digitalis Preparations

The **digitalis** medications are used to increase the vigor of myocardial contractions and treat atrial flutter and fibrillation. The increased vigor of contraction resulting from digitalis preparations may increase work capacity in individuals with poor ventricular function. Digitalis medications are marketed under several trade names, including Lanoxin, Lanoxicaps, Purodigin, and Crystodigin. Cardiac side effects of the digitalis group include premature ventricular contractions, Mobitz Type I AV block, and atrial tachycardia. Digitalis drugs can cause false-positive S–T segment depression during exercise testing. The side effects of the digitalis drugs can be potentiated by Quinidine Sulfate.

Antihypertensives

The class of **antihypertensives** can be broken down into four groups according to the mechanism of action. Drugs in the first group, *diuretics*, work by increasing the excretion of electrolytes and water. This group includes Lasix, Diamox, Diuril, Hygroton, Esidrix, Enduron, Aldactone, Hydrodiuril, and many others. This group is often used as the first treatment for hypertension. Side effects of these medications include *hypokalemia*, or low blood levels of potassium. Hypokalemia can induce arrhythmias and is a potentially serious problem. Diuretic-induced hypokalemia can often be prevented by increasing consumption of fruits, which are high in potassium. If dietary sources of potassium prove to be ineffective, a prescription potassium supplement (K-Tab, Kay Ceil, or Slo-K) can be used.

The second group of antihypertensive medications is the *vasodilators*. These medications decrease blood pressure by relaxing vascular smooth muscle. Some of the brand names in this category are Apresoline, Apresazide, Hydra-Zide, Reserpine, Ser-Ap-As, and Loniten. Side effects associated with these medications include hypotension, dizziness, and tachycardia. The active chemical in Loniten is also marketed under the name Rogaine in the form of a topical solution for use as a hair-growth stimulant in male-pattern baldness. Rogaine has little or no antihypertensive effect.

The third group of antihypertensive medications works through the alpha- and beta-receptors of the autonomic nervous system. This group includes the ß-blockers discussed earlier and the *alpha-stimulators* such as Minipress and Catapres.

The fourth group of antihypertensive medications

works through the renin-angiotensin system. Some of the brand names in this category are Vasotec, Zestril, Zestoretic, and Capoten. These drugs lower blood pressure by inhibiting angiotensin-converting enzyme (ACE), which converts angiotensin I to angiotensin II. They are called ACE-inhibitors for that reason. This class of medications is usually reserved for patients who were unresponsive to the other antihypertensive treatment options.

Lipid-Lowering Medications

These medications (Questran, Atromid-S, Colestid, Lopid, Choloxin, Mevacor, Lorelco) are used to lower cholesterol and triglycerides in individuals who are unable to adequately control lipids through diet and exercise. This class of medications is unlikely to have any substantial effect on exercise testing or training. Patients taking these medications need to be closely followed by their physicians because of potential toxic effects on the liver. Some lipid-lowering agents (Lopid, Atromid-S) can potentiate the effects of anticoagulants and make participants in exercise programs more susceptible to bruising.

Anticoagulants

Anticoagulants are used to delay the clotting process. Oral anticoagulants include Dicumarol, Panwarfin, and Coumadin. These medications are unlikely to have any direct effect on exercise testing or training, but they do increase the risk of bruising. Aspirin and some other medications can potentiate the action of anticoagulants and increase the risk of bruising with minimal trauma.

Nicotine Gums

Nicotine gums contain nicotine and are used as a smoking substitute for individuals who are trying to stop smoking. The drug is in the form of gum, which is chewed. Nicotine is absorbed through the oral mucosa and provides sufficient plasma nicotine concentrations to curb the craving to smoke. Nicotine gum may increase HR, BP, and the incidence of cardiac arrhythmias. Nicotine gums are marketed under names Bantron and Nicorette.

Bronchodilators

Bronchodilators are used to relax smooth muscle surrounding airways in the lungs and relieve the symptoms of asthma, bronchitis, and related lung disorders. These medications can be taken orally or from an inhaler. The inhalers are generally used for acute asthma episodes; long-term bronchodilation is usually obtained with oral preparations. Most of these drugs stimulate the β_2-receptors, which relax bronchial smooth muscle and increase the airway lumen. Because of their ß-adrenergic stimulating effect, these medications can increase HR and BP, although most of their effect is focused on the smooth muscle found in airways. Inhaler brand names include Brethaire Inhaler, Ventolin, Alupent, and Maxair. The oral bronchodilators include Theobid, Aminophyllin, Bronkaid, and Theo-Dur. See chapter 13 for additional information on the asthmatic.

Oral Diabetic Agents

A substantial number of obese participants in fitness programs have *hyperglycemia*, or elevated levels of blood glucose. In this condition, the pancreas is able to produce insulin but is unable to produce sufficient quantities to maintain normal blood glucose control. This condition is called *non–insulin dependent diabetes* and can often be controlled with oral **antiglycemic agents**. The oral antiglycemic medications work by stimulating the pancreas to secrete more insulin, which facilitates tissue uptake of glucose. The stimulating action of the oral antiglycemic medications requires a functioning pancreas. Brand names of the oral antiglycemic agents include Diaßeta, Diabinese, Glucotrol, Micronase, Orinase, Tolinase. A serious side effect of these drugs is *hypoglycemia*, or low blood sugar. Hypoglycemia is potentially dangerous, and the HFI should be alert for changes in alertness and orientation in patients taking any medication that can lower plasma glucose concentrations.

Insulin-dependent diabetes, a more serious disorder of carbohydrate metabolism, is characterized by an absence of insulin and requires frequent insulin injections. Insulin cannot be taken orally, because it is a protein and would be inactivated by the digestive process. When working with an insulin-dependent diabetic, the HFI should be aware of the possibility of hypoglycemia. Signs of hypoglycemia include bizarre or irrational behavior and slurred speech. When individuals with insulin-dependent diabetes are exercising, it is a good idea to have a source of sugar readily available in the event of a hypoglycemic episode. See chapters 13 and 16 for additional details on the diabetic.

SUMMARY

The heart is a muscular organ composed of four chambers—the right atrium, right ventricle, left atrium, and left ventricle. The coronary arteries supply the heart muscle (myocardium) with blood, and the heart meets the increasing oxygen demands by increasing blood flow. Any restriction in blood flow to the myocardium could result in a change in electrical activity across the heart or in damage to the myocardium itself. The pattern of electrical activity across the heart is called the electrocardiogram (ECG). The ECG is recorded with an electrocardiograph and provides information about the rhythm of the heart. The ECG can indicate the presence of inadequate blood flow (ischemia), and it can indicate if a portion of the heart muscle has died (myocardial infarction). Various common ECG abnormalities and their significance are presented. Medications are prescribed for a variety of reasons: high blood pressure, abnormal heart rhythms, and so forth. The HFI must be aware of the most common medications, because they may directly affect the THR or indirectly affect the participant's overall response to exercise training. This chapter summarizes the major classes of cardiovascular medications and indicates what effects they may have on the cardiovascular response to exercise.

CASE STUDIES FOR ANALYSIS

15.1   55-year-old, apparently healthy male is referred to your facility for an exercise program and brings the results of his most recent exercise test. You notice that the subject was taking Coumadin and Inderal when he took his exercise test. Since the test, his physician has stopped the Inderal. What impact, if any, would this change in medication make on the exercise prescription? (See Appendix A.)

15.2 A participant in your exercise program reports that she was given two new prescriptions during her last visit with her physician. Since starting the new medication, she has noticed an increase in the number of "skipped beats" while taking her heart rate during exercise. The two new medications are Nicorette and Atromid-S. Which medication is most likely to be associated with an increase in arrhythmias, and why? (See Appendix A.)

15.3 A participant in your exercise program has been taking a beta-blocking medication for several years without experiencing any significant side effects. She was recently given a prescription for Isordil and now reports that she often becomes dizzy upon standing suddenly. Could this be related to her prescription? If so, why? (See Appendix A.)

REFERENCES

1. Berne and Levy (1977)
2. Chang and Hossack (1982)
3. Duffey, Horwitz, and Brammell (1984)
4. Ellestad (1980)
5. Hossack, Bruce, and Clark (1980)
6. Hurst (1978)
7. Kannel and Abbot (1984)
8. Pratt et al. (1981)
9. Sable et al. (1982)

SUGGESTED READINGS

Ewy and Bressler (1982)
Froelicher (1983)
Goldman (1982)

See the Bibliography at the end of the book for a complete source listing.

Part V

Safe and Effective Programs

Chapter 16

Injury Prevention and Treatment

Sue Carver

OBJECTIVES

The reader will be able to:

- Describe ways to minimize injury risk
- Distinguish between simple muscle soreness and injury
- Identify signs, symptoms, and proper treatment measures for common injuries, including soft-tissue injuries (sprain, strain, contusion, heel bruise), bone injuries (open fracture, simple fracture), wounds (laceration, incision, puncture, abrasion), and excessive bleeding (external and internal hemorrhage)
- Describe the causes of heat-related disorders, how to prevent them, and how to treat them when they occur
- Provide guidelines for fluid replacement before and following exercise
- Identify signs and symptoms of overexertion
- Distinguish the signs and symptoms of diabetic coma from those of insulin shock, and describe the proper treatment for each
- Identify the common signs, symptoms, and management of the following orthopedic problems: shin splints, inflammatory reactions (bursitis, tendinitis, myositis, synovitis, epicondylitis, tenosynovitis, plantar fasciitis, capsulitis), tennis elbow, stress fracture, and low-back pain
- Classify injuries into mild, moderate, and severe, and recommend appropriate modification of exercise programs when the injuries occur
- Demonstrate CPR
- Check vital signs (level of consciousness, respiration, skin color, temperature, ability to move, pulse, bleeding, blood pressure, eye pupil size and response, pain reaction), and recognize normal and abnormal responses
- Explain the need to protect the injured area and the use of rest, ice, compression, and elevation in the initial treatment of injuries, and the application of heat in long-term treatment
- Describe the emergency procedures, first aid equipment, and evacuation procedures needed in fitness testing and exercise areas
- Discuss the risk factors for musculoskeletal injury and cardiovascular complications resulting from exercise training and how such risks might be minimized

TERMS

The reader will be able to define or describe:

Abrasion	Contusion
Acidosis	CPR
Bursitis	Dehydration
Capsulitis	Diabetic coma
Compartment syndrome	Electrolyte
Compound fracture	Emergency medical system

Epicondylitis
Fracture
Heat cramps
Heat exhaustion
Heat stroke
Heat syncope
Heel bruise
Hemorrhage
Incision
Inflammation
Insulin shock
Laceration
Longitudinal arch
Metatarsal arch
Myositis
Neoplasm
Orthopedic
Plantar fasciitis

Pressure points
PRICE
Puncture
Salt tablets
Shin splints
Shock
Simple fracture
Spondylolisthesis
Sprain
Strain
Stress fracture
Tendinitis
Tennis elbow
Thermogram
Tourniquet
Vital signs
Wounds

Certain inherent risks are associated with participation in physical activity. The HFI should be aware of those risks and take steps to control factors that increase the risk of injury. Advance planning, adequate equipment and facilities, and counseling in the selection of activities all help to reduce the possibility of injury. The following is a brief discussion of the factors contributing to injury and steps that can be taken to reduce injury risk.

Activity implies movement, and with increased movement comes a corresponding increase in the risk of injury. In fitness programs, the frequency of injuries increases when the frequency of the exercise sessions increases and when the intensity of the exercise is maintained at the high end of the THR zone (Figure 16.1). The risk of injury is also increased by increased speed of movement, as found in competitive activities; in activities requiring quick changes in direction (e.g., fitness games); and in activities that focus on smaller muscle groups. Finally, environmental conditions such as extreme heat or cold can increase the risk associated with physical activity. Lack of proper adaptation to the environment, as well as lack of education in the prevention, recognition, and methods of dealing with problems associated with these extreme environments, can lead to devastating results (see chapter 9).

Age, gender, and body structure influence the risk of injury. In general, very young and very old people are at the greatest risk, and older individuals usually require longer periods of time for recovery. Because of body structure and strength differences, females are often more susceptible to injury in particular activities than males. For either gender, a lack or an imbalance of muscle strength, a lack of joint flexibility, and poor CRF increase the chance of injury. Obese individuals

not only have low CRF, but excess weight places additional stress on the weight-bearing joints.

The dictum that the rate and risk of injury are lower for people who follow the rules of the game is usually applied to athletic contests. However, in exercise programs where games are used as a part of the aerobic activities, the HFI must instruct the participants to follow whatever rules exist. Games with few rules and in which the HFI controls the tempo help to reduce the chance of injury. The HFI should change the rules to enhance the safety of the games. For example, use of a softer ball and restricting contact would make soccer a safer fitness game (see chapter 14).

Finally, the HFI should encourage participants to seek professional advice regarding the selection and fitting of proper equipment. The equipment most com-

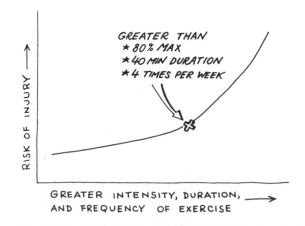

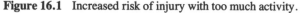

Figure 16.1 Increased risk of injury with too much activity.

monly used, and most widely abused, is footwear (see chapter 14). Inadequate protection of the foot is a major contributor to a variety of leg and low-back problems. Improperly maintained exercise equipment and facilities also contribute to higher overall injury risk (4, 6, 7).

MINIMIZING INJURY RISK

The first thing to do to reduce the chance of a minor or major problem is to screen participants before any physical activity program. The screening should highlight the major areas contributing to increased health risk (see chapter 2 for additional details). Proper screening assists the participant in recognizing problems and alerts the HFI to potential problems that could occur in an exercise session (e.g., asthma attack, diabetic shock). Proper planning for emergency situations contributes to a low overall risk. Individuals who cannot be properly supervised or given adequate care as a result of their physical problems should be referred to a program or facility that can provide the needed services. Policies to handle such referrals and all major emergency situations should be written and communicated to all HFIs involved in a fitness center (see chapter 17 for additional details).

A major factor involved in reducing the risk associated with physical activity is the design and implementation of an individual's exercise program. The program can focus attention on problems encountered in the preliminary tests, which might include

- flexibility measures (chapter 10);
- body-fatness determination (chapter 7);
- evaluation of muscular strength, power, and endurance (chapter 10);
- posture assessment (chapter 10); and
- cardiovascular-fitness evaluation (chapter 9).

The manner in which the HFI conducts the exercise program has a major bearing on the risk of injury to the participant. Figure 16.2 contrasts the "no pain, no gain" performance goal with the "train, don't strain" fitness goal to make this point. Educating participants about the proper intensity of the exercise session (i.e., to stay in the THR zone), and about the recognition of the signs and symptoms of overuse, is important in minimizing injury risk. The HFI should emphasize that the entire program, and each session, is graduated, to avoid doing too much too soon. This is especially true for individuals who have not been involved in a regular exercise program and have a tendency to overestimate their abilities. This can lead to chronic overuse injuries, extreme muscle soreness, and undue fatigue.

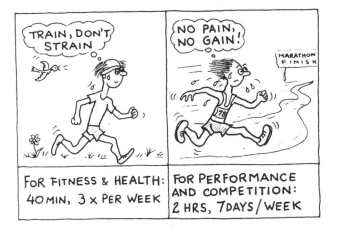

Figure 16.2 Fitness programs versus performance training.

In educating the participants about the signs and symptoms of overuse, the HFI should focus their attention on distinguishing between simple muscle soreness and injury. Muscle soreness tends to peak 24 to 48 hr postexercise and dissipates with use and time. The signs and symptoms of injury include

- exquisite point tenderness,
- pain that persists even when the body part is at rest,
- joint pain,
- pain that does not go away after warming up,
- swelling or discoloration,
- increased pain in weight-bearing or active movement, and
- changes in normal bodily functions.

TREATMENT OF SOFT-TISSUE INJURIES

Sprains (stretching of ligamentous tissue) and **strains** (stretching of muscle or tendon) are common injuries associated with adult fitness programs. Most significant injuries to joint structures or to soft tissue demand *protection*, *rest*, and the immediate application of *ice*, *compression*, and *elevation* (**PRICE**). Usually, a wet wrap is applied first to give compression. Start distal to the injury and wrap toward the heart. Compression should be firm but not tight. If a joint structure is involved, surround the entire area with ice and secure with another elastic wrap. If the injury involves a contusion or strain to a muscle belly, put the muscle on mild stretch before applying ice, and secure in that position if it is feasible to do so. If possible, elevate the injured part above heart level to minimize the effect of gravity and reduce bleeding into tissues. With any injury, the person can go into shock, and the HFI should be prepared to handle this situation, should it occur.

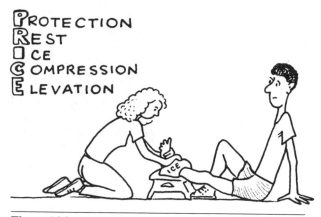

Figure 16.3   The PRICE is right.

In most cases, the participant needs to be informed that the application of ice should be continued anywhere from 24 to 72 hr, depending on the severity of the injury. Ice causes vasoconstriction of the blood vessels, thus helping to control bleeding into tissues. It also reduces the sensation of pain. Standard treatment times with ice are 20 to 30 min, with reapplication hourly or when pain is experienced. In the acute phase, when ice is not being used, the compression bandage should be in place to minimize swelling. Using ice or compression at bedtime is not necessary unless pain interferes with sleeping. If this occurs, frequent application of ice may help to control the pain. Physician referral is recommended in moderate to severe cases.

An injured participant may want to apply heat sooner than warranted. She or he needs to be informed that heat is usually applied in the later stages of an acute injury, when the risk of bleeding into tissues is minimal. The application of heat is a common treatment for chronic inflammatory conditions as well as generalized muscle soreness. Heat causes a vasodilation of the blood vessels and reduces muscle spasm. Standard treatment time for a moist heat pack is 20 to 30 min. When in doubt about which mode of treatment to use, ice is the safer choice.

TREATMENT OF WOUNDS

Another group of common injuries associated with activity programs is **wounds**. The major concern with an open wound is bleeding. Once bleeding is controlled, steps can be taken to give further care. This may consist of treating for **shock** or immediate referral to a physician for suturing. In minor cases, a thorough cleaning and application of a sterile dressing may be all that is needed. Internal bleeding is a very serious condition. The HFI should treat for shock and obtain medical assistance immediately.

Table 16.1 outlines some of the most common injuries encountered in fitness programs, lists the signs and symptoms, and provides guidelines for immediate care.

HEAT ILLNESS

Heat illness can strike anyone. Poor physical condition, although a contributing factor, is not the primary cause. Even the most highly conditioned person can suffer a heat-related disorder. The exercise load and the environment can place large heat loads on an individual. When this occurs, sweat is produced at a high rate, because evaporation of sweat is the major mechanism for heat loss. As a result, large amounts of water may be lost during physical activity. If too much water is lost, circulatory collapse and death can occur. The following information outlines methods of recognizing **dehydration** and presents measures that can be used to prevent heat illness (4).

Water Loss

A water loss equal to 3% of body weight is considered safe. A 5% loss is considered borderline, and an 8% loss is considered dangerous. Water loss can be monitored by weighing participants before and after activity. Individuals who are outside the allowable 3% range from one workout to the next may have an increased risk of heat injury and should be monitored carefully if allowed to participate.

Symptoms of Overexertion

Participants should be educated to recognize symptoms of overexertion: nausea or vomiting, extreme breathlessness, dizziness, unusual fatigue, and headache.

Symptoms of Heat Illness

Participants should be educated to recognize when they are experiencing symptoms related to heat illness: hair standing on end at chest or upper arms, chilling, headache or throbbing pressure, vomiting or nausea, labored breathing, dry lips or extreme cotton mouth, faintness or muscle cramping, and cessation of sweating. If these symptoms are present, the risk for developing **heat exhaustion** or **heat stroke** rises dramatically. The participant should stop the activity and get into the shade. In addition, the participant should be instructed to ask for help if he or she is disoriented or the symptoms are severe. The HFI should provide fluids and encourage the individual to drink.

Table 16.1 Common Injuries

Injury	Signs and symptoms	Immediate care

Sprain—stretching or tearing of ligamentous tissue
 	
Strain—overstretching or tearing of a muscle or tendon
 	
Contusion—impact force that results in bleeding into the underlying tissues
	1st degree—mild injury resulting in stretching or minor tearing of tissue. Range of motion is not limited. Point tenderness is minimal. No swelling.
	2nd degree—moderate injury resulting in partial tearing of tissue. Function is limited. There is point tenderness and probable muscle spasm. Range of motion is painful. Swelling and/or discoloration is probable if immediate first-aid care is not given.
	3rd degree—severe tearing or complete rupture of tissue. Exquisite point tenderness. Immediate loss of function. Swelling and muscle spasm likely to be present with discoloration appearing later. Possible palpable deformity.
		Rest. Ice. Compression. Elevation. Support.
		Usual treatment time:
		  20-30 min—ice bag.
		  5-7 min—ice cup or ice slush.
		How often:
		  Moderate and severe—every hour, or when pain is experienced.
		  Less severe—as symptoms necessitate.
		Continue with ice treatments at least 24 to 72 hours, depending on the severity of the injury.
		Refer to a physician if function is impaired.
		Mild to moderate strains—gradual stretching to the point of pain is recommended.

Heel bruise (stone bruise)—sudden abnormal force to heel area that results in trauma to underlying tissues	Severe pain. Immediate disability. May develop into a chronic inflammatory condition of the periosteum.	Rest. Ice. Compression. Elevation. Support. Pad for comfort when weight bearing is resumed.
Fractures—disruption of bone continuity, ranging from periosteal irritation to complete separation of bony parts **Simple**—bone fracture without external exposure **Compound**—bone fracture with external exposure	Acute: Direct trauma to bone resulting in disruption of continuity and immediate disability. Deformity or bony deviation. Swelling. Pain. Palpable tenderness. Referred pain or indirect point tenderness. Crepitation. False joint. Discoloration—usually becoming apparent later.	Acute: Control bleeding—elevation, pressure points, direct pressure. Treat for shock. If an open fracture, control bleeding and apply a sterile dressing; *do not move bones back into place.* Control swelling with pressure and ice, if wound is closed. Splint above and below the joint and apply traction if necessary. Protect body part from further injury. Refer to physician.
	Chronic: Low-grade inflammatory process causing proliferation of fibroblasts and generalized connective-tissue scarring. Pain progressively worsens until present all of the time. Direct point tenderness.	Chronic: Rest. Heat. Refer to physician.
Laceration—tearing of skin resulting in an open wound with jagged edges and exposure of underlying tissues	Redness. Swelling. Increase in skin temperature. Tender, swollen, and painful lymph glands. Mild fever. Headache.	Soak in antiseptic solution such as hydrogen peroxide to loosen foreign material. Clean with antiseptic soap and water, moving away from injury site. Apply a sterile dressing. Instruct to seek medical attention if signs of infection are recognized. Usually refer to a physician—a tetanus shot may be needed. If injury is extensive, control bleeding, cover with thick sterile bandages, and treat for shock. Refer to physician.

(Cont.)

Table 16.1   (Continued)

Injury	Signs and symptoms	Immediate care
Incision—cutting of skin resulting in an open wound with cleanly cut edges and exposure of underlying tissue		Clean wound with soap and water, moving away from the injury site. Minor cuts can be closed with a butterfly or steri-strip closure. Apply a sterile dressing. Refer to physician if wound may require suturing (i.e., facial cuts and large or deep wounds).
Puncture—direct penetration of tissues by a pointed object	Redness. Swelling. Increase in skin temperature. Tender, swollen, and painful lymph glands. Mild fever. Headache.	If object is imbedded deeply, protect body part and refer to physician for removal and care. Treat for shock. Clean around wound and away from injury site. Allow wound to bleed freely to minimize risk of infection. Apply a sterile dressing. Puncture wounds are usually referred to a physician. A tetanus shot may be needed. Instruct to seek medical attention if signs of infection are recognized.
Abrasion—scraping of tissues resulting in removal of the outermost layers of skin and resulting in the exposure of numerous capillaries		Debride and flush with antiseptic solution such as hydrogen peroxide. Follow with soap-and-water cleansing. Apply a petroleum-based antiseptic agent to keep the wound moist. This allows healing to take place from the deeper layers. Cover with nonadherent gauze. Instruct to seek medical help if signs of infection are recognized.

Excessive bleeding	External hemorrhage
	1. Arterial
	   Color: bright red.
	   Flow: spurts, bleeding is usually profuse.
	2. Venous
	   Color: dark red.
	   Flow: steady.
	3. Capillary
	   Flow: oozing.
		Elevate part above heart level. Put direct pressure over the wound, using a sterile compress if possible. Apply a pressure dressing. Use pressure points. Treat for shock. Refer to a physician.

Individuals Highly Susceptible to Heat Illness

Individuals who have previously suffered from heat stroke may have sustained permanent damage to their thermoregulatory systems. People whose systems are no longer effective in controlling body temperature are highly susceptible to heat injury. Individuals who use medications such as antihistamines or diuretics, use high quantities of salt in their diet, use **salt tablets**, or use alcohol in large quantities (particularly, prior to activity) will have a higher risk of heat injury. Finally,

Table 16.1 (Continued)

Injury	Signs and symptoms	Immediate care
Internal bleeding	Internal hemorrhage—bleeding into chest, abdominal, or pelvic cavity and bleeding of any of the organs contained within these cavities. Generally, there are no external signs. However, any time an individual coughs up blood or finds blood in the urine or feces, internal hemorrhage must be suspected. The following signs are also indicative of internal bleeding: Restlessness. Thirst. Faintness. Anxiety. Skin temperature—cold, clammy. Dizziness. Pulse—rapid, weak and irregular. Blood pressure—significant fall.	Treat for shock. Refer to hospital immediately.
Shock caused by bleeding	Restlessness. Anxiety. Pulse—weak, rapid. Skin temperature—cold, clammy; profuse sweating. Skin color—pale, later cyanotic. Respiration—shallow, labored. Eyes—dull. Pupils—dilated. Thirsty. Nausea and possible vomiting. Blood pressure—marked fall.	Maintain an open airway. Control bleeding. Elevate lower extremities approximately 12 in. (Exceptions: heart problems, head injury or breathing difficulty—place in comfortable position—usually semireclining, unless spinal injury is suspected, in which case *do not move*. Splint any fractures. Maintain normal body temperature. Avoid further trauma. Monitor vital signs and record at regular intervals—every 5 min or so. *Do not* feed or give any liquids.

Note. Adapted from American Medical Association (1966), Arnheim (1987), Henderson (1973), Ritter and Albohm (1987), and Thygerson (1987).

people who participate in physical activity while experiencing fever could elevate their body temperatures to dangerous levels.

Table 16.2 outlines the various stages of heat illness, the signs and symptoms associated with each, and guidelines for immediate care.

PREVENTION OF HEAT INJURY

Be aware of environmental factors such as relative humidity and temperature. The relative humidity can be calculated by measuring dry-bulb and wet-bulb atmospheric temperatures using a sling psychrometer.

See Table 13.6 for classifications of temperature and humidity.

The practical experience of the military and of athletic teams with working in the heat and humidity has led to the development of guidelines to prevent heat injury. The HFI's application of these guidelines (Guidelines for Preventing Heat Injury) to adult fitness programs will enhance the enjoyment and safety of the participants.

Salt and Water Replacement

As mentioned earlier, the evaporation of sweat is a primary means to lose heat during exercise. This fluid loss

Table 16.2   Heat-Related Problems

Heat illness	Signs and symptoms	Immediate care
Heat syncope	Headache Nausea	Normal intake of fluids.

Heat cramps	Muscle cramping
	(calf is very common)
	
	Multiple cramping
	(very serious)
		Isolated cramps:
		    Direct pressure to cramp and release;
		    stretch muscle slowly and gently;
		    gentle massage; ice.
		Multiple cramps:
		    Danger of heat stroke; *treat as heat exhaustion.*

Heat exhaustion	Profuse sweating Cold, clammy skin Normal temperature or slightly elevated Pale Dizzy Weak, rapid pulse Shallow breathing Nausea Headache Loss of consciousness	Move individual out of sun to a well-ventilated area. Place in shock position (feet elevated 12-18 in.); prevent heat loss or gain. Gentle massage of extremities. Gentle range-of-motion movement of the extremities. Force fluids. Reassure. Monitor body temperature and other vital signs. Refer to physician.
Heat stroke	Generally no perspiration Dry skin Very hot Temperature as high as 106 °F Skin color bright red or flushed (blacks—ashen) Rapid and strong pulse Labored breathing—semireclining position	This is an *extreme medical emergency.* Transport to hospital quickly. Remove as much clothing as possible without exposing the individual. Cool quickly, starting at the head and continuing down the body; use any means possible (fan, hose down, pack in ice). Wrap in cold, wet sheets for transport. Treat for shock; if breathing is labored, place in a semireclining position.

Note. Adapted from Arnheim (1987), Ritter and Albohn (1987), Scriber and Burke (1978), and Thygerson (1987).

must be replaced to minimize health risk and maximize safe and enjoyable participation in an exercise program. The following discussion deals with fluid replacement.

When to Drink

For most individuals who participate in CRF programs, thirst is an adequate indicator of when to hydrate. Generally, replacing fluids as they are used is the best way to meet the demands of the body. However, when extreme sweating or dry atmospheric conditions are present, the thirst mechanism may not be able to keep up with the need for fluid intake.

Normal daily intake of fluid for the sedentary individual is between 60 and 80 oz. The actual fluid requirement is dependent on too many factors to establish a single recommendation for maintaining hydration. However, drinking 8 to 10 oz of fluid before heavy exercise, in addition to frequent hydration during activity, helps to prevent heat illness.

Use of Salt Tablets

Loss of salt and other minerals may occur during prolonged exercise, particularly during hot and humid weather. Even so, the use of salt tablets is not recom-

Guidelines for Preventing Heat Injury

The practical experience of the military and athletic teams with working in the heat and humidity has led to the development of guidelines to prevent heat injury. The HFI's application of these guidelines to adult fitness programs will enhance the enjoyment and safety of the participants.

1. Acclimatize to heat and humidity by training over a period of 7 to 10 days.
2. Hydrate prior to activity and frequently during activity.
3. Decrease the intensity of exercise if the temperature or humidity is high; use THR as a guide.
4. Monitor weight loss by weighing before and after workouts. Force fluids if more than 3% of body weight is lost during an activity. Minimize participation until weight is within the 3% range.
5. A diet high in carbohydrates contains a high water content and helps to maintain fluid balance.
6. Wear appropriate clothing for hot or humid weather conditions. Expose as much skin surface as possible. Light-colored clothing does not absorb as much heat as darker clothing. Cotton materials absorb sweat and allow evaporation to occur. Certain synthetic clothing and materials with paint screens do not absorb sweat and should be avoided. Use of sauna suits prevents the evaporation of sweat and should be avoided.

mended unless accompanied by a large intake of water. Water with 0.1% to 0.2% salt solution may be given to individuals with high water loss. However, just increasing the use of table salt along with high intake of water meets the body's need for sodium and fluid replacement.

Plain Water Versus Special Electrolyte Drinks

Most **electrolyte** drinks are diluted solutions of glucose, salt, and other minerals, with added artificial flavoring. Some brands also contain as much as 200 to 300 kcal per quart of solution. Other than sodium, the minerals provided by an electrolyte solution do not provide much benefit. When sweating is profuse, large amounts of electrolyte solution may help to serve the same function as a diluted salt solution. In cases of mild to moderate sweating, the normal intake of salt in food provides adequate sodium replacement.

The main advantage of using a flavored solution is that the participant might drink more than if ingesting plain water or a salt solution. However, considering the prices of commercially prepared electrolyte solutions, plain water or homemade solutions are much more economical (10).

Homemade Electrolyte Solution

1 qt water
1/3 tsp salt
Some sugar for flavoring (0.5 to 1.5 Tbsp)

Fluid Temperature

Fluids at a temperature of 5 to 15 °C (41 to 59 °F) are absorbed faster than fluids at other temperatures.

THE DIABETIC

The HFI should be familiar with the signs and symptoms of diabetic coma and insulin shock (see Table 16.3). When an emergency situation arises with a diabetic and the individual is conscious, she or he is usually able to indicate what the problem is. If the individual cannot, then ask when food was last eaten and whether insulin was taken that day. If the diabetic has eaten but has not taken insulin, the person is probably going into a **diabetic coma**, a condition in which there is too little insulin to fully metabolize the carbohydrates. If the individual has taken insulin but has not eaten, then she or he is probably suffering from **insulin shock**, a condition in which there is too much insulin or not enough carbohydrate to balance the insulin intake.

If the individual lapses into unconsciousness, check for a medic-alert identification tag. This may help to identify the present problem. If you are undecided as to whether the individual is suffering from diabetic coma or insulin shock, give sugar. Brain damage or death can occur quickly if insulin shock is left untreated; it is a far more critical state than diabetic coma. If the problem is insulin shock, the individual should respond quickly—within 1 to 2 min; transport the individual to a hospital as quickly as possible. If the individual is in a diabetic coma, there is little chance of seriously worsening the condition by giving sugar. Several hours of fluid and insulin therapy will be needed, under a physician's direction. Table 16.3 outlines the diabetic reactions, signs, and symptoms, and immediate care of each.

COMMON ORTHOPEDIC PROBLEMS

Many injuries that are commonly referred to an **orthopedic** physician for diagnosis and treatment result from overuse or irritation of a chronic musculoskeletal problem. In most instances, the injuries do not incapacitate the participant immediately. It may be weeks or months after the onset of pain before the participant seeks medical consultation. By this time, the **inflammation** is severe and generally prevents normal function of the part involved. In many cases, a severe injury can be avoided

if proper care is initiated early enough. Table 16.4 outlines common orthopedic problems, their causes, signs, and symptoms, and general treatment guidelines.

Shin Splints

Shin splints is a catch-all expression used to describe a variety of conditions of the lower leg. It is often used to define any pain located between the knee and the ankle. A diagnosis of shin splints should be limited to conditions involving inflammation of the musculo-tendinous unit caused by overexertion of muscles during weight-bearing activity. A more specific diagnosis is preferred over the general term "shin splints." In any event, the physician needs to rule out the following conditions: stress fracture, metabolic or vascular disorder, **compartment syndrome**, and muscular strain. The physical complaints often accompanying shin-splints pain include (4)

- a dull ache in the lower leg region following workouts,

Table 16.3   Diabetic Reactions

Diabetes	Signs and symptoms	Immediate care
Diabetic coma—too little insulin to fully metabolize carbohydrates. Because foods are only partially broken down, they form various acid compounds. This is referred to as *acidosis*.	May complain of a headache. Confused. Disoriented. Stuporous. Nauseated. Coma. Skin color—flushed. Lips—cherry red. Body temperature—decreased; skin—dry. Breath odor—sweet, fruity. Intense thirst. Vomiting common. Abdominal pain is frequently present.	Call for medical assistance. Little can be done unless insulin is at hand. If medical assistance is not quickly available, 1. treat as shock; 2. administer fluids in large amounts by mouth, if individual is conscious; 3. maintain an open airway; 4. if individual is nauseated, turn the head to the side to prevent aspirating vomitus; and 5. do not give sugar, carbohydrates, or fats in any form. Recovery—gradual improvement over 6-12 hr. Fluid and insulin therapy should be directed by a physician.
Insulin shock—too much insulin or not enough carbohydrates to balance insulin intake.	Skin color—pale; (blacks—ashen color). Skin temperature—moist and clammy; cold sweat. Pulse—normal or rapid. Breathing—normal or shallow and slow. No odor of acetone on breath. Intense hunger. Double vision may be present.	Administer sugar as quickly as possible (orange juice, candy, etc.). If individual is unconscious, place sugar granules under tongue. If individual is unconscious or recovery is slow, call for medical assistance. Recovery—generally quick; 1 or 2 min. Refer to physician if unconscious or slow recovery.

Note. Adapted from American Academy of Orthopaedic Surgeons (1977), Arnheim (1987), and Henderson (1973).

Table 16.4   Common Orthopedic Problems

Injury	Common causes	Signs and symptoms	Treatment
Inflammatory reactions— **Bursitis**—inflammation of bursa (sac between a muscle and bone that is filled with fluid; facilitates motion, pads, and helps to prevent abnormal function). **Tendinitis**—inflammation of a tendon (a band of tough inelastic fibrous tissue that connects muscle to bone). **Myositis**—inflammation of voluntary muscle. **Synovitis**—inflammation of the synovial membrane (a highly vascularized tissue that lines articular surfaces). **Epicondylitis**—inflammation of muscles or tendons attaching to the epicondyles of the humerus. **Tenosynovitis**—inflammation of a tendon sheath. **Plantar faciitis**—inflammation of connective tissue that spans the bottom of the foot. **Capsulitis**—inflammation of the joint capsule.	Overuse. Improper joint mechanics. Improper technique. Pathology. Trauma. Infection.	Redness. Swelling. Pain. Increased skin temperature over the area of inflammation. Tenderness. Involuntary muscle guarding.	Ice and rest in the acute stages. Chronic—generally heat is used before exercise or activity, followed by ice after activity. Massage. Muscle strengthening and stretching exercises. Correct the cause of the problem. If correction of cause and symptomatic treatment does not relieve symptoms, referral to a physician is recommended; antiinflammatory medication is usually prescribed. If disease process or infection is suspected, refer to a physician immediately.

(Cont.)

- performance and work-output decrease because of pain,
- soft-tissue pain,
- mild swelling along the area of inflammation,
- slight temperature elevation at the site of inflammation, and
- pain on moving the foot up and down.

The individual usually has no history of trauma. Usually the symptoms start gradually and progress if activity is not reduced. The following is the usual symptomatic treatment:

- Rest in the acute stage; reduce weight-bearing activity.
- In mild cases brought about by overuse, decrease or modify activity for a few days (e.g., swimming or cycle ergometer workouts instead of running).
- Apply heat or ice before activity; use ice after activity. Heat treatments may consist of moist heat packs for 20 min or whirlpool treatments. The temperature of whirlpool water should be approxi-

mately 104 to 106 °F. Treatment time is usually 20 min. Ice application may consist of ice-bag treatments for 20 min or ice massage/ice slush treatments for 5 to 7 min.

Treatment should begin at the first sign of pain. If pain is extreme, medical consultation should be obtained. Determination and treatment of the cause, in addition to symptomatic treatment, is necessary, to prevent a recurrence of the problem. Table 16.5 cites the major causes for shin splints as well as the signs and symptoms accompanying those causes and steps that can be taken to help prevent the onset or recurrence of lower leg pain.

EXERCISE MODIFICATION

Most orthopedic-related injuries can be classified as mild, moderate, or severe. When in doubt, conservative

Table 16.4   (Continued)

Injury	Common causes	Signs and symptoms	Treatment
Tennis elbow—inflammation of the musculotendinous unit of the elbow extensors where they attach on the outer aspect of the elbow (lateral epicondylitis).	Faulty backhand mechanics—faults may include leading with the elbow, using an improper grip, dropping the racket head, or using a topspin backhand with a whipping motion. Improper grip size—usually too small. Racket strung too tightly. Improper hitting—hitting off center, particularly if using wet, heavy balls.	Pain directly over the outer aspect of the elbow in the region of the common extensor origin. Swelling. Increased skin temperature over the area of inflammation. Pain on extension of the middle finger against resistance with the elbow extended. Pain on racket gripping and extension of the wrist.	Ice and rest in the acute stages. Chronic—generally heat is used before exercise or activity, followed by ice after activity. Deep friction massage at the elbow. Strengthening and stretching exercises for the wrist extensors. Correct the cause of the problem: 1. Use proper techniques. 2. Use proper grip size (when racket is gripped, there should be room for one finger to fit in the gap between the thumb and fingers). 3. Racket should be strung at the proper tension (usually between 50 and 55 lb). 4. Avoid stiff rackets that vibrate easily. Keep elbow warm, particularly in cold weather. Use a counterforce brace, a circular band that is placed just below the elbow (serves to reduce the stress at the origin of the extensors). If correction of cause and symptomatic treatment does not relieve symptoms, referral to a physician is recommended; anti-inflammatory medication is usually prescribed.

(Cont.)

treatment is recommended. Any injury resulting in acute pain or affecting performance, and any injury in which the individual hears or feels a pop at the time of injury, should be referred to a physician. Any time conservative measures fail to result in improvement of the condition within a reasonable period of time (2 to 4 weeks), physician consultation is again recommended.

Other conditions may call for a modification of an exercise program. The participant may be obese, arthritic, or possess a history of musculoskeletal problems. Pool work is often employed with these individuals. Warm water is very therapeutic, body weight is supported, and the water generally allows for

a greater range of movement. In any case, the activity should be suited to the condition. Any individual who requires exercise modification should be monitored closely. Table 16.6 summarizes the general guidelines used to classify injuries and offers suggestions for modifying activity.

CPR AND EMERGENCY PROCEDURES

All HFIs should be well-versed in **CPR** techniques. (Courses are generally available through the local Heart

Table 16.4   (Continued)

Injury	Common causes	Signs and symptoms	Treatment
Stress fracture—a bone defect that occurs because of accelerated rate of remodeling that occurs to accommodate the stress to weight-bearing bones. This results in a loss of continuity in the bone and periosteal irritation. Tibial stress fractures are more common in individuals with high-arched feet. Fibula stress fractures are more common in pronators.	Overuse or abrupt change in training program. Change in running surface. Change in running gait.	Referred pain to the fracture site when a percussion test is used. (Example: Hitting the heel may cause pain at the site of a tibial stress fracture). Pain is usually localized to one spot and is exquisitely tender to palpation. Pain is generally present all of the time but increases with weight-bearing activity. Pain does not subside after warm-up.	Referral to physician. X-ray films should be obtained. Usually no crack is detected in bone. A cloudy area becomes visible when the callus begins to form. Often this does not show up until 2-6 weeks after onset of pain. Early detection can usually be made through a bone scan or **thermogram**. If a stress fracture is suspected but not diagnosed, treat as a stress fracture. Running and other high-stress, weight-bearing activities should not be allowed until the fracture has healed and bone is no longer tender to palpation. Tibial stress fractures usually take 8-10 weeks to heal; fibular stress fractures take approximately 6 weeks. When acute symptoms have subsided, bicycling and swimming activities can usually be initiated to maintain cardiovascular levels. This should be cleared with the supervising physician. If a specific cause is attributed to the development of a stress fracture, steps should be taken to correct the cause. (See common causes for shin splints and their prevention.)

(Cont.)

Association or Red Cross.) In an emergency situation, there is little time to think. Most reactions occur automatically. Having a plan of action and running through practice drills on a routine basis help to ensure that proper procedures are followed in an emergency situation.

Be Prepared

Make sure a phone is available for use during the exercise class, and know where the phone is located. If a phone is not available, have an alternative emergency plan in mind. The HFI should identify the **emergency medical system** (EMS) and services that are to be used (ambulance, hospital, doctor, etc.), and have a phone list located in a convenient place. Decide who is to phone for medical help in an emergency situation, and make sure that he or she knows how to direct help to the location of the injured (see chapter 17). All necessary medical information (release forms, medical history forms, etc.) should be readily available, and all emergency equipment and supplies should be easily accessible (stretcher, emergency kit and supplies, splints, ice, money for phone call, blanket, spine board, etc.). The equipment should be checked periodically to ensure that

Table 16.4   (Continued)

Injury	Common causes	Signs and symptoms	Treatment
Mechanical low-back pain—low-back pain which results from poor body mechanics, inflexibility of certain muscle groups, or muscular weakness.	Tight lower-back musculature. Tight hamstrings. Poor posture or habits. Weak trunk musculature, particularly abdominals. Differences in leg length because of a structural or functional problem. Structural abnormality. Obesity.	Generalized low-back pain, usually aggravated by activity that accentuates the curve in the low back (example: hill running). Muscle spasm. Palpable tenderness that is limited to musculature and not located directly over the spine. May see a difference in pelvic height or other signs that would indicate a possible leg-length discrepancy. Muscle tightness, particularly of the hamstrings, hip flexors, and low back.	Acute care of low-back pain or any individual who displays signs of nerve impingement should be referred to a physician for evaluation and X-ray. It is necessary to rule out structural abnormalities such as **spondylolisthesis**, ruptured disc, fractures, **neoplasms**, or possible segmental instability prior to instituting a general exercise program. Further diagnostic procedures may be warranted. Symptomatic treatment consists of ice application and referral to physician in acute cases. Chronic cases are generally treated with moist heat to reduce muscle spasm, and ice after activity. Correct the causes of low-back pain. 1. Stretch tight muscles. 2. Strengthen weak muscles. 3. Proper warm-up prior to activity and proper cool-down following activity. 4. Correct leg-length differences. 5. Emphasize correct postural positions 6. If possible, correct or compensate for structural abnormalities (example: orthotics for a biomechanical problem).

Note. Adapted from American Medical Association (1966), Arnheim (1987), and Henderson (1973).

it is in proper working order, and the supplies should be up-to-date. Finally, know where the fire alarms and fire exits are located.

Remain Calm

Remaining calm reassures the injured person and helps prevent the onset of shock. Clear thinking allows for sound judgment and proper execution of rehearsed plans. In most instances, speed is not necessary. Cases of extreme breathing difficulty, stoppage of breathing or circulation, choking, severe bleeding, shock, head or neck injury, heat illness, and internal injury are exceptions to this and require urgent action. Otherwise, careful evaluation and a deliberate plan of action is desirable. The HFI should have a system for evaluating and dealing with a life-threatening situation. All procedures should be conducted in a calm, professional manner.

Table 16.5   Shin-Splint Syndrome

Injury	Common causes	Signs and symptoms	Prevention
Shin splints—inflammatory reaction of the musculotendinous unit, caused by overexertion of muscles during weight-bearing activity. The following conditions must be ruled out: stress fracture, metabolic or vascular disorder, compartment syndrome, and muscular strain.	Prominent callus in metatarsal region.		Keep callus filed down. Metatarsal arch pad.
	Fallen **metatarsal arch**.		
	Weak **longitudinal arch**.	Lower longitudinal arch on one side in comparison to the opposite side.	Strengthening exercises. Longitudinal arch tape support.
		Tenderness in arch area.	Arch supports.
	Muscular imbalance.		Strengthening exercises; generally weakness of the dorsiflexors and invertors.
	Poor leg, ankle, and foot flexibility.		Exercise to increase range of motion.
	Improper running surface.		Avoidance of hard surfaces. Decrease in hill running. Avoidance of running on uneven terrain. Minimization of changing from one surface to another.
	Improper running shoes.		Selection of shoe with good shock absorbency qualities. Properly fitted shoes.
	Overuse.		Gradual increase in workouts. Flexibility in changing training program if there are signs that much physical stress is occurring. Encourage year-round conditioning. Proper warm-up. Rest when indicated.
	Biomechanical problems or structural abnormalities.	Abnormal wear pattern of shoes.	Refer to podiatrist or professional specializing in foot care; orthotics may be indicated. Design a special training program to allow for individual differences (example: increase intensity of workouts, reduce duration).
	Improper running or skills technique.		Correct technique. Specific stretching or strengthening exercises as well as technique work.
	Training in poor weather conditions.		Use common sense when training in cold or foul weather. Dress properly to maintain warmth. Warm up and cool down properly.

Note. Adapted from Morris (1984).

Table 16.6 Injury Classification Criteria and Exercise Modification

Criteria	Modifications
Mild injury Performance is not affected. Pain is experienced only after athletic activity. Generally, no tenderness on palpation. No or minimal swelling. No discoloration.	Reduce activity level, modify activity to take stress off of the injured part, treat symptomatically, and gradually return to full activity.
Moderate injury Performance mildly affected or not affected at all. Pain is experienced before and after athletic activity. Mild tenderness on palpation. Mild swelling may be present. Some discoloration may be present.	Rest the injured part, modify activity to take stress off of the injured part, treat symptomatically, and gradually return to full activity.
Severe injury Pain is experienced before, during, and after activity. Performance definitely affected because of pain. Normal daily function affected because of pain. Movement limited because of pain. Moderate to severe point tenderness on palpation. Swelling most likely present. Discoloration may be present.	Rest completely and see a physician.

Note. Adapted from Arnheim (1987).

Determine How the Injury Occurred

The history of the injury can be surmised from observation of what happened, the injured person's account of what happened, or by a witness's account of the injury. If the injured person is unconscious or semiconscious, and no cause is determined, check for a medic-alert identification tag.

Check Vital Signs

The HFI should determine the seriousness of the situation by checking **vital signs**: HR, breathing, BP, bleeding, and so on. The outcome of this evaluation will identify a course of action. The following sections describe vital signs, how to monitor each, and a planned course of action to follow.

Level of Consciousness

Is the individual conscious? If not, there may be a possible head, neck, or back injury. If you are unsure why the individual is unconscious, check for a medic-alert identification tag. Assess airway, breathing, and circulation. *Do not use ammonia capsules to arouse*; the individual may suddenly move the head backward in response, causing additional injury.

If breathing has stopped and the individual is in a prone position, she or he should be log-rolled as carefully as possible, keeping the head, neck, and spine in the same relative position, to begin CPR techniques.

If the individual is unconscious but breathing, protect from further injury. Do not move unless the individual's life is in danger. Wait for medical assistance to arrive. Make a systematic evaluation of the entire body and perform necessary first-aid procedures (1, 4, 11).

Respiration

Is the individual breathing? If not, establish an airway and administer artificial respiration. Summon medical help. The following will aid in determining the problem:

- Normal respiration—20 breaths per minute
- Respiration in well-trained individuals—6 to 8 breaths per minute
- Shock—rapid, shallow respiration
- Airway obstruction, heart disease, pulmonary disease—deep, gasping, labored breathing
- Lung damage—frothy sputum with blood at the nose and mouth, accompanied by coughing
- Diabetic **acidosis**—alcoholic or sweet, fruity odor
- Cessation of breathing—note movement of abdomen and chest as well as airflow at nose and mouth

Pulse

Check pulse by using light finger pressure over an artery. The most common sites are the carotid, brachial, radial, and femoral pulses. If there is no pulse and the individual is unconscious, begin CPR (1, 4, 11).

Skin Color

For light-pigmented individuals, assess skin color, fingernail beds, lips, sclera of eyes, and mucous membranes. If these are red, there is the possibility of heat stroke, high blood pressure, or carbon monoxide poisoning. If pale or ashen, it could be due to shock, fright, insufficient circulation, heat exhaustion, insulin shock, or a heart attack. If bluish, the poor oxygenation of the blood could be due to an airway obstruction, respiratory insufficiency, heart failure, or some poisonings. For dark-pigmented individuals, assess nail beds, inside of lips, mouth, and tongue. Pink is the normal color for these. A bluish cast suggests shock. A greyish cast suggests shock from **hemorrhage**. A red flush at the tips of the ears suggests fever.

Body Temperature

Normal body temperature is 98.6 °F. Assess skin by palpation. Record temperature with a thermometer placed under the tongue (for 3 min), axilla (10 min), or in the rectum (1 min). Cool, clammy, damp skin suggests shock and heat exhaustion; cool, dry skin indicates exposure to cold air; and hot, dry skin suggests fever or heat stroke.

Ability to Move

Inability to move (paralysis) suggests injury or illness of the spinal cord or brain.

Bleeding

Is the individual bleeding profusely? If so, control bleeding by elevating the body part, putting direct pressure over the wound and at **pressure points**, and as a last resort, putting on a **tourniquet**. *A tourniquet should only be used in life-threatening situations in which choosing to risk a limb is a reasonable action in order to save a life.* Treat for shock.

Blood Pressure

BP is usually taken at the brachial artery with a blood pressure cuff and sphygmomanometer. The following will aid in determining the problem (1, 4):

- Normal BP—in men, systolic pressure, the pressure during the contraction phase of the heart, is equal to 100 plus the age of the individual up to 140 to 150 mmHg; diastolic pressure, the pressure during the relaxation phase of the heart, is equal to 65 to 90 mmHg. In females, both readings are generally 8 to 10 mmHg lower.
- Severe hemorrhage, heart attack—marked fall (20 to 30 mmHg) in blood pressure.
- Damage or rupture of vessels in the arterial circuit—abnormally high BP (>150/>90).
- Brain damage—rise in systolic pressure with a stable or falling diastolic pressure.

- Heart ailment—fall in systolic pressure with a rise in diastolic pressure.

Eye Pupil Size and Response

Is there evidence of a head injury? This can be determined through a history of a blow to the head or a fall onto the head, deformity of the skull, loss of consciousness, clear or straw-colored fluid coming from the nose or ears, unequal pupil size, dizziness, loss of memory, and nausea. Prevent any unnecessary movement. If it is necessary to move the individual, use a stretcher with the individual's head elevated. If the individual is unconscious, assume that there is also a neck injury. Summon medical help immediately. The following will aid in determining the problem (1, 4, 11):

- Drug addict or nervous system disorder—constricted pupils
- Unconscious, cardiac arrest—dilated pupils
- Head injury—pupils unequal size
- Disease, poisoning, drug overdose, injury—pupils do not react to light
- Death—pupils widely dilated and unresponsive to light

Pain Reaction

Is there evidence of a neck or back injury? The history of the injury may give a clue. Other indications of a possible neck or back injury include pain directly over the spine, burning or tingling in the extremities, and loss of muscle function or strength in the extremities. *When in doubt, assume there is a neck or back injury.* The following will aid in determining the problem (1, 4):

- Probable injury of spinal cord—numbness or tingling in the extremities
- Occlusion of a main artery—severe pain in the extremity, with loss of cutaneous sensation; pulse is absent in the extremity
- Hysteria, violent shock, excessive drug or alcohol use—no pain

Although the following information lists the steps for artificial respiration and cardiopulmonary techniques for adults only, the HFI should review current recommended techniques for all age categories: adults, children, and infants.

Artificial Respiration

If the HFI believes the person has stopped breathing, artificial respiration should be initiated. The following is a list of nine steps to use in mouth-to-mouth resuscitation (2).

1. Determine responsiveness of the individual by shouting "Are you okay?"
2. Position the victim and call for help.
3. Open the airway by using a jaw thrust or head tilt/chin lift.
4. Determine whether the victim is breathing. Listen and feel for air exchange. Look for chest movement.
5. If there is no breathing, give two quick, full ventilations using mouth-to-mouth or mouth-to-nose technique.
6. Determine whether there is a pulse by checking the carotid artery.
7. Implement the emergency medical system—call 911 or the emergency number for your area.
8. If there is a pulse, ventilate once every 5 s for an adult.
9. Assess the victim's condition after 1 min and approximately every 2 to 3 min thereafter.

One-Person CPR

If the HFI finds that breathing has stopped and there is no pulse, she or he should initiate CPR. The following outlines nine steps for one-person CPR.

1. Determine responsiveness of the individual by shouting "Are you okay?"
2. Position the victim and call for help.
3. Open the airway by using a jaw thrust or head tilt/chin lift.
4. Determine whether the victim is breathing. Listen and feel for air exchange. Look for chest movement.
5. Give two ventilations using mouth-to-mouth or mouth-to-nose technique.
6. Determine whether there is a pulse by checking the carotid artery.
7. Implement the emergency medical system—call 911 or the emergency number for your area.
8. If there is no breathing and no pulse, give 15 compressions followed by two ventilations at a rate of 80 compressions per minute for an adult.
9. Assess the victim's condition after 1 min and every 2 to 3 min thereafter.

Two-Person CPR

If the HFI is doing one-person CPR, and another CPR-trained individual appears, two-person CPR can be ini-

tiated. The following outlines the steps in two-person CPR.

1. The second rescuer states that he or she knows CPR and asks to assist. The second rescuer then takes a position at the head when the first rescuer moves down to give chest compressions.
2. The second rescuer checks for a pulse while compressions are being given. This determines the effectiveness of the compressions. The second rescuer then tells the first rescuer to stop compressions and checks again for a pulse.
3. If a pulse is found, respiration should be checked. If there is no respiration, continue ventilation only, once every 5 s.
4. If there is no pulse, the second rescuer tells the first rescuer to continue CPR and then gives one ventilation.
5. The first rescuer follows the ventilation with five chest compressions at a rate of 60 per minute for an adult.
6. The second rescuer gives one ventilation after the last compression.
7. Assess the victim's condition after 1 min and every 2 to 3 min thereafter.

SUMMARY

Certain inherent risks are associated with physical activity. The HFI should be aware of these risks and take steps to minimize them. Advanced planning, proper equipment and facilities, and appropriate exercise recommendations for the participant help to reduce the possibility of injury. These recommendations include participant evaluation, a graduated program of exercises with clear guidelines to follow, and an education program about signs and symptoms of injuries.

When injuries occur, there are clear steps to take to reduce the possibility of more trauma and to aid in the healing process. Protection of the injured area followed by rest, ice, compression, and elevation (PRICE) are the important steps associated with the immediate treatment of most skeletal, muscle, and joint injuries. Heat is used in the later stages of acute injury and as a treatment for muscle soreness and chronic inflammatory conditions. A list of steps for the most common orthopedic injuries is provided.

Heat illness is potentially deadly, and the HFI must be aware of the steps to prevent its occurrence and, simultaneously, be able to recognize the signs of heat illness and act on them. Proper hydration, evaluated through a weight chart, is a good first step in prevention. Gradually acclimatizing the participants to heat and humidity and reducing exposure in extreme heat and humidity are reasonable precautionary guidelines.

The HFI should be able to deal with heart attacks and other emergencies by having a series of steps outlined that will be followed if an emergency occurs. Be prepared, remain calm, determine how the injury occurred, check vital signs, and if appropriate, administer artificial respiration or CPR. HFIs are cautioned to work within the limits of their qualifications to provide assistance and to not hesitate to refer a problem to appropriate professional health care services.

CASE STUDIES FOR ANALYSIS

You are instructing an aerobics class when a participant collapses. On approaching the individual you note that breathing is shallow and slow, and that the skin color is pale, moist, and clammy. The individual is conscious but not alert. She reports double vision and an intense hunger. She is wearing a medical alert tag.

a. What illness do you suspect?
b. What questions would you ask?
c. What action should the HFI take?

(See Appendix A.)

You are leading an aerobics class and a participant collapses. You observe that the individual's skin is dry and red, the breathing is labored, the pulse is rapid and strong. No trauma was experienced.

a. What heat-related illness should be suspected?
b. What is the immediate care?

c. What emergency planning should be in effect?

(See Appendix A.)

REFERENCES

1. American Academy of Orthopaedic Surgeons (1977)
2. American Heart Association (1987b)
3. American Medical Association (1966)
4. Arnheim (1987)
5. Henderson (1973)
6. Klafs and Arnheim (1977)
7. Morris (1984)
8. Ritter and Albohm (1987)
9. Scriber and Burke (1978)
10. Smith (1976)
11. Thygerson (1987)

SUGGESTED READINGS

American College of Sports Medicine (1975)
American Red Cross (1980)
American Red Cross (1981a)
American Red Cross (1981b)
Anderson (1980)
D'Ambrosia and Drez (1982)
Darden (1976)
Fox and Mathews (1974)
Getchell (1976)
Kuland (1982)
O'Donoghue (1984)
Parcel (1986)
Williams (1980)

Chapter 17

Administrative Concerns

OBJECTIVES

The reader will be able to:
- Describe the process of long-range planning
- List the qualifications needed for fitness-program personnel
- Describe the elements of a comprehensive fitness program
- Explain the components of informed consent
- Explain safety and legal concerns for fitness programs
- Describe elements of the budget
- Explain the importance of communication with staff, participants, and the public
- Describe the records that are needed
- Describe the process of evaluation

TERMS

The reader will be able to define or describe:

Budget	Informed consent
Communication	Liability
Cost effectiveness	Long-range goals
Emergency procedures	Negligence
Evaluation	Personnel

In small fitness programs the HFI may be in charge of administering the program, but in most cases a program director has the major administrative responsibilities. However, all staff personnel should have an understanding of the types of decisions that are made and the processes that are used by the program executive.

The key concept to administration is planning. Many different programs and management styles can be successful when carefully planned. On the other hand, almost nothing works well over the long term without prior thought. This chapter deals with the items that need to be considered in establishing a long-range plan for a fitness center, and presents suggestions for dealing with responsibilities that administrators normally have in any type of program.

The program director is normally responsible for

- long-range planning;
- decisions about what specific classes will be offered, when, where, and for whom;
- hiring and evaluating personnel;
- budget;
- communications; and
- quality control.

LONG-RANGE GOALS

Any organization—private, public, for profit, or nonprofit—needs to clearly indicate what it wants to accomplish. The long-range plan includes what goals should be accomplished, what is needed to accomplish these goals, how the organization will move from where it is to where it wants to be, and what processes should be followed to implement the program. The board of directors (governing body) must approve the long-range plan. However, advisory committees (composed of key people in the community and in related groups), staff, and participants (consumers) should all have input concerning the **long-range goals**. The administrator facilitates the establishment of the long-range plan by working with the governing body in defining the areas that should be addressed, seeking input from appropriate individuals and groups, and providing working drafts for reactions and revisions. The program director also helps the governing body by setting realistic timelines for the draft plan, getting reactions, making modifications, and obtaining final approval. The administrator implements the plan, including periodic evaluation. The HFI's role is to provide details concerning possible fitness programs that are consistent with the aims of the fitness center and will be popular with current and potential participants. The HFI works with the fitness director in determining appropriate equipment, facilities, scheduling, personnel, and supplies.

KEY POINT.   Development of long-range goals and plans is essential for a fitness program.

PERSONNEL

The most important aspect of any program is the quality of the staff. The recruitment, hiring, support for, and evaluation of **personnel** to help achieve the organization's goals is essential, time consuming, and often sensitive.

Who Is Needed

The first question is, What types of people are needed to carry out the planned program? Fitness programs need staff personnel who can present and supervise the fitness activities. A typical fitness center needs the following personnel.

Full time:

- Program director
- HFI
- Educational coordinator
- Secretary

Part time:

- Medical adviser
- Fitness leaders
- Nutritionist
- Psychologist
- Physical therapist
- Equipment technician

Qualifications

A related question is, What characteristics are desired for the staff? The qualifications include education, personal qualities, and professional competence. Gettman (1) lists the many administrative responsibilities involved in a fitness program: managing, planning, supervising, educating, leading exercise, motivating, counseling, promoting, assessing, and evaluating.

During the search for specific personnel, decisions are made concerning which of these general responsibilities, and what specific tasks, each person will need to be responsible for. A realistic list of required and preferred qualifications is developed for each staff member. For example, an education requirement is established for each position. Requiring more education than is needed, or failing to require enough, causes problems. For fitness programs, the appropriate ACSM certification can be useful in establishing minimum qualifications. Use the certification that matches the position. For example, the original certifications were aimed at postcardiac programs and include competencies unnecessary for people working with apparently healthy individuals. See the Sample Job Description form.

KEY POINT.   Full- and part-time personnel are needed who are qualified to administer a fitness program, lead exercise, test fitness components, and deal with specific aspects of fitness.

Working Environment

The fitness center should provide a good working environment and accurately describe the working conditions to prospective staff members. The physical environment should be safe, clean, and cheerful, with functioning equipment, available supplies, and quick repairs when needed. The professional environment is one in which the expectations for each staff member are clearly described, and supervision is ample to assist professional growth and ensure quality performance. The psychological environment ensures that employees are valued, with their input being solicited and welcomed. They are communicated with openly and honestly, and feel that they have support for problems that might arise.

Evaluation

A clear job description that is mutually understood pro-

Sample Job Description
Generic Fitness Center

Health Fitness Instructor

Qualifications

BS in physical education or related field (MS preferred)
ACSM Health Fitness Instructor Certification
Experience in testing and leading exercise in adult fitness setting
Ability to relate to people with diverse backgrounds

Responsibilities

Administer physical fitness tests
Lead physical-fitness exercise sessions
Work with Program Director in
    Scheduling fitness programs and staff
    Adding variety to fitness classes
    Training new staff members

Application Process

Send a letter of application, vita, and the names, addresses, and phone numbers
of three references to
    Dr. Drawde Yelwoh, Director
    Generic Fitness Center
    Yarbrogh, MI 22222
To ensure consideration for position, applications should be received by March 1,
1993.

Title and Starting Date

The Health Fitness Instructor will begin September 1, 1993. The 12-month position
includes 2 weeks of vacation and an excellent fringe-benefit package. The salary
will be within the range of $17,500 to $25,000, depending on qualifications.

Affirmative Action

The Generic Fitness Center encourages minority, female, and physically chal-
lenged candidates to apply for this position.

---

vides the basis for periodic **evaluations**. The main purpose of the evaluation is to assist the staff member in
improving herself or himself. However, the evaluation
is also used to determine whether or not employees are
retained in the position, and if so, what merit raises
should be awarded. Evaluation of the HFI includes

- the content of the fitness program;
- the manner in which the program is conducted;
- the HFI's rapport with fitness participants, other
  staff, and the fitness director;
- the HFI's response to emergency and unusual
  situations;
- the HFI's accuracy in collecting and recording test
  data; and
- whether the HFI has a prompt and professional manner of carrying out other assigned responsibilities.

The Sample Evaluation Checklist presents questions
that can be asked in an annual evaluation conference.

KEY POINT.   The working environment (physical,
professional, and psychological) and a clear process for
evaluation are important elements for fitness personnel.

Sample Evaluation Checklist
Generic Fitness Center

Evaluation of a Health Fitness Instructor

Attainment of Current Goals

Did the HFI

Adhere to Center procedures?
Make proper screening decisions?
Administer tests efficiently, with accurate results and good records?
Provide appropriate content for the exercise sessions?
Conduct the sessions with enthusiasm?
Provide a variety of fitness activities?
Relate well with the clients?
Relate well with the staff?
Provide comprehensive training and supervision of new staff members?
Understand and carry out emergency procedures?
Make suggestions for improvement in all aspects of the Center's activities and
    procedures?
Make efforts to improve in identified areas of weakness?
Accomplish things not listed as specific goals for this year?

Evaluation of Past Activities

What responsibilities were carried out (be specific)

Very well?
Adequately, but could be improved?
Below expectations that must be corrected?

Future Goals

What responsibilities should be

Continued?
Added?
Deleted or handled by someone else?

What additional knowledge, skills, and so forth are needed?

How will they be obtained?

How can the evaluation process be improved?

PROGRAM

Painter and Haskell (7) list four aspects of interaction between the fitness program and the participant: screening, individual program development, fitness program implementation, and maintenance.

Criteria for Entry into Program

All participants should be screened before they are placed in appropriate fitness programs. Chapter 2 deals with criteria for admission to various programs. For example, people with known or suspected health problems are not allowed in fitness programs aimed to increase the positive health of apparently healthy people. The administrator ensures that the testing criteria for exclusion or referral is consistently applied and that the staff personnel leading activities are able to recognize signs and symptoms indicative of problems requiring special attention.

Informed Consent

Any fitness program should follow the **informed-consent** procedures established to protect participants. Informed consent has several elements, including

- a clear description of program and procedures,
- a clear description of potential benefits and risks of the program,
- a statement that the participant is participating voluntarily and has the right to withdraw at any time, and
- a statement that each individual's data is confidential.

The first component of informed consent is to clearly describe the fitness program and all of the procedures that will be used. This description should be in writing, and each individual should read and receive a copy. In addition, each person should be given an opportunity to have any questions answered. The second element of this procedure, included in the written description of the program, is a list of the possible benefits and risks of such a program. The fitness benefits are extensive; however, the risk of certain kinds of injuries (e.g., ankle, knee) is increased, and heart attacks do occasionally happen during or after exercise. After reading the description of the program with the potential benefits and risks, the person signs the form indicating that she or he is participating voluntarily, with the provision that tests and all other activities can be stopped at any time without penalty or coercion to continue.

Finally, each individual's data is confidential unless the individual gives permission to release it. People normally agree to have their test scores used in fitness reports and research, but these reports should be presented in such a manner that an individual's test score remains confidential. An exception to this guideline is using test scores to recognize people in newsletters or news releases—in these cases, permission should be obtained (and usually is granted) from the person before publishing the individual scores. A Sample Consent Form that might be used in a fitness program is shown here. Specific procedures need to be modified to fit the particular fitness testing and program.

Scheduling

Although the general types of experiences offered by the organization are determined prior to staff selection, the staff can assist in fine-tuning the specific classes that will be offered to take advantage of the strengths of each staff member and provide the activities needed by the participants. Chapter 14 includes suggestions and examples of activities to be included in the fitness program.

Scheduling of personnel and facilities requires attention to the types of programs being offered, the desires of consumers for specific times, and the optimal work performance from staff. Priorities are established to ensure that the more important objectives receive the needed staff and facilities. Public relations are enhanced by making the facilities available to other groups, although that is usually a lower priority. Guidelines should be established to ensure that the top-priority activities have adequate time. For example, the main exercise room might be scheduled for classes first, then other peak times set aside for members to use it on their own. Community groups can reserve it only during specific nonpeak times of the day. A form like the Sample Form for Use of Facility could be used to lease the facilities to local groups.

Testing Procedures

Fitness participants should be tested to decide whether or not they should be excluded, can enter the program only with medical clearance, or can begin immediately (see chapter 2). For people in the program, testing is important to determine the extent to which their individual objectives are being met. The test results can motivate participants to continue and can provide the basis for activity modification. Fitness-testing procedures are included in chapters 2, 5, 7, 9, and 10.

KEY POINT. Scheduling of the facilities, activities, and appropriate testing are important aspects of the administration of a fitness program.

Sample Consent Form
Generic Fitness Center

Informed Consent for Physical Fitness Test

In order to more safely carry on an exercise program, I hereby consent, voluntarily, to exercise tests. I shall perform a graded exercise test by riding a cycle ergometer or walking/running on a treadmill. Exercise will begin at a low level and be advanced in stages. The test may be stopped at any time because of signs of fatigue. I understand that I may stop the test at any time because of my feelings of fatigue or discomfort or for any other personal reason.

I understand that the risks of this testing procedure may include disorders of heart beats, abnormal blood-pressure response, and, very rarely, a heart attack. I further understand that selection and supervision of my test is a matter of professional judgment.

I also understand that skinfold measurements will be taken at (number) sites to determine percent body fat and that I will complete a sit-and-reach test and a curl up test to evaluate factors related to low-back function.

I desire such testing so that better advice regarding my proposed exercise program may be given to me, but I understand that the testing does not entirely eliminate risk in the proposed exercise program.

I understand that information from my tests may be used for reports and research publications. I understand that my identity will not be revealed.

I understand that I can withdraw my consent or discontinue participation in any aspect of the fitness testing or program at any time without penalty or prejudice toward me.

I have read the statement above and have had all of my questions answered to my satisfaction.

_____
Signed
_____
Witness
_____
Date

(Copy for participant and for program records.)

Safety and Legal Concerns

The main concern for the fitness program is that it be conducted safely for everyone permitted to participate in the program. Fortunately, the same kinds of things done to make the program safe also help protect the program legally. Chapter 16 includes detailed procedures to prevent and deal with injuries and emergencies, including CPR procedures, that are essential for all staff members who will be in contact with fitness participants.

Liability

The program and its staff have a responsibility to perform the procedures as described in a professional man-

ner, watch for any danger signs that might indicate a problem, and take appropriate actions to stop the activity before problems occur. Herbert and Herbert (2) list **common potential liability problems**. These are failure to

- monitor and/or stop a GXT, using professional judgment;
- evaluate participants' physical capabilities or impairments that would need special attention;
- recommend a safe exercise intensity;
- instruct participants adequately on safe activities and proper use of equipment;
- supervise exercise and advise individuals regarding restrictions or modifications needed during unsupervised exercise;

Sample Form for Use of Facility by Outside Group
Generic Fitness Center

Use of Facility

Name of Group:

Person responsible for the group:

   Name:

   Phone:

Purpose for use of building:

Estimated number of participants:

Age range of participants:

Room(s) desired:

Date(s) & Time(s):   Date   Time

   First choice:

   Second choice:

   Third choice:

On behalf of the group desiring to lease a part of the Fitness Center, I have read and agree to follow the regulations for the building. Our group understands that the security deposit may be used for any damage that occurs as a result of our group's activities. In addition, we will reimburse the Generic Fitness Center for any damages that exceed the deposit.

_____

Signed

_____

Witness

_____

Date

- assign participants to levels of monitoring, supervision, and emergency medical support commensurate with health status;
- perform in a nonnegligent manner;
- refrain from giving advice construed to represent diagnosis of a medical condition;
- refer participants to medical or other professionals based on appropriate signs or symptoms; and
- maintain proper and confidential records.

If problems do occur, take the appropriate actions to deal with minor problems and get immediate help for major problems. Professional organizations (e.g., AAHPERD, ACSM) have arrangements with insurance carriers to provide liability insurance available for individuals. Staff members should be encouraged to have this type of insurance. In addition, the organiza-

tion should include liability for the program and facilities in its insurance coverage.

Negligence

No amount of informed-consent procedures can justify **negligence**. Participants and facilities need supervision. Staff personnel need training in appropriate emergency procedures, which need to be followed. Failure to do so, or failure to act in a manner fitting for a fitness professional, constitutes negligence. If injury or death occur as a result of the negligence, then the leader and program are legally liable.

Consent

Although getting the participant's consent does not prevent legal actions or protect against negligence, it does indicate that the program is concerned with the participant and has acted in good faith.

Safety Procedures

Concern for safety includes regular checks of the equipment and facilities and periodic reviews of the procedures used by the staff both in testing and in the classes. Records showing when the review, training, and practice were carried out should be kept in the central office.

Emergency Procedures

A written **emergency procedure** is to be established, and staff members trained to carry out the procedure. Local emergency services to be used are to be contacted to help establish the procedure and comprehend the procedure that is to be followed. The Sample Emergency Procedures form can be modified for a specific situation.

KEY POINT. Detailed safety and emergency procedures need to be established, with proper training of all staff. Participants need to be given good information and advice, facilities and programs need supervision, and unusual events should be responded to professionally.

BUDGET

The **budget** is one aspect of long-range planning. A suggested budget process includes the steps outlined in the Sample Budget Process. The Sample Monthly Budget Report is adapted from (6). A more detailed example of a fitness budget can be found in (8).

Third-Party Payments

Insurance companies have always invested in health by providing health education, supporting research, and providing payment for treatment of health problems (e.g., postcardiac rehabilitation programs). More recently, they have offered incentives for healthy behaviors such as lower premiums for nonsmokers and cash paybacks for people who did not use their medical insurance for a set period of time. Unfortunately, the insurance companies, for the most part, still do not provide payment for preventive programs. With increasing evidence of the health benefits of fitness programs emphasizing a variety of healthy behaviors, the program director should approach insurance companies with proposals for third-party payment for some of the

services and for premium incentives for people engaging in healthy behaviors. Meyers (4) lists public and private agencies that might pay for inpatient and outpatient care.

Personnel

The biggest part of the budget involves salary and benefits for the staff. Relatively high base salaries and benefits, with regular increments based on evaluations, can assist the program in employing people with better qualifications. An attractive salary and benefit package results in higher job satisfaction, higher quality performance, and a lower turnover rate. Administrators attempting to economize in terms of staff salaries, benefits, and raises often find out that it is false economy.

Facilities

There is a regular and ongoing expense in terms of insurance, maintenance, and repair of facilities. People are often tempted to ignore regular maintenance and repair, but keeping the facilities in good shape is more efficient than incurring major expenses as a result of not having done so. New or expanded facilities are usually handled in a separate fundraising campaign and are not part of the normal budget process.

KEY POINT. Financial management is a major part of long-range planning. The budget needs to be based on realistic estimates of income and expenditures, with the flexibility to adjust for unexpected developments.

Equipment

Equipment should be available so participants may accomplish their goals; this equipment should be kept in good condition. However, programs often go beyond what is needed in terms of equipment. For a beginning program, exercise tests can be done without the most expensive treadmill. Gas analysis equipment, necessary for many research projects, is a luxury for a beginning fitness program. Much of the muscular strength and endurance needed for fitness can be gained with strength exercises with minimal weights, thus expensive resistive-exercise machines are not needed. Many program administrators use nice-looking equipment to sell their programs, when the fitness benefits might be accomplished better with activities requiring very little

Sample Emergency Procedures
Generic Fitness Program

Cardiac Emergency

1. Do NOT move the victim, except to try to get him or her into a lying position.
2. Check for breathing and pulse; if absent, begin CPR immediately.
3. Call, or have someone call, the Emergency Room at _____(name)_____ Hospital, _____(phone number)_____ , ext. _____(number)_____ .
4. Read the statement above the phone to the person:

(Statement to be posted by all phones:)

This is _____(name)_____ at the _____(name)_____ Fitness Center. We have a cardiac emergency, please send an ambulance to the _____(name)_____ Street entrance of the _____(name)_____ building, at _____(address)_____ .

5. Send someone to get Dr. _____(name)_____, whose schedule is posted by the phone [this is for Centers that have medical personnel on the site].
6. Continue CPR until medical personnel arrive, then follow their instructions.

Other Serious Accidents or Injuries

For any of the following:

Airway problems of any type
Unconsciousness
Head injury
Bleeding from ear, nose, or mouth
Neck or back injuries
Limb injury with obvious deformity
Severe chest pains

1. Do NOT move the person, except to try to get her or him into a lying position, with feet elevated (unless you suspect back injuries).
2. Contact ambulance and medical personnel—same as cardiac emergencies.
3. Treat for shock.
4. Control bleeding.

Other Injuries or Accidents

1. Do not allow a sick or injured person to sit, stand, or walk until you are sure that his or her condition warrants it.
2. Do not encourage a person who is "feeling bad" to begin or continue working out.
3. Check on people who have questionable symptoms in the locker room.
4. For less serious injuries, a first-aid kit is available at _____(place)_____ .

As soon as the situation is under control, inform _____(person)_____ about the accident, complete accident report, and turn in to _____(name or place)_____ within 24 hr.

Your suggestions for improving these instructions and the emergency procedures are welcome—talk to _____(name)_____ .

Sample Budget Process
Generic Fitness Center

1. What are the purposes of your program?
2. Describe the current program.
3. What are your current expenditures:

   A. Personnel
   B. Facilities

      (1) Loan repayment
      (2) Insurance
      (3) Maintenance and repairs
      (4) Utilities
      (5) Taxes

   C. Supplies
   D. Other

4. What is your current income:

   A. Membership
   B. Insurance
   C. Gifts
   D. Investments
   E. Other

5. A. What changes should be made in your program (e.g., classes, workshops, personnel, facilities, equipment, renovation, repair) over the next 5 years?
   B. For each of these changes, indicate the change in cost and potential income.
   C. Can the changes be phased in logical steps?
6. A. What are potential sources of increased revenue?
   B. What is needed to achieve this increased revenue?
   C. How much will it cost to secure the additional funding?
   D. What will be the net increase for each potential source of money?
7. What is a reasonable estimate for income for each year over the next 5 years?
8. What aspects of the program can be supported with this income for each year?
9. If the income exceeds expectations, what additional aspects of the program should be added?
10. If the income falls short of expectations, what aspects of the program can be reduced or eliminated?

equipment supervised by qualified personnel. Some testing equipment is needed, but once again, inexpensive items are often satisfactory for the essential fitness tests.

Testing

Testing equipment will vary with the specific program options. The list of Testing Equipment (3) presents some suggestions.

Emergency

Emergency equipment in the center will depend on access to medical or other emergency facilities.

Exercise

The list of Exercise Equipment presents suggestions for equipment to be used as part of the fitness conditioning program.

Sample Monthly Budget Report

Item	For June Budgeted	Actual	Year-to-date Budgeted	Actual
Revenues				
Membership				
Cardiac rehab				
Fitness tests				
Wellness programs				
Other				
Total				
Expenses				
Salaries				
Administrative				
Professional				
Clerical				
Commissions				
Materials				
GXT				
Wellness				
Office				
Towels				
Other				
Overhead				
Telephone				
Maintenance				
Heat/air cond				
Rent				
Service Contracts				
Other				
Total				
Balance				
Compared with 1 year ago				

Note. Adapted from Musser, 1988.

Testing Equipment

Area	Minimum	Advanced
Health status	Forms	Microcomputer
Cardiorespiratory	Walking/running track Bench RPE scale	Cycle ergometer Treadmill Oxygen analysis ECG Blood pressure Lipid assays
Relative leanness	Scale Tape measure Skinfold calipers	Underwater tank
Abdominal strength/endurance	Mat	
Midtrunk flexibility	Sit-and-reach box	
Upper body strength/endurance	Modified pull-up bar	Weights, machines

Exercise Equipment

Area	Minimum	Advanced
Cardiorespiratory	Walking/running track Bench	Cycle ergometer Treadmill Pool Stair climbing Rowing machine Skiing machine
Relative leanness		
Abdominal strength/endurance	Mat	
Midtrunk flexibility	Mat	
Upper body strength/endurance	Mat Modified pull-up bar	Free weights Isokinetic machines Pull-up bars Dip bars

Supplies

The supplies for the testing equipment and for the participant's use of the facilities must be kept in stock, with a procedure for identifying what is needed. Normally, one person is designated to be in charge of checking supplies on a regular basis. Other staff members report potential shortages to this one person. Guidelines for ordering equipment and supplies include

- order early;
- order on the basis of accurate inventory and estimate of needs—including replacement of old equipment, new equipment, and supplies for all programs;
- buy from suppliers who have a good record of service; and
- each year, ask all involved personnel in the process to make suggestions to improve the system.

Financial Management

Careful inventory, assessment of needs, and a balance among personnel, equipment, facilities, and other expenses provide the maximum service for the minimum cost.

KEY POINT. Testing and exercise equipment should be carefully selected to provide essential items economically. A process needs to be established to keep needed supplies in stock.

COMMUNICATION

One of the traits of the successful administrator is the quality of **communication** at all levels.

Staff

Open and honest communication is essential so that staff personnel know what is expected and how they are evaluated. The staff personnel need to feel appreciated and encouraged to try to find better ways of accomplishing the goals. Many advances in organizations come from staff personnel who are encouraged to help find better ways to improve the content and procedures of the program.

Participants

The consumers need basic information concerning what the fitness program can (and cannot) do for them, with periodic progress reports and educational information to enhance their positive health knowledge and status. Minilectures during warm-up, bulletin boards, and newsletters all have been used to help educate participants. The information should be accurate, brief, and to the point.

Public

Fitness programs have a responsibility to help educate the public concerning positive health—its definition and components, and recommendations for its achievement. Communicate the beneficial effects of fitness programs on health, with corresponding benefits for the family, community, and work performance, via the mass media and with interested groups such as local industry.

KEY POINT. The fitness program needs to provide clear and helpful information to staff, fitness participants, and the public.

RECORDS

Careful, systematic collection of personal and testing information, properly recorded and filed, provides the basis for much of the communication with the board, staff, and participants. This information can also be used to evaluate the effectiveness of various programs and the extent to which the long-range goals are being met. Keep records of staff training, including a demonstration of competence in emergency and safety procedures.

Data Entry, Storage, and Retrieval

What information is needed? How is it obtained? What forms are used? Where is the information stored? How is it retrieved? When is it used? Who evaluates particular programs? Address these questions before the beginning of the program. After a reasonable amount of time working with the procedure, reevaluate it to determine whether modifications would make it better. Computers are increasingly used for these tasks. It is essential to get professional assistance in setting up the procedures for computer use, so that they can be used effectively.

Accident/Injury Reports

Forms like the Sample Accident/Injury Form can be used to keep a record of all accidents and injuries. Be sure to follow up to determine the status of the individual's recovery. The completed form provides a check on whether staff personnel used appropriate emergency procedures; it is essential to have this record when questions are raised about a particular incident.

KEY POINT. The fitness program should have complete and accurate records of all aspects of the fitness program, including screening, testing, and accidents.

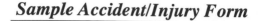

Sample Accident/Injury Form

1. _____ _____
   Name of victim   Date

2. Describe, in detail, the nature of the injury or health problem:

3. Describe, in detail, how the accident occurred:

4. List, in order, the things you or other staff members did in response to the incident:

5. Describe any problems encountered in dealing with the situation:

6. List the names of people who witnessed the accident or emergency procedures being performed:

Turn in this form, within 24 hr of the accident, to _____ (name or place) _____ .

Your suggestions concerning safety, emergency procedures, and/or this form are welcome; please talk to _____ (name) _____ .

EVALUATION

Evaluation has been mentioned throughout this chapter. A value judgment should be based on the best data available concerning the extent to which the program objectives are being reached. How many people are included in the fitness program? What kind of body-composition, CRF, and low-back function changes have been made? Do the participants enjoy the activities? How many dropouts were there? Why? How many injuries? Why? What can be done to help more people make better fitness gains, and decrease the number of dropouts and injuries? Are some staff members better than others in some of these areas? What can be done to help staff personnel maintain their strengths and improve in their weak areas?

In addition to this type of continuing evaluation of the program, it is helpful to have a formal evaluation of the program periodically (e.g., every 3 to 5 years). Mitchell and Blair (4) provide steps and helpful suggestions for developing and conducting a program evaluation. They provide assistance in setting up the evaluation (questions to be asked, evaluation design), collecting, analyzing, and reporting the information.

COST EFFECTIVENESS OF FITNESS PROGRAMS

Good fitness programs cost a substantial amount of money for personnel, facilities, equipment, and supplies, in addition to the cost of clothing, time, and travel

for the participant. Shephard (9) reviews the potential benefits for the individual and for businesses that sponsor fitness program for their employees (see Benefits of a Fitness Program). Shephard (9) summarizes the current research evidence as follows: "The currently available cost–benefit figures are encouraging in suggesting that benefits outweigh immediate program costs by a substantial margin" (p. 57).

KEY POINT.   Evaluation of the program is a continual process to ensure that quality information and inclusive programs are being provided in a cost-effective manner.

QUALITY

The most important element of a program is setting up procedures to try to ensure a high standard of quality in all information, personal contact, and activities that are conducted in the name of the fitness program. One aspect of establishing high standards is to ensure the inclusiveness of the program. All people should feel welcome in the program regardless of gender, ethnic background, or social class. The administrator can do several things to achieve this atmosphere, including

- employing a staff with varied backgrounds,
- training the staff to be sensitive to people from different backgrounds,
- scheduling programs at convenient times and places,

Benefits of a Fitness Program

Individual	*Industry*
Enhanced quality of life	Improvement of
Feeling better	Corporate image
Elevation of mood	Worker satisfaction
Increased range of experiences	Productivity
Improvement of	Decrease in
Personal appearance	Absenteeism
Self-image	Employee turnover
Health	Injury rate
Lower risk of major health problems	Medical cost
Potential increased life span	

Note. Adapted from Shephard (1990).

- contacting various groups within the community,
- providing ways for people with low incomes to participate, and
- implementing a policy where inappropriate (e.g., sexist or racist) comments or actions by staff members or participants will not be tolerated.

SUMMARY

The key to administration is planning. Long-range goals need to be established with input from staff, participants, and the community. The most important aspect of any program is the quality of the staff. Qualified individuals should be selected to do the expected tasks, and they should be evaluated on a regular basis. Scheduling of personnel and facilities revolves around the type of program being offered. Testing procedures need to be established, with criteria for entry into the program developed and applied consistently. Participants should sign an informed-consent form before entering the program. The HFI needs to understand liability and the concept of negligence.

The budget should include realistic estimates of income and expected expenditures for personnel, facilities, equipment, and supplies. Records of testing procedures, activity schedules of the participants, informed-consent forms, and so forth need to be filed for later reference. Accidents and injuries should be recorded on a special form and reported. The quality of the fitness center is enhanced by ensuring that its programs are inclusive.

REFERENCES

1. Gettman (1988)
2. Herbert and Herbert (1988)
3. Howley (1988)
4. Meyers (1988)
5. Mitchell and Blair (1988)
6. Musser (1988)
7. Painter and Haskell (1988)
8. Patton, Corry, Gettman, and Graf (1986)
9. Shephard (1990)

See the Bibliography at the end of the book for a complete source listing.

Chapter 18

Computer Software for the Health Fitness Instructor

James R. Morrow, Jr.

OBJECTIVES

The reader will be able to:

- Have a general, introductory understanding of computer use
- Have a general understanding of several computer software packages that are available
- Know references and sources she or he can turn to when seeking state-of-the-art microcomputer programs to assist in program conduction

TERMS AND DEFINITIONS

We define here a few terms necessary to assist the reader with this chapter.

Apple II family—a series of microcomputers manufactured by Apple Computer, Inc., of Cupertino, CA. Includes the Apple II, Apple II Plus, Apple IIe, and Apple IIgs microcomputers. "Apple" is a registered trademark of Apple Computer, Inc.

Backup—A spare copy of a computer program or of the data generated from a program.

Compatible (IBM compatible)—A microcomputer that can run programs written for the IBM microcomputer.

DOS (Disk Operating System)—The software that resides in the computer's memory when you turn the computer on. It gives the user the opportunity to read, write, generate, print, compute, and so on.

DOS 3.3—The disk operating system used by older members of the Apple II family of computers (e.g., Apple II and Apple II Plus).

Floppy disk—A "disk," typically 3.5 or 5.25 inches in diameter, that contains either a computer program or data to input to, or that was written from a microcomputer. Information is magnetically stored on the disk in the same way that information is stored on audio tapes.

Hardware—The physical computer device and associated peripherals. Differentiated from software.

IBM—International Business Machines of Endicott, NY.

Input—To enter data into a computer; also, the data that is entered.

Macintosh (Mac)—A microcomputer line manufactured by Apple Computer, Inc., of Cupertino, CA. A number of computers are included (e.g., Mac Plus, Mac Classic, Mac SE, Mac II series). "Macintosh" is a registered trademark of Apple Computer, Inc.

Microcomputer—A relatively small, but powerful, computer that typically can reside on a desk. The typical microcomputer (and necessary peripherals) can cost between $500 and $10,000.

Modem—Acronym for MOdulator/DEModulator, which is a peripheral device that permits a computer to send and receive messages (data) over telephone lines.

MS-DOS (Microsoft Disk Operating System)—The operating system that controls the IBM-PC and compatibles. "MS-DOS" is a registered trademark of Microsoft Corporation. See *DOS*.

Operating system—The system that controls the operation of the microcomputer. See *DOS, MS-DOS, DOS 3.3,* and *ProDos.*

Output—What is received when a computer program is run. Output may be received on a number of different devices (e.g., screen, printer, plotter, disk, tape).

Peripheral—A device associated with (and sometimes required for) particular hardware or software. For example, some programs require you to have a printer, and others may permit (or require) a plotter.

ProDos (Professional Disk Operating System)—The operating system used by newer members of the Apple II family of computers (e.g., Apple IIe and Apple IIgs).

Random access memory (RAM)—That portion of the computer's memory where the computer program is retained while the program is running. The program no longer exists in RAM once the machine is turned off.

Read-only memory (ROM)—That portion of the computer that retains instructional code even when the machine is turned off. Built in when the computer was manufactured, ROM permits the computer to perform computing functions.

Software (computer program or application)—The computer code generated to cause the computer to perform various functions. For example, a computer software program can be written to estimate percent body fat from skinfold measurements. Word-processing packages are also software. Differentiated from hardware.

Computers have transformed many aspects of everyday life, and they can significantly influence the Health Fitness Instructor's work. Tasks that previously were arduous, time consuming, confusing, and laborious can now be accomplished in a matter of minutes or seconds. The variety of convenient forms of output (e.g., on-screen, printed, or plotted) can be a great help in communicating with clients and supervisors and can generally enhance your services and relations with others. Of course, computers are a tremendous boon for clinical and research work.

The development of artificial intelligence systems permits physicians to enter physiological and symptomatic characteristics into a machine that can then develop a diagnosis based on known probabilities. Prescriptions can be computer-generated based on these results. Similar capabilities exist for the Health Fitness Instructor. A computer can let you quickly and accurately determine an individualized exercise prescription based on a person's present physiological condition, interest levels, time schedule, and commitment. The computer can then be used to track the person's progress and develop modified prescriptions based on changes in physical condition.

When the Health Fitness Instructor develops an individualized exercise prescription, she or he is basically following a set of ordered instructions for developing the plan based on test results. Microcomputers were developed precisely to perform such rule-governed functions. Once guidelines had been established for determining exercise prescriptions based on fitness evaluations, computer programmers became able to develop software packages (programs or applications) that swiftly produce individualized exercise prescriptions and spare you much work that was formerly time-consuming. You do not have to be a computer programmer to use these programs. You only need enough computer literacy to be able to enter data. You simply access software that others have already developed, and you're on your way.

The purpose of this chapter is to provide a brief description of available software related to the topics presented in this book. Hardware is not our topic here. We have focused on software that is relatively inexpensive; occasionally more expensive software packages are mentioned for contrast. Some sources offer only a single program. Others have developed many different programs that reside on a single disk, are interrelated, and are accessed through a single computer menu (or many submenus). Larger companies have developed and marketed programs that are quite expensive. However, the primary programs described throughout this chapter are relatively inexpensive and readily available.

If you are interested in more expensive and more advanced software, the American College of Sports Medicine's annual meeting has software vendors who demonstrate very sophisticated (and often expensive) software with capabilities exceeding the software described in this chapter. These more expensive packages often have highly integrated components that permit data analysis, storage, and retrieval capabilities for many operations and data sources (e.g., word processing, mailing capabilities, dietary analyses, membership directories, etc.) in addition to the more simplified examples provided here. Contact some of the developers of the more fully integrated systems if your group has the resources for such programs. The annual meetings of the American Alliance for Health, Physical Education, Recreation and Dance and Association for Fitness in Business are also excellent resources for such software.

Computers and computer interfaces are becoming very sophisticated. Those who can afford expensive integrated hardware and software can now have breath-by-breath (nearly "real time") analyses of oxygen uptake during rest or a fitness examination; computer control of every aspect of fitness evaluations or graded exercise testing (e.g., treadmill speed, elevation, cycle workload, gas collection and analyses, test cessation, etc.); tracking of workouts and caloric expenditure; recording and analysis of data from remote sites; and so on. But most HFIs do not have such resources available and are not engaged in research. The software described herein is primarily inexpensive and requires the user to input data rather than having data recorded "online." It is software that is generally available to the typical "small business" Health Fitness Instructor and geared to clinical or service work rather than research.

SOURCES FOR SOFTWARE

Various sources list computer software specifically for health and fitness. Major Sources of Computer Programs in Exercise, Health, and Fitness provides a listing of a few major sources. Current information regarding additional sources and recent software development can be obtained from software vendors' catalogs, libraries, microcomputer centers, university computer science departments, microcomputer stores, and local schools.

CHOOSING SOFTWARE

Some general Considerations When Purchasing Software follow. In general, it is extremely important to be certain that

- the software does what you need to have accomplished,
- it meets your needs and abilities, and
- you are aware of the hardware needed to support the software before purchasing it.

Some vendors let you review software before purchasing it or provide you with an inexpensive "demo" disk to help you learn the software's capabilities.

SOFTWARE PACKAGES

The list of Various Software Sources Available to the Health Fitness Instructor provides a schematic representation of available software discussed in this chapter. Vendor names, addresses, and telephone numbers are presented in the sources section at the end of the chapter.

Fitness, Lifestyle, and Health—the Evaluation of Health Status

Several large companies offer computer-based "Health Risk and Lifestyle Assessments" for a fee. The price depends on the extent of the questionnaire completed and whether physiological measures are also obtained, but usually HFIs cannot obtain the actual computer programs and instead must submit completed questionnaires to such services and contract to receive computerized evaluations from them.

However, health status and lifestyle (see chapter 2) can be evaluated by a variety of available software packages. Many of these programs are physical-fitness oriented, and others address medical aspects of health status. In general, these programs require the user to input a variety of "measured variables" that could be the results of a physiological examination (e.g., systolic and diastolic blood pressure, cholesterol level, etc.) and/or lifestyle behaviors (whether the subject wears seat belts, eating habits, exercise habits, etc.). More sophisticated programs require users to complete an exhaustive "health risk appraisal" (which may or may not include a physician's examination). The software

---

Major Sources of Computer Programs in Exercise, Health, and Fitness

Directory of Computer Software with Application to Sport Science, Health, and Dance II is available from AAHPERD. This 87-page booklet describes dozens of software packages of particular interest to the Health Fitness Instructor.

Softshare is coordinated by Sally Ayer of California State University, Fresno. Cosponsored by the California State University at Fresno and Western Society for Physical Education of College Women, Softshare makes inexpensive, practical software available for Health Fitness Instructors. Most programs sell for less than $10.00. However, some of the Softshare programs are not professionally prepared, and although they are representative examples, they might not be appropriate for professional use. Oftentimes these programs are modifiable. Other programs are professionally prepared and could be used immediately.

Human Kinetics Publishers, Inc. is a publisher with several computer software programs developed for the Health Fitness Instructor.

Comptech Systems Design has developed a wide range of software and peripherals for use in exercise science, sport, physical education, and health.

The most widely used youth-fitness tests also have computer software available with them. These include

- **Fitnessgram**—available from the Institute for Aerobics Research,
- AAHPERD's **Physical Best**—available from AAHPERD,
- **Fit Youth Today**—available from the American Health and Fitness Foundation, and
- PCPFS's **President's Challenge**—currently under development by the President's Council on Physical Fitness and Sports.

The American Alliance for Health, Physical Education, Recreation and Dance's annual meeting has provided software developers the opportunity to demonstrate their programs for the past few years.

The American College of Sports Medicine's annual meeting has software vendors who demonstrate very sophisticated and powerful (but some quite expensive) software.

The annual meeting of the Association for Fitness in Business has software vendors who demonstrate very sophisticated and powerful (but some quite expensive) software.

---

generates an appraisal of health and fitness based on the data that is input. Results may include relative risks of developing certain diseases, dying as a result of an accident, expected longevity, and so on.

The American Heart Association distributes "**Risko**," a noncomputerized, simple appraisal that assesses cardiovascular disease risk from lifestyle behaviors and physiological variables. Some smaller computer programs in this area are available from Softshare, though none of these programs are particularly extensive nor do they assess *all* aspects of risk. The American Cancer Society has computer software that addresses smoking behaviors and various types of cancer risk. **Cardiovascular Risk Evaluation** is available from Softshare to evaluate risk of

cardiovascular disease based on data from the Framingham studies. **Fitness & Wellness Software** provides relatively inexpensive and fairly comprehensive software that evaluates health status. **Cardio Stress's** programs also evaluate health status.

Exercise Science—Kinesiology, Anatomy, and Exercise Physiology

Few inexpensive software packages are available that teach the exercise physiology concepts presented in this book (chapter 3). The **Bone Box** is a HyperCard-based tutorial program on the human skeleton (chapter 4), in

---

Considerations When Purchasing Software

What operating system is used? Do you have it? Do you have the appropriate machines with which to run the software?

What are the hardware requirements for the software? Are particular peripherals required to run the software? Do you need a particular printer, plotter, and so on? Are special graphics capabilities necessary?

Does the software do what you need to have accomplished? Nothing is more frustrating than to purchase software (even inexpensively) incapable of meeting your needs.

Is the software modifiable? Can the computer code be accessed and changed if desired?

What documentation is available for the software? Some of the more inexpensive software packages do not have documentation because they are so "user friendly" anyone can run them. But this may not be the case once you run into a problem. If documentation is available, is it readable and helpful?

Is technical support available if (when!) you run into a problem?

Is the software copyable, and are you permitted to make backup copies?

Are licensing arrangements available if you have more than one machine or location?

---

which 65 drawings of the human skeleton can be studied from multiple views. Educational software catalogs list a variety of "general science" software packages on biology and chemistry. **Simulated Exercise Physiology Laboratories** is a teaching tool for cognitive concepts of exercise physiology consisting of 20 simulated laboratory lessons (oxygen uptake, cardiac output, blood pressure, training heart rate, etc.) and a lab manual. The user inputs for various parameters and then estimates outcomes based on the relationships among these variables before actually obtaining results. Parameters can then be manipulated and the impact of the manipulation observed.

Many biomechanics/kinesiology programs have been developed within biomechanics laboratories. However, most of these address film analyses and utilize digitizing capabilities to evaluate movement. Aside from being quite expensive, most of these programs are of little use to the typical HFI. Softshare has a number of programs available in this area. Be certain to determine hardware needs (e.g., digitizer) before purchasing such software.

Calculation of Oxygen Uptake and Carbon Dioxide Production

Several available programs can calculate oxygen consumption, carbon dioxide production, and the energy cost of activity (see chapters 3 and 8). Programs from Softshare require the user to input obtained variables (expired volumes, fractional concentrations, barometric pressure, gas temperature, heart rate, etc.). **MaxVO$_2$ and Body Composition: Laboratory and Field Methods** also completes these calculations. **Simulated Exercise Physiology Laboratories** has a lab session specifically related to teaching the calculations involved in oxygen uptake. **Oxycalc** is a Macintosh program that can be used to calculate oxygen uptake.

Energy Cost of Activity

Programs that estimate caloric expenditure during physical activity are generally limited in the types of activities for which calculations can be made (e.g., walking, running, cycling, swimming). The outcomes are only estimates and are open to considerable error because of the relatively large variation in caloric cost for any activity, from one individual to another. For these programs, the user inputs weight, type of activity, and number of minutes of exercise completed. These values are used to estimate caloric expenditure (and caloric balance, if caloric intake is also entered) and potential weight loss. **Kcal Expenditure** provides the user with 90 activity choices for which caloric expenditure is estimated. See chapter 8 for a list of caloric expenditures associated with a wide range of activities.

Various Software Sources Available to the Health Fitness Instructor

Program	Type[a]	Exercise prescription	Body composition	Aerobic fitness	Strength	Stress	Record keeping	Disease risk	Diet analysis	Other
Body Composition Estimation in Children	A, I									
Bone Box	M		x							x
Cardio Stress Incorporated	I	x	x	x	x		x	x	x	x
Comptech Systems Design Programs	A, I, M	x	x	x	x		x			
Diet Analysis	A, I							x	x	
Dine System	A, I								x	
Fit-n-dex	A, I		x	x	x				x	
Fitness & Wellness Software	I					x		x	x	x
Fitnessgram	A, I	x	x	x	x		x			
Fitscan	I	x	x	x	x		x			
Fit Youth Today	A, I	x	x	x	x		x			
Human Kinetics Publishers	A, I	x	x	x	x					
Kcal Expenditure	I									
Max $\dot{V}O_2$ & Body Composition: Lab & Field	A, I		x	x						x
Oxycalc	M									
Simulated Exercise Physiology Laboratories	A, I									x
Softshare Programs	A, I, M	x	x	x	x	x	x	x	x	x
Y's Way to Physical Fitness	I	x	x	x	x		x	x	x	x
YMCA Diet Analysis	A, I								x	

[a]A is Apple II family, I is IBM and compatibles, M is Apple Macintosh.

Diet and Nutrition

Diet and nutrition programs are used to evaluate an individual's current dietary status and provide healthy meals based on typical caloric expenditure, eating habits, and likes and dislikes (see chapter 6). The user generally inputs the amounts and types of foods eaten for a number of meals, and the program determines the caloric and nutritional content of the foods. Several programs are available that conduct dietary analyses. As you might well imagine, such a program has to be of considerable size to include a wide range of foods and their nutrient characteristics. Softshare has software in this area, but the food choices are somewhat limited. The **Dine System**, which is moderately priced, may be the most valuable dietary analysis program available. It has a large list of foods and has received positive evaluations. **Diet Analysis** is an inexpensive dietary analysis program available from Human Kinetics. The **YMCA Diet Analysis Software** is an inexpensive package that compares diet with recommended daily allowances.

Relative Leanness

This is probably the area for which the largest number of inexpensive programs are available. There are many software packages for anthropometric and body-composition assessment; some of these permit storage and retrieval of data, and others only generate a written or screen output. Programs have been written for the numerous equations developed for skinfold and anthropometric assessment of body composition (see chapter 7). These programs are relatively easy to prepare and have been used in numerous computer course assignments. In general, the user inputs a series of variables (e.g., gender, height, weight, skinfolds, age), although some programs require you to have access to an underwater weighing tank and a means of measuring residual volume. Measured variables (e.g., hydrostatic weight, body volume, residual volume) are input, and the output consists of weight, lean body weight (or lean body mass), relative fatness (percent fat), ideal weight, and comparisons with normative or criterion-referenced standards. Some packages are written for evaluating children only (e.g., **Body Composition Estimation for Children**). Most of the youth-fitness programs evaluate body-composition characteristics based on criterion-referenced standards. **Max$\dot{V}O_2$ and Body Composition: Laboratory and Field Methods** computes body fatness and lean body tissue, in addition to providing the user the option of estimating desired (and optimal) body weight. **Simulated Exercise Physiology Laboratories** has a program that calculates weight loss based on caloric balance.

Softshare offers many inexpensive body-composition programs. These typically work well and are technically accurate, but in some the screen presentation and output are poor, which is aesthetically unappealing and makes their use awkward for novice users. However, many of the Softshare programs are modifiable, and programmers can "clean them up."

Cardiorespiratory Fitness

Most of the programs that have been developed for estimating cardiorespiratory fitness in children and adults (see chapter 9) permit estimation of oxygen consumption from running, cycle ergometer, and treadmill tests. There are probably more computer programs available for this area than for any other except for percent body fat. **Max$\dot{V}O_2$ and Body Composition: Laboratory and Field Methods** permits the user to obtain on-screen and printed output estimates of $\dot{V}O_2$max using seven different methods (expired air, single- and double-stage cycle and treadmill, and Bruce and Balke treadmill protocols). **Fitscan** is a more expensive package that provides a wide range of programs that can be useful in a corporate fitness center. Softshare also has a number of inexpensive programs that assess aerobic endurance.

Strength, Endurance, and Flexibility

Programs in this area typically require the user to input measured strength and/or flexibility test results (see chapter 10). The obtained results are then compared to age- and gender- specific normative data for evaluative purposes. There are few inexpensive packages available in this area for adult populations. The package from **Cardio Stress**, which is expensive but fully integrated, permits data entry, tracking, and reporting on predetermined parameters as well as permitting entry of user-defined specific variables assessed at each site. **Fit-n-dex** is a moderately priced program that provides assessment of aerobic endurance, strength, flexibility, pulmonary function, and body composition. Each of the school-age-youth-fitness packages (**Fitnessgram**, AAHPERD's **Physical Best, Fit Youth Today**) provides a means of assessing and reporting muscular strength and endurance, aerobic endurance, and flexibility, and reports data in a criterion-referenced format.

Relaxation, Arousal, and Behavior Modification

The few inexpensive programs that are available in this area assess an individual's degree of stress or arousal by having the subject complete a series of stress-related questions, the answers to which reflect the degree of stress evident in the respondent's life (see chapter 11). Output includes an estimation of the degree of stress and recommendations for stress reduction (relaxation techniques, exercise, etc.). **Stress and Shrink** (available from Softshare) is used to determine stress level. **Fitness & Wellness Software** contains an evaluation of tension and stress. Some rather expensive biofeedback systems are available for research purposes, but such software is not generally accessible or useful to the Health Fitness Instructor.

Exercise Prescription and Programming

These programs could well be the most valuable to the HFI. All clients like the idea of having an individualized exercise prescription developed for them based on their current level of fitness and fitness objectives (see chapter 13). Software in this area lets the HFI produce IEPs quickly and easily. The user inputs fitness test data (aerobic power, anaerobic power, strength, flexibility, etc.), and the software develops an individualized program based on these data.

Some of the more elaborate software for exercise programs provide a training schedule that can be printed for a week or month at a time, allowing the individual to see the changes that can be expected (or that have taken place) as a result of training. The **Cardio Stress** program provides an excellent, albeit rather expensive, means to develop individualized exercise programs. **Fitness & Wellness Software** provides exercise prescriptions with a wide range of options, including cardiovascular fitness, cancer risk, tension and stress, dietary analysis, and exercise logging. The **Y's Way to Physical Fitness** is a moderately priced package available to those seeking a full-function program. The **Fit Youth Today** youth-physical-fitness program also provides an excellent exercise prescription based on the student's fitness test performance.

Administrative Concerns

Client billing, addresses, locker assignments, record keeping, and other administrative responsibilities are important to the HFI (see chapter 17). General-purpose word-processing and data-based management systems are often used for these purposes. Perhaps the best program developed specifically for billing, tracking, and administrative functions in the health/fitness industry is the **Cardio Stress** software. This software was specifically developed with a fitness-club orientation. There are some large-scale data-base programs that specifi-

cally address these management issues, but not with the health/fitness industry in mind, although an HFI could certainly use them to build a data-base system that would be sufficient for data tracking.

FUTURE DEVELOPMENTS

New and better programs are constantly being developed, but there is no single reference listing for newly developed software for use by the HFI. The annual meeting of the American Alliance for Health, Physical Education, Recreation and Dance has provided program developers the opportunity to demonstrate their software for the past few years and is likely to continue this practice as more and more individuals become aware of the capabilities and helpfulness of computers. Likewise, the annual meetings of the American College of Sports Medicine and the Association for Fitness in Business provide the opportunity to review the latest software developed for exercise, health, and fitness. To remain up to date about new software and stay current with the latest research in the profession, become active in these organizations.

SOFTWARE SOURCES

American Alliance for Health, Physical Education, Recreation and Dance. Microcomputer software is demonstrated at the annual meeting. Contact AAHPERD at 1900 Association Drive, Reston, VA 22091 (703-476-3400).

American College of Sports Medicine. Microcomputer software is demonstrated at the annual meeting. Contact ACSM at P.O. Box 1440, Indianapolis, IN 46202 (317-637-9200).

Association for Fitness in Business. 310 North Alabama, Suite A100, Indianapolis, IN 46204 (317-636-6621).

Body Composition Estimation for Children. (1987). Authored by T.G. Lohman. Available from Human Kinetics Publishers, Box 5076, Champaign, IL 61820 (1-800-342-5457).

Bone Box. (1989). Available from New Visions Software, 1108 Hazel Road, Burlington, NC 27215.

Cardio Stress Incorporated. 15425 North Freeway, Houston, TX 77090 (713-872-0984).

Comptech Systems Design. Markets a wide array of microcomputer hardware and software related to exercise, health, and fitness. 1722 Vermillion Street, Hastings, MN 55033. (612-437-1350).

Diet Analysis. Available from Human Kinetics Publishers, Box 5076, Champaign, IL 61820 (1-800-342-5457).

Dine System. Available through AAHPERD, Reston, VA.

Directory of Computer Software with Application to Sport Science, Health, and Dance II (2nd ed.). Baumgartner, T.A., & Cicciarella, C.F. (Eds.). Reston, VA: AAHPERD (703-476-3400).

Fit-n-dex. Cramer Educational Services Department, P.O. Box 1001, Gardner, KS 66030.

Fitness & Wellness Software. (1989). Developed by W. and S. Hoeger of Boise State University, Boise, ID. Available from the authors.

Fitnessgram. (1987). Dallas: Institute for Aerobics Research.

Fitscan. (1990). Available from ARA Human Factors, 15312 Spencerville Court, Burtonsville, MD 20866.

Fit Youth Today. (1986). 6225 U.S. Highway 290E, Suite 114, Austin, TX 78723: American Health and Fitness Foundation.

Health Education. October 1983 issue.

Health Education. December 1987/January 1988 issue.

Human Kinetics Publishers, Inc. Markets a number of software packages in exercise, health, and fitness. Box 5076, Champaign, IL 61820 (1-800-342-5457).

HyperCard is a product of Apple Computer, Inc.

Journal of Nutrition Education. June 1984 issue.

Journal of Physical Education, Recreation and Dance. November/December 1983 issue.

Kcal Expenditure. (1990). Authored by M.B. Broskusk, J.R. Morrow, Jr., J.M. Pivarnik, and T.J. Michael. University of Houston, Houston, TX. Available from the authors.

MaxVO$_2$ and Body Composition: Laboratory and Field Methods. (1987). Authored by J.R. Morrow, Jr., J.M. Pivarnik, and A.S. Jackson of the University of Houston, Houston, TX. Available from the authors.

Oxycalc. Available from Exeter Research, RFD 1, Rte 125, Brentwood, NH 03833 (603-642-7055).

Physical Best. (1988). Reston, VA: AAHPERD.

President's Challenge. (1987). Washington, DC: President's Council on Physical Fitness and Sports.

Simulated Exercise Physiology Laboratories. (1989). Authored by J.R. Morrow, Jr. and J.M. Pivarnik. Available from Human Kinetics Publishers, Champaign, IL 61820 (1-800-342-5457).

Softshare. Department of Physical Education and Human Performance, California State University, Fresno, CA 93740-0028 (209-278-2650).

YMCA Diet Analysis Software. Available from Human Kinetics Publishers, Champaign, IL 61820 (1-800-342-5457).

Y's Way to Physical Fitness. Available from Human Kinetics Publishers, Champaign, IL 61820 (1-800-342-5457).

Appendix A

Case Study Prescriptions and Answers

2.1 Encourage the woman to begin low-intensity exercise, using the walking program in chapter 14. Recommend that she get a health screening, including body composition, blood pressure, and blood profile. If the breathlessness continues or gets worse with regular exercise, she should see her personal physician. After she reaches the final stage of the walking program, recommend that she have physical-fitness testing to determine appropriate moderate-intensity exercise.

2.2 It appears that this may be an anxious response to a new environment. Talk with him about the kinds of activities he enjoys. Explain the procedures of the GXT, indicating again that he can stop whenever he wants to and that the fitness center has never had problems on the test. Have him walk around the center to look at the various fitness stations. When he returns, have him sit, and show him how to relax when he exhales. Retake his HR and BP. If they are lower, then continue with the GXT, giving him extra attention (e.g., frequently asking how he is doing during the test). If HR and BP remain high, ask him to come back for a second visit at a time that is convenient for him when the center will not be busy. Give him a relaxation program to try at home.

4.1 Explain to the exerciser that the same muscles that are used to push against the weights, the knee and hip extensor muscles, are working to control the descent. The press requires concentric contraction; the return requires an eccentric contraction. Both kinds of contraction can lead to increases in strength.

4.2 The gastrocnemius muscle crosses both the ankle joint and the knee joint; the soleus only crosses the ankle joint. When knees are kept extended during wall stretches, the gastrocnemius is in a lengthened position; if the knee is in a flexed position, the length of the gastrocnemius is too short and cannot be stretched by just the ankle position. By flexing the knee however, the position of the ankle joint is not restricted by the gastrocnemius, and the soleus muscle can be better stretched.

7.1 With 1 in. added to account for heels, the height/weight chart recommends 178-199 lb, with a midpoint of 188.5 lb.

$$RW = \frac{220}{188.5} \times 100\% = 116.7\%$$

RW greater than 110% is overweight. RW greater than 120% is obese.

$$74 \text{ in.} \times \frac{2.54 \text{ cm}}{\text{in.}} \times \frac{1 \text{ m}}{100 \text{ cm}} = 1.8796 \text{ m}$$

$$220 \text{ lb} \times \frac{0.454 \text{ kg}}{\text{lb}} = 99.88 \text{ kg}$$

$$BMI = \frac{\text{Weight (kg)}}{\text{Height}^2 \text{ (m)}} = \frac{99.88 \text{ kg}}{(1.8796 \text{ m})^2} = 28.27 \text{ kg/m}^2$$

Desirable BMI for men is 22 to 24. For men, obesity begins at 28.3. With a BMI of 28.27 kg/m², this individual is at greater risk of cardiovascular disease and diabetes.

Body density

$$= \frac{\text{Weight in air}}{\dfrac{\text{Weight in air} - \text{Weight in water}}{\text{Density of water}} - RV}$$

$$= \frac{99.88 \text{ kg}}{\dfrac{99.88 \text{ kg} - 3.0 \text{ kg}}{.9965 \text{ kg} \cdot \text{L}^{-1}} - 0.90 \text{ L}}$$

$$= 1.0369572 \text{ kg} \cdot \text{L}^{-1} \text{ or g} \cdot \text{cc}^{-1}$$

Using the equation:

$$\text{Percent fat} = \left(\frac{4.570}{\text{density}} - 4.142\right) \times 100\%$$

$$= \left(\frac{4.570}{1.0369572} - 4.142\right) \times 100\%$$

$$= 26.5\%$$

1) Fat weight = 220 lbs $\times \dfrac{26.5\%}{100\%}$ = 58.3 lb

2) Lean body weight = 220 lbs − 58.3 lbs = 161.7 lb

3) Desirable weight = $\dfrac{161.7\,\text{lb}}{1 - \dfrac{18\%}{100\%}}$ = 197.2 lb

4) Desirable adipose tissue loss = 220 lb − 197.2 lb

   = 22.8 lb

5) The average caloric deficit is 750 kcal/day.

   22.8 lbs $\times \dfrac{3,500\,\text{kcal}}{\text{lb}}$ = 79,800 kcal

   79,800 kcal $\times \dfrac{\text{day}}{750\,\text{kcal}}$ = 106.4 days

---

7.2

$$\text{WHR} = \frac{36\,\text{in.}}{42\,\text{in.}} = 0.86$$

This woman would be considered at increased risk of cardiovascular disease due to a high percentage of body fat and a WHR greater than 0.80.

9.1 The requirement that sedentary middle-aged participants take a maximal, unmonitored test at the beginning of their fitness program is inappropriate. You might suggest, in place of the 1.5-mi run, the use of the 1-mi-walk test, which should be used *after* the participants have demonstrated that they can comfortably walk one mile.

9.2 37.8 ml•kg^{-1}•min^{-1}.

11.1 You need to approach this situation from several different directions. First of all, talk with Jim privately, indicating that you are glad about his running interest but that he should not commit the center or other participants to participation in road races without checking with you and the others. Explain that some of the members might enjoy running if the emphasis is on finishing the race, not winning, and that others will not have any interest in road races. In the class, you should encourage those who have been running several miles per week at the THR to consider entering one road race just to try it. Their emphasis should be on setting their own paces, and their goal should be to finish the race. Finally, make it clear that running in road races is not for everyone—it is not necessary for fitness improvement, and in fact it falls into the performance category, just

like playing racquetball, tennis, soccer, or some other sport. These are good options for persons who enjoy them, but they are not essential for fitness goals, and they involve higher risks of injury.

11.2 You might guess that Jennifer's days are full of interaction with people—children, employees, employers, and the public. The walking and jogging programs provided her with some time to be alone with her own thoughts without dealing with other people. You might start the conversation by telling Jennifer that you have missed her the past couple of weeks. Ask her what she liked about the first few months of the fitness program, what her fitness goals are, and what could be done to help her. If your guess about her wanting to be alone is correct, then emphasize that to continue in the running program is a good option for her exercise. You might suggest that she try cycling or swimming laps just for variety for some of her workouts. It is important for her to realize that it's OK for her to choose to have her individual exercise schedule.

12.1 The HFI at the sixth health/fitness center, Naomi Barnes, had been a HFI for 5 years. She claimed that for some people to develop successful exercise programs, social factors need to be considered. When Naomi began to work with Sara, she treated Sara as a new friend. They spent time talking about common interests such as books recently read and places to go on vacation. Naomi also made it a point to introduce Sara to other participants at the center. The main motivating factor that encouraged Sara to go to the fitness center was to be with friends. There was a good deal of encouragement given and received among the center participants. For Sara, new friendships and encouragement were the keys to long-term participation in an exercise program.

12.2 Carl's sister, after talking with the HFI, suggested a contract to Carl. She suggested that Carl suggest to Terry that if Carl could quit smoking entirely for 1 year, Terry would agree to marry him. Terry readily agreed to the plan. A contract was written, signed by Carl and Terry and witnessed by the sister. A year later, Terry and Carl were married, and Carl had given up smoking for good. Carl related that the main reason the contract worked was his strong desire to marry Terry, in combination with his longstanding wish to quit anyway. It was critical that the marriage was contingent on stopping smoking.

14.1 Topics to address include

- attention to signs and symptoms that indicate problems and directions to act on them with a visit to their physician,
- proper shoes,
- clothing appropriate for the season,
- site (surface, lighting, etc.),
- buddy system where possible to encourage participation, and
- alternate place in poor weather (shopping mall).

14.2 The appropriate transition from a walking program would be into a low-intensity, low-impact aerobics class. The participant should stay at the low end of the THR zone during this transition period and increase the intensity of the class only after these low intensity, low-impact sessions can be comfortably completed.

15.1 The person's maximal heart rate measured during the exercise test would be lower, due to the effect of Inderal, than it is now. His target heart rate range established at the time of the exercise test would no longer be useful.

15.2 The Nicorette would be the probable cause of the skipped beats since the drug contains nicotin which can alter heart rate and blood pressure and cause arrhythmias.

15.3 Isordil contains nitroglycerine and is used to reduce the chance of having an angina attack. The drug relaxes vascular smooth muscle and might cause the pooling of blood in the extremities. This pooling could cause a decrease in blood pressure and result in symptoms of dizziness.

16.1 a. Suspect insulin shock.
   b. Ask the following questions: What happened? Are you a diabetic? Have you taken your insulin today? Have you eaten?
   c. Check medic alert tag. If insulin shock is still suspected, administer sugar (orange juice, candy, sugar granules). If unconscious or slow recovery (greater than 1 to 2 minutes), refer to physician.

16.2 a. Suspect heat stroke.
   b. Implement EMS—911. This is a **medical emergency**. Cool quickly starting at the head and work down. Expose as much skin surface as possible. Monitor vital signs. Treat cramps by stretching, application of ice, direct pressure, and gentle massage. Treat for shock. Wrap in cold wet sheets for transport.
   c. Emergency plans and materials should include
   - access to cooling agents, such as water, ice, ice towels, cool environment;
   - access to phone, with knowledge of EMS;
   - knowledge of roles in emergency: person in charge, who assists person in charge, person responsible for making emergency phone call, who is to meet and direct the emergency vehicle to the injured; and
   - knowledge of rules to move person if necessary.

Appendix B

Calculation of Oxygen Uptake and Carbon Dioxide Production

CALCULATION OF OXYGEN CONSUMPTION ($\dot{V}O_2$)

The air we breathe is composed of 20.93% oxygen (O_2), 0.03% carbon dioxide (CO_2), and the balance, 79.04%, nitrogen. When we exhale, the fraction of the air represented by O_2 is decreased and the fraction represented by CO_2 is increased. To calculate the volume of O_2 used by the body ($\dot{V}O_2$), we simply subtract the number of liters of O_2 exhaled from the number of liters of O_2 inhaled. Equation (1) summarizes these words.

(1) Oxygen consumption =

[Volume of O_2 inhaled]

   − [Volume of O_2 exhaled]

Now, using $\dot{V}O_2$ to mean volume of *oxygen* used, V_I to mean volume of *air* inhaled, V_E to mean volume of *air* exhaled, F_{IO_2} to mean fraction of oxygen in inhaled air, and F_{EO_2} to mean fraction of oxygen in exhaled air, equation (1) can be written:

(2) $\dot{V}O_2 = [V_I \cdot F_{IO_2}] - [V_E \cdot F_{EO_2}]$

You know that $F_{IO_2} = 0.2093$ and F_{EO_2} will be determined on an oxygen analyzer. Consequently, you are left with only two unknowns, the volume of air (liters) inhaled (V_I) and the volume of air (liters) exhaled (V_E). It appears that you must measure both volumes, but fortunately, this is not necessary. It was determined years ago that N_2 is neither used nor produced by the body. Consequently, the number of liters of N_2 inhaled must equal the number of liters of N_2 exhaled. Equation (3) states this equality using the symbols mentioned earlier.

(3) $V_I \cdot F_{IN_2} = V_E \cdot F_{EN_2}$

This is a very important relationship because it permits you to calculate V_E when V_I is known or vice versa. Using equation (3) here are two formulas, one to give V_E when V_I is known, and one to give V_I when V_E is known.

$$V_I = \frac{V_E \cdot F_{EN_2}}{F_{IN_2}} \qquad V_E = \frac{V_I \cdot F_{IN_2}}{F_{EN_2}}$$

Now that you know how to do this, there is only one other piece to the puzzle needed to permit you to calculate $\dot{V}O_2$. The value for F_{IN_2} is constant (0.7904) so we must determine F_{EN_2}. When the expired gas sample is analyzed you will obtain a value for F_{EO_2} and F_{ECO_2}, but not F_{EN_2}. However, since all the gas fractions must add up to 1.0000, you can calculate F_{EN_2}. (In the same way, we calculated F_{IN_2}: $1.0000 - .0003$ (CO_2) − .2093 (O_2) $= .7904$).

Problem: Calculate F_{EN_2} when $F_{EO_2} = .1600$ and $F_{ECO_2} = .0450$

Answer: $F_{EN_2} = 1.0000 - .1600 - .0450 = .7950$

The following problem shows how these equations are used. Given that V_I equals 100 liters, $F_{EO_2} = .1600$, and $F_{ECO_2} = .0450$, calculate V_E.

$$V_E \cdot F_{EN_2} = V_I \cdot F_{IN_2}, \text{ so } V_E = \frac{V_I \cdot F_{IN_2}}{F_{EN_2}}$$

$F_{IN_2} = .7904$ and

   $F_{EN_2} = 1.0000 - .1600 - .0450 = .7950$

$V_E = 100 \text{ liters} \cdot \dfrac{.7904}{.7950} = 99.4 \text{ liters}$

At this point, the equation for $\dot{V}O_2$ can be rewritten, using V_I, V_E, F_{IO_2}, and F_{EO_2}.

$\dot{V}O_2 = V_I \cdot F_{IO_2} - V_E \cdot F_{EO_2}$

Assuming that you measure only V_I this formula is rewritten:

$$\dot{V}O_2 = V_I \cdot F_{IO_2} - \frac{V_I \cdot F_{IN_2}}{F_{EN_2}} \cdot F_{EO_2}$$

V_I can be factored out of this equation, so:

$$\dot{V}O_2 = V_I[F_{IO_2} - \frac{F_{IN_2}}{F_{EN_2}} \cdot F_{EO_2}]$$

We will repeat the last two steps assuming that V_E is the volume that is measured and then factor out V_E.

$$\dot{V}O_2 = \frac{V_E \cdot F_{EN_2}}{F_{IN_2}} \cdot F_{IO_2} - V_E \cdot F_{EO_2}$$

$$= V_E[\frac{F_{EN_2}}{F_{IN_2}} \cdot F_{IO_2} - F_{EO_2}]$$

At this point you know how to calculate $\dot{V}O_2$. If you ever get stuck, always go back to the formula: $VO_2 = V_I \cdot F_{IO_2} - V_E \cdot F_{EO_2}$ and simply substitute for V_E or V_I, depending on what was measured.

Some comments:

1. You must always match the volume measurement with the F_{EO_2} and F_{ECO_2} values measured in that expired volume. If you measure V_I for two minutes, you must have a single two-minute bag of expired gas to get F_{EO_2} and F_{ECO_2} values. If you measure a 30-second volume your expired bag must be collected over those 30 seconds.

2. $\dot{V}O_2$ and $\dot{V}CO_2$ are usually expressed in liters/min: the *rate* at which O_2 is used or CO_2 is produced per minute. To signify this *rate*, we write $\dot{V}O_2$ (read Vee dot). You would convert 30-second or 2-minute volumes to one-minute values before making calculations of $\dot{V}O_2$.

Sample problem:

$\dot{V}_I = 100$ L/min, $F_{EO_2} = .1600$, $F_{ECO_2} = .0450$

Calculate $\dot{V}O_2$:

$$\dot{V}O_2 = \dot{V}_I \cdot F_{IO_2} - V_E \cdot F_{EO_2}$$

$$\dot{V}_E = \frac{\dot{V}_I F_{IN_2}}{F_{EN_2}}$$

$$\dot{V}O_2 = \dot{V}_I \cdot F_{IO_2} - \frac{\dot{V}_I F_{IN_2}}{F_{EN_2}} \cdot F_{EO_2}$$

$$= \dot{V}_I [F_{IO_2} - \frac{F_{IN_2}}{F_{EN_2}} \cdot F_{EO_2}]$$

$$F_{EN_2} = 1.0000 - .1600 - .0450 = .7950$$

$$\dot{V}O_2 = 100 \text{ L/min } [.2093 - \frac{.7904}{.7950} - .1600]$$

$$= 5.02 \text{ L/min}$$

The volume (let's assume that V_E was measured) used in the above equations was measured at room temperature (23 °C) and at the barometric pressure of that moment (740 mmHg). The environmental conditions under which the volume was measured are called ambient conditions. If this volume of gas were transported to 10,000 feet above sea level, where the barometric pressure is lower, the volume would increase because of the reduced pressure. The volume of a gas varies inversely with pressure (at a constant temperature). Another factor influencing the volume of a gas is the temperature. If that volume, measured at 23 °C, were placed in a refrigerator at 0 °C, the volume of gas would decrease. The volume of gas varies directly with the temperature (at constant pressure).

Since the volume ($\dot{V}_E$) is influenced by both pressure and temperature, the value measured as O_2 used ($\dot{V}O_2$) might reflect changes in pressure or temperature, rather than a change in workload, training, and so on. Consequently, it would be convenient to express $\dot{V}_E$ in such a way as to make measurements comparable when they are obtained under different environmental conditions. This is done by standardizing the temperature, barometric pressure, and water vapor pressure at which the volume is expressed. By convention, volumes are expressed at Standard Temperature and Pressure, Dry (STPD): 273 °K (equals 0 °C), 760 mmHg pressure (sea level), and with no water vapor pressure. When $\dot{V}O_2$ is expressed STPD you can calculate the number of molecules of oxygen actually used by the body because *at STPD one mole of oxygen equals 22.4 liters.*

Let's make the correction to STPD one step at a time. Let's assume that a volume (V_E) was measured at 740 mmHg, 23 °C and equaled 100 L/min. This *expired* volume is *always* saturated with water vapor.

To correct for temperature you use 273 °K as the standard (0 °C).

$$\text{Volume} \times \frac{273 \text{ °K}}{273 \text{ °K} + x \text{ °C}} = \frac{273 \text{ °K}}{273 + 23}$$

$$100 \text{ L/min} \times \frac{273 \text{ °K}}{296 \text{ °K}} = 92.23 \text{ L/min}$$

When we make corrections for pressure we must remove the effect of water vapor pressure because the gas volume is adjusted on the basis of the standard pressure (760 mmHg) which is a dry pressure.

To correct the volume to the standard 760 mmHg pressure (dry) use:

Volume $\times$

$$\frac{\text{barometric pressure} - \text{water vapor pressure}}{760 \text{ mmHg (dry)}}$$

Water vapor pressure is dependent on two things: the temperature and the relative humidity. In expired gas the gas volume is saturated (100% relative humidity). Consequently, you can obtain a value for water vapor pressure directly from a table:

Temperature (°C)	Saturation water vapor pressure (mmHg)
18	15.5
19	16.5
20	17.5
21	18.7
22	19.8
23	21.1
24	22.4
25	23.8
26	25.2
27	26.7

Going back to our pressure correction:

$$92.23 \text{ L/min} \times \frac{740 - 21.1}{760}$$

$$= 87.24 \text{ L/min (STPD)}$$

To combine the temperature and pressure correction:

$$100 \text{ L/min} \times \frac{273 \text{ °K}}{273 \text{ °K} + 23} \times \frac{740 - 21.1}{760}$$

$$= 87.24 \text{ L/min (STPD)}$$

A special note must be made here. If you are using an inspired (inhaled) volume ($\dot{V}_I$), you are rarely dealing with a gas saturated with water vapor. Consequently, when you correct for pressure you must find what the water vapor is in the inspired air. You do this by finding the relative humidity of the air. You then multiply this value by the water vapor pressure value for saturated air at whatever the temperature is. To clarify, if our volume in the above example was $\dot{V}_I$ and had a relative humidity of 50%, the pressure correction would have been:

$$\text{Volume} \times \frac{740 - (.50 \times 21.1 \text{ mmHg})}{760 \text{ mmHg}}$$

While this may seem like a minor point, it is critical to the accurate measurement of $\dot{V}O_2$ that the proper water vapor correction be used. When you do calculations for $\dot{V}O_2$ you usually find the STPD factor first since you will be multiplying this factor by each volume measured.

Problem: Given $\dot{V}_I$ = 100 L/min, F_{EO_2} = .1700, F_{ECO_2} = .0385. The temperature = 20 °C, barometric pressure = 740 mmHg, and the relative humidity = 30%.
Answer:

$$\text{STPD factor} = \frac{740 \text{ mmHg} - (.30)17.5 \text{ mmHg}}{760}$$

$$\times \frac{273 \text{ °K}}{273 \text{ °K} + 20 \text{ °C}} = .900$$

$$100 \text{ L/min} \times .900 = 90 \text{ L/min STPD}$$

$$\dot{V}O_2 = \dot{V}_{I_{STPD}} [F_{IO_2} - \frac{F_{IN_2}}{F_{EN_2}} \cdot F_{EO_2}]$$

$$\dot{V}O_2 = 90 \text{ L/min} [.2093 - \frac{.7904}{.7915} \cdot .1700]$$

$$\dot{V}O_2 = 3.56 \text{ L/min}$$

CARBON DIOXIDE PRODUCTION ($\dot{V}CO_2$)

When O_2 is used, CO_2 is produced. The ratio of CO_2 production ($\dot{V}CO_2$) to O_2 consumption ($\dot{V}O_2$) is an important measurement in metabolism. This ratio ($\dot{V}CO_2 \div \dot{V}O_2$) is called the respiratory exchange ratio and is abbreviated as "R."

How do we measure $\dot{V}CO_2$? We start at the same step as for $\dot{V}O_2$:

$$\dot{V}CO_2 = \text{liters of } CO_2 \text{ expired} - \text{liters of } CO_2 \text{ inspired} = \dot{V}_E \cdot F_{ECO_2} - \dot{V}_I F_{ICO_2}$$

The steps to follow are the same as for measuring $\dot{V}O_2$. Always use an STPD volume in your calculations. The following is the equation to use when $\dot{V}_I$ is measured:

$$\dot{V}CO_2 = \dot{V}_{I_{STPD}} [\frac{F_{IN_2}}{F_{EN_2}} \cdot F_{ECO_2} - F_{ICO_2}]$$

The following steps summarize the calculations for $\dot{V}CO_2$ and R for the previous problem.

$$\dot{V}CO_2 = 90 \text{ L/min} [\frac{.7904}{.7915} \cdot .0385 - .0003]$$

$$= 3.43 \text{ L/min}$$

$$R = \dot{V}CO_2 \div \dot{V}O_2 = 3.43 \text{ L/min} \div 3.56 \text{ L/min}$$

$$R = .96$$

Appendix C

Recommended Dietary Allowances and Intakes

Estimated Safe and Adequate Daily Dietary Intakes of Selected Vitamins and Minerals[a]

Category	Age (years)	Vitamins		Trace elements[b]				
		Biotin (μg)	Pantothenic acid (mg)	Copper (mg)	Manganese (mg)	Fluoride (mg)	Chromium (μg)	Molybdenum (μg)
Infants	0-0.5	10	2	0.4-0.6	0.3-0.6	0.1-0.5	10-40	15-30
	0.5-1	15	3	0.6-0.7	0.6-1.0	0.2-1.0	20-60	20-40
Children and adolescents	1-3	20	3	0.7-1.0	1.0-1.5	0.5-1.5	20-80	25-50
	4-6	25	3-4	1.0-1.5	1.5-2.0	1.0-2.5	30-120	30-75
	7-10	30	4-5	1.0-2.0	2.0-3.0	1.5-2.5	50-200	50-150
	11+	30-100	4-7	1.5-2.5	2.0-5.0	1.5-2.5	50-200	75-250
Adults		30-100	4-7	1.5-3.0	2.0-5.0	1.5-4.0	50-200	75-250

[a]Because there is less information on which to base allowances, these figures are not given in the main table of RDA and are provided here in the form of ranges of recommended intakes.

[b]Because the toxic levels for many trace elements may be only several times usual intakes, the upper levels for the trace elements given in this table should not be habitually exceeded.

Reprinted with permission from *Recommended Dietary Allowances, 10th Edition*. © 1989 by the National Academy of Sciences. Published by National Academy Press.

Food and Nutrition Board, National Academy of Sciences—National Research Council Recommended Dietary Allowances,[a] Revised 1989[*] (Designed for the maintenance of good nutrition of practically all healthy people in the United States)

Age (years) or condition	Weight[b] (kg)	Weight[b] (lb)	Height[b] (cm)	Height[b] (in.)	Protein (g)	Fat-soluble vitamins				Water-soluble vitamins							Minerals						
						Vitamin A (μg R.E.)[c]	Vitamin D (μg)[d]	Vitamin E (mg α-T.E.)[e]	Vitamin K (μg)	Vitamin C (mg)	Thiamin (mg)	Riboflavin (mg)	Niacin (mg N.E.)[f]	Vitamin B_6 (mg)	Folate (μg)	Vitamin B_{12} (μg)	Calcium (mg)	Phosphorus (mg)	Magnesium (mg)	Iron (mg)	Zinc (mg)	Iodine (μg)	Selenium (μg)
Infants																							
0.0-0.5	6	13	60	24	13	375	7.5	3	5	30	0.3	0.4	5	0.3	25	0.3	400	300	40	6	5	40	10
0.5-1.0	9	20	71	28	14	375	10	4	10	35	0.4	0.5	6	0.6	35	0.5	600	500	60	10	5	50	15
Children																							
1-3	13	29	90	35	16	400	10	6	15	40	0.7	0.8	9	1.0	50	0.7	800	800	80	10	10	70	20
4-6	20	44	112	44	24	500	10	7	20	45	0.9	1.1	12	1.1	75	1.0	800	800	120	10	10	90	20
7-10	28	62	132	52	28	700	10	7	30	45	1.0	1.2	13	1.4	100	1.4	800	800	170	10	10	120	30
Males																							
11-14	45	90	157	62	45	1,000	10	10	45	50	1.3	1.5	17	1.7	150	2.0	1,200	1,200	270	12	15	150	40
15-18	66	145	176	69	59	1,000	10	10	65	60	1.5	1.8	20	2.0	200	2.0	1,200	1,200	400	12	15	150	50
19-24	72	160	177	70	58	1,000	10	10	70	60	1.5	1.7	19	2.0	200	2.0	1,200	1,200	350	10	15	150	70
25-50	79	174	176	70	63	1,000	5	10	80	60	1.5	1.7	19	2.0	200	2.0	800	800	350	10	15	150	70
51+	77	170	173	68	63	1,000	5	10	80	60	1.2	1.4	15	2.0	200	2.0	800	800	350	10	15	150	70
Females																							
11-14	46	101	157	62	46	800	10	8	45	50	1.1	1.3	15	1.4	150	2.0	1,200	1,200	280	15	12	150	45
15-18	55	120	163	64	44	800	10	8	55	60	1.1	1.3	15	1.5	180	2.0	1,200	1,200	300	15	12	150	50
19-24	58	128	164	65	46	800	10	8	60	60	1.1	1.3	15	1.6	180	2.0	1,200	1,200	280	15	12	150	55
25-50	63	138	163	64	50	800	5	8	65	60	1.1	1.3	15	1.6	180	2.0	800	800	280	15	12	150	55
51+	65	143	160	63	50	800	5	8	65	60	1.0	1.2	13	1.6	180	2.0	800	800	280	10	12	150	55
Pregnant					60	800	10	10	65	70	1.5	1.6	17	2.2	400	2.2	1,200	1,200	320	30	15	175	65
Lactating 1st 6 months					65	1,300	10	12	65	95	1.6	1.8	20	2.1	280	2.6	1,200	1,200	355	15	19	200	75
2nd 6 months					62	1,200	10	11	65	90	1.6	1.7	20	2.1	260	2.6	1,200	1,200	340	15	16	200	75

[a]The allowances, expressed as average daily intakes over time, are intended to provide for individual variations among most normal persons as they live in the United States under usual environmental stresses. Diets should be based on a variety of common foods in order to provide other nutrients for which human requirements have been less well defined. See text for detailed discussion of allowances and of nutrients not tabulated.

[b]Weights and heights of reference adults are actual medians for the U.S. population of the designated age, as reported by NHANES II. The median weights and heights of those under 19 years of age were taken from Hamill et al. (1979). The use of these figures does not imply that the height to weight ratios are ideal.

[c]Retinol equivalents. 1 retinol equivalent = 1 μg retinol or 6 μg β-carotene. See text for calculation of vitamin A activity of diets as retinol equivalents.

[d]As cholecalciferol, 10 μg cholecalciferol = 400 I.U. of vitamin D.

[e]α–Tocopherol equivalents. 1 mg d-α tocopherol = 1 α-T.E. See text for variation in allowances and calculation of vitamin E activity of the diet as α-tocopherol equivalents.

[f]1 N.E. (niacin equivalent) is equal to 1 mg of niacin or 60 mg of dietary tryptophan.

[*]Reprinted with permission from *Recommended Dietary Allowances, 10th Edition.* © 1989 by the National Academy of Sciences. Published by National Academy Press.

Estimated Sodium, Chloride, and Potassium Minimum Requirements of Healthy Persons[a]

Age	Weight (kg)[a]	Sodium (mg)[ab]	Chloride (mg)[ab]	Potassium (mg)[c]
Months				
0-5	4.5	120	180	500
6-11	8.9	200	300	700
Years				
1	11.0	225	350	1,000
2-5	16.0	300	500	1,400
6-9	25.0	400	600	1,600
10-18	50.0	500	750	2,000
> 18[d]	70.0	500	750	2,000

[a]No allowance has been included for large, prolonged losses from the skin through sweat.

[b]There is no evidence that higher intakes confer any health benefit.

[c]Desirable intakes of potassium may considerably exceed these values (~3,500 mg for adults).

[d]No allowance included for growth. Values for those below 18 years assume a growth rate at the 50th percentile reported by the National Center for Health Statistics (Hamill et al., 1979) and averaged for males and females.

Reprinted with permission from *Recommended Dietary Allowances, 10th Edition*. © 1989 by the National Academy of Sciences. Published by National Academy Press.

Food Exchanges for 1,800 Calories

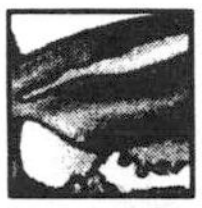

1 Starches and Breads

One portion of each food in this list contains about 15 g carbohydrate, 3 g protein, a trace of fat, and 80 calories. To choose a similar portion of a starch or bread not listed, follow these general rules:
- Cereal, grain, pasta — ½ cup
- Bread product — 1 oz

Breads	Portion
Bagel	½ (1 oz)
Bun (hamburger, hot dog)	½ (1 oz)
English muffin	½
Pita (6″ across)	½
Tortilla, flour or corn (6″ across)	1
Whole wheat, rye 🌾, white, pumpernickel, raisin (no icing)	1 slice (1 oz)

Cereals/Grains/Pasta	
Bran cereal 🌾, concentrated, such as Bran Buds®, All-Bran®	⅓ cup
Bran cereal 🌾, flaked	½ cup
Cooked cereal, grits, bulgur	½ cup
Grapenuts®	3 Tbsp
Macaroni, noodles, spaghetti (cooked)	½ cup
Puffed cereal	1½ cup
Ready-to-eat cereal, unsweetened	¾ cup
Rice, white or brown	⅓ cup
Shredded wheat	½ cup
Wheat germ 🌾	3 Tbsp

Crackers/Snacks	
Graham cracker (2½″ square)	3
Matzo	¾ oz
Melba toast	5 slices
Oyster crackers	24
Popcorn, popped, no fat added	3 cups
Pretzels	¾ oz
Rye crisp (2″ x 3½″)	4

Starchy Vegetables	
Beans 🌾, baked	¼ cup
Corn 🌾	½ cup or 6″ cob
Lentils 🌾, beans, or peas (dried), such as kidney, white, split, black-eyed	⅓ cup
Lima beans 🌾	½ cup
Peas 🌾, green (canned or frozen)	½ cup
Potato, baked	1 small (3 oz)
Potato, mashed	½ cup
Winter squash (acorn, butternut)	¾ cup
Yam or sweet potato, plain	⅓ cup

Starch Foods Prepared With Fat
(Count as 1 starch/bread exchange and 1 fat exchange)

Biscuit (2½″ across)	1
Chow mein noodles	½ cup
Corn bread (2″ cube)	1 (2 oz)
Cracker, round butter type	6
French fried potatoes (2″-3½″ long)	10 (1½ oz)
Muffin (small, plain)	1
Taco shell (6″ across)	2

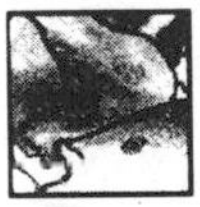

2 Meats and Meat Substitutes

One portion of each food in this list contains about 7 g protein. **Lean meats and meat substitutes** have about 55 calories per serving; other meat items have 78 to 100 calories per serving. To follow a diet low in cholesterol and saturated fat, choose the **lean meats, fish,** and other items that appear in **bold type.** Portions are weighed after cooking and with skin, bones, and fat removed.

Beef	Portion
Lean cuts, such as **USDA Good/Choice round, sirloin, or flank steak, tenderloin, chipped beef** 🐟	1 oz
All other cuts	1 oz

Cheese	
Cottage or ricotta	¼ cup
Diet (less than 55 calories per oz)	1 oz
Parmesan, grated	2 Tbsp
Other cheese (except cream cheese)	1 oz

Eggs	
Egg substitute (less than 55 calories per ¼ cup)	¼ cup
Egg white	3
Egg, whole*	1

<u>List 2</u> (continued)   <u>Portion</u>

Fish and Seafood
All fresh or frozen fish . . . . 1 oz
Clams, crab, lobster, shrimp,
    scallops . . . . 2 oz
Herring, smoked . . . . 1 oz
Oysters . . . . 6 medium
Sardines (canned) . . . . 2 medium
Tuna (water-packed) 🔻 . . . . . ¼ cup
Salmon (canned) 🔻 . . . . ¼ cup

Miscellaneous
Hot dog† 🔻 (10 per lb) 1
Lamb (all cuts) . . . . 1 oz
Liver,* heart,* kidney,*
    sweetbreads* . . . . 1 oz

Luncheon meats — **95% fat
    free**; all others . . . . 1 oz
Peanut butter . . . . 1 Tbsp
Sausages 🔻 , such as
    Polish, Italian, smoked . . . . . 1 oz

Pork
Lean cuts, such as **Canadian
    bacon**🔻**; fresh ham;
    canned, cured, boiled
    ham**🔻**; tenderloin** . . . . 1 oz
Other cuts . . . . 1 oz

Poultry
**Chicken, turkey, Cornish
    hen (skin removed)** . . . . . . 1 oz

Veal
Lean chops and roasts . . . . . 1 oz
Cutlets . . . . 1 oz

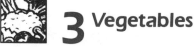

3 Vegetables

One portion of each vegetable in this list contains about 5 g carbohydrate, 2 g protein, and 25 calories. If no portion size is listed, the following measurements should be used:
- Cooked vegetables or juice — ½ cup
- Raw vegetables — 1 cup

Check Free Foods (List 7) and Starches/Breads (List 1) for vegetables not listed here.

Asparagus	Okra
Beans (green, wax, Italian)	Onion
	Pea pods (snow peas)
Bean sprouts	Peppers (green)
Beets	Sauerkraut 🔻
Broccoli	Spinach (cooked)
Brussels sprouts	Summer squash
Cabbage (cooked)	(crookneck)
Carrots	Tomato (1 large)
Cauliflower	Tomato or vegetable
Eggplant	juice 🔻
Greens (collard, mustard, etc)	Turnip
	Water chestnuts
Mushrooms (cooked)	Zucchini (cooked)

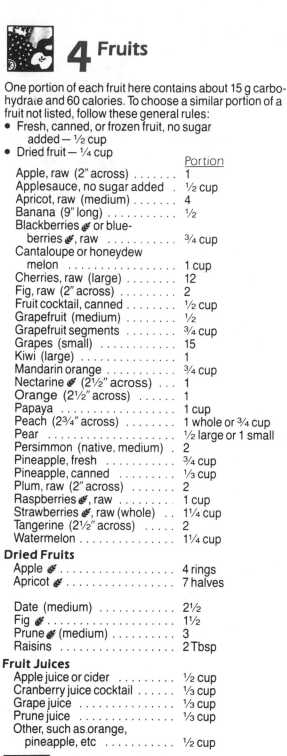

4 Fruits

One portion of each fruit here contains about 15 g carbohydrate and 60 calories. To choose a similar portion of a fruit not listed, follow these general rules:
- Fresh, canned, or frozen fruit, no sugar added — ½ cup
- Dried fruit — ¼ cup

	<u>Portion</u>
Apple, raw (2" across)	1
Applesauce, no sugar added .	½ cup
Apricot, raw (medium)	4
Banana (9" long)	½
Blackberries 🌿 or blueberries 🌿, raw	¾ cup
Cantaloupe or honeydew melon	1 cup
Cherries, raw (large)	12
Fig, raw (2" across)	2
Fruit cocktail, canned	½ cup
Grapefruit (medium)	½
Grapefruit segments	¾ cup
Grapes (small)	15
Kiwi (large)	1
Mandarin orange	¾ cup
Nectarine 🌿 (2½" across) . . .	1
Orange (2½" across)	1
Papaya	1 cup
Peach (2¾" across)	1 whole or ¾ cup
Pear	½ large or 1 small
Persimmon (native, medium) .	2
Pineapple, fresh	¾ cup
Pineapple, canned	⅓ cup
Plum, raw (2" across)	2
Raspberries 🌿, raw	1 cup
Strawberries 🌿, raw (whole) . .	1¼ cup
Tangerine (2½" across)	2
Watermelon	1¼ cup

Dried Fruits
Apple 🌿	4 rings
Apricot 🌿	7 halves
Date (medium)	2½
Fig 🌿	1½
Prune 🌿 (medium)	3
Raisins	2 Tbsp

Fruit Juices
Apple juice or cider	½ cup
Cranberry juice cocktail	⅓ cup
Grape juice	⅓ cup
Prune juice	⅓ cup
Other, such as orange, pineapple, etc	½ cup

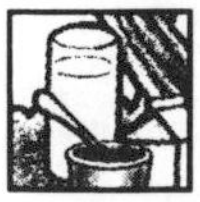

5 Milk and Milk Products

One portion of each milk or milk product on this list contains about 12 g carbohydrate and 8 g protein. These foods also contain 1 to 8 g fat and 90 to 150 calories per serving, depending on their butterfat content. Choose foods from the skim and lowfat milk groups as often as possible, because they contain less butterfat than do whole milk products.

Skim and Very Lowfat Milk   <u>Portion</u>
  Skim, ½%, or 1% milk . . . . .   1 cup
  Buttermilk, lowfat . . . .   1 cup
  Evaporated skim milk . . . . .   ½ cup
  Nonfat dry milk . . . .   ⅓ cup
  Nonfat yogurt, plain . . . .   8 oz

Lowfat Milk
(Count as 1 milk exchange and 1 fat exchange)
  2% milk . . . .   1 cup
  Lowfat yogurt, plain (with
    added nonfat milk solids) .   8 oz

Whole Milk
(Count as 1 milk exchange and 2 fat exchanges)
  Whole milk . . . .   1 cup
  Evaporated whole milk . . . .   ½ cup
  Whole yogurt, plain . . . .   8 oz

6 Fats

One portion of each food on this list contains about 5 g fat and 45 calories. Choose unsaturated fats instead of saturated fats as often as possible.

Unsaturated Fats   <u>Portion</u>
  Almonds, dry roasted . . . . . .   6 whole
  Avocado (medium) . . . .   ⅛
  Margarine . . . .   1 tsp
  Margarine, diet . . . .   1 Tbsp
  Mayonnaise . . . .   1 tsp
  Oil (corn, cottonseed,
    olive, peanut, safflower,
    soybean, sunflower) . . . . .   1 tsp
  Olives ◀ . . . .   10 small or 5 large
  Peanuts . . . .   20 small or 10 large
  Pecans or walnuts . . . .   2 whole
  Salad dressing,
    mayonnaise-type . . . .   2 tsp
  Salad dressing, other
    varieties . . . .   1 Tbsp
  Sunflower seeds . . . .   1 Tbsp

Saturated Fats
  Bacon ◀ . . . .   1 slice
  Butter . . . .   1 tsp
  Coconut, shredded . . . .   2 Tbsp
  Coffee whitener, liquid . . . . .   2 Tbsp
  Coffee whitener, powdered .   4 tsp
  Cream (light, coffee,
    table, sour) . . . .   2 Tbsp
  Cream (heavy, whipping) . .   1 Tbsp
  Cream cheese . . . .   1 Tbsp

7 Free Foods

Each free food or drink contains fewer than 20 calories per serving. You may eat as much as you want of free foods that have no portion size given; you may eat two or three servings per day of free foods that have portions listed. Be sure to spread your servings throughout the day.

Drinks
  Bouillon ◀ or broth,
    no fat
  Cocoa powder,
    unsweetened
    baking type
    (1 Tbsp)
  Coffee or tea
  Soft drinks, calorie-
    free, including
    carbonated drinks

**Vegetables
(raw, 1 cup)**
  Cabbage
  Celery
  Cucumber
  Green onion
  Hot peppers
  Mushrooms
  Radishes
  Salad greens (as
    desired):
    Lettuce
    Romaine
    Spinach (raw)

  Zucchini ✔

Fruits
  Cranberries or
    rhubarb, no sugar
    (½ cup)

Sweet Substitutes
  Gelatin, sugar-free
  Jam or jelly, sugar-free
    (2 tsp)
  Whipped topping
    (2 Tbsp)

Condiments
  Catsup (1 Tbsp)
  Dill pickles ◀,
    unsweetened
  Horseradish
  Hot sauce
  Mustard
  Salad dressing, low-
    calorie, including
    mayonnaise-type
    (2 Tbsp)
  Taco sauce (1 Tbsp)
  Vinegar

Seasonings can be used as desired. If you are following a low-sodium diet, be sure to read the labels and choose seasonings that do not contain sodium or salt.

  Flavoring extracts
    (vanilla, almond,
    butter, etc)
  Garlic or garlic powder
  Herbs, fresh or dried
  Lemon or lemon
    juice
  Lime or lime juice

  Onion powder
  Paprika
  Pepper
  Pimento
  Spices
  Soy sauce ◀
  Worcestershire sauce

✔ High in fiber.
◀ High in sodium.
*High in cholesterol.
†Count as 1 meat exchange and 1 fat exchange.

Note. From *Meal Plan/1,800 Calories.* Lilly Leadership in Diabetes Care. Eli Lilly Company, Indianapolis, IN 46285.

Glossary

The following list of words are terms related to physical fitness with which the HFI will come into contact. Many of these words have more general alternative meanings. The health and fitness implications of appropriate terms are noted. The chapters in which the terms are used are indicated (with the exception of standard weight measurements).

Abdominal muscular endurance (chapter 10)—The ability of the muscles in the abdominal area to continue to contract without fatigue. Abdominal muscular endurance appears to be an important element in the prevention of low-back pain.

Abnormal (chapter 5)—Not typical. Abnormal is often defined as one, two, or three standard deviations above or below the mean for a test score including about 68%, 96%, and 99% of the population, respectively. An abnormal score may be related to positive health (e.g., low resting heart rate due to a high level of physical condition) or negative health (e.g., high percent of body fat).

Abrasion (chapter 16)—A superficial injury to skin, usually scraping a surface.

Acclimatization (chapter 13)—A physiological adaptation to a new environment. For example, a person can do the same work with less effort and can do more total work after becoming acclimatized to a higher altitude (or temperature).

Accommodating (variable) resistance (chapter 10)—Providing resistance so that maximal force can be applied throughout the complete range of motion.

Acidosis (chapter 3)—A disturbance in the acid–base balance of the body tissues in which the tissues become more acidic (pH is lowered).

Acromion (chapter 4)—A bony process on the superior lateral aspect of the scapula (shoulder blade).

Actin (chapter 4)—Thin protein constituent of the myofibril contractile structure; binds to myosin to form cross-bridges to facilitate muscle contraction.

Action potential (chapter 15)—A change in electrical potential at the surface of a nerve or muscle cell, occurring at the moment of its excitation.

Activity revision (chapter 13)—Recommending changes in the level (e.g., frequency, intensity, duration) and/or type of physical activity for better fitness results.

Actomyosin (chapter 3)—The active form of myosin that can release the energy contained in the crossbridge.

Acute injury (chapter 16)—An injury that has just occurred, needing immediate attention.

Acute stressor (chapter 11)—A situation or condition that causes an immediate and temporary physiological reaction in excess of what is needed to carry out the task.

Adaptation (chapter 11)—The ability to adjust mentally and physically to circumstances or a changing situation. Acclimatization is one example of adaptation.

Adenosine diphosphate (ADP) (chapter 3)—One of the chemical products resulting from the breakdown of ATP (e.g., during muscle contraction).

Adenosine triphosphate (ATP) (chapter 3)—A high-energy compound from which the body derives energy.

Adherence (chapter 12)—State of continuing. Often used to describe people who continue to participate in a physical fitness program.

Adipose tissue (chapter 7)—A connective tissue in which fat is stored.

Adrenal glands (chapter 3)—Endocrine glands directly above each kidney, composed of the medulla (which secretes the hormones epinephrine and norepinephrine) and the cortex (which secretes cortisol, aldosterone, androgens, and estrogens).

Adrenalin—See *epinephrine*.

Aerobic activities (chapter 13)—The activities of moderate intensity that use large muscle groups with energy (ATP) supplied aerobically.

Aerobic metabolism (chapter 3)—Processes in which energy (ATP) is supplied when oxygen is utilized while a person is working.

Aerobic power (chapter 9)—The maximal oxygen uptake, or the rate at which oxygen can be utilized during maximal physical work.

Aggression (chapter 11)—High levels of animosity or hostility, often unprovoked, which sometimes result from frustration or a feeling of inferiority.

Aging (chapters 1, 3, 9, 11, 13)—The process of becoming older. Changes associated with aging are caused by various factors, including the lapse of time. These factors include decreased physical activity and an increased number and severity of health problems.

Agonist (chapter 4)—A muscle that is the prime mover in a contraction.

Alkalosis (chapter 3)—An increase of pH of the body, caused by excessive alkaline substances such as bicarbonate or by a removal of acids or chlorides from the blood.

Altitude (chapters 3, 13)—The height above sea level for a given point. A person has a lower maximal aerobic power with increasing altitudes because of the decreased partial pressure of oxygen in the air.

Alveolus (plural, alveoli) (chapter 4)—A tiny air sac of the lungs where carbon dioxide and oxygen are exchanged with the surrounding pulmonary capillaries.

American Alliance of Health, Physical Education, Recreation and Dance—An organization of professionals interested in these fields.

American College of Sports Medicine—An organization of professionals interested in the relationship of sport (and other physical activity) to medicine (and health and performance).

Amino acid (chapter 3)—A compound present in proteins from which the body builds tissue. Amino acids can be used for energy.

Amphiarthrodial joint (chapter 4)—A type of joint that allows slight movement.

Anaerobic activities (chapter 3)—High-intensity activities during which energy demands exceed the ability to work aerobically.

Anaerobic metabolism (chapter 3)—Energy supplied without oxygen, causing an oxygen debt; creatine phosphate and glycolysis supply ATP without O_2.

Anaerobic threshold (chapter 3)—The sudden increase in lactic acid in the blood during a graded exercise test.

Anatomy (chapter 4)—The science that deals with the structure of the human body.

Android-type obesity (chapter 7)—Upper body obesity; associated with cardiovascular and metabolic diseases.

Aneurysm (chapter 2)—A spindle-shaped or saclike bulging of the wall of a blood-filled vein, artery, or ventricle.

Anger (chapter 11)—A strong emotion of displeasure or antagonism, which is often excited by a sense of injury or insult and frequently paired with a desire to retaliate.

Angina, angina pectoris (chapter 15)—Severe cardiac pain that may radiate to the jaw, arms, or legs. Angina is caused by myocardial ischemia, which can be induced by exercise in susceptible individuals. Exercise should be stopped, and the person should be referred for medical attention.

Angular momentum (chapter 4)—The quantity of rotation. Angular momentum is the product of the rotational inertia and angular velocity.

Anorexia, anorexia nervosa (chapter 6)—An abnormal lack of appetite. Self-induced weight loss with excessive concern for body fatness.

Antagonist (chapter 4)—A muscle that causes movement at a joint in a direction opposite to that of its agonist (prime mover).

Anthropometry (chapter 7)—The measurement of the body and its parts.

Anticoagulant (chapter 15)—A drug that delays blood clotting.

Anxiety (chapter 11)—Feeling of fear, apprehension, and dread, often without apparent cause.

Aorta (chapter 15)—The main artery coming out of the left ventricle.

Aponeurosis (chapter 4)—Broad, flat, tendinous sheath attaching muscles to each other.

Apoplexy, stroke (chapter 3)—The loss of consciousness and paralysis caused by an inadequate blood supply to a portion of the brain.

Apparently healthy (chapter 2)—A term used to describe people without a known disease or illness. These people may vary widely in terms of levels of physical fitness and numbers of risk factors.

Apple II family (chapter 18)—A series of microcomputers manufactured by Apple Computer, Inc., of Cupertino, CA. Includes the Apple II, Apple II Plus, Apple IIe, and Apple IIgs microcomputers.

Aquatics (chapter 14)—Physical activities performed on or in water.

Arousal (chapter 11)—The act of becoming excited, causing a stress response (i.e., a greater physiological response than is needed to perform the task). Arousal often occurs in competitive situations.

Arteriosclerosis (chapter 2)—An arterial disease characterized by the hardening and thickening of vessel walls.

Articular cartilage (chapter 4)—Cartilage covering bone surfaces that articulate with other bone surfaces.

Asthma (chapter 13)—Wheezing, coughing, and shortness of breath caused by constriction of the pulmonary pathways. May be initiated by exercise, allergies, or other irritants.

Atherosclerosis (chapter 2)—A form of arteriosclerosis in which fatty substances deposit in the inner walls of the arteries.

Athlete's foot (chapter 16)—A foot fungus, often accompanied by a bacterial infection, that causes itching, redness, and a rash on the soles, toes, or between toes.

Atrioventricular (chapter 15)—Pertaining to the atria and the ventricles of the heart, such as a node, a tract, and a valve.

Atrioventricular node (chapter 15)—The origin of the bundle of His in the right atrium of the heart. Normal electrical activity of the heart passes through the AV node prior to depolarization.

Atrium, also called auricle (plural is atria, adjective is atrial) (chapter 15)—One of the two (i.e., left and right) upper cavities of the heart.

Atrophy (chapter 10)—A reduction in the size of a muscle or other body part. Atrophy is often caused by disuse.

Autonomic nervous system (chapter 3)—The nerves that innervate the heart, viscera, and glands and control their involuntary functions. The autonomic nervous system consists of sympathetic and parasympathetic divisions.

AV block (chapter 15)—Obstruction of the nerve impulse at the AV node.

Background information (chapter 2)—Health problems, characteristics, lifestyle, habits, signs, and symptoms of a person (and family) that are related to positive health and risks of health problems.

Backup (chapter 18)—A spare copy of a computer program or of the data generated from a program.

Ballistic movement (chapter 4)—A rapid movement with three phases: an initial concentric muscle contraction by agonists to begin movement, a coasting phase, and a deceleration by the eccentric contraction of the antagonist muscles.

Baroreceptors (chapter 3)—Receptor that monitors arterial blood pressure.

Basal metabolic rate (BMR) (chapter 7)—The minimum energy expenditure required for life in the resting, postabsorptive state.

Basic Four Food Groups (chapter 6)—Foods can be placed into four groups: meat, fish and poultry; milk and milk products; breads and cereals; and fruits and vegetables.

Behavior (chapters 2, 12)—The manner of conducting oneself, often in relation to others or in a particular environment. Behavior usually refers to a person's activities (rather than his or her thoughts or intentions).

Behavior contract (chapter 12)—An agreement (usually written) made with a friend or helper pledging to modify behavior—for example, to stop smoking.

Bench (chapter 9)—A step used to test cardiorespiratory function. The height of the bench and the number of steps per minute determine the intensity of the effort.

Beta-adrenergic (chapter 15)—Receptors in the heart and lungs that respond to catecholamines (epinephrine and norepinephrine).

Bigeminy (chapter 15)—On ECG, alternating normal and premature ventricular contractions.

Blood chemistry (chapter 2)—The analysis of the content of the blood, used to determine the levels of substances related to health (e.g., cholesterol) or performance (e.g., lactic acid).

Blood pressure (chapter 2)—The pressure exerted by the blood on the vessel walls, measured in millimeters of mercury by the sphygmomanometer. The systolic pressure (SBP, when the left ventricle is in maximal contraction) is the first sound, followed by the diastolic pressure (DBP, when the left ventricle is at rest), which is recorded when there is a change of tone of the sound (4th phase, depending on rest or exercise).

Blood-pressure cuff (chapter 9)—The cuff that is wrapped around the arm and pumped up to block off the artery. The pressure in the cuff is then slowly released to determine SBP and DBP. It is important to have the right size cuff for the arm, because improper-sized cuffs may result in inaccurate readings (e.g., too small a cuff will provide an artificially elevated blood pressure).

Blood profile (chapter 2)—Assessment of health-related variables found in the blood, such as cholesterol.

Blood vessel (chapter 15)—Any vessel (i.e., artery, vein, or capillary) through which blood circulates.

Body composition (chapter 7)—The relative amounts of muscle, bone, and fat in the body. Body composition is usually divided into fatness (% body fat) and lean body (% lean body mass).

Body density (chapter 7)—The relative weight of the body compared to an equal volume of water, or weight of the body per unit volume. Body density can be used to estimate percent fat.

Body mass index (BMI) (chapter 7)—An index of body fatness equal to kilograms of body mass divided by the height squared (expressed in meters): $kg \cdot m^{-2}$.

Bradycardia (chapter 15)—Slow heart rate, below 60 beats·min^{-1} at rest. Bradycardia is healthy if it is the result of physical conditioning.

Breathlessness (chapter 2)—The inability to breathe without difficulty. Breathlessness may indicate a pulmonary disorder or a risk of CHD if it occurs with mild exertion; a person with this condition should be referred to medical personnel.

Bronchiole (chapter 4)—A small branch of the airway. A bronchiole sometimes undergoes a spasm and makes breathing difficult, such as in exercise-induced asthma.

Bronchitis (chapter 2)—The inflammation of the bronchi. Symptoms are a productive cough, wheezy breathing, and varying degrees of breathlessness.

Buffer (chapter 3)—A substance in blood that binds with hydrogen ions to minimize changes in the acid-base balance.

Bulimia, bulimia nervosa (chapter 6)—A condition characterized by binge eating and vomiting, with perception of lack of control. Includes use of self-induced vomiting, laxatives, fasting, and exercise to prevent weight gain.

Bundle branch block (chapter 15)—A heart block caused by a lesion in one of the branches of the bundle of His.

Bundle of His (chapter 15)—The bundle of nerve fibers between atria and ventricles that conducts impulses into both ventricles.

Bursa (chapter 4)—A fibrous sac lined with synovial membrane that contains a small quantity of synovial fluid. Bursae are found between tendon and bone, skin and bone, and between muscle and muscle. Their function is to facilitate movement without friction between these surfaces.

Bursitis (chapter 16)—The inflammation of a bursa.

Calibrate (chapter 5)—To determine the accuracy of an instrument, by measurement of its variation from a standard.

Calisthenics (chapter 10)—Exercise without equipment, performed for flexibility or muscular development.

Caloric cost (chapter 8)—The number of calories used for a specific task, normally reported in C or kcal·min^{-1}.

Calorie (chapters 6, 8)—1 calorie = the amount of heat required to raise the temperature of 1 g of water 1 °C; 1,000 calories = 1 kilocalorie.

Calorimetry (chapter 8)—The method used to measure the number of calories in something.

Capillary (chapter 3)—The smallest blood vessel; the link between the end of the arteries and the beginning of the veins.

Capsular ligament (chapter 4)—The ligament lined with synovial membrane surrounding the diarthrodial or synovial joints.

Capsulitis (chapter 16)—The inflammation of a capsule.

Carbohydrate (chapter 6)—A group of chemical compounds containing only carbon, hydrogen, and oxygen; sugars, cellulose, and starches are carbohydrates.

Carbon dioxide (chapter 15)—A gas; a waste product of many forms of combustion and metabolism, excreted via the lungs.

Carbon monoxide (chapter 13)—A pollutant derived from the incomplete combustion of fossil fuels; binds hemoglobin to reduce oxygen transport, and reduces maximal aerobic power.

Cardiac cycle (chapter 3)—One total heart beat with one complete contraction (systole) and relaxation (diastole) of the heart.

Cardiac output (chapter 3)—The amount of blood circulated by the heart each minute; cardiac output = heart rate × stroke volume.

Cardiac rehabilitation (chapter 13)—A program designed to help cardiac patients return to normal lives with reduced risk of additional health problems.

Cardiopulmonary resuscitation (CPR) (chapter 16)—A method to restore normal pulse and breathing by mouth-to-mouth respiration and rhythmical compression on the chest. People working in fitness programs should be certified in CPR.

Cardiorespiratory function (chapter 9)—Pertaining to the heart and respiration.

Cardiovascular (chapter 9)—Pertaining to the heart and blood vessels.

Carotid artery (chapter 15)—The principal artery in each side of the neck.

Catecholamines (chapter 3)—Epinephrine and norepinephrine.

Catharsis (chapter 11)—Purification of the emotions through action.

Cellulite (chapter 6)—A label given to lumpy deposits of fat commonly appearing on the back and front of the legs and buttocks in overweight individuals.

Center of gravity (chapter 4)—The theoretical point about which the entire weight of the body (or body part) can be considered to be acting.

Cerebral vascular disease (chapter 2)—A disease of the blood vessels of the brain.

Certification (chapter 14)—A document that serves as evidence of a certain status or qualification. For example, several groups certify that people are qualified to conduct specific aspects of a fitness program.

Chest pain (chapter 2)—A tightness, compression, or sharp sensation in the chest, which may be caused by myocardial ischemia. People with chest (arm, shoulder, or jaw) pain should be referred for medical attention.

Cholesterol (chapter 2)—A fat-like substance found in animal tissues. High-density lipoprotein cholesterol (HDL-C) is protective against the development of CHD, in that it helps transport cholesterol to the liver, where it is eliminated. Thus *low* levels of HDL-C are a high risk of CHD. Low-density lipoprotein cholesterol (LDL-C) is responsible for the buildup of plaque in the inner wall of the arteries (atherosclerosis). Thus *high* levels of LDL-C are a high risk of CHD. The normal plasma level of total cholesterol is considered to be less than 200 mg per 100 ml.

Chronic injury (chapter 16)—An ongoing injury that lasts for an extended period of time.

Chronic obstructive pulmonary disease (COPD) (chapter 13)—A term used to describe a number of specific diseases that cause a chronic unremitting obstruction to flow of air in the airways of the lungs.

Chronic stressor (chapter 11)—A continuing condition or situation that causes physiological responses in excess of those needed to complete a task. For example, excess fat causes chronic stress responses at rest and during exertion.

Circuit training (chapter 14)—A sequence of exercises done one after the other in the same workout.

Circulation (chapters 3, 15)—The continuous movement of blood through the heart and blood vessels.

Cirrhosis (chapter 2)—The hardening of an organ. The term is applied almost exclusively to degenerative changes in the liver with resulting fibrosis. Damage to liver cells can be by virus, microbes, toxic substances, or dietary deficiencies interfering with the nutrition of the cells—often as a result of alcoholism.

Claudication (chapter 2)—Interference with the blood supply to the legs, often resulting in limping.

Closed-circuit spirometry (chapter 8)—The subject breathes 100% oxygen from a "bell" while carbon dioxide is absorbed; loss of volume of oxygen from bell is proportional to oxygen consumption.

Coagulation, blood clotting (chapter 3)—The formation of fibrin, a threadlike clot or clump of solid material in the blood.

Collateral circulation (chapter 3)—Additional, supplementary, or substitute vessels that increase circulation to a part of the tissue, such as in the heart.

Collection bag (chapter 3)—Airtight container used to store expired air during an exercise-tolerance test. Samples of air in bags are analyzed for percentages of oxygen and carbon dioxide.

Compatible (IBM compatible) (chapter 18)—A microcomputer that can run programs written for the IBM microcomputer.

Compound fracture (chapter 16)—Bone fracture with external exposure.

Concentric contraction (chapter 4)—A shortening of the muscle as a result of its contraction.

Concussion (chapter 2)—A condition resulting from a violent jar or shock. A concussion is associated with the brain and may result in loss of consciousness, pallor, coldness, and an increase in heart rate.

Conditioning (chapter 1)—Exercise conducted on a regular basis over a period of time. Also called training.

Conduction (chapter 15)—The transmission of energy, heat, electricity, or sound. For example, conduction is the passage of electrical currents and nerve impulses through body tissues.

Confidentiality (chapter 17)—The act of keeping information about an individual private. One of the elements of "informed consent" of fitness participants is that the information and data will be kept in a secure place and not shared with anyone without the individual's permission.

Congestive heart failure (chapter 2)—Failure of the heart, caused by its inability to pump a sufficient proportion of the blood it contains, with subsequent congestion.

Constant resistance (chapter 10)—Weight-training program in which the resistance is constant throughout the range of motion, as when using free weights; old term is *isotonic weight training*.

Contractility (chapter 4)—The ability (e.g., of a muscle) to shorten in response to a stimulus.

Contraindication (chapter 13)—A sign or symptom suggesting that a certain activity should be avoided.

Control (chapter 11)—The power to influence the outcome. The perception of control of a situation is one of the key elements in coping with potentially stressful conditions. In an experimental sense, control refers to the extent to which related variables are accounted for so that the result is the effect of the experimental treatment. Often the experimental control is in the form of one or more control groups.

Contusion (chapter 16)—A bruise; slight bleeding into tissues while the skin remains unbroken.

Cool-down, taper-down (chapter 13)—A period of light activity following moderate to heavy exercise.

The cool-down period is important because it allows the leg muscles to continue to pump blood back to the heart, whereas stopping immediately after exercise causes pooling of the blood in the legs and a lack of venous return.

Cope (chapter 11)—To struggle or strive to deal with a difficult situation with some degree of success.

Core temperature (chapter 3)—The temperature of the central portion of the body, usually estimated by a rectal probe.

Coronary arteries (chapter 15)—Blood vessels that supply the heart muscle.

Coronary artery bypass surgery (chapter 15)—Arteries or veins are sutured above and below a blocked coronary artery to restore adequate blood flow to that portion of the myocardium.

Coronary artery thrombosis (chapter 15)—An occlusion of a coronary vessel by a blood clot.

Coronary heart disease (CHD) (chapter 2)—Atherosclerosis of the coronary arteries. Also called coronary artery disease (CAD).

Coronary occlusion (chapter 15)—The blockage of a coronary artery.

Coronary-prone personality (chapter 11)—A person with Type A behavior (e.g., hard-driving, impatient, time-conscious). Someone with a coronary-prone personality may have a higher risk of CHD.

Coronary sinus (chapter 15)—The channel into which most cardiac veins empty; leads to the right atrium.

Coronary thrombosis (chapter 15)—Blockage of a coronary artery by a blood clot.

Cortisol (chapter 3)—A hormone released from the adrenal cortex in response to stress; involved in glucose metabolism and inflammation reactions.

Cost effectiveness (chapter 17)—Assessment of the cost versus the benefits of a program.

Creatine phosphate (chapter 3)—A high-energy phosphate compound that represents the primary immediate anaerobic source of ATP at the onset of exercise; important in all-out activities lasting seconds.

Criteria for entry into program (chapter 17)—Standards for deciding which people should be referred for medical attention and which should be allowed to participate in fitness testing and activities.

Cross-adaptation (chapter 11)—The transfer of increased adaptation from one stimulus (or stressor) to another stimulus. For example, some have claimed that increased adaptation to physical work from physical conditioning carries over to better adaptation to mental or emotional stressors. The evidence is inconclusive.

Cyanosis (chapter 16)—A bluish tinge frequently observed under the nails, lips, and skin, caused by lack of oxygen. If found, the exercise test or activity should be stopped.

Cycle ergometer (chapter 9)—A one-wheeled stationary cycle with adjustable resistance used as a work task for exercise testing or conditioning.

Defibrillator (chapter 15)—Any agent or measure, such as an electric shock, that stops an uncoordinated contraction of the heart muscle and restores a normal heartbeat.

Degenerative disease (chapter 2)—A disease involving gradual deterioration and impairment of a tissue or organ.

Dehydration (chapter 3)—The excessive loss of body fluids.

Denial (chapter 11)—Refusal to acknowledge a truth. In fitness programs, people sometimes deny pain and discomfort—they need to be cautioned about doing too much.

Depolarization (chapter 15)—The change of polarity, specifically the electrical stimulus changing the atrium or ventricle from the resting to the working state.

Depression (chapter 11)—Emotional dejection greater than that warranted by any objective reasons, often with symptoms such as insomnia, headaches, exhaustion, anorexia, irritability, loss of interest, impaired concentration, feelings that life is not worth living, and suicidal thoughts.

Detrained (chapters 3, 13)—The result of becoming sedentary after a physical conditioning program. The effects (e.g., increased fat, decreased CRF) are opposite those of conditioning.

Development . . . deterioration (chapter 11)—A continuum describing the effects of stress. Positive stress results are found toward the development end of the continuum and negative stress results are near the deterioration end.

Diabetes (chapters 13, 16)—A metabolic disorder characterized by an inability to oxidize carbohydrates because of inadequate insulin (TYPE I) or a resistance to insulin (TYPE II).

Diabetic coma (chapter 16)—A lack of consciousness caused by lack of insulin, associated with extreme hyperglycemia.

Diagnosed medical problem (chapter 2)—Any health problem that has been recognized by a person in the medical profession.

Diaphysis (chapter 4)—The shaft of a long bone.

Diarthrodial joint, or synovial joint (chapter 4)—A

freely moving joint characterized by its synovial membrane and capsular ligament.

Diastolic blood pressure (DBP) (chapters 2, 9)—The pressure exerted by the blood on the vessel walls during the resting portion of the cardiac cycle, measured in millimeters of mercury by a sphygmomanometer.

Diet (chapter 6)—The food eaten by an individual. Diet sometimes refers to a special selection of food.

Dietary exchange lists (chapter 6)—Lists of foods containing similar quantities of nutrients and calories that are effective in planning diets for weight control and the management of diabetes.

Digitalis (chapter 15)—A drug that augments the contraction of the heart muscle and slows the rate of conduction of cardiac impulses through the AV node.

Dimethyl sulfoxide (DMSO) (chapter 15)—A controversial drug originally used by veterinarians to reduce joint inflammation in animals and presently used by some athletes for joint and soft-tissue injuries.

Direct calorimetry (chapter 8)—A method of measuring the metabolic rate, using a closed chamber in which a subject's heat loss is picked up by water flowing through the wall of a chamber; the gain in temperature of the water, plus that lost in evaporation, determine the metabolic rate.

Diurnal variation (chapter 3)—A daily variation or change.

Dizziness (chapter 2)—Unsteadiness, with the tendency to stagger or fall.

DOS—disk operating system (chapter 18)—The software that resides inside the computer's memory when you turn the computer on. It gives the user the opportunity to read, write, generate, print, compute, etc.

DOS 3.3 (chapter 18)—The disk operating system used by older members of the Apple II family of computers (e.g., Apple II and Apple II plus).

Double product (chapter 3)—The product of the heart rate and systolic blood pressure; indicative of the heart's oxygen requirement during exercise. Also called the rate-pressure product.

Drugs (chapter 15)—A substance (other than food) that, when taken into the body, produces a change in it. If the change helps the body, the drug is a medicine. If the change is harmful, the drug is a poison. Drugs are often addictive.

Dry-bulb temperature (chapter 13)—The temperature of the air measured by an ordinary thermometer.

Duration (chapter 13)—The length of time for a fitness workout. Guidelines often include 15 to 30 min of aerobic work at a target heart rate; however, more importantly, the total work accomplished (e.g., distance covered) should be emphasized.

Dyspnea (chapter 9)—Difficult or labored breathing beyond what is expected for the intensity of work. The exercise test or activity should be stopped.

Eccentric contraction (chapter 4)—A lengthening of the muscle during its contraction; resists movement caused by another force.

Ectopic ventricular complex (chapter 15)—A ventricular contraction originating at some point other than the sinoatrial node.

Efficiency (chapter 3)—The ratio of energy expenditure to work output.

Ejection fraction (chapter 15)—The fraction of the end diastolic volume ejected per beat (stroke volume divided by end diastolic volume).

Electrocardiogram (ECG) (chapter 15)—A tracing of the electrical activity of the heart during a complete contraction/relaxation cycle, including the depolarization of the atrium (P wave) and the depolarization (QRS) and repolarization (T wave) of the ventricle.

Electrode (chapter 15)—A conductor of electrical activity, specifically a plate attached to various parts of the body to receive and transmit the heart's electrical activity to a recorder.

Electrophysiology (chapter 15)—The study of electrical activity in the body as it relates to functional aspects of health.

Embolism (chapter 2)—The obstruction of a blood vessel by a foreign object, such as a loose blood clot.

Emotion (chapter 11)—A strong feeling, often accompanied by stress reactions and behaviors.

Empathy (chapter 11)—Identification with thoughts or feelings of another person.

End diastolic volume (chapter 3)—The volume of blood in the heart just prior to ventricular contraction; a measure of the stretch of the ventricle.

Endocardium (chapter 15)—The membrane lining that covers the chambers of the heart, including the valves.

Endorphins (chapter 11)—A group of hormones that are similar in composition to morphine and normally produced and released by the pituitary gland to help reduce great pain, anxiety, and stress.

End point (chapter 9)—The point at which an exercise test is changed to the taper-down or stopped.

Endurance run (chapter 9)—A race of a set distance (for time) or set time (for distance). Normally used to determine a person's cardiorespiratory endurance. Runs of at least 1 mi or 6 min should be used.

Energy (chapter 8)—The capacity for performing work, often measured in terms of oxygen consumption.

Enjoyable . . . Unpleasant (chapter 11)—One of the continuums used to describe a stressful condition.

Enlarged heart (chapter 2)—A heart bigger than average size. If an enlarged heart is the result of pathological conditions, then it is weak and unhealthy. If it results from physical conditioning, then it is strong and healthy.

Environmental factors (chapter 13)—Aspects of the surroundings (e.g., heat, altitude, pollution) that influence the response to exercise.

Enzyme (chapter 3)—An organic catalyst that aids many body processes, such as digestion and oxidation.

Epicardium (chapter 15)—The layer of the pericardium attached to the heart.

Epicondylitis (chapter 16)—Inflammation of muscles or tendons attaching to the epicondyles of the humerus.

Epidemiological studies (chapter 1)—Long-term studies of the distribution of diseases in whole populations. Those characteristics, signs, and symptoms that are related to major health problems based on epidemiological studies are called risk factors.

Epilepsy (chapter 13)—A nervous disorder resulting from disordered electrical activity of the brain, often resulting in a seizure.

Epimysium (chapter 4)—The connective-tissue sheath surrounding a muscle.

Epinephrine, adrenaline (chapter 3)—A chemical liberated from the adrenal medulla and from sympathetic nerve endings. Effects include cardiac stimulation and constriction of blood vessels, and mobilization of glucose and free fatty acids.

Epiphyseal plates (chapter 4)—The sites of ossification in long bones.

Epiphyses (chapter 4)—The ends of long bones.

Erythrocytes (chapter 3)—The red blood cells.

Etiology (chapter 2)—The study of the causes of disease.

Euphoria (chapter 11)—An exaggerated sense of well-being.

Evaluation (chapters, 5, 17)—The determination or judgment of the value or worth of something or someone. In a fitness setting, an evaluation determines the health or fitness status of an individual based on his or her characteristics, signs, symptoms, behaviors, and test results.

Evaporation (chapter 13)—Conversion from the liquid to the gaseous state by means of heat, as in evapora-

tion of sweat; results in the loss of 580 kcal per liter of sweat evaporated.

Exercise (chapter 1)—Physical activity, the purpose of which is to improve some component(s) of physical fitness.

Exercise components (chapter 14)—Warm-up, main body of exercise, and taper-down (cool-down).

Exercise-induced asthma (chapter 13)—A form of asthma induced by exercise; can be prevented with medication.

Exercise modification (chapters 13, 16)—Adjustment of a person's exercise program in terms of type of activity, intensity, frequency, and/or total work accomplished to more nearly achieve the fitness goals.

Exercise prescription (chapter 13)—A recommendation for a fitness program in terms of types of activities, intensity, frequency, and total amount of work aimed at producing or maintaining desirable fitness objectives.

Exercise progression (chapter 13)—The increase in total work and/or intensity as a person gradually goes from a sedentary lifestyle to the recommended levels of physical activity.

Exercise Specialist (Introduction)—A person certified by the American College of Sports Medicine to work in exercise rehabilitation settings with high-risk or diseased populations.

Exercise Technologist (Introduction)—A person certified by the American College of Sports Medicine to conduct graded exercise stress tests for a variety of populations.

Expiration (chapter 3)—Exhalation of air from the lungs.

Expired gas (chapter 9)—The air that is exhaled from the lungs, often analyzed to determine oxygen and carbon dioxide concentrations.

Extension (chapter 10)—Increasing the angle at a joint, such as straightening the elbow.

Extensor (chapter 4)—A muscle that extends a joint.

Extrinsic (chapter 11)—External, as in extrinsic motivation (e.g., reward) to begin or continue exercise.

Extrovert (chapter 11)—A person who regulates self-behavior in response to others.

Facility (chapter 17)—Something designed, built, or installed to serve a specific function, such as the facilities for a fitness program.

Family history (chapters 1, 2)—The major health problems that have been found in a person's grandparents, parents, uncles, aunts, and siblings. Heart disease in a person's family is a secondary risk factor for CHD.

Fartlek (chapter 14)—A form of physical conditioning, also known as speed play, which alternates fast and slow running over varied terrain for 3 to 4 mi.

Fasciculus (chapter 4)—A bundle of muscle fibers surrounded by perimyseum.

Fast-twitch fiber (chapter 4)—A muscle fiber characterized by its fast speed of contraction.

Fat (chapters 1, 7)—A compound containing glycerol and fatty acids that is used as a source of energy and can be stored in the body.

Fat-free weight, also lean body weight (chapter 7)—The amount of total body weight that is free of fat, calculated by total body weight minus fat weight.

Fat-soluble vitamin (chapter 6)—Vitamins that are stored in fat tissue (vitamins A, D, E, and K).

Fatty acid (chapter 6)—Molecules 16 to 18 carbons in length, such as stearic, palmitic, or oleic acid. Circulating fatty acids can be used for energy.

Fat weight (chapter 7)—The absolute amount of total body weight that is body fat, calculated by total body weight times percent fat.

Fear (chapter 11)—A distressing emotion aroused by impending pain, danger, and so forth.

Field tests (chapter 9)—Tests that can be used in mass testing situations.

First-degree AV block (chapter 15)—The delayed transmission of impulses from atria to ventricles (in excess of 0.21 s).

Fitness (chapter 1)—A state of health characteristics, symptoms, and behaviors enabling a person to have the highest quality of life. Increases in fitness components are related to positive health, whereas decreases in fitness components increase the risk of major health problems.

Fitness activities (chapter 14)—Actions that lead to increased fitness.

Fitness continuum (chapter 1)—A continuum that extends from death to severe disease, to lack of disease, to optimal capacity to accomplish a person's goals.

Fitness Instructor (Introduction)—A person who assists people in evaluating and improving fitness. Certification is offered by the American College of Sports Medicine for those HFIs who work with apparently healthy populations.

Fitness program (chapters 14, 17)—An organized series of activities aimed at promoting increased fitness.

Fitness testing (chapters 2, 7, 9, 10)—The measurement and evaluation of the status of all fitness components.

Fitness workout (chapter 13)—A specific fitness session.

Fixator muscle (chapter 4)—The muscle that stabilizes a joint to prevent undesirable joint movement.

Flexibility (chapter 10)—The ability to move a joint through the full range of motion without discomfort or pain.

Flexion (chapter 4)—The movement of a limb caused by concentric muscular contraction, resulting in a decrease in the angle of a joint.

Floppy disk (chapter 18)—A round "disk," typically 3.5 or 5.25 inches in diameter, that contains either a computer program or data to input to or that was written from a microcomputer. Information is magnetically stored on the disk in the same way that information is stored on audio tapes.

Flow meter (chapter 9)—An instrument that measures the rate of air movement (e.g., liters of air moved per minute) in a graded exercise test.

Fracture (chapter 16)—A break in a bone.

Frequency (chapter 13)—How often a person has a fitness workout (usually days per week).

Friction massage (chapter 16)—A form of massage in which the stroking motion of the hands builds up heat on the surface of the skin overlying a tight or sore muscle.

Frostbite (chapter 13)—Freezing of the skin and superficial tissues, resulting from exposure to extreme cold.

Function . . . Severe stress (chapter 11)—A continuum describing the response to a stimulus.

Functional (chapter 11)—Pertaining to function. The response to a stimulus can be subdivided into the functional response needed to do the task and the stress response beyond what is essential for that task.

Functional capacity (chapter 9)—Maximal oxygen uptake, expressed in milliliters of oxygen per kilogram of body weight per minute, or in METs.

Fun run (chapter 14)—A race with an emphasis on participation (as opposed to winning).

Game (chapter 14)—A form of playing for amusement. Games may be cooperative or competitive, involving a few or many people. Games can also be used to achieve fitness improvements.

Gas analyzer (chapter 9)—An instrument that measures components of air. In the case of maximal oxygen uptake, a gas analyzer is used to measure oxygen and carbon dioxide in expired air.

Genetic potential (chapter 1)—The possibilities and limits imposed by a person's inherited genes.

Glucose (chapters 2, 6)—A carbohydrate that is transported in the blood stream and metabolized by the cell as a primary energy source.

Glycogen (chapter 6)—The form in which glucose is stored in the body.

Glycolysis (chapter 3)—The metabolic pathway producing ATP from the anaerobic breakdown of glucose; the short-term source of ATP that is important in all-out activities lasting less than 2 min.

Goal orientation (chapter 11)—The tendency of a person to behave on the basis of her or his goals.

Graded exercise test (GXT) (chapter 9)—A multistage test that determines a person's physiological responses to different intensities of exercise and/or the person's peak aerobic capacity.

Gram (g)—A basic unit of mass in the metric system. 1,000 g = 1 kg.

Gynoid-type obesity (chapter 7)—Lower body obesity that does not carry the same disease risk as upper body obesity.

Hamstring (chapter 4)—The tendon in the back of the knee. A hamstring is also a large muscle group at the back of the thigh that crosses both the knee and hip joints.

Hardware (chapter 18)—Hardware is the physical computer device and associated peripherals. Differentiated from software.

Health (chapter 1)—Being alive with no major health problem, also called apparently healthy.

Health Fitness Instructor (HFI) (Introduction)—A person who is certified by the American College of Sports Medicine and is thus qualified to assist in the evaluation and improvement of health and fitness in normal populations.

Health history (chapter 2)—Information about a person's past health record.

Health-related attitudes (chapter 2)—A manner of thinking associated with healthy behaviors.

Health-related behavior (chapter 2)—A person's actions that are associated with positive or negative health.

Health-related sign (chapter 2)—Evidence of something with a potential health consequence.

Health-related symptom (chapter 2)—A sensation that arises from or accompanies a particular disease or disorder and serves as an indicator of it.

Health status (chapter 2)—Current level of disease and fitness.

Healthy behavior (chapters 2, 12)—Activities, habits, and avoidances that are related to total fitness and low risk of developing major health problems. These behaviors include exercise, healthy diet, nonsmoking, no or slight use of alcohol, no use of nonessential drugs, adequate sleep, ability to relax and cope with stressors, and safety habits.

Healthy life (chapter 2)—A lifestyle including behaviors related to enhanced fitness and excluding harmful behaviors.

Heart attack (chapter 15)—A general term used to describe an acute episode of heart disease; common name for myocardial infarction.

Heart disease (chapter 2)—A general term used to describe any of several abnormalities of the heart that make the heart unable to function properly.

Heart rate (chapters 2, 9, 13)—The number of beats of the heart per minute.

Heart-rate reserve (chapter 13)—The difference between maximal and resting heart rates.

Heart rhythm (chapter 15)—The regularity of the heart beat, or components of the cardiac cycle.

Heat cramps (chapter 16)—A spasmodic contraction of a muscle or group of muscles that is caused by working in extreme heat.

Heat exhaustion (chapter 16)—Collapse, with or without loss of consciousness, suffered in conditions of heat and high humidity, largely resulting from the loss of fluid and salt by sweating.

Heat illness (chapters 9, 16)—A general term denoting problems caused by activity in high temperatures.

Heat stroke (chapter 16)—The final stage in heat exhaustion. When the body is unable to lose heat, hyperpyrexia occurs, and death may ensue.

Heat syncope (chapter 16)—Fainting or sudden loss of strength because of excessive heat gain.

Heel bruise (chapter 16)—An injury in which the skin is not broken but the periosteum is inflamed; often caused by a foot landing on a sharp object.

Hematocrit (chapter 3)—The volume of red blood cells per unit volume of blood, usually about 40% to 45%.

Hemoglobin (chapter 3)—The respiratory pigment in the red blood corpuscles. It has the reversible function of combining with and releasing oxygen.

Hemorrhage (chapter 16)—The escape of blood from a vessel.

Heredity (chapter 1)—The transmission of genetic characters from parents to offspring.

High blood pressure, hypertension (chapters 2, 13)—Blood pressure in excess of normal values for a specific age and gender.

High-calorie diet (chapter 6)—Food consumption of which the caloric value exceeds the total daily energy requirement, resulting in increased adipose tissue.

High-density lipoprotein cholesterol (HDL-C) (chapters 2, 6)—A plasma lipid-protein complex containing relatively more protein and less cholesterol and triglycerides. Low levels of HDL-C are associated with CHD.

High-intensity exercise (chapter 1)—Activity at 80% to 120% of functional capacity, recommended only for those interested in high-level performance after medical screening.

Homeostasis (chapter 11)—The tendency of the body to maintain internal equilibrium of temperature, fluid content, and so forth by the regulation of its bodily processes.

Hormone (chapter 3)—A chemical product produced by an endocrine gland and secreted into the blood; exerts a distinct and usually powerful effect on some body function or organ.

Hostile (chapter 11)—Antagonistic, unfriendly.

Humidity (chapter 13)—The amount of moisture in the atmosphere.

Hydrostatic weighing (chapter 7)—Underwater weighing; body density is estimated by the loss of weight when submerged in water, and the value is converted to percent body fat.

Hypercholesterolemia (chapter 2)—An excess of cholesterol in the blood.

Hyperglycemia (chapter 3)—An elevation of blood glucose that can occur in the diabetic who does not achieve a proper balance between dietary intake and injected insulin.

Hyperlipoproteinemia (chapter 6)—An increase in the concentration of the three fatty substances of the blood: cholesterol, phospholipids, and triglycerides.

Hyperplasia (chapter 6)—New fat-cell formation.

Hypertension (chapters 2, 13)—High blood pressure. Normally systolic blood pressure exceeds 140 mmHg or diastolic pressure exceeds 90 mmHg in someone who has hypertension.

Hyperthermia (chapter 13)—An elevation of the core temperature; if unchecked, can lead to heat exhaustion or heat stroke and death.

Hypertrophy (chapter 4)—An increase in the size of a muscle, organ, or other body part caused by an enlargement of its constituent cells.

Hyperventilation (chapter 3)—A level of ventilation beyond that needed to maintain the arterial carbon dioxide level; can be initiated by a sudden increase in the hydrogen ion concentration due to lactic acid production during a progressive exercise test.

Hypervitaminosis (chapter 6)—A condition in which the level of a vitamin in the blood or tissues is high enough to cause undesirable effects.

Hypoglycemia (chapter 2)—Low blood sugar, attended by anxiety, excitement, perspiration, delirium, or coma.

Hypokinetic disease (chapter 1)—A disease that relates to or is caused by the lack of regular physical activity.

Hypothermia (chapter 13)—Below-normal body temperature.

H zone (chapter 3)—The mid-area of the sarcomere containing only myosin.

I band (chapter 3)—An area of the sarcomere that is bisected by the Z line and is composed of actin; the I band decreases during muscle shortening as the actin slides over the myosin.

IBM (chapter 18)—International Business Machines of Endicott, NY.

Iliac crest (chapter 7)—The large bony prominence at the top of each side of the hips.

Incision (chapter 16)—A cut into body tissue using a sharp instrument.

Increment (chapter 9)—A degree of increase. In a graded exercise test, a work increment exists between stages.

Inderal, propranolol (chapter 15)—A drug-blocking beta-receptor activation in the heart, aimed at reducing cardiac arrhythmias and dysrhythmias.

Indirect calorimetry (chapter 8)—The estimation of energy production on the basis of oxygen consumption.

Infarction (chapter 15)—Death of a section of tissue due to lack of blood flow, as in myocardial infarction.

Inferior vena cava (chapter 15)—The large vein that discharges blood from the lower half of the body into the right atrium of the heart.

Inflammation (chapter 16)—A reaction to injury; signs include heat, redness, pain, and swelling.

Informed consent (chapters 9, 17)—A procedure used to obtain a person's voluntary permission to participate in a program. Informed consent requires a description of the procedures to be used, the potential benefits and risks, and written consent.

Injury (chapter 17)—Damage to a bodily part.

Inotropic (chapter 4)—Affecting the force or energy of muscular contraction.

Input (chapter 18)—To enter data into a computer; or, the data entered.

Inspiration (chapter 3)—The drawing of air into the lungs.

Insulin (chapter 3)—A pancreatic hormone, secreted into the blood, that influences carbohydrate metabolism by stimulating the transport of glucose into cells.

Insulin shock (chapter 16)—A shock-like state resulting from an overdose of insulin.

Intensity (chapter 13)—The magnitude of energy required for a particular activity, often referred to in terms of percentage of maximum ($\dot{V}O_2$ or HR) or METs.

Intermittent work (chapter 14)—Exercises performed with alternate periods of harder and lighter physical work, or work and rest, rather than continuous work.

Interval training (chapter 14)—A fitness workout that alternates harder and lighter work.

Intrinsic (chapter 11)—Belonging to a thing by its very nature (e.g., people continue to be active based on intrinsic motivation).

Introvert (chapter 11)—A person concerned primarily with his or her own thoughts and feelings.

Ion (chapter 15)—An electrified or charged (positive or negative) particle.

Iron-deficiency anemia (chapter 6)—Anemia brought on by a chronic deficiency in iron intake; the most common mineral deficiency in women.

Ischemia (chapter 15)—Inadequate blood supply to the heart.

Isocaloric balance (chapter 6)—The state achieved when the calories consumed equal the energy expended.

Isoelectric (chapter 15)—Baseline, as in an ECG.

Isokinetic contraction (chapter 4)—A muscle contraction with controlled speed, allowing maximal force to be applied throughout the range of motion.

Isometric contraction (chapter 4)—A muscle contraction in which the muscle length is unchanged.

Isotonic contraction (chapter 4)—A muscle contraction in which the force of the muscle is greater than the resistance, resulting in joint movement with shortening of the muscle.

Jogging (chapter 14)—Slow running.

Joint (chapter 4)—The articulation of two or more bones.

Joint cavity (chapter 4)—The space between bones enclosed by the synovial membrane and articular cartilage.

J point (chapter 15)—On an ECG, the point at which the S wave ends and the S–T segment begins.

Ketosis (chapter 6)—A condition brought about by restricted carbohydrate intake, resulting in excessive acetones or other ketones being secreted by the liver; stored fat becomes more available for energy.

Kidneys (chapter 2)—Two glands situated in the upper, posterior abdominal cavity, one on either side of the vertebral column. Their function is to maintain water and electrolyte balance and to secrete urine.

Kilocalorie (kcal) or Calorie (Cal) (chapter 8)—The amount of heat required to raise the temperature of 1 kg of water 1°C. This is the ordinary calorie discussed in food or exercise energy-expenditure tables.

Kilogram (kg) (chapter 9)—A metric unit of mass; 1 kg = 1,000 g.

Kilopond meters per minute (kpm·min^{-1}), kilogram meters per minute (kgm·min^{-1}) (chapter 9)—In a normal gravitational field, these are identical. This is a measure of power used to describe the external work rate, often on a cycle ergometer.

Krebs cycle (chapter 3)—A series of chemical reactions occurring in mitochondria in which carbon dioxide is produced and hydrogen ions and electrons are removed from carbon atoms (oxidation). The Krebs cycle is also referred to as the tricarboxyclic acid cycle, or citric acid cycle.

Kyphosis (chapter 10)—An excessive posterior curvature of the upper (thoracic) spine.

Laceration (chapter 16)—A wound with rough edges.

Lactate (chapter 3)—An end product of the anaerobic metabolism of glucose; the dissociated form of lactic acid.

Lactate threshold (chapter 3)—The point during a graded exercise test at which the blood lactate concentration suddenly increases; a good indicator of the highest sustainable work rate.

Leadership (chapter 14)—The ability to influence and motivate people in a group to make decisions and to act on the basis of those decisions.

Lean body weight (chapter 7)—The portion of the body that is not fat tissue. Lean body weight is often used to refer to all nonfat weight.

Leukocytes (chapter 3)—White blood cells.

Liability (chapter 17)—Legal responsibility.

Life events (chapter 11)—Situations that cause stress reactions; they may be enjoyable (e.g., a vacation) or sad (e.g., the death of a loved one).

Lifestyle (chapters 2, 11, 12)—A person's general pattern of living, including healthy and unhealthy behaviors.

Ligament (chapter 4)—The connective tissue that attaches bone to bone.

Limiting factor (chapter 3)—A physiological characteristic that establishes the upper limit of performance (e.g., muscle fiber type, maximal cardiac output, maximal oxygen uptake).

Lipid (chapter 6)—A fatty substance.

Lipoprotein (chapter 6)—A complex consisting of lipid and protein molecules bound together. Cholesterol and triglycerides are transported in the bloodstream in the form of lipoproteins.

Liter—A unit of volume in the metric system.

Longitudinal arch (chapter 16)—The long arch along the medial aspect of the foot.

Lordosis (chapter 10)—An excessive forward curvature of the lumbar spine.

Low-back function (chapter 10)—The ability to carry on normal activities without back pain.

Low-back pain (chapter 10)—Strong discomfort in the low-back area, often caused by lack of muscular endurance and flexibility in the midtrunk region, or improper posture or lifting.

Low blood sugar—See *hypoglycemia*.

Low-calorie diet (chapter 6)—Food intake of which the caloric value is below the total energy requirement, resulting in a loss of weight.

Low-density lipoprotein cholesterol (LDL-C) (chapters 2, 6)—A plasma protein containing relatively more cholesterol and triglycerides and less protein. High levels are associated with an increased risk of CHD.

Low-intensity exercise (chapter 2)—Exercise of less than 50% of functional capacity, with little increase in respiration and no discomfort. This exercise can be universally recommended, except for individuals with extreme disease or physical impairment, to expend calories and lower the risk of health problems.

Low-organized games (chapter 14)—Games with simple rules not requiring high levels of skill.

Lumbar (chapter 4)—Pertaining to the low back; five lumbar vertebrae are located just below the thoracic vertebrae and just above the sacrum.

Macintosh (Mac) (chapter 18)—A microcomputer manufactured by Apple Computer, Inc., of Cupertino, CA. A number of computers are included (e.g., Mac Plus; Mac SE; Mac II series).

Macrominerals (chapter 6)—The major dietary minerals, including calcium, phosphorus, potassium, sulfur, sodium, chloride, and magnesium.

Maintenance load (chapter 13)—The amount of exercise that enables an individual to maintain her or his present level of fitness.

Malnutrition (chapter 6)—Poor or improper nutrition, usually associated with undernutrition.

Mast cell (chapter 13)—A cell in the bronchial tube that releases histimine and other chemicals in response to certain stimuli; involved in an asthmatic attack.

Maximal (chapter 9)—The highest level possible, such as maximal heart rate or oxygen uptake.

Maximal aerobic power (chapter 3)—The maximal rate at which oxygen can be used by the body during maximal work; related directly to the maximal capacity of the heart to deliver blood to the muscles.

Maximal heart rate (HRmax) (chapter 13)—The highest heart rate attainable. A person's maximal heart rate can be estimated by subtracting his or her age from 220. The normal variation in this estimate (S.D.)=± 11 beats$\cdot$min^{-1}.

Maximal oxygen uptake ($\dot{V}O_2$max) (chapter 3)—The greatest rate of oxygen utilization attainable during heavy work, expressed in L$\cdot$min^{-1}, or ml$\cdot$kg$^{-1}\cdot$min^{-1}.

Maximal tests (chapter 9)—Tests that continue until a person has reached a maximal level (e.g., $\dot{V}O_2$max) or voluntary exhaustion.

Max $\dot{V}O_2$—See *maximal oxygen uptake*.

Medical clearance (chapter 2)—An indication by medical personnel that an individual can safely engage in specified activities.

Medical history (chapter 2)—A person's previous health problems, signs, and characteristics.

Medical physical exam (chapter 2)—The systematic examination of the different parts of the body, used to determine a person's health status.

Medical referral (chapter 2)—A recommendation that a person get medical attention, tests, or an opinion about a characteristic, symptom, or test result to determine if medical treatment is needed, and/or to determine whether it is safe to participate in specified activities.

Medical supervision (chapter 2)—The presence of qualified medical personnel during a fitness test or workout.

Medication, medicine (chapter 15)—A therapeutic substance.

Menisci (chapter 4)—Partial discs between the femur and tibia and the knee.

Metabolic load (chapter 8)—The energy required to complete a task.

Metabolism (chapter 3)—The process of chemical changes by which energy is provided for the maintenance of life.

Metatarsal arch (chapter 16)—The arch of the foot located between the "balls" of the foot.

METs (chapter 8)—Multiples of resting metabolism [1 MET is about 3.5 ml(kg$\cdot$min)$^{-1}$].

Microcomputer (chapter 18)—A relatively small, but powerful, computer that typically can reside on a desk. The typical microcomputer (and necessary peripherals) can cost between \$500 and \$10,000.

Micromineral (chapter 6)—Trace dietary minerals, including iron, zinc, copper, iodine, manganese, selenium, chromium, molybdenum, cobalt, arsenic, nickle fluoride, and vanadium.

Millisecond—One one-thousandth (.001) of a second.

Mineral (chapter 6)—An inorganic, metallic substance necessary for proper cell functioning (e.g., iron, calcium).

Mitochondria (chapter 3)—Subcellular structures responsible for the production of most of the ATP in the cell with the consumption of oxygen (aerobic metabolism).

Mobitz Type I AV block (chapter 15)—On an ECG, P–R interval progressively increasing until the P wave is not followed by a QRS complex. The site of the block is the AV node.

Mobitz Type II block (chapter 15)—On an ECG, a constant P–R interval, with some but not all P waves followed by QRS. The site of the block is the bundle of His.

Modem (chapter 18)—An acronym for MOdulator/DEModulator, which is a peripheral device that permits a computer to send and receive messages (data) over telephone lines.

Moderate-intensity exercise (chapter 1)—Exercise at 60% to 85% of functional capacity that causes mild breathlessness and some perspiration. If unaccustomed to it, there may be some discomfort and later soreness. This activity is recommended for optimal cardiorespiratory benefits after health-status evaluation.

Moment arm (force, resistance arm) (chapter 4)—The shortest or perpendicular distance from the point of force application to the axis or joint.

Monosaccharide (chapter 6)—A simple sugar, such as glucose.

Motivation (chapter 11)—An incentive that prompts a person to act with a sense of purpose.

Motor unit (chapter 4)—The functional unit of muscular contraction that includes a motor nerve and the muscle fibers that its branches innervate.

Movement forms (chapter 14)—Types of physical activity, such as aquatics, dance, exercise, games, gymnastics, and sports.

MS-DOS (chapter 18)—Microsoft Disk Operating System is the operating system that controls the IBM-PC and compatibles. See *DOS*.

Muscle fiber (chapter 4)—Muscle cell; contains myofibrils that are composed of sarcomeres; uses chemical energy of ATP to generate tension, which, when greater than the resistance, results in movement.

Muscle group (chapter 4)—A group of specific muscles that are responsible for the same action at the same joint.

Myocardial infarction (MI) (chapter 15)—Death to a section of heart tissue in which the blood supply has been cut off.

Myocardial ischemia (chapter 15)—A lack of oxygen for heart function.

Myocardium (chapter 15)—The middle layer of the heart wall; involuntary, striated muscle innervated by autonomic nerves.

Myofibril (chapter 3)—Found inside muscle fibers; composed of a long string of sarcomeres, the basic unit of muscle contraction.

Myosin (chapter 3)—A contractile protein in sarcomere that can bind actin and split ATP to generate cross-bridge movement and the development of tension.

Myositis (chapter 16)—Inflammation of a muscle.

Negative energy balance (chapter 6)—A condition in which less energy is consumed than is expended, resulting in a decrease in body weight.

Negative health (chapter 11)—The presence of characteristics and behaviors that prevent optimal functional capacity and increase risks of serious health problems.

Negligence (chapter 17)—The failure to provide reasonable care, or the care required by the circumstances. The person and/or program is legally liable for injury that results from this.

Neoplasm (chapter 16)—New or abnormal growth.

Neutralizer (chapter 4)—A muscle that counteracts an undesirable action of another muscle.

Newton (N)—A unit of measure of force.

Nitrates (chapter 15)—A class of drugs used to prevent and stop angina pectoris; side effects include headaches, dizziness, and hypotension.

Nitroglycerin (chapter 15)—A vasodilator drug used to treat angina pectoris.

Nonfunctional stressor (chapter 11)—A stimulus or situation that causes an arousal (stress) that exceeds the physiological response needed for the task.

Noradrenalin—See *Norepinephrine*.

Norepinephrine (chapter 3)—One of the adrenal medullary hormones similar in action to epinephrine. Norepinephrine is also secreted by sympathetic nervous system nerve endings.

Nutrient density (chapter 6)—A measure of the amounts of proteins, carbohydrates, fats, vitamins, and minerals per 100 kcal of food.

Nutrients (chapter 6)—Compounds and elements contained in foods and needed by the body.

Nutrition (chapter 6)—The study of foods and their use in the body.

Obesity (chapter 7)—The accumulation and storage of excess body fat. Obese people have an increased risk of CHD, diabetes, and hypertension.

Objectivity (chapter 5)—The degree to which different scorers obtain the same result.

Obsession (chapter 11)—An idea or emotion that persists in an individual in spite of any conscious attempts to remove it.

One-repetition maximum (1 RM) (chapter 10)—The maximal force that can be exerted in a single contraction by a muscle group.

Open-circuit spirometry (chapter 3)—The method of measuring oxygen consumption by breathing in room air, while collecting and analyzing the expired air.

Operating system (chapter 18)—The system that controls the operation of the microcomputer. See *DOS, MS-DOS, DOS 3.3,* and *ProDos.*

Orthopedic (chapter 13)—Skeletal problem, disease, or deformity.

Orthopedically disabled (chapter 13)—A disorder of some aspect of the locomotor system.

Ossification (chapter 4)—The replacement of cartilage by bone.

Osteoporosis (chapter 6)—The thinning and weakening of the bones; found mainly in postmenopausal women.

Output (chapter 18)—What is received when a computer program is run. Output may be received on a number of different devices (e.g., screen, printer, plotter, disk, tape).

Overfat (chapter 7)—An accumulation of more than the desirable amount of fat.

Overload (chapter 13)—To place greater than usual demands upon some part of the body, (e.g., picking up more weight than normal overloads the muscles involved). Chronic overloading leads to increased strength and function.

Overweight (chapter 7)—Weight that is greater than expected for the person's height.

Oxygen (chapter 3)—A colorless, odorless, gaseous element; necessary for life and combustion.

Oxygen consumption—See *oxygen uptake.*

Oxygen cost (chapter 8)—The amount of oxygen used by body tissues during an activity.

Oxygen debt (chapter 3)—The amount of oxygen used during recovery from work that exceeds the amount needed for rest.

Oxygen deficit (chapter 3)—The difference between the theoretical oxygen requirement of a physical activity and the measured oxygen uptake.

Oxygen requirement (chapter 8)—The rate of oxygen utilization needed for an activity.

Oxygen uptake (chapter 3)—The rate at which oxygen is utilized during a specific level of an activity.

Ozone (chapter 13)—An active form of oxygen formed in reaction to UV light and as an emission from internal combustion engines; exposure can decrease lung function.

Pallor (chapter 9)—Unnatural paleness. Exercise should be stopped.

Palpation (chapter 9)—Examination by touch, as in determining HR by feeling the pulse at the wrist or neck.

Palpitation (chapter 2)—A rapid, forceful beating of the heart of which the person is aware.

Papillary muscles (chapter 15)—Cardiac muscles that originate at the walls of the heart ventricles and attach to AV valves.

Parasympathetic nervous system (chapter 3)—A portion of the autonomic nervous system, derived from some of the cranial and sacral nerves belonging to the central nervous system; the system produces such involuntary responses as blood vessel dilation, increased digestive organ, reproductive organ, and gland activity, eye pupil contraction, decreased heart rate, and others; effects are opposite those of the sympathetic nervous system.

Partial pressure of gas (chapter 3)—Pressure exerted by oxygen, carbon dioxide, nitrogen, or water. The sum of these partial pressures equals the barometric pressure.

Peak heart rate (chapter 13)—The highest heart rate occurring during a specific activity.

Perceived exertion (chapter 9)—A subjective rating of intensity of a particular task, normally rated on one of the Borg scales for rating perceived exertion.

Percent fat (chapter 7)—The percentage of total body weight that is fat.

Percent maximal heart rate (%HRmax) (chapter 9)—Submaximal heart rate divided by maximal heart rate [e.g., 70% maximal heart rate in a person with a maximal heart rate of 200 beats$\cdot$min^{-1} = 140 beats/minute (200$\cdot$0.7)].

Percent $\dot{V}O_2$max (%$\dot{V}O_2$max) (chapter 9)—Submaximal oxygen uptake divided by maximal oxygen uptake; e.g., 60% maximal oxygen uptake in a person with a maximal oxygen uptake of 3 L$\cdot$min^{-1} = 1.8 L$\cdot$min^{-1} (3$\cdot$0.6).

Perception (chapter 11)—A conscious impression of objects or situations. The stressfulness of a situation depends largely on the way it is perceived by the individual.

Percussion test (chapter 16)—A tapping test used in the evaluation of a broken bone.

Percutaneous transluminal coronary angioplasty (chapter 13)—A procedure in which a catheter is inserted in a blocked artery and a balloon is inflated to push the plaque back toward the wall to open the artery.

Performance (chapter 1)—The ability to perform a task or sport at a desired level. Also called motor fitness, or physical fitness.

Perimyseum (chapter 4)—The connective tissue surrounding fasciculi within a muscle.

Periosteum (chapter 4)—The connective tissue surrounding all bone surfaces except the articulating surfaces.

Peripheral (chapter 18)—A device associated with (and sometimes required for) particular hardware or software. For example, some programs require you to have a printer, and others may permit (or require) a plotter.

Peripheral resistance (chapter 3)—The resistance offered by the arterioles and capillaries to the flow of blood from the arteries to the veins. An increase in peripheral resistance causes a rise in blood pressure.

pH (chapter 3)—The symbol for hydrogen ion concentration, or degree of acidity; 7.0 is neutral, below 7.0 is acid, and above 7.0 is alkaline.

Phases of activities (chapter 13)—The sequence of exercise recommended to progress from a sedentary to an active lifestyle, including a gradual progression to walking 4 mi, jogging 3 mi, and including a variety of sports and games.

Phlebitis (chapter 2)—The inflammation of a vein.

Physical activity (chapter 1)—Any movement of the body (or substantial parts of the body) produced by skeletal muscles, resulting in energy expenditure.

Physical conditioning (chapter 13)—Chronic regular exercise aimed at obtaining or maintaining high levels of components of fitness.

Physical fitness (chapter 1)—Optimal physical quality of life, including obtaining criterion levels of physical fitness test scores, and low risk of developing health problems. Also called health-related physical fitness, or physiological fitness.

Physical fitness tests (chapters 2, 7, 9, 10)—Ways to measure and evaluate the components of physical fitness.

Physical inactivity (chapter 1)—A sedentary lifestyle.

Physical stimulus (chapter 11)—A situation or task, such as exercise, heat, or high altitude, that requires a physiological response greater than rest.

Physical work capacity (chapter 9)—The capacity to perform physical work, usually measured in oxygen uptake or kilopond meters per minute, while at a set heart rate (e.g., PWC−150).

Physiological response (chapter 11)—The reaction of the physiological systems to a task, condition, or stressor.

Plantar fasciitis (chapter 16)—The inflammation of connective tissue that spans the bottom of the foot.

Plaque (chapter 6)—Strands of fibrous tissue that attach to the inside of arteries to form soft and mushy (if fat) or hard (if scar tissue) atheromatous buildup. Also, bacteria that form on the teeth.

Plasma (chapter 3)—The solvent or liquid portion of the blood.

Play (chapter 14)—Physical activity for amusement or recreation.

Playfulness (chapter 14)—An attitude of fun.

Plyometric (chapter 10)—The eccentric or lengthening contraction of a muscle; usually referring to the lengthening of a muscle before its concentric contraction.

Polarization (chapter 15)—A changing of electrical state. An ECG reflects depolarization and repolarization of atria and ventricles.

Pollution (chapter 13)—Potentially toxic waste products found in water and air.

Polysaccharide (chapter 6)—A complex sugar that yields three or more monosaccharides when hydrolyzed.

Polyunsaturated fats (chapter 6)—Fats derived from vegetables, lean poultry, fish, and cereal.

Positive energy balance (chapter 6)—A condition in which more energy is consumed than is expended, resulting in an increase in body weight.

Positive health (chapter 1)—A move toward optimal functional capacity; more than a mere absence of disease.

Postabsorptive (chapter 6)—A condition in which all food in the gastrointestinal tract has been absorbed into the blood.

Postexercise energy expenditure (chapter 3)—The amount of energy expended, above resting levels, following exercise.

Postprandial (chapter 6)—Occurring after a meal.

Posture (chapter 10)—The position or carriage of the body as a whole. Improper posture is related to low-back pain.

Potential benefits and risks (chapter 17)—A description of the relative gains and dangers of a procedure or program; one aspect of informed consent for fitness participants.

Predicted maximum heart rate (chapter 9)—An estimate of HRmax; 220 minus a person's age.

Premature atrial contraction (PAC) (chapter 15)—On an ECG, the rhythm is irregular, and the R–R interval is short; the origin of the beat is somewhere other than the SA node.

Premature junctional contraction (chapter 15)—On an ECG, the ectopic pacemaker in the AV junctional area that causes a QRS complex, frequently seen with inverted P waves.

Premature ventricular contraction (PVC) (chapter 15)—On an ECG, the QRS interval is longer than 0.12 s, and the T wave is usually in the opposite direction; the origin is in the His-Purkinje system.

Preparticipation physical (chapter 16)—A medical physical examination prior to an increase in physical activity.

Prescribed exercise (chapter 13)—A recommendation of type, intensity, frequency, duration, and total work needed to accomplish fitness objectives.

Pressure points (chapter 16)—The point of application of pressure over major arteries to control bleeding.

PRICE (chapter 17)—The suggested treatment for minor sprains and strains: *p*rotection, *r*est, *i*ce, *c*ompression, and *e*levation.

Primary risk factor (chapter 1)—A characteristic or behavior that is associated with a major health problem regardless of other factors. For example, smoking is a primary risk factor of CHD.

Prime mover (chapter 4)—A muscle that is effective in causing a joint movement.

P–R interval (chapter 15)—The time interval between the beginning of the P wave and the QRS complex. The upper limit is 0.2 s. This segment is normally used as the isoelectric baseline.

Private speech (chapter 12)—Talking to oneself in order to prepare for or cope with a stressor.

ProDos (chapter 18)—Professional Disk Operating System is the operating system used by newer members of the Apple II family of computers (e.g., Apple IIe and Apple IIgs).

Program Director (Introduction)—The administrator of a program. Program Directors are certified by the American College of Sports Medicine in postcardiac rehabilitation and health fitness programs.

Progression (chapter 13)—A gradual increase from a current level to a desired level. For example, a sedentary person may gradually increase walking and jogging until she or he is able to jog 3 mi continuously without discomfort over an 8-month period of time.

Progressive resistance exercise (chapter 10)—A descriptive term for strength-training programs in which a muscle adapts to a resistance, and a greater resistance is chosen to overload the muscle, and continue to increase strength.

Proprioceptive neuromuscular facilitation (chapter 10)—A stretching procedure in which a muscle-tendon unit is put on stretch; the subject does an isometric contraction with that muscle against a resistance applied by a helper; the subject relaxes, and the stretch is moved farther into the range of motion by the helper.

Protein (chapter 6)—A compound composed of amino acids that provides the basic structural properties of cells.

Psychological stressor (chapter 11)—A mental condition that causes physiological arousal beyond what is needed to accomplish a task.

Pulmonary artery (chapter 15)—The artery that carries venous blood directly from the right ventricle of the heart to the lungs.

Pulmonary function (chapter 3)—The capacity of the respiratory system to move air.

Pulmonary valve (chapter 15)—A set of three crescent-shaped flaps at the opening of the pulmonary artery; the semilunar valves.

Pulmonary veins (chapter 15)—Four veins that carry oxygenated blood directly from the lungs to the left atrium of the heart.

Purkinje fibers (chapter 15)—The muscle-cell fibers found beneath the endocardium of the heart; the impulse-conducting network of the heart.

P wave (chapter 15)—On an ECG, a small positive deflection preceding a QRS complex, indicating atrial depolarization, normally less than 0.12 s with an amplitude of 0.25 mV or less.

QRS complex (chapter 15)—The largest complex on an ECG, indicating a depolarization of the left ventricle, normally less than 0.1 s.

QRS interval (chapter 15)—The time interval from the beginning to the end of the QRS complex.

Q–T interval (chapter 15)—The time interval from the beginning of the QRS complex to the end of the T wave. The Q–T interval reflects the electrical systole of the cardiac cycle.

Quadriceps (chapter 4)—The large muscle group at the front of the thigh, responsible for extending the knee joint.

Quality of life (chapter 1)—Those aspects of living that are important to meaning and enjoyment.

Q wave (chapter 15)—The initial negative deflection of the QRS complex on an ECG.

Radial pulse (chapter 9)—A pulse taken at the wrist.

Radiation (chapter 3)—The process of losing heat from surface of one object to the surface of another object; the heat loss is dependent on a temperature gradient between the surfaces of the objects.

Random access memory (RAM) (chapter 18)—That portion of the computer's memory where the computer program is retained while the program is running. The program no longer exists in RAM once the machine is turned off.

Rate-pressure product (chapter 3)—The product of heart rate and systolic blood pressure; indicative of the oxygen requirement of the heart during exercise; also called the double product.

Rating of perceived exertion (RPE) (chapter 9)—A scale, by Borg, used to quantify the subjective feeling of physical effort. The original scale was 6—20; the revised scale is 0—10.

Rationalization (chapter 11)—The process of inventing plausible explanations for acts or opinions that actually have other causes.

Read-only memory (ROM) (chapter 18)—That portion of the computer that retains instructional code even when the machine is turned off. Built in when the computer was manufactured, ROM permits the computer to perform computing functions.

Recommended dietary allowance (RDA) (chapter 6)—The quantities of daily specified vitamins, minerals, and proteins needed for good nutrition.

Recruitment (chapter 4)—Stimulation of additional motor units to increase the strength of a muscle contraction.

Referral (chapter 2)—A recommendation that a person consult with a professional about a particular characteristic, sign, symptom, or test result.

Regional fat distribution (chapter 7)—Evaluation of the tendency of an individual to deposit fat above or below the waist; the waist-to-hip ratio is used to measure this, with a high ratio being associated with greater risk of coronary heart disease and diabetes.

Rehabilitation (chapter 13)—A planned program in which disabled people progress toward, or maintain, the maximum degree of physical and psychological independence they are capable of.

Relative humidity (chapter 3)—A measure of the dryness of the air; the ratio of the amount of water vapor in the air to the maximum the air can hold at that temperature times 100%.

Relative weight (RW) (chapter 7)—An estimate of body fatness; the ratio of a person's weight to the midpoint of the weights for a medium-framed individual of the same height; a value of 1.10 indicates overweight, 1.20 indicates obesity.

Relax (chapter 11)—To loosen or make less stiff or gain relief from work or tension.

Reliability (chapter 5)—The degree to which the same test score will be achieved on separate administrations of a test.

Repetitions (chapter 10)—The number of consecutive contractions performed.

Repetitions maximum (chapter 10)—The number of repetitions that can be done without stopping.

Repolarization (chapter 15)—In the heart, the change from a working to a resting state. The T wave on an ECG reflects the repolarization of the ventricle at the end of the systole and the beginning of the diastole.

Reproducibility (chapter 5)—The degree to which a person is able to replicate performance exactly. For example, a reproducible work task is important in order to determine the progress a person makes as a result of a fitness program.

Residual volume (chapter 7)—The volume of air remaining in the lungs at the end of maximal expiration.

Resistance (chapter 10)—The amount of force applied opposite a movement.

Respiration (chapter 3)—The act of breathing.

Respiratory exchange ratio; respiratory quotient (RQ) (chapter 3)—The ratio of the volume of carbon dioxide produced to the volume of oxygen utilized during a given period of time (VCO_2/VO_2).

Resting metabolic rate (RMR) (chapter 7)—The measure of the amount of energy expended at rest; represents about 70% of an individual's total daily energy expenditure.

Reversibility (chapter 13)—A corollary to the principle of overload; loss of a training effect with disuse.

Rhythm (chapter 15)—In terms of the cardiac cycle, the sequence and regularity of an occurrence of events.

Risk factor (chapter 2)—A characteristic, sign, symptom, or test score that is associated with increased probability of developing a health problem. For example, people with hypertension have increased risks of developing CHD.

Role model (chapter 14)—Someone who sets an example for similar people by behaving in accordance with the highest standards for a particular position.

Rotation (chapter 4)—The movement of a bone around its longitudinal axis.

Rotational inertia (chapter 4)—Reluctance to rotate; proportional to the mass and distribution of the mass around the axis.

R-R interval (chapter 15)—The time interval from the peak of the QRS of one cardiac cycle to the peak of the QRS of the next cycle; 60/R-R interval = HR, $b \cdot min^{-1}$.

Runner's high (chapter 11)—A special emotional experience that transcends normal sensations; reported by some runners.

Running (chapter 14)—Moving the whole body quickly by propelling the body off the ground during part of the movement.

Running shoes (chapter 14)—Special athletic shoes offering good support and cushioning in the heel area to minimize trauma at impact.

R wave (chapter 15)—The positive deflection of the QRS complex in the ECG.

Salt (chapter 6)—A crystalline compound of sodium and chlorine, occurring as a mineral. High levels of salt intake have been associated with hypertension.

Salt tablets (chapter 13)—Generally not recommended as means to increase salt in the diet; if used, they must be taken with large amounts of water.

Sarcomeres (chapter 3)—The basic units of muscle contraction; contain actin and myosin; tension is developed as the myosin cross-bridges pull the actin toward the center of the sarcomere.

Sarcoplasmic reticulum (chapter 3)—The network of membranes that surround the myofibril; stores calcium needed for muscle contraction.

Saturated fat (chapter 6)—A fat that is not capable of absorbing any more hydrogen. These fats are solid at room temperature and are usually of animal origin, such as the fats in milk, butter, and meat.

Saturation pressure (chapter 3)—Water vapor pressure that exists at a particular temperature when the air is saturated with water.

Scoliosis (chapter 10)—An abnormal lateral curvature of the spine.

Screening (chapter 2)—An examination used to select or reject. In fitness programs, potential participants are screened to determine whether they should be referred for medical attention prior to engaging in exercise.

Secondary risk factor (chapter 1)—A characteristic, sign, symptom, or test score that has a weak independent association with a health problem but increases the risk when other risk factors are present.

Second-degree AV block (chapter 15)—On an ECG, some but not all P waves precede the QRS complex.

Second wind (chapter 3)—A phenomenon characterized by a sudden transition from a feeling of distress or fatigue during the early portion of a workout to a more comfortable, less stressful feeling later in the exercise.

Sedentary (chapter 2)—An inactive lifestyle, characterized by a lot of sitting.

Sequence of testing (chapter 9)—The logical order in which tests are conducted.

Set (chapter 10)—A designated number of repetitions.

Shin splints (chapter 16)—An inflammatory reaction of the musculotendinous unit of the anterior aspect of the lower leg caused by overexertion of muscles during weight-bearing activities.

Shock (chapter 16)—A circulatory disturbance produced by severe injury or illness and largely caused by a reduction in blood volume, characterized by a fall in blood pressure, a rapid pulse, pallor, restlessness, thirst, and cold clammy skin. A discrepancy exists between the circulating blood volume and the capacity of the vascular bed. The initial cause of shock is a reduction in the circulating blood volume; continuation is caused by vasoconstriction.

Sinus (chapter 15)—On an ECG, refers to a regular sequence of electrical activity (i.e., SA node, atrium, AV node, ventricle).

Sinus arrhythmia (chapter 15)—A normal variant with sinus rhythm in which the R–R interval varies by more than 10% per beat.

Sinus bradycardia (chapter 15)—The normal rhythm (i.e., the sinus node is the pacemaker) and sequence, with slow heart rate (below 60 beats$\cdot$min^{-1} at rest). The occurrence of sinus bradycardia may be indicative of a high level of fitness, or of a mental problem such as depression.

Sinus node (chapter 15)—A mass of tissue in the right atrium of the heart, near the vena cava, that initiates the heartbeat.

Sinus rhythm (chapter 15)—The normal timing and sequence of the cardiac events, with the sinus node as a pacemaker; resting rate is between 60 beats$\cdot$min^{-1} and 100 beats$\cdot$min^{-1}.

Sinus tachycardia (chapter 15)—The normal rhythm and sequence, with a fast heart rate (above 100 beats$\cdot$min^{-1} at rest). The occurrence of sinus tachycardia may be indicative of illness or stress.

Skinfold caliper (chapter 7)—An instrument used to measure the thickness of folds of fat that have been pinched away from the body.

Sliding filament theory (chapter 3)—The theory that muscular tension is generated when the actin in the sarcomere slides over the myosin due to the action of the myosin cross-bridges.

Slow-twitch fiber (chapter 4)—A muscle fiber characterized by its slow speed of contraction.

Software (computer program or application) (chapter 18)—The computer code generated to cause the program to perform various functions. For example, a computer software program can be written to estimate percent body fat from skinfold measurements. Word processing packages are also software. Differentiated from hardware.

Spasm (chapter 16)—A sudden involuntary muscular contraction.

Special populations (chapter 13)—People with physical or mental characteristics requiring special attention, often needing modified activities.

Specificity (chapter 13)—Belonging to and characteristic of a particular thing. For example, skill is specific to a certain aspect of a sport.

Spondylolisthesis (chapter 10)—The vertebral body and transverse processes slip anteriorly (forward) on the vertebral body below; common for L4 to slip over L5.

Spot reducing (chapter 7)—An effort to reduce fat at one site by doing calisthenics at that site. No research evidence supports this concept.

Sprain (chapter 16)—Stretching or tearing of ligamentous tissues surrounding a joint, resulting in discoloration, swelling, and pain.

Stability (chapter 4)—The ease with which balance is maintained.

Stage (chapter 9)—In exercise testing, a step in the levels of work going from light to hard.

Standard deviation (chapter 5)—An indication of the variability of test scores based on the difference of each score from the group average.

State (chapter 11)—A temporary condition. For example, a person's emotional state may change rapidly depending on the particular situation, as contrasted to a personality trait that is consistent and does not change quickly.

Static stretching (chapter 10)—Flexing or extending a body part to the limit of its range of motion and holding it in that position.

Steady state (chapters 3, 8)—Unchanging, or changing very little. For example, during submaximal exercise, a person reaches a steady state (a leveling-off of $\dot{V}O_2$, HR, etc.) after a few minutes.

Stethoscope (chapter 5)—An instrument with earpieces attached to a microphone used for listening to various body sounds, such as heart rate or the sound over the brachial artery while taking blood pressure.

Stimulus (chapter 11)—Something that causes a physiological or psychological response.

Stone bruise (chapter 16)—A discoloration of the skin caused by blood in the underlying tissues, without abrasion of the skin, often located on the heel of the foot and usually caused by stepping on a sharp object while walking or running.

Strain (chapter 16)—The overstretching or tearing of a muscle or tendon.

Strength (chapter 10)—The amount of force that can be exerted by a muscle group against a resistance.

Stress (chapter 11)—A physiological or psychological response to a stressor beyond what is needed to accomplish a task.

Stress continuum (chapter 11)—A characteristic extending along a continuous line from one extreme to another. Three continuums appear to help describe stress, namely, *functional response . . . severe stress; enjoyable . . . unpleasant*; and *results in development . . . deterioration*.

Stress fracture (chapter 16)—A defect in a bone that occurs because of an accelerated rate of remodeling to accommodate the stress of weight-bearing bones; results in a loss of continuity in the bone and periosteal irritation.

Stress management (chapter 11)—The ability to cope with potential stressors so that there is a minimum stress response.

Stressor (chapter 11)—A stimulus that causes a stress response.

Stretching (chapter 10)—Extending the limbs through a full range of motion.

Stroke, apoplexy (chapter 2)—A vascular accident (embolism, hemorrhage, or thrombosis) in the brain, often resulting in sudden loss of body function.

Stroke volume (chapter 3)—The amount of blood pumped from the left ventricle each time the heart contracts.

S–T segment (chapter 15)—The part of the ECG between the end of the QRS complex and beginning of the T wave. Depression below (or elevation above) the isoelectric line indicates ischemia.

S–T segment displacement (chapter 15)—On an ECG, the depression or elevation of the portion of the ECG between the end of the QRS complex and the beginning of the T wave; S–T segment displacement may indicate the development of myocardial ischemia.

Submaximal (chapter 9)—Less than maximal (e.g., an exercise that can be performed with less than maximal effort).

Substrate (chapter 8)—A foodstuff used for energy metabolism.

Sulfur dioxide (chapter 13)—A pollutant that can cause bronchoconstriction in asthmatics.

Summation (chapter 10)—An increased rate of stimulation to increase force of muscle contraction.

Superior vena cava (chapter 15)—The upper main vein that discharges blood from the upper half of the body into the right atrium of the heart.

Supervised fitness program (chapter 2)—A group of fitness activities conducted with instructor present.

Support (chapters 11, 17)—To uphold and aid. An important element in changing behavior or coping with stress is to have a group that provides encouragement. In an organization, the support-staff personnel provide needed technical and clerical assistance.

S wave (chapter 15)—On an ECG, the last negative portion of the QRS complex, representing the final portion of the depolarization of the left ventricle.

Sweat, perspiration (chapter 3)—Moisture coming through the pores of the skin from the sweat glands, usually as a result of heat, exertion, or emotion.

Sympathetic nervous system (chapter 3)—Part of the autonomic nervous system consisting of two groups of ganglia connected by nerve cords, one on either side of the spinal cord; it releases substances that cause a physiological arousal, such as increased heart rate and decreased activity of the digestive and reproductive organs—the opposite of the parasympathetic nervous system.

Symptom (chapter 2)—A noticeable change in the normal working of the body that indicates or accompanies disease or sickness.

Synovial membrane (chapter 4)—The inner lining of the joint capsule.

Synovitis (chapter 16)—Inflammation of the synovial membrane.

Systolic blood pressure (SBP) (chapter 2)—The pressure exerted on the vessel walls during ventricular contraction, measured in millimeters of mercury by the sphygmomanometer.

Tachycardia (chapter 15)—A heart rate greater than 100 beats$\cdot$min^{-1} at rest. Tachycardia may be seen in deconditioned people or people who are apprehensive about a situation (e.g., an exercise test).

Taper-down; cool-down (chapter 13)—Light activity after a workout, allowing a gradual return to normal, with leg muscles continuing to pump blood back to the heart, thus preventing pooling of blood in the lower extremities.

Target heart rate (THR) (chapter 13)—The heart rate recommended for fitness workouts.

Ta wave (chapter 15)—On an ECG, the result of atrial depolarization. The Ta wave is not normally seen, because it occurs during ventricular depolarization and is hidden by the larger electrical forces generated by the ventricles (QRS).

Tendinitis (chapter 16)—Inflammation of a tendon.

Tendon (chapter 4)—A band of tough, inelastic, fibrous connective tissue that attaches muscle to bone.

Tennis elbow (chapter 16)—Inflammation of the musculotendonous unit of the elbow extensors where they attach on the outer aspect of the elbow (lateral epicondylitis).

Tenosynovitis (chapter 16)—Inflammation of a tendon sheath.

Testing protocol (chapter 9)—A particular testing scheme, often the starting level, timing, and increments for each stage of an exercise tolerance test.

Thermogram (chapter 16)—Infrared measure of surface of body to locate "hot" spots associated with inflammation due to trauma.

Third-degree AV block (chapter 15)—On an ECG, the QRS appears independently, P–R varies with no regular pattern, rate less than 45 beats$\cdot$min^{-1}.

Third-party payments (chapter 17)—Reimbursement for services rendered by someone else. Third-party payments are usually some form of insurance payment.

Threshold (chapter 13)—The minimum level needed for a desired effect. Often used to refer to the minimum level of exercise intensity needed for improvement in cardiorespiratory function.

Thrombosis (chapter 2)—A blood clot in a blood vessel.

Tidal volume (TV) (chapter 3)—The volume of air inspired or expired per breath.

Timed vital capacity (chapter 2)—The amount of the vital capacity that can be expelled in a certain time, usually 1 s.

Time to exhaustion (chapter 9)—The time interval from the beginning of an exercise test until the participant is unable or unwilling to continue.

Torque (chapter 4)—The effect produced by a force causing rotation; the product of the force and length of force arm.

Total cholesterol (chapters 2, 6)—This is the sum of all forms of cholesterol. Because LDL-C is the primary factor in the total amount, a *high* level of total cholesterol is also a risk factor for CHD.

Total cholesterol/HDL-C ratio (chapter 2)—One of the best ways to determine risk of CHD in terms of cholesterol. *High* ratios of total cholesterol to HDL-C are indicative of high risk of CHD.

Total fitness (chapter 1)—Optimal quality of life, including social, mental, spiritual, and physical components. Also called wellness, or positive health.

Total lung capacity (TLC) (chapter 3)—The sum of the vital capacity and the residual volume.

Total work (chapter 13)—The amount of work accomplished during a workout.

Training (chapter 3)—Physical conditioning through repeated bouts of exercise.

Trait (chapter 11)—A semipermanent characteristic that generally is true about a person and is resistant to change.

Transfer of angular momentum (chapter 4)—Transfer of angular momentum from one body segment to another can be achieved by stabilizing the initial moving part at a joint.

Transverse tubule (chapter 3)—Connects the sarcolemma (muscle membrane) to the sarcoplasmic reticulum; action potentials move down the transverse tubule to cause the sacroplasmic reticulum to release calcium to initiate muscle contraction.

Treadmill (chapter 9)—A machine with a moving belt that can be adjusted for speed and grade, allowing a person to walk or run in place. Treadmills are widely used for exercise-tolerance testing.

Tricuspid valve (chapter 15)—A valve located between the right atrium and ventricle of the heart.

Trigeminy (chapter 15)—In an ECG, every third beat is a premature ventricular contraction.

Triglyceride (chapters 2, 6)—A compound consisting of three molecules of fatty acid and glycerol. A triglyceride is the main type of lipid found in adipose tissue and the main dietary lipid. When hydrolyzed, a triglyceride releases free fatty acids into the blood stream. A high level of triglycerides in serum is a secondary risk factor of CHD.

Tropomyosin (chapter 3)—A protein in muscle that regulates muscle contraction; works with troponin.

Troponin (chapter 3)—Binds calcium released from the sarcoplasmic reticulum and works with tropomyosin to allow the myosin cross-bridge to interact with actin and initiate cross-bridge movement.

T wave (chapter 15)—On an ECG, follows the QRS complex and represents ventricular repolarization.

Twelve-lead ECG (chapter 15)—A record of the electrical activity of the heart from different directions, with six limb leads and six chest leads.

Twelve-min run (chapter 9)—A field test for cardiorespiratory endurance, scored by the distance run in 12 min.

Two-mi run (chapter 9)—A field test for cardiorespiratory endurance, scored by the time it takes to complete 2 mi.

Type A behavior (chapter 11)—A label denoting a person who is hard-driving, time conscious, and impatient. Some evidence suggests that this type of behavior is a secondary risk factor of CHD. Type A is the opposite of Type B.

Type B behavior (chapter 11)—The opposite of Type A behavior.

Type I (slow oxidative) fiber (chapter 3)—A slow-contracting fiber generating small amount of tension with most of the energy coming from aerobic processes; active in light to moderate activities and possesses great endurance.

Type IIa (fast oxidative, glycolytic) fiber (chapter 3)—A fast-contracting muscle generating great tension that can produce energy aerobically as well as anaerobically; adds to Type I fiber's tension as exercise intensity increases.

Type IIb (fast glycolytic) fiber (chapter 3)—A fast-contracting muscle generating great tension; produces energy by anaerobic metabolism; fatigues quickly.

U.S. Recommended Dietary Allowances (U.S. RDAs) (chapter 6)—Standards used in labeling nutritional content of foods; the U.S. RDA values exceed the requirements of most people.

Unsaturated fatty acid (chapter 6)—The molecules of a fat that have one or more double bonds and are thus capable of absorbing more hydrogen. These fats are liquid at room temperature and usually are of vegetable origin.

Unsupervised program (chapter 13)—A group of fitness activities conducted without qualified fitness personnel, for people with a low risk of health problems.

U wave (chapter 15)—On an ECG, the wave occasionally seen after T wave. The origin of the U wave is unclear, and it is normally not a factor in interpreting the ECG for exercise prescription.

Validity (chapter 5)—Evaluation of a test to determine if it measures what it is supposed to measure. Validity includes test consistency (reliability) and tester consistency (objectivity). Validity is determined by logic (content), comparison with a valid test (criterion), ability to accurately predict (predictive), and theoretical means (construct).

Valsalva maneuver (chapter 3)—Increased pressure in the abdominal and thoracic cavities caused by breath holding and extreme effort.

Vasoconstriction (chapter 3)—The narrowing of a blood vessel.

Vasodilation (chapter 3)—The opening or widening of a blood vessel.

Vein (chapter 3)—A blood vessel that returns blood to the heart.

Velocity (chapter 4)—The rate of motion of a body in a certain direction.

Ventilation (chapter 3)—The process of oxygenating the blood through the lungs.

Ventilatory threshold (chapter 3)—The intensity of work at which the rate of ventilation sharply increases.

Ventricle (chapter 15)—The two (left and right) lower muscular chambers of the heart.

Ventricular arrhythmias (chapter 15)—Irregular waveforms on the ECG caused by contractions originating in the ventricle rather than from the SA node.

Ventricular fibrillation (chapter 15)—The heart contracts in an unorganized, quivering manner, with no discernible P or QRS complexes; requires immediate emergency attention.

Ventricular tachycardia (chapter 15)—An extremely dangerous condition in which three or more consecutive premature ventricular contractions occur. Ventricular tachycardia may degenerate into ventricular fibrillation.

Vertigo (chapter 2)—Dizziness.

Very low-density lipoproteins (VLDL) (chapters 2, 6)—Mainly triglycerides, a secondary risk factor for CHD.

Vigorous (chapter 13)—Of sufficient intensity to result in cardiorespiratory improvements if done on a regular basis.

Viscoelastic (chapter 10)—The characteristic that allows a tissue to return to its original length following a quick stretch but to adapt when placed under prolonged slow stretch.

Vital capacity (chapter 2)—The amount of air that can be expelled from the lungs after a maximal inspiration.

Vital signs (chapter 16)—The measurable essential bodily functions, such as pulse rate and temperature.

Vitamins (chapter 6)—Organic substances that are present in small amounts of food and that are necessary for the normal functioning of the cells. Vitamins are classified as water soluble and fat soluble.

$\dot{V}O_2max$ (chapter 3)—The highest amount of oxygen that can be utilized by the body during hard work.

Waist-to-hip ratio (chapter 7)—A measure of body-fat distribution; used as another indicator of health risk associated with coronary heart disease and diabetes.

Walking (chapter 14)—Moving the body in a set direction while maintaining contact with the ground or floor.

Warm-up (chapter 13)—Physical activity of light to moderate intensity prior to a workout.

Water-soluble vitamins (chapter 6)—Vitamins that are carried in water (B complex and C).

Water vapor pressure gradient (chapter 13)—The tendency for water to evaporate is dependent on the gradient between the water vapor pressure on the skin and the water vapor pressure in the air.

Weight (chapter 7)—Heaviness of the whole body.

Wenchebach AV block—See *Mobitz Type I AV Block*.

Wet-bulb temperature (chapter 13)—Air temperature measured with a thermometer whose bulb is surrounded by a wick wetted with water; an indication of the ability to evaporate moisture from the skin.

Windchill (chapter 13)—The coldness felt on exposed human flesh by a combination of temperature and wind velocity.

Work (chapter 9)—The movement of a force through a distance; measured as foot-pound or kilogram-meter, as in the cycle ergometer.

Workout (chapter 13)—An exercise bout aimed at improving fitness or performance.

Work rate (chapter 9)—Power, or work done per unit of time (e.g., kilogram-meters per minute; watts).

Work/relief (chapter 13)—The ratio of time spent in more- and less-intense exercise in an interval type of workout.

Z line (chapter 3)—The connective tissue of a sarcomere, the basic unit of muscle contraction.

Bibliography

Adrian, M.J., & Cooper, J.M. (1989). *Biomechanics of Human Movement*. Indianapolis: Benchmark Press.

Allen, D.L., & Iwata, B. (1980). Reinforcing exercise maintenance using existing high-rate activities. *Behavior Modification*, **4**(3), 337-354.

American Academy of Orthopaedic Surgeons. (1977). *Emergency care and transportation of the sick and injured* (2nd ed.). WI: George Banta.

American Alliance for Health, Physical Education, Recreation and Dance. (1984). *Technical manual: Health-related physical fitness*. Reston, VA: Author.

American Alliance for Health, Physical Education, Recreation and Dance. (1988). *Physical best*. Reston, VA: Author.

American College of Sports Medicine. (1975). Prevention of heat injuries during distance running. *Medicine and Science in Sports*, **7**, vii-viii.

American College of Sports Medicine. (1983). Proper and improper weight-loss programs. *Medicine and Science in Sports and Exercise*, **15**, ix-xiii.

American College of Sports Medicine. (1985). The prevention of thermal injuries during distance running. *Medicine and Science in Sports and Exercise*, **19**, 529-533.

American College of Sports Medicine. (1990). The recommended quantity and quality of exercise for developing and maintaining cardiorespiratory and muscular fitness in healthy adults. *Medicine and Science in Sports and Exercise*, **22**, 265-274.

American College of Sports Medicine. (1991). *Guidelines for exercise testing and prescription* (4th ed.). Philadelphia: Lea & Febiger.

American Diabetes Association. (1985). *Fact sheet on diabetes*. Alexandria, VA: Author.

American Diabetes Association. (1987). Position statement: Nutritional recommendations and principles for individuals with diabetes mellitus: 1986. *Diabetes Care*, **10**, 126-132.

American Dietetic Association. (1987). Nutrition for physical fitness and athletic performance for adults. *ADA Reports*, **87**, 933-939.

American Heart Association. (1987a). *Diet and coronary heart disease*. Dallas: Author.

American Heart Association. (1987b). *Heartsaver manual: A student handbook for cardiopulmonary resuscitation*. Dallas: Author.

American Heart Association. National Cholesterol Education Program. (1988). *Physician's cholesterol education handbook*. Dallas, TX: Author.

American Heart Association. (1989). *1989 heart facts*. Dallas: Author.

American Heart Association Committee on Stress, Strain, and Heart Disease. (1977). Report. *Circulation*, **55**, 1-11.

American Heart Association Committee Report. (1982). Rationale of the diet-heart statement of the American Heart Association. *Nutrition Today*, Sept./Oct.: 16-20; Nov./Dec.: 15-19.

American Heart Association. Joint National Committee on Detection, Evaluation, and Treatment of High Blood Pressure. (1987). *Recommendation for human blood-pressure determination by sphygmomanometers*. Dallas: Author.

American Medical Association. (1966). *Standard nomenclature of athletic injuries*. Chicago: Author.

American Red Cross. (1980). *Red cross CPR module: Respiratory and circulatory emergencies*. Washington, DC: Author.

American Red Cross. (1981a). *American Red Cross multimedia standard first-aid student workbook*. Washington, DC: Author.

American Red Cross. (1981b). *Standard first aid and personal safety* (2nd ed.). New York: Doubleday.

Anderson, B. (1980). *Stretching*. Bolinas, CA: Shelter.

Andrew, G.M., Oldridge, N.B., Parker, J.O., Cunningham, D.A., Rechnitzer, P.A., Jones, N.L., Buck, C., Kavanagh, T., Shephard, R.J., & Sutton, J.R. (1981). Reasons for dropout from exercise programs in post-coronary patients. *Medicine and Science in Sports and Exercise*, **13**, 164-168.

Arnheim, D. (1987). *Essentials of athletic training*. St. Louis: Times Morrow/Mosby College Publishing.

A Roundtable: Physiological adaptations to chronic endurance exercise training in patients with coronary artery disease. (1987). *The Physician and Sports-medicine*, **15**(9), 129-156.

Åstrand, I. (1960). Aerobic work capacity in men and women with special reference to age. *Acta Physiologica Scandinavica*, **49**, Suppl. 169.

Åstrand, P.O. (n.d.). *Work tests with the bicycle ergometer*. Verberg, Sweden: Monark-Crescent AB.

Åstrand, P.O. (1952). *Experimental studies of physical working capacity in relation to sex and age*. Copenhagen: Manksgaard.

Åstrand, P.O. (1984). Principles of ergometry and their implications in sport practice. *International Journal of Sports Medicine*, **5**, 102-105.

Åstrand, P.O., & Rodahl, K. (1970, 1977, 1986). *Textbook of work physiology* (1st, 2nd, and 3rd eds.). New York: McGraw-Hill.

Åstrand, P.O., & Rhyming, I. (1954). A nomogram for calculation of aerobic capacity (physical fitness) from pulse rate during submaximal work. *Journal of Applied Physiology*, **7**, 218-221.

Åstrand, P.O., & Saltin, B. (1961). Maximal oxygen uptake and heart rate in various types of muscular activity. *Journal of Applied Physiology*, **16**, 977-981.

Averill, J.R. (1982). *Anger and aggression*. New York: Springer-Verlag.

Balke, B. (1963). A simple field test for assessment of physical fitness. *Civil Aeromedical Research Institute Report*, 63-66. Oklahoma City, OK: Civil Aeromedical Research Institute.

Balke, B. (1970). *Advanced exercise procedures for evaluation of the cardiovascular system* (Monograph). Milton, WI: Burdick.

Balke, B., & Ware, R.W. (1959). An experimental study of "physical fitness" of air force personnel. *Armed Forces Medical Journal*, **10**, 675-688.

Bandura, A. (1969). *Principles of behavior modification*. New York: Holt, Rinehart & Winston.

Barham, J. (1978). *Mechanical kinesiology*. St. Louis: Mosby.

Basmajian, J.V., & MacConaill, M.A. (1977). *Muscles and movements—A basis for human kinesiology*. Huntington, NY: Kreiger.

Bassett, D.R., & Zweifler, A.J. (1990). Risk factors and risk factor management. In G.B. Zelenock, L.G. D'Alecy, J.C. Fantone, III, M. Shlafer, & J.C. Stanley (Eds.), *Clinical Ischemic Syndromes* (pp. 15-46). St. Louis: Mosby.

Baumgartner, T.A., & Jackson, A.S. (1987). *Measurement for evaluation in physical education and exercise science* (3rd ed.). Dubuque, IA: Brown.

Bayless, M.A., & Adams, S.H. (1985). A liability checklist. *Journal of Physical Education, Recreation, and Dance*, **36**, 49.

Ben-Sira, Z. (1982). The health-promoting function of mass media and reference groups: Motivating or reinforcing of behavior change. *Social Science Medicine*, **16**, 825-834.

Benson, H. (1975). *The relaxation response*. New York: Morrow.

Berg, K.E. (1986). *Diabetic's guide to health and fitness*. Champaign, IL: Life Enhancement.

Berger, M., & Kemmer, F.W. (1990). Discussion: Exercise, fitness, and diabetes. In C. Bouchard, R.J. Shephard, T. Stephens, J.R. Sutton, & B.D. McPherson (Eds.), *Exercise, fitness, and health* (pp. 491-495). Champaign, IL: Human Kinetics.

Berman, L.B., & Sutton, J.R. (1986). Exercise and the pulmonary patient. *Journal of Cardiopulmonary Rehabilitation*, **6**, 52-61.

Bernacki, E.J., & Baun, W.B. (1984). The relationship of job performance to exercise adherence in a corporate fitness program. *Journal of Occupational Medicine*, **16**(7), 529-531.

Berne, R.M., & Levy, M.N. (1977). *Cardiovascular Physiology* (3rd ed.). St. Louis: Mosby.

Bjorntrop, P. (1985). Regional patterns of fat distribution. *Annals of Internal Medicine*, **103**, 994-995.

Blair, S.N., Jacobs, D.R., & Powell, K.E. (1985). Relationships between exercise or physical activity and other health behaviors. *Public Health Reports*, **100**, 180-188.

Blair, S.N., Kohl, H.W., III, Paffenbarger, R.S., Jr., Clark, D.G., Cooper, K.H., & Gibbons, L.W. (1989). Physical fitness and all-cause mortality. *Journal of the American Medical Association*, **262**, 2395-2401.

Blair, S.N., Painter, P., Pate, R.R., Smith, L.K., & Taylor, C.B. (Eds.) (1988). *Resource manual for guidelines for exercise testing and prescription*. Philadelphia: Lea & Febiger.

Bogduk, N., & Macintosh, J.E. (1984). The applied anatomy of the thoracolumbar fascia. *Spine*, **9**, 164.

Bonge, D., & Donnelly, J.E. (1989). Trials to criteria for hydrostatic weighing at residual volume. *Research Quarterly for Exercise and Sport*, **60**, 176-179.

Booth, D.A. (1980). Acquired behavior controlling energy intake and output. In A.J. Stunkard (Ed.), *Obesity* (pp. 101-143). Philadelphia: Saunders.

Borg, G.A.V. (1982). Psychological bases of physical exertion. *Medicine and Science in Sports and Exercise*, **14**(5), 377-381.

Bouchard, C. (1990). Discussion: Heredity, fitness, and health. In C. Bouchard, R.J. Shephard, T. Stephens, J.R. Sutton, & B.D. McPherson (Eds.), *Exercise, fitness, and health* (pp. 147-153). Champaign, IL: Human Kinetics.

Bouchard, C., Lesage, R., Lortie, G., Simoneau, J., Hamel, P., Boulay, M., Perusse, L., Theriault, G., & Leblank, C. (1986). Aerobic performance in brothers, dizygotic and monozygotic twins. *Medicine and Science in Sports and Exercise*, **18**, 639-646.

Bouchard, C., Shephard, R.J. Stephens, T., Sutton, J.R., & McPherson, B.D. (Eds.) (1990a). *Exercise, fitness, and health: A consensus of current knowledge*. Champaign, IL: Human Kinetics.

Bouchard, C., Shephard, R.J., Stephens, T., Sutton, J.R., & McPherson, B.D. (1990b). Exercise, fitness, and health: The consensus statement. In C. Bouchard, R.J. Shephard, T. Stephens, J.R. Sutton, & B.D. McPherson (Eds.), *Exercise, fitness, and health* (pp. 3-28). Champaign, IL: Human Kinetics.

Bowers, D.G. (1976). *Systems of organization*. Ann Arbor: University of Michigan Press.

Brancazio, P.J. (1984). *Sportscience*. New York: Simon & Schuster.

Bransford, D.R., & Howley, E.T. (1977). The oxygen cost of running in trained and untrained men and women. *Medicine and Science in Sports*, **9**, 41-44.

Bray, G.A. (1990). Exercise and Obesity. In C. Bouchard, R.J. Shephard, T. Stephens, J.R. Sutton, & B.D. McPherson (Eds.), *Exercise, fitness, and health* (pp. 497-510). Champaign, IL: Human Kinetics.

Brehm, B.A. (1988). Elevation of metabolic rate following exercise: Implications for weight loss. *Sport Medicine*, **6**, 72-78.

Breslow, L. (1990). Lifestyle, fitness, and health. In C. Bouchard, R.J. Shephard, T. Stephens, J.R. Sutton, & B.D. McPherson (Eds.), *Exercise, fitness, and health* (pp. 155-163). Champaign, IL: Human Kinetics.

Broer, M.R., & Zernicke, R.F. (1979). *Efficiency of human movement*. Philadelphia: Saunders.

Brooks, G.A. (1985). Anaerobic threshold: Review of the concept, and directions for future research. *Medicine and Science in Sports and Exercise*, **17**, 22-31.

Brooks, G.A., & Fahey, T.D. (1987). *Fundamentals of human performance*. New York: Macmillan.

Brown, D.R. (1990). Exercise, fitness, and mental health. In C. Bouchard, R.J. Shephard, T. Stephens, J.R. Sutton, & B.D. McPherson (Eds.), *Exercise, fitness, and health* (pp. 607-626). Champaign, IL: Human Kinetics.

Brownell, K.D. (1988). Weight management and body composition. In S.N. Blair, P. Painter, R.R. Pate, L.K. Smith, & C.B. Taylor (Eds.), *Resource manual for guidelines for exercise testing and prescription*. Philadelphia: Lea & Febiger.

Brownell, K.D., Stunkard, A.J., & Albaum, J.M. (1980). Evaluation and modification of exercise patterns in natural environment. *American Journal of Psychiatry*, **137**, 1540-1545.

Brozek, J., Grande, F., Anderson, J.T., & Keys, A. (1963). Densitometric analysis of body composition: Revision of some quantitative assumptions. *Annals of the New York Academy of Science*, **110**, 113-140.

Bruce, R.A. (1972). Multistage treadmill test of submaximal and maximal exercise. In American Heart Association, *Exercise testing and training of apparently healthy individuals: A handbook for physicians* (pp. 32-34). New York: American Heart Association.

Bubb, W.J., Martin, A.D., & Howley, E.T. (1985). Predicting oxygen uptake during level walking at speeds of 80 to 130 meters per minute. *Journal of Cardiac Rehabilitation*, **5**(10), 462-465.

Burchfield, S.R. (1979). The stress response: A new perspective. *Psychosomatic Medicine*, **41**, 661-672.

Burton, A.C., & Edholm, O.G. (1955). *Man in a cold environment*. London: Edward Arnold.

Buskirk, E.R. (1987). Obesity. In J.S. Skinner, *Exercise testing and exercise prescription for special cases*. Philadelphia: Lea & Febiger.

Buskirk, E.R., & Bass, D.E. (1974). Climate and exercise. In W.R. Johnson & E.R. Buskirk (Eds.), *Science and medicine of exercise and sport* (pp. 190-205). New York: Harper & Row.

Buskirk, E.R., & Hodgson, J.L. (1987). Age and aerobic power: The rate of change in men and women. *Federation Proceedings*, **46**, 1824-1829.

Cady, L.D., Bischoff, D.P., O'Connell, E.R., Thomas, P.C., & Allom, J.H. (1979). Strength and fitness and subsequent back injuries in firefighters. *Journal of Occupational Medicine*, **21**, 269.

Calabrese, L.H. (1990). Exercise, immunity, cancer, and infection. In C. Bouchard, R.J. Shephard, T. Stephens, J.R. Sutton, & B.D. McPherson (Eds.), *Exercise, fitness, and health* (pp. 567-579). Champaign, IL: Human Kinetics.

Caldwell, F., & Jopke, T. (1985). Questions and answers: ACSM 1985. *The Physician and Sportsmedicine*, **13**(8), 145-151.

Calliet, R. (1981). *Low-back pain* (3rd ed.). Philadelphia: Davis.

Cantu, D.C. (1982). *Diabetes and exercise*. Ithaca, NY: Mouvement.

Cappozzo, A. (1983). Force actions in the human trunk during running. *Journal of Sports Medicine*, **23**, 14-22.

Caspersen, C.J., & Heath, G.W. (1988). The risk-factor

concept of coronary heart disease. In S.N. Blair, P. Painter, L.K. Smith, & C.B. Taylor (Eds.), *Resource manual for guidelines for graded exercise testing and prescription* (pp. 111-125). Philadelphia: Lea & Febiger.

Chang, K., & Hossack, K.F. (1982). Effect of diltiazem on heart-rate responses and respiratory variables during exercise: Implications for exercise prescription and cardiac rehabilitation. *Journal of Cardiac Rehabilitation*, **2**, 326-332.

Chusid, E.L. (Ed.) (1983). *The selective and comprehensive testing of adult pulmonary function*. Mount Kisco, NY: Futura.

Claytor, R.P. (1985). Selected cardiovascular, sympathoadrenal, and metabolic responses to one-leg exercise training. Unpublished doctoral dissertation, University of Tennessee, Knoxville.

Cooper, K.H. (1977). *The aerobics way*. New York: Bantam Books.

Cooper, K.H., & Collingwood, T.R. (1984). Physical fitness: Programming issues for total well-being. *Journal of Physical Education, Recreation, and Dance*, **35**(6), 44.

Cooper, K.H., & Glassow, R.B. (1982). *Kinesiology*. St. Louis: Mosby.

Cormier, W.H., & Cormier, L.S. (1979). *Interviewing strategies for helpers: A guide to assessment, treatment, and evaluation*. Monterey, CA: Brooks/Cole.

Costill, D.L. (1988). Carbohydrates for exercise: Dietary demands of optimal performance. *International Journal of Sports Medicine*, **9**, 1-18.

Coyle, E.F., Hemmert, M.K., & Coggan, A.R. (1986). Effects of detraining on cardiovascular responses to exercise: Role of blood volume. *Journal of Applied Physiology*, **60**, 95-99.

Coyle, E.F., Martin, W.H., III, Bloomfield, S.A., Lowry, O.H., & Holloszy, J.O. (1985). Effects of detraining on responses to submaximal exercise. *Journal of Applied Physiology*, **59**, 853-859.

Coyle, E.F., Martin, W.H., III, Sinacore, D.R., Joyner, M.J., Hagberg, J.M., & Holloszy, J.O. (1984). Time course of loss of adaptation after stopping prolonged intense endurance training. *Journal of Applied Physiology*, **57**, 1857-1864.

Coyle, E.F. (1988). Detraining and retention of training-induced adaptations. In S.N. Blair, P. Painter, R.R. Pate, L.K. Smith, & C.B. Taylor (Eds.), *Resource manual for guidelines for exercise testing and prescription*. Philadelphia: Lea & Febiger.

Cureton, K.J., Sparkling, P.B., Evans, B.W., Johnson, S.M., Kong, U.D., & Purvis, J.W. (1978). Effect of experimental alterations in excess weight on aerobic capacity and distance-running performance. *Medicine and Science in Sports*, **10**, 194-199.

Cureton, T.K. (1965). *Physical fitness and dynamic health*. New York: Dial Press.

D'Ambrosia, R.D., & Drez, D. (1982). *Prevention and treatment of running injuries*. Thorofare, NJ: Slack.

Danaher, B.G. (1977). Research on rapid smoking. An interim summary and recommendations. *Addictive Behaviors*, **2**, 151-166.

Daniels, J.T. (1985). A physiologist's view of running economy. *Medicine and Science in Sports and Exercise*, **17**, 332-338.

Daniels, J., Oldridge, N., Nagle, F., & White, B. (1978). Differences and changes in $\dot{V}O_2$ among young runners 10-18 years of age. *Medicine and Science in Sports*, **10**, 200-203.

Darden, E. (1976). *Nutrition and athletic performance*. Pasadena: Athletic Press.

Davidson, P.O., & Davidson, S.M. (Eds.) (1980). *Behavioral medicine: Changing health lifestyles*. New York: Brunner/Mazel.

Davis, J.H. (1985). Anaerobic threshold: Review of the concept and directions for future research. *Medicine and Science in Sports and Exercise*, **17**, 6-18.

Dehn, M.M., & Mullins, C.B. (1977). Physiologic effects and importance of exercise in patients with coronary artery disease. *Cardiovascular Medicine*, **2**, 365.

deVries, H.A. (1980). *Physiology of exercise for physical education and athletics* (3rd ed.). Dubuque, IA: Brown.

Dill, D.B. (1965). Oxygen cost of horizontal and grade walking and running on the treadmill. *Journal of Applied Physiology*, **20**, 19-22.

Dishman, R.K. (1990). Determinants of participation in physical activity, In C. Bouchard, R.J. Shephard, T. Stephens, J.R. Sutton, & B.D. McPherson (Eds.), *Exercise, fitness, and health* (pp. 75-101). Champaign, IL: Human Kinetics.

Dishman, R.K., & Gettman, L.R. (1980). Psychobiologic influences on exercise adherence. *Journal of Sport Psychology*, **2**, 295-310.

Dishman, R.K., Ickes, W., & Morgan, W.P. (1980). Self-motivation and adherence to habitual physical activity. *Journal of Applied Social Psychology*, **10**, 115-132.

Dodd, S., Powers, S.K., Callender, T., & Brooks, E. (1984). Blood lactate disappearance at various intensities of recovery exercise. *Journal of Applied Physiology*, **57**, 1462-1465.

Doxey, G.E., Fairbanks, B., Housh, T.H., Johnson, G.O., Katch, F., & Lohman, T. (1987). Body composition roundtable: Part 1. Scientific considerations. *National Strength and Conditioning Association Journal*, **9**, 14-15.

Drinkwater, B.L., Denton, J.E., Kupprat, I.C., Talag, T.S., & Horvath, S.M. (1976). Aerobic power as a factor in women's response to work within hot environments. *Journal of Applied Physiology*, **41**, 815-821.

Duffey, D.J., Horwitz, L.D., & Brammell, H.L. (1984). Nifedipine and the conditioning response. *American Journal of Cardiology*, **53**, 908-911.

Edington, D.W., & Edgerton, V.R. (1976). *The biology of physical activity*. Boston: Houghton Mifflin.

Eggleston, P.A. (1986). Pathophysiology of exercise-induced asthma. *Medicine and Science in Sports and Exercise*, **18**, 318-321.

Einkauf, D.K., Gohdes, M.L., Jensen, G.M., & Jewell, M.J. (1987). Changes in spinal mobility with increasing age in women. *Physical Therapy*, **67**, 370-375.

Ekblom, B., Åstrand, P.O., Saltin, B., Stenberg, J., & Wallstrom, B. (1968). Effect of training on circulatory response to exercise. *Journal of Applied Physiology*, **24**, 518-528.

Ellestad, M. (1980). *Stress testing: Principles and practice*. Philadelphia: Davis.

Epstein, L.H., Masek, B.J., & Marshall, W.R. (1978). The effects of prelunch exercise on lunchtime caloric intake. *The Behavior Therapist*, **1**, 3-15.

Epstein, L.H., Wing, R.R., Thompson, J.K., & Griffen, W. (1980). Attendance and fitness in aerobics exercise: The effects of contract and lottery procedures. *Behavior Modification*, **4**, 465-479.

Etnyre, B.R., & Abraham, L.D. (1986). Gains in range of ankle dorsiflexion using three popular stretching techniques. *American Journal of Physical Medicine*, **65**, 189-196.

Etnyre, B.R., & Lee, E.J. (1987). Comments on proprioceptive neuromuscular facilitation stretching techniques. *Research Quarterly for Exercise and Sport*, **58**, 184-188.

Ewy, G.A., & Bressler, R. (1982). *Current cardiovascular therapy*. New York: Raven Press.

Faulkner, J.A., Roberts, D.E., Elk, R.L., & Conway, J. (1971). Cardiovascular responses to submaximum and maximum effort cycling and running. *Journal of Applied Physiology*, **30**, 457-461.

Faulkner, R.A., Sprigings, E.S., McQuarrie, A., & Bell, R.D. (1988). *Partial curl-up research project final report*. Report submitted to the Canadian Fitness and Lifestyle Research Institute.

Flaxman, J. (1978). Quitting smoking now or later: Gradual, abrupt, immediate, and delayed quitting. *Behavior Therapy*, **9**, 260-270.

Fleck, S.J., & Dean, L.S. (1987). Resistance-training experience and the pressor response during resistance exercise. *Journal of Applied Physiology*, **63**, 116-120.

Folinsbee, L.J. (1990). Discussion: Exercise and the environment. In C. Bouchard, R.J. Shephard, T. Stephens, J.R. Sutton, & B.D. McPherson (Eds.), *Exercise, fitness, and health* (pp. 179-183). Champaign, IL: Human Kinetics.

Food and Nutrition Board. (1989). *Recommended dietary allowances*. Washington, DC: National Academy of Sciences, National Research Council.

Foster, C., Hare, J., Taylor, M., Goldstein, T., Anholm, J., & Pollock, M.L. (1984). Prediction of oxygen uptake during exercise testing in cardiac patients and healthy volunteers. *Journal of Cardiac Rehabilitation*, **4**, 537-542.

Fox, E.L., Bowers, R.W., & Foss, M.L. (1988). *The physiological basis of physical education and athletics* (4th ed.). New York: Saunders College Publishing.

Fox, E.L., & Mathews, D.K. (1974). *Interval training: Conditioning for sports and general fitness*. Philadelphia: Saunders.

Fox, E.L., & Mathews, D.K. (1981). *The physiological basis of physical education and athletics* (3rd ed.). Philadelphia: Saunders.

Franklin, B.A. (1978). Motivating and educating adults to exercise. *Journal of Physical Education and Recreation*, **49**, 13-17.

Franklin, B.A. (1985). Exercise testing, training, and arm ergometry. *Sports Medicine*, **2**, 100-119.

Franklin, B.A., Hellerstein, H.K., Gordon, S., & Timmis, G.C. (1986). Exercise prescription of the myocardial infarction patient. *Journal of Cardiopulmonary Rehabilitation*, **6**, 62-79.

Franklin, B.A., Oldridge, N.B., Stoedefalke, K.G., & Loechel, W.E. (1990). *On the ball*. Carmel, IN: Benchmark Press.

Franklin, B., Vanders, L., Wrisley, D., & Rubenfire, M. (1983). Aerobic requirements of arm ergometry: Implications for exercise testing and training. *The Physician and Sportsmedicine*, **11**(10), 81-90.

Franks, B.D. (1983). Warm-up. In M. Williams (Ed.), *Ergogenic aids in sport* (pp. 340-375). Champaign, IL: Human Kinetics.

Franks, B.D. (1984a). Physical activity and stress: Part 1. Acute effects. *International Journal of Physical Education*, **21**(4), 9-12.

Franks, B.D. (1984b). Physical activity and stress: Part 2. Chronic effects. *International Journal of Physical Education*, **21**(4), 13-16.

Franks, B.D. (1989). *YMCA youth fitness test*. Champaign, IL: Human Kinetics.

Franks, B.D., & Deutsch, H. (1973). *Evaluating performance in physical education*. New York: Academic Press.

Franks, B.D., & Howley, E.T. (1989). *Fitness leaders's handbook*. Champaign, IL: Human Kinetics.

Franks, C.M., Wilson, C.T., Kendal, P.C., & Brownell, K.D. (Eds.) (1982). *Annual review of behavior therapy: Theory and practice* (Vol. 8). New York: Guilford.

Franz, M.J. (1987). Exercise and the management of diabetes mellitus. *Journal of the American Dietetic Association*, **87**, 872-880.

Froelicher, V.F. (1983). *Exercise testing and training*. Chicago: Year Book Medical.

Frohlich, E.D., Grim, C., Labarthe, D.R., Maxwell, M.H., Perloff, D., & Weidman, W.H. (1988). Recommendations for human blood-pressure determination by sphygmomanometers. *Circulation*, **77**, 501A-514A.

Garfinkel, P.E., & Coscina, D.V. (1990). Discussion: Exercise and obesity. In C. Bouchard, R.J. Shephard, T. Stephens, J.R. Sutton, & B.D. McPherson (Eds.), *Exercise, fitness, and health* (pp. 511-516). Champaign, IL: Human Kinetics.

Garrick, J.G., & Requa, R.K. (1988). Aerobic dance—a review. *Sports Medicine*, **6**, 169-179.

Gauthier, M.M. (1986). Guidelines for exercise during pregnancy: Too little or too much. *The Physican and Sportsmedicine*, **14**(4), 162-169.

Gerhard, H., & Schachter, E.N. (1980). Exercise-induced asthma. *Postgraduate Medicine*, **67**, 91-102.

Getchell, B. (1976). *Physical fitness: A way of life*. New York: Wiley.

Gettman, L.R. (1988). Fitness testing. In S.N. Blair, P. Painter, R. Pate, L.K. Smith, & C.B. Taylor (Eds.), *Resource manual guidelines for exercise testing and prescription* (pp. 161-170). Philadelphia: Lea & Febiger.

Gettman, L.R. (1988). Management skills required for exercise programs. In S.N. Blair, P. Painter, R. Pate, L.K. Smith, & C.B. Taylor (Eds.), *Resource manual guidelines for exercise testing and prescription* (pp. 377-389). Philadelphia: Lea & Febiger.

Gettman, L.R., Pollock, M.L., & Ward, A. (1983). Adherence to unsupervised exercise. *The Physician and Sportsmedicine*, **11**, 56-64.

Giese, M.D. (1988). Organization of an exercise session. In S.N. Blair, P. Painter, R. Pate, L.K. Smith, & C.B. Taylor (Eds.), *Resource manual guidelines for exercise testing and prescription* (pp. 244-247). Philadelphia: Lea & Febiger.

Gisolfi, C., & Wenger, C.B. (1984). Temperature regulation during exercise: Old concepts, new ideas. In R. Terjung (Ed.), *Exercise and sports science reviews* (Vol. 12, pp. 339-372). Lexington, MA: Collamore Press.

Gisolfi, G.V., & Cohen, J. (1979). Relationships among training, heat acclimation, and heat tolerance in men and women: The controversy revisited. *Medicine and Science in Sports*, **11**, 56-59.

Golding, L.A., Myers, C.R., & Sinning, W.E. (1989). *The Y's way to physical fitness*. Champaign, IL: Human Kinetics.

Goldman, L., & Cook, E.F. (1984). The decline in ischemic heart disease mortality rates. *Annals of Internal Medicine*, **101**, 825-836.

Goldman, M.J. (1982). *Principles of clinical electrocardiography*. Cambridge, MD: Lange Medical.

Goodrick, G.K., & Iammarino, N.K. (1982). Teaching aerobic lifestyles: New perspectives. *Journal of Physical Education, Recreation, and Dance*, **53**, 48-50.

Gormally, J., & Rardin, D. (1981). Weight loss and maintenance and changes in diet and exercise for behavioral counseling and nutrition education. *Journal of Counseling Psychology*, **28**(4), 295-304.

Gowitzke, B.A., & Milner, M. (1988). *Scientific bases of human movement* (3rd ed.). Baltimore: Williams & Wilkins.

Gracovetsky, S., & Farfan, H. (1986). The optimum spine. *Spine*, **11**, 543-572.

Gray, H. (1966). *Anatomy of the human body*. Philadelphia: Lea & Febiger.

Grover, R., Reeves, J., Grover, E., & Leathers, J. (1967). Muscular exercise in young men native to 3,100 m altitude. *Journal of Applied Physiology*, **22**, 555-564.

Habgerg, J.M. (1990). Exercise, fitness, and hypertension. In C. Bouchard, R.J. Shephard, T. Stephens, J.R. Sutton, & B.D. McPherson (Eds.), *Exercise, fitness, and health* (pp. 455-466). Champaign, IL: Human Kinetics.

Hagberg, J.M., Mullin, J.P., Giese, M.D., & Spitznagel, E. (1981). Effect of pedaling rate on submaximal exercise responses of competitive cyclists. *Journal of Applied Physiology*, **51**, 447-451.

Hage, P. (1983). Prescribing exercise: More than just a running program. *The Physician and Sportsmedicine*, **11**(5), 123-133.

Hall, D. (1978). Changing attitudes by changing behavior. *Journal of Physical Education and Recreation*, **49**, 20-21.

Halpern, A.A., & Bleck, E.E. (1979). Sit-up exercises: An electromyographic study. *Clinical Orthopedics*, **145**, 172-178.

Hanson, P. (1988). Clinical Exercise Testing. In S.N. Blair, P. Painter, R. Pate, L.K. Smith, & C.B. Taylor (Eds.), *Resource manual for guidelines for exercise testing and prescription* (pp. 205-222). Philadelphia: Lea & Febiger.

Hanson, P.G., & Zimmerman, S.W. (1979). Exertional heatstroke in novice runners. *Journal of the American Medical Association*, **242**, 154-157.

Hardy, J.D., & Bard, P. (1974). Body temperature regulation. In V.B. Mountcastle (Ed.), *Medical physiology* (13th ed., Vol. 2, pp. 1305-1342). St. Louis: Mosby.

Hardy, L. (1985). Improving active range of hip flexion. *Research Quarterly for Exercise and Sport*, **56**, 111-114.

Harkcom, T.M., Lampman, R.M., Banwell, B.F., & Castor, C.W. (1985). Therapeutic value of graded aerobic exercise training in rheumatoid arthritis. *Arthritis Rheumatism*, **28**, 32.

Hartley-O'Brien, S.J. (1980). Six mobilization exercises for active range of hip flexion. *Research Quarterly for Exercise and Sport*, **51**(4), 625-635.

Haskell, W.L. (1978). Design and implementation of cardiac conditioning programs. In N.K. Wenger & H.K. Hellerstein (Eds.), *Rehabilitation of the coronary patient* (pp. 203-241). New York: Wiley.

Haskell, W.L. (1984). The influence of exericse on the concentrations of triglyceride and cholesterol in human plasma. In R.L. Terjung (Ed.), *Exercise and sports sciences reviews* (Vol. 12, pp. 205-244). Lexington, MA: Collamore.

Haskell, W.L., Montoye, H.J., & Orenstein, D. (1985). Physical activity and exercise to achieve health-related physical fitness components. *Public Health Reports*, **100**, 202-212.

Haskell, W.L., Savin, W., Oldridge, N., & DeBusk, R. (1982). Factors influencing estimated oxygen uptake during exercise testing soon after myocardial infarction. *American Journal of Cardiology*, **50**, 299-304.

Hau, M.L., & Fischer, J. (1974). Self-modification of exercise behavior. *Journal of Behavioral Therapy and Experimental Psychiatry*, **5**, 213-214.

Hay, J.G., & Reid, J.G. (1982). *The anatomical and mechanical bases of human motion*. Englewood Cliffs, NJ: Prentice Hall.

Hayes, S.G., Feinleib, M., & Kannel, W.B. (1980). The relationship of psychosocial factors to coronary heart disease in the Framingham study. Part III. Eight-year incidence of coronary heart disease. *American Journal of Epidemiology*, **111**(1), 37-58.

Hayward, M.G., & Keatinge, W.R. (1981). Roles of subcutaneous fat and thermoregulatory reflexes in determining ability to stabilize body temperature in water. *Journal of Physiology (London)*, **320**, 229-251.

Heaney, R.P. (1987). The role of calcium in prevention and treatment of osteoporosis. *The Physician and Sportsmedicine*, **15**(11), 83-88.

Hellerstein, H.K., & Franklin, B.A. (1984). Exercise testing and prescription. In N.K. Wenger & H.K. Hellerstein (Eds.), *Rehabilitation of the coronary patient* (2nd ed., pp. 197-284). New York: Wiley.

Henderson, J. (1973). *Emergency medical guide* (3rd ed.). St. Louis: McGraw-Hill.

Herbert, W.G., & Herbert, D.L. (1988). Legal considerations. In S.N. Blair, P. Painter, R. Pate, L.K. Smith, & C.B. Taylor (Eds.), *Resource manual for guidelines for exercise testing and prescription* (pp. 395-399). Philadelphia: Lea & Febiger.

Hettinger, T. (1961). *Physiology of strength*. Springfield, IL: Thomas.

Hickson, R.C., Bomze, H.A., & Holloszy, J.O. (1977). Linear increase in aerobic power induced by a strenuous program of endurance exercise. *Journal of Applied Physiology: Respiratory, Environmental, and Exercise Physiology*, **42**, 372-376.

Hickson, R.C., Bomze, H.A., & Holloszy, J.O. (1978). Faster adjustment of O_2 uptake to the energy requirement of exercise in the trained state. *Journal of Applied Physiology: Respiratory, Environmental, and Exercise Physiology*, **44**, 877-881.

Hickson, R.C., Foster, C., Pollock, M.L., Galassi, T.M., & Rich, S. (1985). Reduced training intensities and loss of aerobic power, endurance, and cardiac growth. *Journal of Applied Physiology*, **58**, 492-499.

Hickson, R.C., Kanakis, C., Jr., Davis, J.R., Moore, A.M., & Rich, S. (1982). Reduced training duration effects on aerobic power, endurance, and cardiac growth. *Journal of Applied Physiology*, **53**, 225-229.

Hickson, R.C., & Rosenkoetter, M.A. (1981). Reduced training frequencies and maintenance of increased aerobic power. *Medicine and Science in Sports and Exercise*, **13**, 13-16.

Hinson, M.M. (1981). *Kinesiology*. Dubuque, IA: Brown.

Holloszy, J.O., & Coyle, E.F. (1984). Adaptations of skeletal muscle to endurance exercise and their metabolic consequences. *Journal of Applied Physiology: Respiratory, Environmental, and Exercise Physiology*, **56**, 831-838.

Holmer, I. (1979). Physiology of swimming man. In R.S. Hutton & D.I. Miller (Eds.), *Exercise and sport sciences reviews* (Vol. 7, pp. 87-123). Salt Lake City: Franklin Institute.

Holmes, T.H., & Rahe, H. (1967). The social readjustment rating scale. *Journal of Psychosomatic Research*, **11**, 213-218.

Holmgren, A. (1967). Cardiorespiratory determinants of cardiovascular fitness. *Canadian Medical Association Journal*, **96**, 697-702.

Horan, J.J., Linberg, S.E., & Hackett, G. (1977). Nicotine poisoning and rapid smoking. *Journal of Consulting and Clinical Psychology*, **45**, 344-347.

Horvath, S.M. (1981). Exercise in a cold environment. In D.I. Miller (Ed.), *Exercise and sport sciences reviews* (Vol. 9, pp. 221-263). Salt Lake City: Franklin Institute.

Horvath, S.M., Raven, P.R., Dahms, T.E., & Gray, D.J. (1975). Maximal aerobic capacity of different levels of carboxyhemoglobin. *Journal of Applied Physiology*, **38**, 300-303.

Hossack, K.F., Bruce, R.A., & Clark, L.J. (1980). Influence of propranolol on exercise prescription of training heart rates. *Cardiology*, **65**, 47-58.

Howley, E.T. (1980). Effect of altitude on physical performance. In G.A. Stull & T.K. Cureton (Eds.), *Encyclopedia of physical education, fitness, and sports: Training, environment, nutrition, and fitness* (pp. 177-187). Salt Lake City: Brighton.

Howley, E.T. (1988). The Exercise Testing Laboratory. In S.N. Blair, P. Painter, R.R. Pate, L.K. Smith, & C.B. Taylor (Eds.), *Resource manual for guidelines for exercise testing and prescription* (pp. 406-413). Philadelphia: Lea & Febiger.

Howley, E.T., & Glover, M.E. (1974). The caloric costs of running and walking 1 mile for men and women. *Medicine and Science in Sports*, **6**, 235-237.

Howley, E.T., & Martin, D. (1978). Oxygen uptake and heart-rate responses measured during rope skipping. *Tennessee Journal of Health, Physical Education and Recreation*, **16**, 7-8.

Hubert, H.B., Feinleib, M.N., McNamara, P.M., & Castelli, W.P. (1983). Obesity as an independent risk factor for cardiovascular disease: A 26-year follow-up of participants in the Framingham heart study. *Circulation*, **26**, 968-977.

Hubley-Kosay, C.L., & Stanish, W.D. (1984). Can stretching prevent athletic injuries? *Journal of Musculoskeletal Medicine*, **1**, 25-32.

Huelster, L.J. (1982). Social relevance perspective for sport and physical education. In E.F. Zeigler (Ed.), *Physical education and sport: An introduction* (pp. 1-22). Philadelphia: Lea & Febiger.

Hughson, R.L., Green, H.J., Houston, M.E., Thompson, J.A., MacLean, D.R., & Sutton, J.R. (1980). Heat Injuries in Canadian mass-participation runs. *Canadian Medicine Medical Association Journal*, **122**, 1141-1144.

Hultman, E. (1967). Physiological role of muscle glycogen in man, with special reference to exercise. *Circulation Research*, **20-21**(Suppl. 1), 99-114.

Hurst, J.W. (1978). *The heart*. New York: McGraw-Hill.

Hussina, R.A., & Lawrence, P.S. (1978). The reduction test, state, and trait anxiety by test-specific and generalized stress-inoculation training. *Cognitive Therapy and Research*, **2**, 25-38.

Ike, R.W., Lampman, R.M., & Castor, C.W. (1989). Arthritis and aerobic exercise: A review. *The Physician and Sportsmedicine*, **17**, 128-138.

Imrie, D., & Barbuto, L. (1988). The back-power program. Toronto: Stoddart. In S.N. Blair, P. Painter, R.R. Pate, L.K. Smith, & C.B. Taylor (Eds.), *Resource manual for guidelines for exercise testing and prescription*. Philadelphia: Lea & Febiger.

Issekutz, B., Birkhead, N.C., & Rodahl, K. (1962). The use of respiratory quotients in assessment of aerobic power capacity. *Journal of Applied Physiology*, **17**, 47-50.

Jackson, A.S., & Pollock, M.L. (1978). Generalized equations for predicting body density for men. *British Journal of Nutrition*, **40**, 497-504.

Jackson, A.S., Pollock, M.L., Graves, J.E., & Mahar, M. (1988). Comparison of the reliability and validity of total-body electrical impedance and anthropometry in determining body composition. *Journal of Applied Physiology*, **62**, 529-534.

Jackson, A.S., Pollock, M., & Ward, A. (1980). Generalized equations for predicting body density for women. *Medicine and Science in Sports and Exercise*, **12**, 175-182.

Jackson, A.W., & Baker, A.A. (1986). The relationship of sit-and-reach test to criterion measures of hamstring and back flexibility in young females. *Research Quarterly for Exercise and Sport*, **57**, 183.

Jacobsen, E. (1938). *Progressive relaxation*. Chicago: University of Chicago Press.

Jarvik, M.E., Cullen, T.W., Gritz, E.R., Vogt, T.M., & West, L.S. (Eds.) (1977). Research on smoking behavior (DHHS Publication No. ADM 78-581). Washington, DC: U.S. Government Printing Office.

Jellinek, E.M. (1960). *The disease concept of alcoholism*. New Brunswick, NJ: Hillhouse Press.

Jensen, C.R., Schultz, G.W., & Bangerter, B.L. (1983). *Applied kinesiology and biomechanics*. New York: McGraw-Hill.

Johnson, C.C., & Slemenda, C. (1987). Osteoporosis: An overview. *The Physician and Sportsmedicine*, **15**(11), 65-68.

Johnson, D.W. (1981). *Reaching out: Interpersonal ef-*

fectiveness and self-actualization (2nd ed.). Englewood Cliffs, NJ: Prentice-Hall.

Jones, N.L., Berman, L.B., Bartkiewig, P.D., & Oldridge, N.B. (1987). Chronic obstructive respiratory disorders. In J.S. Skinner (Ed.), *Exercise testing and exercise prescription for special cases* (pp. 175-187). Philadelphia: Lea & Febiger.

Kannel, W.B. (1979). Nutrition and atherosclerosis. In D.T. Mason & H. Guthrie (Eds.), *The medicine called nutrition*. Englewood Cliffs, NJ: Best Foods.

Kannel, W.B. (1990). Contribution of the Framingham study to preventive cardiology. *Journal of the American College of Cardiology*, **15**, 206-211.

Kannel, W.B., & Abbot, R.D. (1984). Incidence and prognosis of unrecognized myocardial infarction. *New England Journal of Medicine*, **311**, 1144-1147.

Kannel, W.B., & Gordon, T. (1979). Physiological and medical concomitants of obesity: The Framingham study. In *Obesity in America* (NIH Publication No. 79-359, pp. 125-143). Washington, DC: Department of Health, Education, and Welfare.

Kaplan, N.M. (1986). *Clinical hypertension* (4th ed.). Baltimore: Williams & Wilkins.

Karvonen, M.J., Kentala, E., & Mustala, O. (1957). The effects of training heart rate: A longitudinal study. *Annales Medicinae Experimentalis et Biologiae Fenniae*, **35**, 307-315.

Kasch, F.W., Boyer, J.L., Van Camp, S.P., Verity, L.S., & Wallace, J.P. (1990). The effects of physical activity and inactivity on aerobic power in older men (a longitudinal study). *The Physican and Sportsmedicine*, **18**(4), 73-83.

Kasch, F.W., Wallace, J.P., & Van Camp, S.P. (1985). Effects of 18 years of endurance exercise on the physical work capacity of older men. *Journal of Cardiopulmonary Rehabilitation*, **5**, 308-312.

Kasch, F.W., Wallace, J.P., Van Camp, S.P., & Verity, L.S. (1988). A longitudinal study of cardiovascular stability in active men aged 45 to 65 yrs. *The Physician and Sportsmedicine*, **16**(1), 117-126.

Katz, R.M. (1986). Prevention with and without the use of medications for exercise-induced asthma. *Medicine and Science in Sports and Exercise*, **18**, 331-333.

Katz, R.M. (1987). Coping with exercise-induced asthma in sports. *The Physician and Sportsmedicine*, **15**(July), 100-112.

Keefe, F.J., & Blumenthal, J.A. (1980). The life fitness program: A behavioral approach to making exercise a habit. *Journal of Behavioral Therapy and Experimental Psychiatry*, **11**, 31-34.

Keeley, J., Mayer, T.G., Cox, R., Gatchel, R.J., Smith, J., & Mooney, V. (1986). Quantification of lumbar function—part 5: Reliability of range-of-motion measures in the sagittal plane and an invivo torso rotation measurement technique. *Spine*, **11**, 31-37.

Kendall, F.P., & McCreary, E.K. (1983). *Muscles testing and function* (3rd ed.). Baltimore: Williams & Wilkins.

Kendall, P.C., & Hollon, S.D. (Eds.) (1979). *Cognitive-behavioral interventions: Theory, research, and procedures*. New York: Academic Press.

Kincey, J. (1983). Compliance with a behavioral weight-loss programme: Target setting and locus of control. *Behavior Research Therapy*, **21**(2), 109-114.

King, J.C., Cohenour, S.H., Corruccini, C.G., & Schneeman, P. (1978). Evaluation and modification of the basic four food group guide. *Journal of Nutrition Education*, **10**, 27-29.

Kippers, V., & Parker, A.W. (1987). Toe-touch test—a measure of its validity. *Physical Therapy*, **67**, 1680-1684.

Kirkendall, W.M., Feinlieb, M., Freis, E.D., & Mark, A.L. (1980). Recommendations for human blood-pressure determination by sphygmomanometers. *Circulation*, **62**, 1146A-1155A.

Kisselle, J., & Mazzeo, K. (1983). *Aerobic dance*. Englewood, CO: Morton.

Klafs, C.E., & Arnheim, D.D. (1977). *Modern principles of athletic training*. St. Louis: Mosby.

Kline, G.M., Porcari, J.P., Hintermeister, R., Freedson, P.S., Ward, A., McCarron, R.F., Ross, J., & Rippe, J.M. (1987). Estimation of $\dot{V}O_2$max from a 1-mile track walk, gender, age, and body weight. *Medicine and Science in Sports and Exercise*, **19**, 253-259.

Knoebel, L.K. (1984). Energy metabolism. In E. Selkurt (Ed.). *Physiology* (5th ed.). Boston: Little, Brown.

Krasevec, J.A., & Grimes, D.C. (1984). *Hydroaerobics*. New York: Leisure Press.

Kraus, H., & Raab, W. (1961). *Hypokinetic disease*. Springfield, IL: Thomas.

Kreighbaum, E., & Barthels, K.M. (1990). *Biomechanics*. Minneapolis: Burgess.

Krumboltz, J.D., & Thoresen, C.E. (Eds.) (1976). *Counseling methods*. New York: Holt, Rinehart & Winston.

Kuland, D.N. (1982). *The injured athlete*. Philadelphia: Lippincott.

Lamb, D. (1984). *Physiology of exercise*. New York: Macmillan.

Laporte, R.E., Adams, L.L., Savage, D.D., Brenes, G., Dearwater, S., & Cook, T. (1984). The spectrum of physical activity, cardiovascular disease, and health: An epidemiologic perspective. *American Journal of Epidemiology*, **120**, 507-517.

Leblanc, C., Bouchard, C., Godbout, P., & Mondor, J. (1981). Specificity of submaximal working capacity. *Journal of Sports Medicine*, **21**, 15-19.

Leveille, G.A., & Dean, A. (1979). Choosing foods for health. In D.T. Mason and H. Guthrie (Eds.), *The medicine called nutrition*. Englewood Cliffs, NJ: Best Foods.

Liemohn, W.P. (1990). Exercise and the back. In T.C. Namey (Ed.), *Rheumatic disease clinics of North America: Vol. 16 Exercise and Arthritis* (pp. 945-970). Philadelphia: Saunders.

Liemohn, W.P., Sharpe, G.L., & Wasserman, J. (1990). The ubiquitous sit-and-reach. Unpublished manuscript.

Liemohn, W.P., Snodgrass, L.B., & Sharpe, G.L. (1988). Unresolved controversies in back management—a review. *Journal of Orthopaedic and Sports Physical Therapy*, **9**, 239-244.

Lind, A.R., & McNicol, G.W. (1967). Muscular factors which determine the cardiovascular responses to sustained and rhythmic exercise. *Canadian Medical Association Journal*, **96**, 706-713.

Lindsay, R. (1987). Estrogen and osteoporosis. *The Physician and Sportsmedicine*, **15**(11), 105-108.

Logan, G.A., & McKinney, W.C. (1982). *Anatomical kinesiology*. Dubuque, IA: Brown.

Lohman, T.G. (1985). Research related to assessment of skeletal status. In A.F. Roche (Ed.), *Body composition assessments in youth and adults* (pp. 38-41). Columbus, OH: Ross Laboratories.

Lohman, T.G. (1986). Applicability of body composition techniques and constants for children and youth. In K.B. Pandolf (Ed.), *Exercise and sport science reviews* (Vol. 14, pp. 325-357). New York: Macmillan.

Londeree, B.R., & Ames, S.A. (1976). Trend analysis of the %$\dot{V}O_2$max–HR regression. *Medicine and Science in Sports*, **8**, 122-125.

Londeree, B.R., & Moeschberger, M.L. (1982). Effect of age and other factors on maximal heart rate. *Research Quarterly for Exercise and Sport*, **53**, 297-304.

Lotgering, F.K., Gilbert, R.D., & Longo, L.D. (1984). The interactions of exercise and pregnancy: A review. *American Journal of Obstetrics and Gynecology*, **149**, 560-568.

Lotgering, F.K., Gilbert, R.D., & Longo, L.D. (1985). Maternal and fetal responses to exercise during pregnancy. *Physiological Reviews*, **65**, 1-36.

Luttgens, K., & Well, K.F. (1982). *Kinesiology—scientific basis of human motion*. Philadelphia: Saunders College.

MacDougall, J.D., Tuxen, D., Sale, D.G., Moroz, J.R., & Sutton, J.R. (1985). Arterial blood-pressure response to heavy resistance exercise. *Journal of Applied Physiology*, **58**, 785-790.

Marcotte, B., & Price, J.H. (1983). The status of health promotion programs at the worksite—a review. *Health Education*, **14**(4), 4-9.

Margaria, R., Carretelli, P., Aghemo, P., & Sassi, J. (1963). Energy cost of running. *Journal of Applied Physiology*, **18**, 367-370.

Martin, J.E. (1982). Exercise and health: The adherence problem. *Behavioral Medicine Update*, **14**, 16-24.

Martin, J.E., & Dubbert, P.M. (1982). Exercise applications and promotion in behavioral medicine: Current status and future directions. *Journal of Consulting and Clinical Psychology*, **50**(6), 1004-1017.

Mason, J.W. (1975a). A historical view of the stress field. Part 1. *Journal of Human Stress*, **1**(1), 6-12.

Mason, J.W. (1975b). A historical view of the stress field. Part 2. *Journal of Human Stress*, **1**(2), 22-36.

Mathews, D.K., & Fox, E.L. (1976). *The Physiological Basis of Physical Education and Athletics* (2nd ed.). Philadelphia: Saunders.

Mayer, T.G. (1990). Discussion: Exercise, fitness, and back pain. In C. Bouchard, R.J. Shephard, T. Stephens, J.R. Sutton, & B.D. McPherson (Eds.), *Exercise, fitness, and health* (pp. 541-546). Champaign, IL: Human Kinetics.

Mayer, T.G., Smith, S.S., Keeley, J., & Mooney, V. (1985). Quantification of lumbar function. Part 2: Sagittal-plane trunk strength in chronic low-back pain patients. *Spine*, **10**, 765-772.

Mazzeo, J.W. (1984). *Shape-up*. Englewood, CO: Morton.

McArdle, W.D., Katch, F.I., & Katch, V.L. (1991). *Exercise physiology* (3rd ed.). Philadelphia: Lea & Febiger.

McArdle, W.D., Katch, F.I., & Pechar, G.S. (1973). Comparison of continuous and discontinuous treadmill and bicycle tests for max $\dot{V}O_2$. *Medicine and Science in Sports*, **5**(3), 156-160.

McArdle, W.D., & Magel, J.R. (1970). Physical work capacity and maximum oxygen uptake in treadmill and bicycle exercise. *Medicine and Science in Sports*, **2**(3), 118-123.

McArdle, W.D., Magel, J.R., Gergley, T.J., Spina, R.J., & Toner, M.M. (1984). Thermal adjustment to cold-water exposure in resting men and women. *Journal of Physiology: Respiratory Environment Exercise Physiology*, **56**, 1565-1571.

McArdle, W.D., Magel, J.R., Spina, R.J., Gergley, T.J., & Toner, M.M. (1984). Thermal adjustment to cold-water exposure in exercising men and women. *Journal of Applied Physiology: Respiratory Environmental and Physiology*, **56**, 1572-1577.

McKenzie, R. (1981). Exercises. In R.McKenzie (Ed.), *The lumbar spine—mechanical diagnosis and therapy* (p. 49). Upper Hutt, New Zealand: Spinal.

Meyers, G.C. (1988). Reimbursement for clinical exercise programs. In S.N. Blair, P. Painter, R. Pate, L.K. Smith, & C.B. Taylor (Eds.), *Resource manual for guidelines for exercise testing and prescription* (pp. 400-405). Philadelphia: Lea & Febiger.

Middleton, E. (1980). A rational approach to asthma therapy. *Postgraduate Medicine*, **67**, 107-123.

Miller, W.R. (Ed.) (1980). *The addictive behaviors: Treatment of alcoholism, drug abuse, smoking, and obesity*. New York: Pergamon.

Miracle, V.A. (1986). Pulmonary exercise program: A model for pulmonary rehabilitation. *Journal of Cardiopulmonary Rehabilitation*, **6**, 368-371.

Mitchell, B.S., & Blair, S.N. (1988). Evaluation of preventive and rehabilitation exercise programs. In S.N. Blair, P. Painter, R. Pate, L.K. Smith, & C.B. Taylor (Eds.), *Resource manual for guidelines for exercise testing and prescription* (pp. 414-420). Philadelphia: Lea & Febiger.

Montgomery, D.L. (1983). Physical fitness over a 10-year period—a longitudinal comparison of exercisers and dropouts. *Medicine and Science in Sports and Exercise*, **15**, 109.

Montoye, H.J. (1975). *Physical activity and health: An epidemiologic study of an entire community*. Englewood Cliffs, NJ: Prentice Hall.

Montoye, H.J., & Ayen, T. (1986). Body-size adjustment for oxygen requirement in treadmill walking. *Research Quarterly for Exercise and Sport*, **57**, 82-84.

Montoye, H.J., Ayen, T., Nagle, F., & Howley, E.T. (1986). The oxygen requirement for horizontal and grade walking on a motor-driven treadmill. *Medicine and Science in Sports and Exercise*, **17**, 640-645.

Morgan, W.P. (1985). Affective beneficence of vigorous physical activity. *Medicine and Science in Sports and Exercise*, **17**, 94-100.

Morris, A.F. (1984). *Sports medicine: Prevention of athletic injuries*. Iowa: Brown.

Murphy, J.K., Williamson, D.A., Buxton, A.E., Moody, S.C., Abshker, N., & Warner, M. (1982). The long-term effects of spouse involvement upon weight loss and maintenance. *Behavior Therapy*, **13**, 681-693.

Murphy, L.R. (1984). Occupational stress management: A review and appraisal. *Journal of Occupational Psychology*, **57**, 1-15.

Musser, J.W. (1988). Budget considerations. In S.N. Blair, P. Painter, R. Pate, L.K. Smith, & C.B. Taylor (Eds.), *Resource manual for guidelines for exercise testing and prescription* (pp. 390-394). Philadelphia: Lea & Febiger.

Nachemson, A. (1975). Towards a better understanding of the low-back pain: A review of the mechanics of the lumbar disc. *Rheumatology and Rehabilitation*, **14**, 129-143.

Nachemson, A.L. (1990). Exercise, fitness, and back pain. In C. Bouchard, R.J. Shephard, T. Stephens, J.R. Sutton, & B.D. McPherson (Eds.), *Exercise, fitness, and health* (pp. 533-540). Champaign, IL: Human Kinetics.

Nagle, F.J., Balke, B., Baptista, G., Alleyia, J., & Howley, E. (1971). Compatibility of progressive treadmill, bicycle, and step tests based on oxygen-uptake responses. *Medicine and Science in Sport*, **3**, 149-154.

Nagle, F.J., Balke, B., & Naughton, J.P. (1965). Gradational step tests for assessing work capacity. *Journal of Applied Physiology*, **20**, 745-748.

National Dairy Council. (1989). *Calcium: A summary of current research for the health professional* (2nd ed.). Rosemont, IL: Author.

National Institute on Alcohol Abuse and Alcoholism. (1971). *Alcohol and health. Report to the U.S. Congress*. Washington, DC: U.S. Government Printing Office.

National Institute on Alcohol Abuse and Alcoholism. (1974). *Alcohol and health. Report to the U.S. Congress*. Washington, DC: U.S. Government Printing Office.

National Institute on Alcohol Abuse and Alcoholism. (1978). *Alcohol and health. Report to the U.S. Congress*. Washington, DC: U.S. Government Printing Office.

Naughton, J.P., & Haider, R. (1973). Methods of exercise testing. In J.P. Naughton, H.R. Hellerstein, & L.C. Mohler (Eds.), *Exercise testing and exercise training in coronary heart disease* (pp. 79-91). New York: Academic Press.

New Games Foundation. (1976). *The new games book*. Garden City, NY: Dolphin Books.

Nieman, D.C. (1990). *Fitness and sports medicine: An introduction*. Palo Alto, CA: Bull.

Noble, B.J. (1986). *Physiology of exercise and sport*. St. Louis: Times Mirror/Mosby College.

Noble, B.J., Borg, G.A.V., Cafarelli, E., Robertson, R.J., & Pandolf, K.B. (1982). Symposium on recent advances in the study and clinical use of perceived exertion. *Medicine and Science in Sports and Exercise*, **14**, 376-411.

Nutrition and your health: Dietary guidelines for Americans. (1980). Washington, DC: U.S. Department of Agriculture and U.S. Department of Health and Human Services.

Nutter, P. (1988). Aerobic exercise in the treatment and prevention of low-back pain. *Occupational Medicine: State of the Art Reviews*, **3**, 137.

O'Connell, A., & Gardner, E. (1972). *Understanding the scientific bases of human movement*. Baltimore: Williams & Wilkins.

O'Donoghue, D.H. (1984). *Treatment of injuries to athletes* (4th ed.). Philadelphia: Saunders.

Oldridge, N.B. (1979). Compliance of post myocardial infarction patients to exercise programs. *Medicine and Science in Sports*, **11**(4), 373-375.

Oldridge, N.B. (1988). Qualities of an exercise leader. In S.N. Blair, P. Painter, R.R. Pate, L.K. Smith, & C.B. Taylor (Eds.), *Resource manual for guidelines for exercise testing and prescription* (pp. 239-243). Philadelphia: Lea & Febiger.

Oldridge, N.B., Haskell, W.L., & Single, P. (1981). Carotid palpation, coronary heart disease, and exercise rehabilitation. *Medicine and Science in Sports and Exercise*, **13**, 6-8.

Oldridge, N.B., & Steiner, D.L. (1985). Health locus of control and compliance with cardiac exercise rehabilitation. *Medicine and Science in Sports and Exercise*, **17**, 181.

Oldridge, N.B., Donner, A.P., Buck, C.W., Jones, N.L., Andrew, G.M., Parker, J.D., Cunningham, D.A., Kavanaugh, T., Rechnitzer, P.A., & Sutton, J.R. (1983). Predictors of dropout from cardiac exercise rehabilitation. *American Journal of Cardiology*, **51**, 70-74.

Paffenbarger, R.S., Hyde, R.T., & Wing, A.L. (1986). Physical activity, all-cause mortality, and longevity of college alumni. *New England Journal of Medicine*, **314**(March 6), 605-613.

Paffenbarger, R.S., Jr., Hyde, R.T., & Wing, A.L. (1990). Physical activity and physical fitness as determinants of health and longevity. In C. Bouchard, R.J. Shephard, T. Stephens, J.R. Sutton, & B.D. McPherson (Eds.), *Exercise, fitness, and health* (pp. 33-48). Champaign, IL: Human Kinetics.

Painter, P., & Haskell, W.L. (1988). Decision making in programming exercise. In S.N. Blair, P. Painter, R.R. Pate, L.K. Smith, C.B. Taylor (Eds.), *Resource manual for guidelines for exercise testing and prescription* (pp. 256-262). Philadelphia: Lea & Febiger.

Parcel, G. (1986). *Basic emergency care of the sick and injured* (3rd ed.). St. Louis: Times Mirror/Mosby College.

Pate, R.R. (1983). A new definition of youth fitness. *The Physician and Sportsmedicine*, **11**, 77-83.

Pattison, E.M., Sobell, M.B., & Sobell, L.C. (1977). *Emerging concepts of alcohol dependence*. New York: Springer.

Patton, R.W., Corry, J.M., Gettman, L.R., & Graf, J. (1986). *Implementing health/fitness programs*. Champaign, IL: Human Kinetics.

Peters, T.J., & Waterman, R.H. (1982). *In search of excellence*. New York: Warner Books.

Pierson, W.E., Covert, D.S., Koenig, J.Q., Namekta, T., & Shin Kim, Yoon. (1986). Implications of air pollution effects on athletic performance. *Medicine and Science in Sports and Exercise*, **18**, 322-327.

Pollock, M.L., Broida, J., Kendrick, Z., Miller, H.S., Janeway, R., & Linnerud, A.C. (1972). Effect of training 2 days per week at different intensities on middle-aged men. *Medicine and Science in Sports*, **4**, 192-197.

Pollock, M.L., Gettman, L.R., Mileses, C.A., Bah, M.D., Durstine, J.L., & Johnson, R.B. (1977). Effects of frequency and duration of training on attrition and incidence of injury. *Medicine and Science in Sports*, **9**, 31-36.

Pollock, M.L., & Wilmore, J.H. (1990). *Exercise in health and disease* (2nd ed.). Philadelphia: Saunders.

Pollock, M.L., Wilmore, J.H., & Fox, S.M. (1984). *Exercise in health and disease*. Philadelphia: Saunders.

Polly, S., Turner, R.D., & Sherman, A.R. (1976). A behavioral approach to individualized exercise programming. In J.D. Krumboltz & C.E. Thoreser (Eds.), *Counseling methods* (pp. 106-116). New York: Holt, Rinehart & Winston.

Powell, K.E., & Paffenbarger, R.S. (1985). Workshop on epidemiologic and public health aspects of physical activity and exercise: A summary. *Public Health Reports*, **100**, 118-126.

Powers, S., Dodd, S., Deason, R., Byrd, R., & McKnight, T. (1983). Ventilatory threshold, running economy, and distance-running performance of trained athletes. *Research Quarterly for Exercise and Sport*, **54**, 179-182.

Powers, S.K., Dodd, S., & Beadle, R.E. (1985). Oxygen-uptake kinetics in trained athletes differing in VO$_2$max. *European Journal of Applied Physiology*, **54**, 306-308.

Powers, S.K., & Howley, E.T. (1980). *Exercise physiology*. Dubuque, IA: Brown.

Powers, S., Riley, W., & Howley, E. (1990). A comparison of fat metabolism in trained men and women during prolonged aerobic work. *Research Quarterly for Exercise and Sport*, **52**, 427-431.

Pratt, C.M., Welton, D.E., Squires, W.G., Kirby, T.E., Hartung, G.H., & Miller, R.R. (1981). Demonstration of training effect during chronic ß-adrenergic blockade in patients with coronary artery disease. *Circulation*, **64**, 1125-1129.

Pugh, L.G.C. (1964). Deaths from exposure in Four Inns Walking Competition, March 14-15, 1964. *Lancet*, **1**, 1210-1212.

Pugh, L.G.C., & Edholm, O.G. (1955). The physiology of Channel swimmers. *Lancet*, **2**, 761-768.

Quinton Instruments Instruction Manual—Model 24-72. (1970). Seattle, WA: Quinton Instruments.

Rabkin, S.W., Mathewson, F.A.L., & Hsu, P. (1977). Relation of body weight to development of ischemic heart disease in a cohort of young North American men after a 26-year observation period: The Manitoba study. *American Journal of Cardiology*, **39**, 452-458.

Ragg, K.E., Murray, T.F., Karbonit, L.M., & Jump, D.A. (1980). Errors in predicting functional capacity from a treadmill exercise stress test. *American Heart Journal*, **100**, 581-583.

Rasch, P.J., & Burke, R.K. (1986). *Kinesiology and applied anatomy: The science of human movement*. Philadelphia: Lea & Febiger.

Raven, P.B. (1974). Effect of carbon monoxide and peroxacetyl nitrate on man's maximal aerobic capacity. *Journal of Applied Physiology*, **36**, 288-293.

Raven, P.B. (1980). Effects of air pollution on physical performance. In *Encyclopedia of physical education: Physical fitness, training, environment and nutrition related to performance* (Vol. 2, pp. 201-216). Salt Lake City: Brighton.

Raven, P.B., Drinkwater, B.L., Ruhling, R.O., Bolduan, N., Taguchi, S., Gliner, J., & Horvath, S.M. (1974). Effect of carbon monoxide and peroxyacetyl nitrate on man's maximal aerobic capacity. *Journal of Applied Physiology*, **36**, 288-293.

Rechnitzer, P.A. (1990). Discussion: Exercise, fitness, and coronary heart disease. In C. Bouchard, R.J. Shephard, T. Stephens, J.R. Sutton, & B.D. McPherson (Eds.), *Exercise, fitness, and health* (pp. 451-453). Champaign, IL: Human Kinetics.

Richter, E.R., & Galbo, H. (1986). Diabetes, insulin, and exercise. *Sports Medicine*, **3**, 275-288.

Riddle, P.K. (1980). Attitudes, belief, behavioral intentions, and behaviors of women and men toward regular jogging. *Research Quarterly for Exercise and Sport*, **51**(4), 663-674.

Rimm, A.A., & White, P.L. (1979). Obesity: Its risks, and hazards. In *Obesity in America*, (NIH Publication No. 79-359, pp. 103-124). Washington, DC: Department of Health, Education, and Welfare.

Rimm, D.C., & Masters, J.C. (1974). *Behavior therapy: Techniques and empirical findings*. New York: Academic Press.

Ritter, M.A., & Albohm, M.J. (1987). *Your inquiry: A commonsense guide to sports injuries*. Indianapolis: Benchmark Press.

Robertson, L.D., & Magnusdottir, H. (1987). Evaluation of criteria associated with abdominal fitness testing. *Research Quarterly for Exercise and Sport*, **58**, 355-359.

Robinson, D. (1990, July 22). Stressbusters. *Parade Magazine*, p. 12.

Roskies, E. (1980). Considerations in developing a treatment program for the coronary-prone (Type A) behavior pattern. In P.O. Davidson & S.M. Davidson (Eds.), *Behavioral medicine: Changing health lifestyles* (pp. 299-333). New York: Brunner/Mazel.

Rowell, L.B. (1986). *Human circulation-regulation during physical stress*. New York: Oxford University Press.

Saal, J.A., & Saal, J.S. (1989). Nonoperative treatment of herniated lumbar intervertebral disc with radiculpathy—an outcome study. *Spine*, **14**, 341.

Sable, D.L., Brammel, H.L., Sheehan, M.W., Nies, A.S., Gerber, J., & Horwitz, L.D. (1982). Attenuation of exercise conditioning by beta-adrenergic blockade. *Circulation*, **65**, 679-684.

Sachs, M.L. (1982). Compliance and addiction to exercise. In R.C. Cantu (Ed.), *The exercising adult*. Boston: Collamore Press.

Safrit, M.J. (1986). *Introduction to measurement in physical education and exercise science*. St. Louis: Times Mirror/Mosby.

Sale, D.G. (1987). Influence of exercise and training on motor unit activation. In K.B. Pandolf (Ed.), *Exercise and sport sciences reviews* (Vol. 15, pp. 95-151). New York: MacMillan.

Saltin, B. (1969). Physiological effects of physical conditioning. *Medicine and Science in Sports*, **1**, 50-56.

Saltin, B., Henriksson, J., Nygaard, E., Anderson, P., & Jansson, E. (1977). Fiber types and metabolic potentials of skeletal muscles in sedentary man and endurance runners. *Annals of the New York Academy of Science*, **301**, 3-29.

Saltin, B., & Gollnick, P.D. (1983). Skeletal muscle adaptability: Significance for metabolism and performance. In L.D. Peachey, R.H. Adrian, & S.R. Geiger (Eds.), *Handbook of physiology* (Section 10: "Skeletal muscle," ch. 19). Baltimore: Williams & Wilkins.

Saltin, B., & Hermansen, L. (1966). Esophageal, rectal, and muscle temperature during exercise. *Journal of Applied Physiology*, **21**, 1757-1762.

Sawka, M.N., Francesconi, R.P., Young, A.J., & Pandolf, K.B. (1984). Influence of hydration level and body fluids on exercise performance in the heat. *Journal of the American Medical Association*, **252**(9), 1165-1169.

Sawka, M.N., Young, A.J., Francesconi, R.P., Muza,

S.R., & Pandolf, K.B. (1985). Thermoregulatory and blood responses during exercise at graded hypohydration levels. *Journal of Applied Physiology*, **59**, 1394-1401.

Schull, W.J. (1990). Heredity, fitness, and health. In C. Bouchard, R.J. Shephard, T. Stephens, J.R. Sutton, & B.D. McPherson (Eds.), *Exercise, fitness and health* (pp. 137-145). Champaign, IL: Human Kinetics.

Schutte, S.A., & Linkswiler, H.M. (1984). Calcium. In R.E. Olson, H.P. Broquist, C.O. Chichester, W.I. Darby, A.C. Kolbye, & R.M. Staley. *Nutrition Reviews' present knowledge in nutrition* (5th ed., pp. 400-412). *Washington, DC: The Nutrition Foundation*.

Schwade, J., Blomqvist, C.G., & Shapiro, W. (1977). A comparison of the response to arm and leg work in patients with ischemic heart disease. *American Heart Journal*, **94**, 203-208.

Schwartz, G.E., Weinberger, D.A., & Singer, J.A. (1981). Cardiovascular differentiation of happiness, sadness, anger, and fear following imagery and exercise. *Psychosomatic Medicine*, **43**, 343-364.

Scriber, K., & Burke, E. (Eds.) (1978). *Relevant topics in athletic training*. New York: Mouvement.

Sedlock, D.A., Knowlton, R.G., Fitzgerald, P.I., Tahamont, M.V., & Schneider, D.A. Accuracy of subject-palpated carotid pulse after exercise. *The Physician and Sportsmedicine*, **11**(4), 106-116.

Segal, K.R., Gutin, B., Presta, E., Wang, J., & Van Itallie, T.B. (1985). Estimation of human body composition by electrical impedance methods: A comparative study. *Journal of Applied Physiology*, **58**, 1565-1571.

Selye, H. (1956). *Stress of life*. New York: McGraw-Hill.

Selye, H. (1974). *Stress without distress*. Toronto: McCelland & Stewart.

Selye, H. (1975). Confusion and controversy in the stress field. *Journal of Human Stress*, **1**(2), 37-44.

Selye, H. (1976). Stress and physical activity. *McGill Journal of Education*, **11**, 3-14.

Serfass, R.C., & Gerberich, S.G. (1984). Exercise for optimal health: Strategies and motivational considerations. *Preventive Medicine*, **13**, 79-99.

Sharkey, B.J. (1984). *Physiology of fitness* (2nd ed.). Champaign, IL: Human Kinetics.

Sharkey, B.J. (1990). *Physiology of fitness* (3rd ed.). Champaign, IL: Human Kinetics.

Sharpe, G.L., Liemohn, W.P., Wasserman, J.F., Hungerford, J.C., & Lewis, J.L. (1990). *The effect of different levels of muscular strength on body posturing in a manual lifting task*. Abstracts of Platform and Poster Presentations, 65th Annual Conference of the American Physical Therapy Association, Anaheim, CA.

Shephard, R.J. (1976). Exercise and chronic obstructive lung disease. In J. Keogle & R.S. Hutton (Eds.), *Exercise and Sport Sciences Reviews* (Vol. 4, pp. 263-296). Santa Barbara, CA: Journal Publishing Affiliates.

Shephard, R.J. (1984). Tests of maximal oxygen uptake: A critical review. *Sports Medicine*, **1**, 99-124.

Shephard, R.J. (1985). Motivation: The key to fitness compliance. *The Physician and Sportsmedicine*, **13**, 88-101.

Shephard, R.J. (1988). PAR-Q, Canadian home fitness test, and exercise screening alternatives. *Sports Medicine*, **5**, 185-195.

Shephard, R.J. (1990). Costs and benefits of an exercising versus a nonexercising society. In C. Bouchard, R.J. Shephard, T. Stephens, J.R. Sutton, & B.D. McPherson (Eds.), *Exercise, fitness, and health* (pp. 49-60). Champaign, IL: Human Kinetics.

Sheppard, C.S., & Carroll, D.C. (1980). *Working in the twenty-first century*. New York: Wiley.

Sherman, W.M. (1983). Carbohydrates, muscle glycogen, and muscle glycogen super compensation. In M.H. Williams (Ed.), *Ergogenic aids in sports* (pp. 3-26). Champaign, IL: Human Kinetics.

Sime, W.E. (1990). Discussion: Exercise, fitness, and mental health. In C. Bouchard, R.J. Shephard, T. Stephens, J.R. Sutton, & B.D. McPherson (Eds.), *Exercise, fitness, and health* (pp. 627-633). Champaign, IL: Human Kinetics.

Sime, W.E., & McKinney, M.E. (1988). Stress management applications in the prevention and rehabilitation of coronary heart disease. In S.N. Blair, P. Painter, R.R. Pate, L.K. Smith, & C.B. Taylor (Eds.), *Resource manual for guidelines for exercise testing and prescription* (pp. 367-374). Philadelphia: Lea & Febiger.

Siri, W.E. (1956). Gross composition of the body. In J.H. Lawrence & C.A. Tobias (Eds.), *Advances in biological and medical physics* (Vol. 4, pp. 239-280). New York: Academic Press.

Siscovick, D.S. (1990). Risks of exercising: Sudden cardiac death and injuries. In C. Bouchard, R.J. Shephard, T. Stephens, J.R. Sutton, & B.D. McPherson (Eds.), *Exercise, fitness, and health* (pp. 707-713). Champaign, IL: Human Kinetics.

Sly, R.M. (1986). History of exercise-induced asthma. *Medicine and Science in Sports and Exercise*, **18**, 314-317.

Smith, E.L. (1984). Special considerations in developing exercise programs for the older adult. In J.D. Matarazzo, N.E. Miller, S.M. Weiss, J.A.

Herd, & S.M. Weiss (Eds.), *Behavioral health: A handbook of health enhancement and disease prevention* (pp. 525-546). New York: Wiley.

Smith, E.L., & Gilligan, C. (1987). Effects of inactivity and exercise on bone. *The Physician and Sportsmedicine, 15*(11), 91-102.

Smith, E.L., Smith, K.A., & Gilligan, C. (1990). Exercise, fitness, osteoarthritis, and osteoporosis. In C. Bouchard, R.J. Shephard, T. Stephens, J.R. Sutton, & B.D. McPherson (Eds.), *Exercise, fitness, and health* (pp. 517-528). Champaign, IL: Human Kinetics.

Smith, E.L. & Stoedefalke, K.G. (1978). *Aging and Exercise*. Unpublished. Copyright by Author.

Smith, N.J. (1976). *Food for sport*. Palo Alto, CA: Bull.

Sobell, M.B., & Sobell, L.C. (1978). *Behavioral treatment of alcoholic problems: Individualized therapy and controlled drinking*. New York: Plenum.

Sonstroem, R.J. (1978). Physical estimation and attraction scales: Rationale and research. *Medicine and Science in Sport, 10*(2), 97-102.

Sonstroem, R.J. (1984). Exercise and self-esteem. In R.L. Terjung (Ed.), *Exercise and sport sciences reviews* (Vol. 12, pp. 123-156). Lexington, MA: Collamore Press.

Sphygmomanometers, Principles and Precepts. (1961). New York: Baum.

Spielberger, C.D., Gorsuch, R.L., & Lushene, R.E. (1970). *The state-trait anxiety inventory*. Palo Alto, CA: Consulting Psychologists Press.

Spielberger, C., & Sarason, I. (Eds.) (1975). *Stress and anxiety* (Vol. 2). New York: Wiley.

Stalonas, P.M., Johnson, W.G., & Christ, M. (1978). Behavior modification for obesity: The evaluation of exercise, contingency management, and program adherence. *Journal of Consulting and Clinical Psychology, 46*, 463-469.

Stephens, T. (1990). Discussion: Behavioral adaptations to physical activity. In C. Bouchard, R.J. Shephard, T. Stephens, J.R. Sutton, & B.D. McPherson (Eds.), *Exercise, fitness, and health* (pp. 399-405). Champaign, IL: Human Kinetics.

Stockdale-Woolley, R., Haggerty, M.C., & McMahon, P.M. (1986). The pulmonary rehabilitation program at Norwalk Hospital. *Journal of Cardiopulmonary Rehabilitation, 6*, 505-518.

Strauss, W.E., Scaramuzzi, M.S., Panton-Lapsley, D., & McIntyre, K. (1988). Emergency plans and procedures for an exercise facility. In S.N. Blair, P. Painter, R.R. Pate, L.K. Smith, & C.B. Taylor (Eds.), *Resource manual for guidelines for exercise testing and prescription* (pp. 278-284). Philadelphia: Lea & Febiger.

Stuart, R.B., & Davies, B. (1971). *Slim change in a fat world: Behavioral control of obesity*. Champaign, IL: Research Press.

Stunkard, A.J. (1984). *Eating and its disorders*. New York: Raven Press.

Surburg, P.R. (1983). Flexibility exercises re-examined. *Athletic Training, 18*, 37-39.

Sutton, J.R. (1990). Exercise and the environment. In C. Bouchard, R.J. Shephard, T. Stephens, J.R. Sutton, & B.D. McPherson (Eds.), *Exercise, fitness, and health* (pp. 165-178). Champaign, IL: Human Kinetics.

Tanaka, K., & Matsuura, Y. (1984). Marathon performance, anaerobic threshold, and onset of blood lactate accumulation. *Journal of Applied Physiology, 57*, 640-643.

Tanii, K., & Masuda, T. (1985). A study by EMG stick diagrams of the muscular activities in the trunk flexion and extension movement. *Ergonomics, 28*, 895.

Taylor, C.B., & Miller, N.H. (1988). Basic psychologic principles related to group exercise programs. In S.N. Blair, P. Painter, R.R. Pate, L.K. Smith, & C.B. Taylor (Eds.), *Resource manual for guidelines for exercise testing and prescription* (pp. 329-334). Philadelphia: Lea & Febiger.

Taylor, H.L., Buskirk, E.R., & Henschel, A. (1955). Maximal oxygen intake as an objective measure of cardiorespiratory performance. *Journal of Applied Physiology, 8*, 73-80.

Thaxton, L. (1982). Physiological and psychological effects of short-term exercise addiction on habitual runners. *Journal of Sport Psychology, 4*, 73-80.

The fad-free diet: How to take weight off (and keep it off) without getting ripped off. *FDA Consumer*, (1985, July/Aug). pp. 26-29.

Thompson, C.E., & Wankel, L.M. (1980). The effects of perceived activity choice upon frequency of exercise behavior. *Journal of Applied Social Psychology, 10*, 436-443.

Thompson, C.W. (1988). *Manual of structural kinesiology*. St. Louis: Mosby.

Thompson, P.D. (1988). The safety of exercise testing and participation. In S.N. Blair, P. Painter, R.R. Pate, L.K. Smith, & C.B. Taylor (Eds.), *Resource manual for guidelines for exercise testing and prescription* (pp. 273-277). Philadelphia: Lea & Febiger.

Thygerson, A.L. (1987). *First aid and emergency care workbook*. Boston: Jones & Bartkett.

Tommaso, C.L., Lesch, M., & Sonnenblick, E.H. (1984). Alterations in cardiac function in coronary heart disease, myocardial infarction, and coronary bypass surgery. In N.K. Wenger & H.K. Hellerstern (Eds.), *Rehabilitation of the coronary patient* (pp. 41-66). New York: Wiley.

U.S. Department of Health and Human Services. (1980). *Promoting health/preventing disease: Objectives for the nation.* Washington, DC: U.S. Government Printing Office.

U.S. Department of Health and Human Services. (1981). *Exercise and your heart* (NIH Publication 81 1677). Washington, DC: U.S. Government Printing Office.

U.S. Department of Health and Human Services, Public Health Service (1990). *The 1990 Health objectives for the nation: A midcourse review.* Washington, DC: U.S. Government Printing Office.

U.S. Department of Health and Human Services, Public Health Service (1981). *Work practices guide for manual lifting.* Washington, DC: U.S. Government Printing Office.

U.S. Department of Health and Human Services, Public Health Service, Office on Smoking and Health. (1983). *The health consequences of smoking: Cardiovascular disease, a report of the Surgeon General* (DHEW Publication No. PHS 79-50066). Washington, DC: U.S. Government Printing Office.

U.S. Public Health Service. (1985). Public health aspects of physical activity and exercise. *Public Health Reports,* **100**(2), 118-124.

U.S. Public Health Service. (1990). *Healthy people 2000.* Washington, DC: Author.

U.S. Senate Select Committee on Nutrition and Human Needs. (1977). *Dietary goals for the U.S.* (2nd ed.). Washington, DC: U.S. Government Printing Office.

Vander, A.J., Sherman, J.H., & Luciano, D.S. (1985). *Human physiology.* (4th ed.). New York: McGraw-Hill.

Van Itallie, T.B. (1988). Topography of body fat: Relationship to risk of cardiovascular and other diseases. In T. Lohman, A.F. Roche, & R. Martorell (Eds.), *Anthropometric standardization reference manual.* Champaign, IL: Human Kinetics.

Voy, R.O. (1986). The U.S. Olympic Committee experience with exercise-induced bronchospasm—1984. *Medicine and Science in Sports and Exercise,* **18**, 328-330.

Vranic, M., & Berger, M. (1979). Exercise and diabetes mellitus. *Diabetes,* **28**, 147-163.

Vranic, M., & Wasserman, D. (1990). Exercise, fitness, and diabetes. In C. Bouchard, R.J. Shephard, T. Stephens, J.R. Sutton, & B.D. McPherson (Eds.), *Exercise, fitness, and health* (pp. 467-490). Champaign, IL: Human Kinetics.

Wadden, T.., Van Itallie, T.B., & Blackburn, G.L. (1990). Responsible and irresponsible use of very-low-calorie diets in the treatment of obesity. *Journal of the American Medical Association,* **263**, 83-85.

Watson, D.L., & Tharp, R.G. (1977). *Self-directed behavior: Self-modification for personal adjustment* (2nd ed.). Monterey, CA: Brooks/Cole.

Wenger, N.K., & Hellerstein, H.K. (1984). *Rehabilitation of the coronary patient* (2nd ed.). New York: Wiley.

Wenger, N.K., & Hurst, J.W. (1984). Coronary bypass surgery as a rehabilitative procedure. In N.K. Wenger & H.K. Hellerstein (Eds.), *Rehabilitation of the coronary patient.* (pp. 115-132). New York: Wiley.

White, A.A., & Panjabi, M.M. (1978). Kinematics of the spine. In *Clinical biomechanics of the spine* (pp. 61-90). Philadelphia: Lippincott.

Willerson, J.T., & Dehmer, G.J. (1981). Exercise stress laboratories in the future—what should their capabilities be? *Chest,* **80**(1), 1-2.

Williams, J.G.P. (1980). *A color atlas of injury in sport.* Chicago: Year Book Medical Publishers, Inc.

Williams, P.C. (1974). *Low back and neck pain.* Springfield, IL: Thomas.

Williams, R.L., & Long, J.D. (1983). *Toward a self-managed life style.* Boston: Houghton Mifflin.

Williford, H.N., Scharff-Olson, M., & Blessing, D.L. (1989). The physiological effects of aerobic dance—a review. *Sports Medicine,* **8**, 335-345.

Wilmore, J.H. (1982). *Training for sport and activity: The physiological basis of the conditioning process.* Boston: Allyn & Bacon.

Wood, P.E., & Stefanick, M.L. (1990). Exercise, fitness, and atherosclerosis. In C. Bouchard, R.J. Shephard, T. Stephens, J.R. Sutton, & B.D. McPherson (Eds.), *Exercise, fitness, and health* (pp. 409-423). Champaign, IL: Human Kinetics.

World Health Organization. (1985). Report of a joint FAO/WHO Expert Consultation. Energy and Protein Requirements. Rome: Food and Agriculture Organization of the United Nations.

World Health Organization. (1986). Guidelines for the treatment of mild hypertension. *Hypertension,* **8**, 957-961.

World Health Organization Expert Committee. (1982). *Prevention of coronary heart disease.* Geneva: World Health Organization.

Wysocki, T., Hall, G., Iwata, B., & Riordan, M. (1979). Behavioral management of exercise contracting for aerobic points. *Journal of Applied Behavior Analysis,* **12**(1), 55-64.

Zuti, W.B., & Golding, L.A. (1976). Comparing diet and exercise as weight-reduction tools. *The Physician and Sportsmedicine,* **4**, 49-53.

Index

Author Biographies

About the Authors

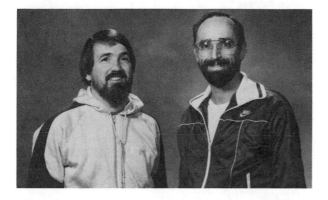

Edward T. Howley received his BS degree in physical education at Manhattan College in New York City and his MS and PhD degrees in physical education at the University of Wisconsin, Madison. His current research interests include the role of exercise in the treatment of obesity and hypertension. He is a professor at the University of Tennessee, where he has received the Alumni Association's Outstanding Teacher Award. He has been active in the American College of Sports Medicine both as a Fellow and as President of the Southeast Chapter. He has also served on the ACSM Preventive and Rehabilitative Committee that developed the college's various certification programs. He enjoys soccer and paddleball and is still on the rising portion of the learning curve in golf.

B. Don Franks grew up in Arkansas and received his BS and MEd degrees in physical education from the University of Arkansas, Fayetteville. He received his PhD in physical education from the University of Illinois at Urbana-Champaign in 1967 and served on the faculty there until 1970. He has also served on the faculty at Paine College in Augusta, Georgia; Temple University in Philadelphia; and the University of Tennessee, Knoxville. He is currently professor and chair of the Department of Kinesiology at Louisiana State University, Baton Rouge. His research interest is in the cardiovascular response to exercise and psychological stressors. He is a Fellow of the American Academy of Physical Education, the ACSM, and the Research Consortium of the American Alliance for Health, Physical Education, Recreation and Dance. He has been President of the AAHPERD Research Consortium where he has advocated the "health-related" approach to physical fitness. He enjoys and participates in many forms of physical activity.

About the Contributing Authors

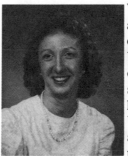

Wendy J. Bubb received BS and MS degrees in physical education from Lock Haven University and the University of Tennessee, Knoxville, respectively. She also received her PhD in physiology from the University of Tennessee and is an assistant professor there in the Department of Human Performance and Sport Studies. While a student, Dr. Bubb received a chancellor's citation for extraordinary professional promise, and in 1991 she received an award for excellence in teaching. Her research interests are in metabolic factors related to obesity. In her leisure time, she jogs, plays tennis, and enjoys her friendships with international students from many parts of the world.

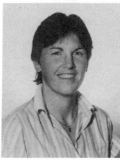

Sue Carver received her MS degree in physical education with a specialization in athletic training from Indiana University in 1978. She obtained her N.A.T.A. Certification the same year. She served as the Women's Athletic Trainer at the University of Tennessee from 1978-1982 before accepting a position in the Sports Treatment and Rehabilitation (STAR) Center at Fort Sanders Regional Medical Center in Knoxville. In 1986, Carver left Fort Sanders to pursue a Master's degree in physical therapy at Emory University. She graduated in 1987 and returned to the STAR Clinic. In October of 1989, Carver accepted a position with Physiotherapy Associates as Director of Little Rock Sports Therapy in Little Rock, Arkansas. Carver has also worked at the Olympic Training Center in Colorado Springs and was selected to work at the 1985 National Sports Festival in Baton Rouge. She was certified as a Fitness Instructor by the American College of Sports Medicine in 1985.

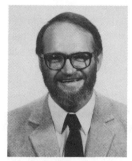

Mark A. Hector received a doctorate in counseling from Michigan State University in 1973. Since then he has been a professor in the Educational and Counseling Psychology Department at the University of Tennessee. His main teaching responsibilities are in the areas of counseling practice and research methods of problem solving. Dr. Hector is also interested in cross-cultural issues and has spent four years teaching in West Africa. For recreation, he plays paddleball and squash several times a week.

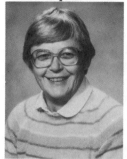

Jean Lewis received her doctorate in education (physical education with an emphasis in exercise physiology) from the University of Tennessee, Knoxville, where she now teaches. She was involved in the establishment of undergraduate major concentrations in physical fitness and exercise physiology and has also developed courses in applied anatomy, applied kinesiology, and weight control, fitness, and exercise. Dr. Lewis is known for her innovative teaching methods, which help physical education majors understand how to apply kinesiological concepts. She has experience in playing and coaching several team sports. Hiking in the Smoky Mountains and bicycling are her current favorite recreational activities.

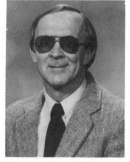

Wendell Liemohn received his BA from Wartburg College and his MA from the University of Iowa. After a few years coaching and teaching on the collegiate level, he returned to the University of Iowa and completed his PhD. He was on the faculty at Indiana University (IU) for 7 years and has been a professor at the University of Tennessee (UT) for the past 13 years. Most of his research at IU and his first few years at UT was related to studying psychomotor functioning in special populations. More recently he has spent more time studying exercise as it relates to low-back function, an interest that originated while he worked with low-back pain patients as a doctoral student at the University of Iowa. He is active in the American Alliance for Health, Physical Education, Recreation and Dance, including being President of the Research Consortium of AAHPERD. He is an avid runner (sometimes a road racer) and cross country skier (usually limited to workouts on the Nordic Track).

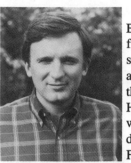

Daniel Martin earned his BS degree in physical therapy from the University of Tennessee Center for Health Science and his PhD in education from the University of Tennessee. He worked for several years with Dr. Joe Acker in the Cardiac Rehabilitation Program at Fort Sanders Regional Medical Center, Knoxville. Dr. Martin is currently an associate professor of physical therapy at the University of Florida. His research interests include pulmonary function in athletes and the effects of exercise on bone density in women. He is a member of the American College of Sports Medicine and the American Physical Therapy Association. A former All-American javelin thrower at Tennessee, he now enjoys fishing in the Gulf of Mexico.

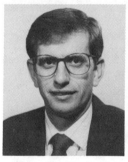

James R. Morrow, Jr. received his BS degree in health and physical education from the University of West Florida. He received his MS in physical education and PhD in research and evaluation methodology from the University of Colorado. Dr. Morrow is a professor in the Department of Health and Human Performance at the University of Houston, Texas, where he has been a faculty member since 1976. He serves as the editor-in-chief of the *Research Quarterly for Exercise and Sport* and has published more than 50 manuscripts, made more than 100 presentations at professional meetings, and authored six microcomputer programs in exercise science, physiology, and youth fitness testing. He is a Fellow in the American College of Sports Medicine and AAHPERD's Research Consortium.

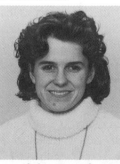

Gina Sharpe received her PhD with an emphasis in exercise science from the University of Tennessee, Knoxville, in 1989. Dr. Sharpe is currently an assistant professor of physical education and Director of the Health-Related Fitness Program at Berry College in Rome, Georgia. Her research interests focus on the kinesiological factors pertaining to exercise prescription and the prevention of low-back pain, and she has presented papers on this topic at national meetings. She received the 1989 Young Scholar Award for the Southern Association for Physical Education of College Women.